AF775367

Nanotechnology Science and Technology Series

Nanostructured Materials for Electrochemical Biosensors

NANOTECHNOLOGY SCIENCE AND TECHNOLOGY SERIES

National Nanotechnology Initiative: Assessment and Recommendations
Jerrod W. Kleike (Editor)
2009. ISBN 978-1-60692-727-4

Nanotechnology Research Collection - 2009/2010. DVD edition
James N. Ling (Editor)
2009. ISBN 978-1-60741-293-9

Nanotechnology Research Collection - 2009/2010. PDF edition
James N. Ling (Editor)
2009. ISBN 978-1-60741-292-2

Safe Nanotechnology
Arthur J. Cornwelle (Editor)
2009. ISBN 978-1-60692-662-8

Safe Nanotechnology in the Workplace
Nathan I. Bialor (Editor)
2009. ISBN 978-1-60692-679-6

Strategic Plan for NIOSH Nanotechnology Research and Guidance
Martin W. Lang (Author)
2009. ISBN: 978-1-60692-678-9

Nanotechnology in the USA: Developments, Policies and Issues
Carl H. Jennings (Editor)
2009. ISBN: 978-1-60692-800-4

New Nanotechnology Developments
Armando Barrañón (Editor)
2009. ISBN: 978-1-60741-028-7

Electrospun Nanofibers and Nanotubes Research Advances
A. K. Haghi (Editor)
2009. ISBN: 978-1-60741-220-5

Nanostructured Materials for Electrochemical Biosensors
Umasankar Yogeswaran, S. Ashok Kuma and Shen-Ming Chen
2009. ISBN: 978-1-60741-706-4

Nanotechnology Science and Technology Series

NANOSTRUCTURED MATERIALS FOR ELECTROCHEMICAL BIOSENSORS

YOGESWARAN UMASANKAR
S. ASHOK KUMAR
AND
SHEN-MING CHEN
EDITORS

Nova Science Publishers, Inc.
New York

Copyright © 2009 by Nova Science Publishers, Inc.

All rights reserved. No part of this book may be reproduced, stored in a retrieval system or transmitted in any form or by any means: electronic, electrostatic, magnetic, tape, mechanical photocopying, recording or otherwise without the written permission of the Publisher.

For permission to use material from this book please contact us:
Telephone 631-231-7269; Fax 631-231-8175
Web Site: http://www.novapublishers.com

NOTICE TO THE READER

The Publisher has taken reasonable care in the preparation of this book, but makes no expressed or implied warranty of any kind and assumes no responsibility for any errors or omissions. No liability is assumed for incidental or consequential damages in connection with or arising out of information contained in this book. The Publisher shall not be liable for any special, consequential, or exemplary damages resulting, in whole or in part, from the readers' use of, or reliance upon, this material. Any parts of this book based on government reports are so indicated and copyright is claimed for those parts to the extent applicable to compilations of such works.

Independent verification should be sought for any data, advice or recommendations contained in this book. In addition, no responsibility is assumed by the publisher for any injury and/or damage to persons or property arising from any methods, products, instructions, ideas or otherwise contained in this publication.

This publication is designed to provide accurate and authoritative information with regard to the subject matter covered herein. It is sold with the clear understanding that the Publisher is not engaged in rendering legal or any other professional services. If legal or any other expert assistance is required, the services of a competent person should be sought. FROM A DECLARATION OF PARTICIPANTS JOINTLY ADOPTED BY A COMMITTEE OF THE AMERICAN BAR ASSOCIATION AND A COMMITTEE OF PUBLISHERS.

LIBRARY OF CONGRESS CATALOGING-IN-PUBLICATION DATA

Nanostructured materials for electrochemical biosensors / [edited by] Umasankar Yogeswaran, S. Ashok Kumar, Shen-Ming Chen.
p. cm.
Includes index.
ISBN 978-1-60741-706-4 (hardcover)
1. Biosensors. 2. Electrochemical sensors. 3. Nanostructured materials. I. Yogeswaran, Umasankar. II. Kumar, S. Ashok. III. Chen, Shen-Ming.
R857.B54N36 2009
610.28--dc22

2009015626

Published by Nova Science Publishers, Inc. ✢ New York

CONTENTS

PREFACE

Electrochemical biosensors are portable devices that permit rapid analysis of substances. They are most useful in detection and monitoring of biological, chemical and toxic agents. Briefly, with the help of transducer, the generated electrical signals from the responses to change in the bioactive layers are used for the interpretation. Similarly, nanomaterials have number of features that make them ideally suited for sensor applications, such as, its high surface area, high reactivity, easy dispersability and rapid fabrication. This collected work composed of the expert knowledge of many specialists in the construction and use of electrochemical biosensors made of nanostructured materials. This includes nanomaterials such as dendrimers, polymers, nanoparticles, nanotubes, oxides, enzymes and their hybrids as catalyst for various sensors such as glucose sensors, DNA sensors, neurotransmitters sensors, etc. This collected work provides new methodological advancements related to and correlated with the measurement of interested species in biomedical samples. Many studies are also included to illustrate the range of application and importance of the electrochemical biosensors. This provides the unique opportunity for readers to choice a new methods and applications of new electrochemical biosensors.

Chapter 1 - Dendrimers represent a unique class of synthetic, highly-branched, monodisperse macromolecules with well-defined architecture of nanometer dimensions.Their highly desirable physicochemical and biological properties make them suitable for a variety of applications including catalysis, photochemical molecular devices, electroluminescent devices, sensors and biomedical devices. Potential applications of dendrimers in electrochemistry are imminent. Especially, the rapid advancements in the synthesis of redox active dendrimers along with their ability to provide a suitable microenvironment for the immobilization of biomolecules retaining their biological activity have given great scope for their exploitation in electrochemical biosensors. The recent advances on the applications of dendrimers in electrochemical biosensors are presented in this chapter. Several methodologies from simple to very versatile fabrication of the dendrimer-bio interfaces have been demonstrated in literature. In particular, the layer-by-layer method has been found to be very effective and successful in preparing the dendrimer- bionanocomposites. Hybrid materials of dendrimers with metal nanoparticles, conjugated polymers and carbon nanotubes have also been developed for this application. The favorable characteristics of the bionanocomposites of dendrimers in the electrochemical sensing of glucose, glutamate, alcohol and pesticides are discussed. This chapter also provides a brief account of the performance of dendrimer-modified electrodes in the detection of DNA hybridization and in affinity biosensors.

Chapter 2 - This chapter summarizes some procedures for intrinsic functionalization, doping and preparation, analysis and biosensor applications of polyaniline nano-composite materials. Details of the synthesis of four novel nanostructured polymeric composites formed with pristine or substituted polyanilines and sulfonated polyanion, as well as their microscopy, spectroscopy, electrochemistry and multifunctional properties in enzyme electrodes, are presented. In the case of the pristine polyaniline (PANI) and poly(dimethoxy aniline) (PDMA), the polyelectrolyte dopants used were polyvinyl sulfonate (PVS) and polystyrene sulfonic acid (PSS). No dopant was used in conjunction with poly(8-anilino naphthalene sulfonic acid) (PANSA) – a self-doping conducting polymer. A final section deals with the application of the resulting nanocomposites as enzyme-immobilization and conducting platforms in amperometric biosensors involving two oxidoreductase enzymes (horseradish peroxidase and cytochrome P450-2D6). The analytical performances of the resulting biosensors in batch operation mode with regard to their responses to standard samples of selected clinical and environmental analytes, including drugs (e.g. sertraline and fluoxetine), hydrogen peroxide (a strategic biomedical analyte) and some pesticides (e.g., glufosinate and glyphosate) are described. The chapter also demonstrates the application of cyclic voltammetry, scanning electron microscopy, uv-visible spectroscopy and infrared spectroscopy in the development and analysis of biosensors based on functionalized polyaniline nanomaterials.

Keywords: polyaniline; hydrogen peroxide, nanomaterials; glufosinate ; glyphosate; sertraline; fluoxetine; pesticide; anti-depressant; horseradish peroxidase; Cytochrome P450-2D6.

Chapter 3 - Recent electrochemical research interest in nanomaterials modified electrodes is focused on the fabrication of new direct electrocatalytic and electrochemical sensing devices using potentially useful metal nanoparticles embedded in suitable support matrices. In recent times, the simple fabrication of direct electrocatalytic and electrochemical sensor devices by employing metal (platinum (Pt) and gold (Au)) nanoparticles (Pt_{nano}, and Au_{nano}) embedded in matrices such as Nafion (Nf) and functionalized silicate sol-gel (SG) network (Nf/Pt_{nano} and $SG\text{-}Au_{nano}$) for the detection and determination of biomolecules such as dopamine (DA), ascorbic acid (AA), serotonin (5-HT), uric acid (UA) and toxic chemicals such as hydrazine, sulfite and nitrite was reported from authors laboratory. In direct electrocatalysis and electrochemical detection systems, metal nanoparticles at the modified electrodes play a major role as mediator and catalyst for the direct oxidation/reduction of substrates. The mediators, such as enzymes or similar molecules, free modified electrodes prepared using metal nanoparticles are a reagentless electrochemical sensor and exhibit low operating potential for substrates reaction at the modified electrode. These electrodes are simple to design, cost-effective, and require no external modification to metal nanoparticles or layer by layer modification. The embedded metal nanoparticles in matrix improve the transducer property of the sensor by providing the necessary electronic conduction pathway and facilitating the electron transfer events between the analyte and electrode surface in the absence of any other external electron transfer mediator. The metal nanoparticles embedded matrix networks are characterized by scanning electron micrograph (SEM), atomic force micrographs (AFM), X-ray photoelectron spectroscopy (XPS), X-ray diffraction (XRD), optical and electrochemical techniques. The simultaneous and selective detection and determination of chemically and biologically important molecules are achieved at the metal nanoparticles based electrochemical sensors. Such simple sensor devices designed from

Nf/Pt_{nano} and $SG\text{-}Au_{nano}$ are expected to play an important role in clinical diagnostics and environmental monitoring and in ensuring authors food safety. Such protocols may be used to design simple sensor devices for routine diagnostic applications, which is only a matter of time.

Chapter 4 - Biomolecules are chemical compounds found in living organisms which are the building blocks of life and perform important functions. Fluctuation from the normal concentration of these biomolecules in living system leads to several disorders. Thus the exact determination of them in human fluids is essential in the clinical point of view. High performance liquid chromatography, flow injection analysis, capillary electrophoresis, fluorimetry, spectrophotometry, electrochemical and chemiluminescence techniques were usually used for the determination of biologically important molecules. Among these techniques, electrochemical determination of biomolecules has several advantages over other methods viz., simplicity, selectivity and sensitivity. In the past two decades, electrodes modified with polymer films, self-assembled monolayers containing different functional groups and carbon paste have been used as electrochemical sensors. But in recent years, nanomaterials based electrochemical sensors play an important role in the improvement of public health because of its rapid detection, high sensitivity and specificity in clinical diagnostics. To date gold nanoparticles (AuNPs) have received arousing attention mainly due to their fascinating electronic and optical properties as a consequence of their reduced dimensions. These unique properties of AuNPs make them as an ideal candidate for the immobilization of enzymes for biosensing. Further, the electrochemical properties of AuNPs reveal that they exhibit interesting properties by enhancing the electrode conductivity, facilitating electron transfer and improving the detection limit of biomolecules. In this chapter, authors summarized the different strategies used for the attachment of AuNPs on electrode surfaces and highlighted the electrochemical determination of glucose, ascorbic acid (AA), uric acid (UA) and dopamine derivatives using the AuNPs modified electrodes.

Chapter 5 - Seed-mediated growth of metal nanoparticles on electrode surfaces has been introduced. Using this wet chemical method, gold nanoparticles were successfully deposited on various electrode substrates such as indium tin oxide (ITO) and glassy carbon. The as-prepared gold nanoparticle-modified electrodes showed catalytic activity toward the oxidation of small biomolecules such as dopamine, ascorbic acid, uric acid, epinephrine and norepinephrine, which could improve the sensitivity or selectivity of bioelectroanalysis. The deposited gold nanoparticles were also biocompatible for immobilization of biomacromolecules, namely hemoglobin and myoglobin, on which the direct electron transfer of redox proteins was realized and reagentless H_2O_2 biosensors were provided.

On the other hand, liquid phase deposition (LPD) has been demonstrated as a flexible wet chemical method for preparing metal oxide nanostructured films on electrode surfaces. By the LPD process, electroactive titanium dioxide (TiO_2) films were prepared on graphite, glassy carbon and ITO. The electrochemical properties of such LPD TiO_2 films were dependent upon the film thickness controlled by the deposition time. The LPD technique was easily combined with other techniques, e.g., seed-mediated growth, which could provide metal/metal oxide composite nanomaterials. Moreover, hybrid nanostructured films were facilely obtained by doping dyes, surfactants and other materials into the LPD films. These dopants improved the electron transfer kinetics at LPD films by reducing the film resistance and thus making the hybrid films useful for bioelectroanalysis.

Chapter 6 - The immobilization of biomolcules especially, enzymes on electrode surfaces is one of the main factor that affects the performance of biosensors. To improve the characteristics of an enzyme sensor, such as sensitivity, response time, dynamic range, enzymes should be deposited on the electrode substrate as an ultrathin film. Different materials and several methodologies have been used for immobilization of thin enzyme films on the electrode surfaces. Due to advantageous of nanomaterials such as, high surface area, favorable electronic properties and electrocatalytic effect they have been considerable attention for construction of electrochemical enzyme biosensors. Among the inorganic materials, metal oxide nanoparticles are suitable matrixes and novel candidates for immobilization of enzymes and proteins due to their high electrical conductivity, wide electrochemical working window, high biocompatibility, excellent substrate adhesion and stable chemical, electrochemical and physical properties.This review discusses main techniques and methods which use for preparation different nanoscale metal oxides and their applications for construction of electrochemical biosensors. Various applications of the metal-oxide nanoparticles based biosensors for detection different analytes are described.

Chapter 7 - Nanotechnology is playing an increasing important role in the development of biosensors. In recent years, electrochemical biosensors based on nanostructured metal oxides gained much attention in the field of health care for the management of various important analytes in a biological system. This article provides a comprehensive review of current research activities relating to nanostructured metal oxide based electrochemical biosensors. The unique properties of nanostructured metal oxides offer excellent prospects for interfacing biological recognition events with electronic signal transduction and for designing a new generation of bioelectronic devices. In this Chapter, authors address various nanostructured metal oxides for fabrication of electrochemical biosensor and assembling procedures of these nanosensors. The authors discuss as to how these materials can be used for detection of various biological molecules and how such devices can be used to achive improved biosensing chrcateristics such as high sensitivity, selectivity and low detection limits.

Chapter 8 - The electrochemical biosensor with a well-aligned nanotube array structure has been developed for amperometric detection and quantitative determination on the basis of bioelectrocatalysis mechanism. The independent and free-standing titania nanotube array has been successfully fabricated through an electrochemical anodization process of titanium sheet precursor in a fluoride-containing electrolyte, which can act well as a suitable electrode material for the biosensor application due to its high surface area and superior biocompatibility. In view of a more feasible loading of enyzme probes in accessible tubular channels, nanotube morphologies have been promoted by expanding tube diameter from 60 to 110 nm and increasing tube length from 520 nm to above 920 nm when anodization process at voltage of 20 V in acidic aqueous electrolyte has been adjusted into that at 60 V in neutral ethylene glycol/glycerol electrolyte. The functionalization modification of the titania nanotube array has been sequentially achieved by filling highly-bioactive glucose oxidases into as-formed nanotubes and then electropolymerizing pyrrole monomer into conductive polypyrrole for an interfacial immobilization of these bioactive enzymes. Morphology & microstructure characterization, electrochemical properties and bioelectrocatalytic reactivities of composite electrodes have been fully investigated. Electrochemical impedance spectroscopy has been employed to investigate the electrical conductivity and capacitance analysis. The direct amperometric detection of hydrogen peroxide through a direct electro-reduction reaction can be well fulfilled on bare titania nanotube array with a detection limit up to 2.0×10^{-4} mM for ordinary nanotubes and 2.2×10^{-4} mM for long nanotubes. A nano-array biosensor based on the glucose oxidase-titania/titanium composite electrodes have been assembled in a conventional three-electrode system for amperometric detection and quantitative determination of glucose concentration in a pH 6.8 phosphate buffer solution at a potentiostatic condition of -0.4 V vs. the saturated calomel electrode. The glucose oxidase biosensor with a well-constructed nanotube array structure show an excellent performance with a high detection sensitivity of 45.5 μA mM^{-1} cm^{-2}, a fast responding time of 5.6 s and a very low detection limit of 2.0×10^{-3} mM. A good operational reliability has also been achieved with a relative standard deviation below 3.0 %. Such a well-designed biosensor with a desired nanotube array structure can consequentially contribute to the potential application of molecule detection and quantitative determination.

Keywords: Biosensor; Titania nanotube array; Hydrogen peroxide; Amperometric detection

Chapter 9 - Although nanostructured alumina was successfully fabricated by electrochemical anodization decades ago, it is only until recently that the electrochemically anodized TiO_2 begins to attract more and more research interest and is now becoming an emerging area of a wide range of important applications, such as, gas sensing, self cleaning, antifogging, water purification, anticorrosion, solar cell, lithium batteries, electrochemical supercapacitors, photo cleavage of water, antibacterial coating, and the improvement of biocompatibility, etc. This is due fundamentally to the fact that TiO_2 is a semiconductor with reactivity or photoreactivity closely related to its defect structure. A variety of attractive functional properties of TiO_2 are the result of its unique electronic band structure which can also be easily tuned by defects. In this article authors will give a detailed review on recent progress in the fabrication of anodic TiO_2 nanostructure, the control of its morphology by varying anodization conditions, and the microstructure related properties. The authors will also review the recent research efforts in various practical applications of anodic TiO_2 with dopants or modifications. Potential future applications of anodic TiO_2 with highly ordered nanostructures are also suggested.

Chapter 10 - In the past decades, development of electrochemical enzyme sensors is of much interest, since they posse's great compatibility, good stability with much low cost of production. This review majorly focuses on nanomaterial based acetylcholinesterase (AChE) sensors which belongs to the category of pesticide sensors in which the enzyme AChE is immobilized either onto glassy carbon, screen printed carbon, gold or graphite electrode surfaces. The enzyme activity is majorly affected by the traces of organophosphorus (OP) and carbamate (CA) pesticides existing in the environment. Detection of these pesticides in trace amounts is essential and it is achieved efficiently by the use of AChE sensors. These pesticide compounds are detected quantitatively by measure of AChE inhibition activity. This is usually carried out by measuring the electrooxidation current of thiocholine generated by the AChE catalyzed hydrolysis of acetylthiocholine (ATCh). In few sensors, residual activity of the enzyme is compared with the initial activity. The working electrode surface shows a dramatic enhancement with lowest detection limit of pesticides when modified with carbon nano tubes (CNTs), gold nano particles, silica nano particles and sol-gel matrix respectively.

Keywords: acetylcholinesterase, electrochemical sensors, organophosphate, carbamate, pesticide, thiocholine, acetylthiocholine, nano materials

Chapter 11 - Mesoporous silicas (MPS) have been widely used as electrode modifier for electrochemical biosensors due to their attractive properties such as unique structure and high pore volume containing large number of widely accessible active centers, tailored pore size for different biomolecules, and good biocompatibility. These properties have been intelligently combined to improve the response and sensitivity of the resulting modified electrodes and to design novel electrochemical biosensor for electrocatalytic reaction and detection. This up-to-date review summarizes the recent progresses made in the electrochemical biosensors by application of MPS modified electrodes and introduces advantages (for examples, their novel structure, functionalized by different organic or inorganic groups with different pore size that can simultaneously fit with different proteins etc) of some novel MPS that have been synthesized in literature. The outlook and successful realization for the development of MPS in electrochemical biosensors requires proper control of their chemical and physical properties and surface functionalization.

Keywords: Mesoporous silica; Enzyme; Redox protein; Modified electrode; Biosensor

Chapter 12 - Electroanalytical chemistry has been widely applied to the study of neurochemical systems. This feasibility stems from the ease of oxidative detection of many neurotransmitters, the small dimensions of electrodes and their inherent fast response time.

Dopamine is a neurotransmitter that has long been of interest to both chemists and neuroscientists. For instance, a loss of dopamine-containing neurons or its transmission is related to a number of illnesses and conditions including Parkinson's disease and schizophrenia. It is therefore of interest to perform quantitative and qualitative determination of dopamine in the extracellular fluid in animals in order to gain an understanding of the neurotransmission processes. Such a study will also aid in correlating neurochemistry with behaviour.

Among the electroanalytical techniques, fast-scan cyclic voltammetry is often used to detect dopamine *in vivo*. Detection of dopamine is further enhanced when fast-scan cyclic voltammetry is conducted at probes with a micrometer-dimension. A review of common materials and techniques for fabricating physically small electrodes is therefore presented in this chapter. Unfortunately, detecting dopamine at naked electrodes is challenging partly because of overlapping oxidation signals from interferents of high concentrations in the brain. Furthermore, electrode fouling caused by adsorption of biological molecules is another common problem encountered in detecting dopamine *in vivo*. In this chapter, a number of approaches including electrode surface modification and diamond electrodes used to minimize these shortcomings have also been reviewed.

In: Nanostructured Materials for Electrochemical Biosensors ISBN: 978-1-60741-706-4
Editors: U. Yogeswaran; S. Kumar; S. Chen ©2009 Nova Science Publishers, Inc.

Chapter 1

DENDRIMERS IN ELECTROCHEMICAL BIOSENSORS

Ramiah Saraswathi*[*1] and Shen-Ming Chen[2]
[1]Department of Materials Science, School of Chemistry,
Madurai Kamaraj University, Madurai, India
[2]Department of Chemical Engineering & Biotechnology,
National Taipei University of Technology, Taipei, Taiwan

ABSTRACT

Dendrimers represent a unique class of synthetic, highly-branched, monodisperse macromolecules with well-defined architecture of nanometer dimensions.Their highly desirable physicochemical and biological properties make them suitable for a variety of applications including catalysis, photochemical molecular devices, electroluminescent devices, sensors and biomedical devices. Potential applications of dendrimers in electrochemistry are imminent. Especially, the rapid advancements in the synthesis of redox active dendrimers along with their ability to provide a suitable microenvironment for the immobilization of biomolecules retaining their biological activity have given great scope for their exploitation in electrochemical biosensors. The recent advances on the applications of dendrimers in electrochemical biosensors are presented in this chapter. Several methodologies from simple to very versatile fabrication of the dendrimer-bio interfaces have been demonstrated in literature. In particular, the layer-by-layer method has been found to be very effective and successful in preparing the dendrimer-bionanocomposites. Hybrid materials of dendrimers with metal nanoparticles, conjugated polymers and carbon nanotubes have also been developed for this application. The favorable characteristics of the bionanocomposites of dendrimers in the electrochemical sensing of glucose, glutamate, alcohol and pesticides are discussed. This chapter also provides a brief account of the performance of dendrimer-modified electrodes in the detection of DNA hybridization and in affinity biosensors.

* Email: saraswathir@yahoo.com

I. INTRODUCTION

Dendrimers are perfect monodisperse macromolecules of nanometric dimensions with a regular and highly-branched three-dimensional architecture. A dendrimer can be defined by a central core and branching units with closely packed surface groups (Fig.1). Dendrimers possess a globular structure having internal voids or cavities or channels. The cavities can be used for the entrapment of guest molecules or engineered for other applications. Dendrimers are often represented with a generation number (G). The number of branching points when going from the core towards the dendrimer surface is the generation number. Dendron is the term used to describe a dendritic wedge without the core.

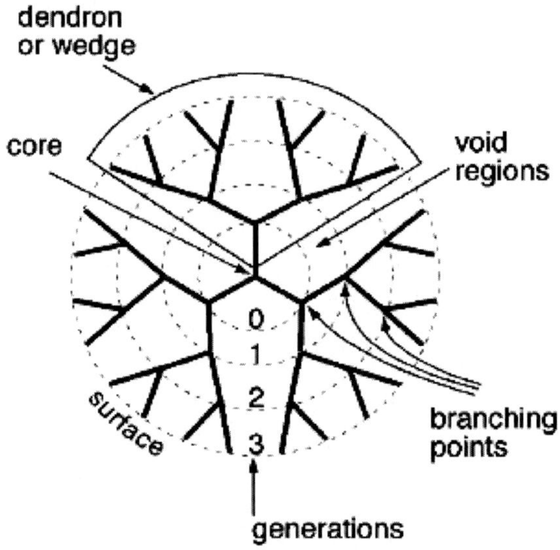

Figure 1. Schematic representation of the structure of a dendrimer

Since the first synthesis of a dendrimer by Buhleier et al in 1978 [1], the science of dendrimers has grown gradually enriching all fields including chemistry, materials science, chemical biology, and medical diagnostics. There are several excellent books and reviews on dendrimers detailing their synthesis, structures, properties and applications [2-23]. This chapter is the first state-of-the-art report on the applications of dendrimers in electrochemical biosensors. A brief overview of the basic aspects of dendrimers is presented below for a comprehensive reading.

II. BASICS OF DENDRIMERS

(a) Structure and Nomenclature

Some of the commonly known dendrimers are shown in Fig.2. Considering the size and complexity of dendrimers, the depiction of their structures cannot be done by conventional chemical structures [15]. Two methods of representing the structures are generally followed *viz.* an abbreviated form and a cartoon representation (Fig.3). The abbreviated form takes advantage of the high symmetry and repetitive nature of a dendrimer. It relies upon drawing just one moiety from each generation. However, its use is only possible when all monomer units in each generation are identical. In the cartoon form each monomer is depicted as a shaded block. The surface groups are shown as circles.

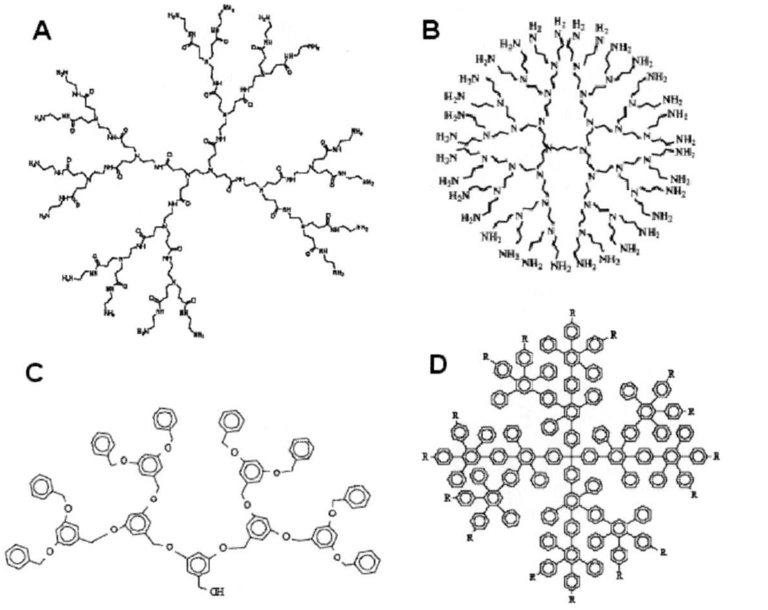

Figure 2. Structures of some commonly known dendrimers: A. Polyamidoamine (G2); B. Poly(propylene imine) (G4) ; C. Benzyl ether monodendron (G3) and D. Poly(phenylene) dendrimer (G2). (G represents the generation number)

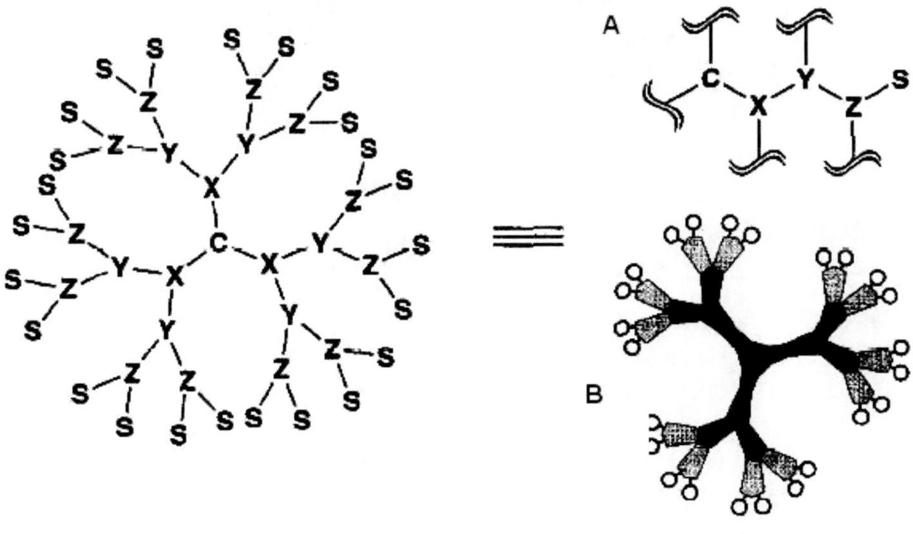

Figure 3 A. Abbreviated and B. Cartoon representations of the dendritic structure on the left showing the core (C/dark), surface (S/circles) and branching (X,Y,Z /wedge) (Adapted from Ref.[15]).

(b) Synthesis

Since the first synthesis of a poly(propylene imine) (PPI) dendrimer [1], several families of dendrimers have been prepared including the poly(amidoamines) (PAMAM), polyethers, poly(phenylenes), poly(phenylacetylenes), polysilanes, silicon, phosphorus and nitrogen-based dendrimers

The concepts surrounding the dendrimer synthesis have been lucidly presented [15, 22]. The general synthetic strategy involves the repetitive alternation of a growth reaction and an activation reaction. Often these reactions have to be performed at many sites on the same molecule simultaneously. The growth reaction dictates the way by which the branching is introduced into a dendrimer. Many dendrimer syntheses rely upon traditional reactions, such as the Michael reaction or the Williamson ether synthesis while others involve the use of solid-phase synthesis or organotransition metal chemistry [1, 24]

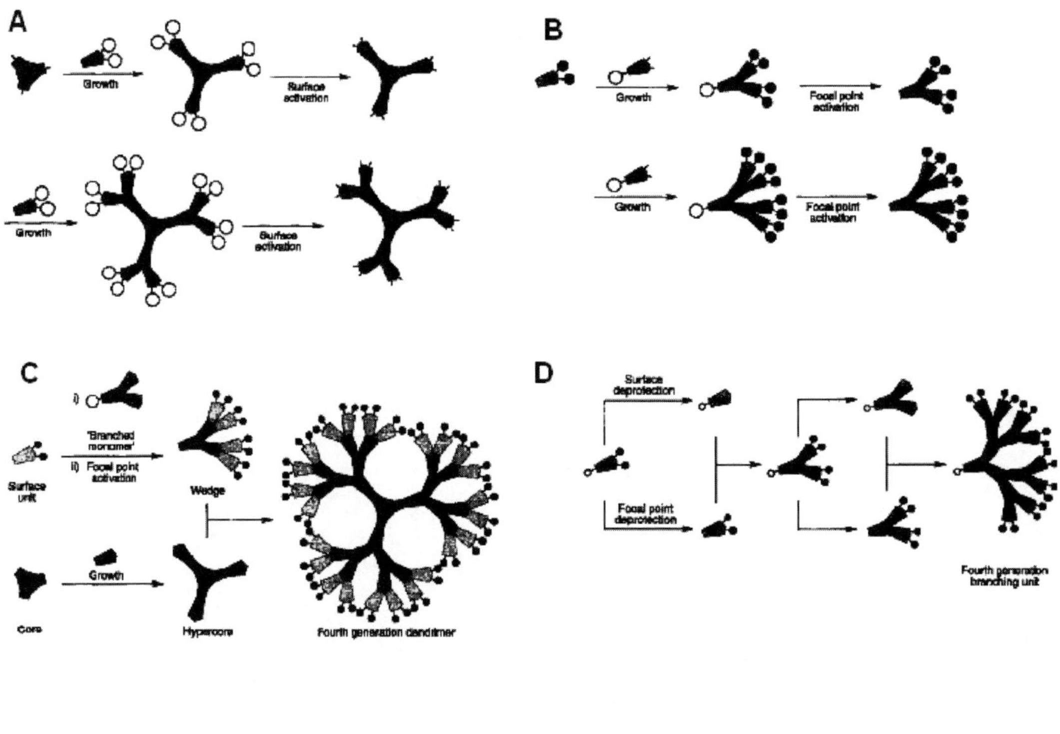

Figure 4. Schematic of dendrimer synthetic strategies : A. Divergent growth ; B. Convergent growth ; C. Hypercore growth ; D. Double exponential and mixed growth (Adapted from Ref.[15]).

The various synthetic strategies are schematically depicted in Fig.4. Divergent synthesis (Fig.4A) is one of the first methods arising from the seminal works of Vogtle's and Tomalia's groups [1, 24-26]. The dendrimer is induced to grow outwards from the core, diverging into space. The convergent method (Fig.4B), first reported by Hawker and Frechet in 1990 [27] begins at what ultimately becomes the surface of the dendrimer and works inwards by gradually linking surface units together with more monomers. The divergent and covergent methods are complementary in that the former is useful in preparing large quantities of the product at the cost of purity whereas the latter yields pure product. The hypercore synthesis

(Fig.4C) involves the pre-assembly of oligomeric species, which can then be linked together to give dendrimers in fewer steps of higher yields, taking advantage of the best points of both convergent and divergent techniques [28]. The double exponential and mixed growth (Fig.4D), employs an AB_2 monomer where the functional groups A and B are both protected [29, 30]. The fully protected monomer is deprotected selectively at the surface and at the branch point in separate reactions to give a convergent-type monomer and a divergent-type monomer. These two products are then reacted together to give an orthogonally protected trimer which may be used to repeat the growth process again. The dendrimer crowding factor, which is defined as the ratio of its total molecular volume to conformationally available volume, limits the synthesis of dendrimers with higher generations. The maximum theoretical value for the dendrimer crowding factor is 1 [15].

Over the years, molecular design has allowed the synthesis of functional dendrimers possessing metal and semiconductor nanoparticles, metal complexes and macrocycles, dyes and biologically important carrier molecules in various parts of the dentritic structures [31-39]. Such dendrimers incorporating functional units are considered as supramolecular species [16, 21]. Functional dendrimers have been proved to be very useful for specific applications [40, 41]. Some examples of functional dendrimers are shown in Fig.5.

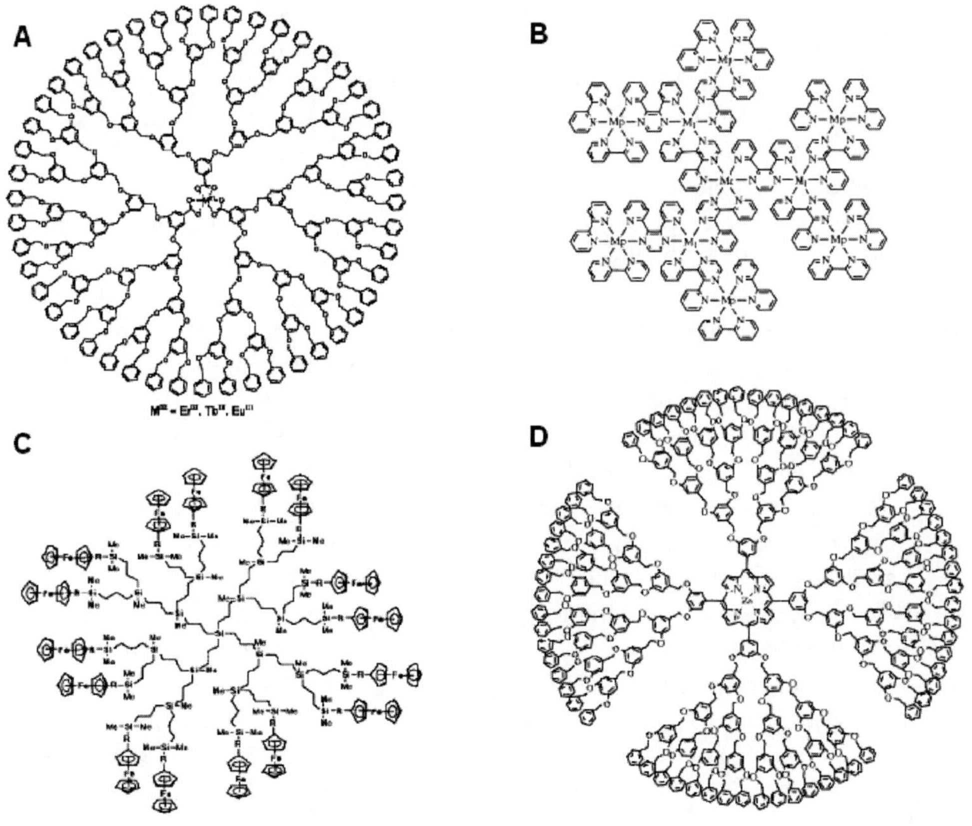

Figure 5. Structures of some functional dendrimers A. Dendrimer with lanthanide ion as the central core with dendrons as ligands ; B. Dendrimer based on metal complex ; C. Silicon-based ferrocenyl dendrimer and D. Dendrimer with zinc-porphyrin core

(c) Characterization

Several analytical techniques can be used for the characterization of the chemical composition, morphology, shape and structural homogeneity of dendrimers [42]. ^{1}H and ^{13}C NMR spectra are useful to follow the structural transformations during the synthesis. For dendrimers containing heteroatom, the resonance of the heteroatom can provide very valuable information. For example, signals of heteroatoms like, ^{31}P, ^{29}Si, ^{11}B, ^{19}F ^{195}Pt and ^{119}Sn have been used in the characterization of the dendrimer derivatives. The spin-lattice relaxation and spin-spin relaxation times of protons of the dendrimer in solution can give information about the variation in the compactness of the interior core and the peripheral segment density with respect to their generation number. Infra-red spectroscopy has been used to derive information about the presence of hydrogen bonding, to follow the chemical transformations at the surface and also to characterize any interactions between end groups in the dendrimers. The UV–visible spectroscopy is a valuable technique to characterize functional dendrimers. The intensity of the absorption maximum is proportional to the number of chromophoric groups and can be used as a test for the purity of dendrimer. Fluorescence spectroscopy is of immense use in characterizing the structure of dendrimers having photochemical probes [40,43]. Circular dichroism and optical rotatory dispersion techniques throw light on the conformations of dendrimers containing chiral groups [44]. Classical mass spectroscopy can be used for the characterization of lower generation dendrimers whose mass is < 3000 D. The matix-assisted laser desorption/ionization–time-of-flight and electrospray mass spectrometry offer the best evidence for dendritic structures, particularly when the NMR spectroscopy is ambiguous [45-47]. Small angle X-ray scattering and small angle neutron scattering techniques are often employed to derive information about the radius of gyration of dendrimers. The latter also gives precise information about the internal structure and molecular weight [48,49]. Dynamic light scattering is mainly used for the detection of aggregates of dendrimers [50]. Similarly, gel permeation chromatography provides information on the polydispersity in dendrimers. Transmission electron microscopy and atomic force microscopy are used for imaging individual dendrimer molecules and their aggregates [51,52]. Electrochemical techniques can also offer information about the structure of dendrimers [42]. Exhaustive coulometry can be used to measure the number of electroactive groups [53]. The degree of encapsulation of electroactive groups can be detected by cyclic voltammetry. Also, any possible interaction between electroactive groups can be detected [54]. Gel electrophoresis is recommended for studying the interaction between positively charged dendrimers and DNA [55].

The cavities and voids inside dendritic structures are of great importance, particularly in the study of supramolecular systems. The nature of this void, how it is affected by dendrimer size, constitution and solvent are of supreme importance in relation to potential applications [15]. It is therefore necessary to discover ways to characterize the microenvironment in the dendrimer. Many investigators have made use of functional probes in order to study dendritic microenvironments [56,57]. These probes are either attached covalently to the dendrimer or introduced as guest species and the effects of solvent and dendrimer size on the microenvironment are then studied.

(d) Salient Properties

The general properties of the dendrimers have been widely discussed [15,22,58-60]. Dendrimers are more soluble in common solvents compared to their analogous linear polymers [61-63]. The solubility characteristics depend predominantly on the properties of their surface groups. For example, dendrimers with very hydrophobic interiors such as polyethers and polycarbosilanes can be made water soluble by introducing hydrophilic groups into their surface. Oppositely, water soluble dendrimers can be made hydrophobic by converting their surface groups into hydrophobic units. The ability to modify a dendrimer surface groups clearly offers alternative opportunities for making it suitable for an application. Dendrimers are considered to be model systems of classical micelles [64]. There are a variety of amphiphilic dendrimers including poly(amidoamines), polyamides, polyethers and polyesters. Like micelles, the amphiphilic dendrimers possess the capability to solubilize insoluble organic substrate in aqueous medium. But unlike the normal micelles that are affected by factors like pH, concentration, ionic strength and temperature, the dendrimer micelle structure is stable under normal conditions. Some dendrimers are considered to be model compounds for biological systems [65].

An important feature of dendrimers is that their viscosity in solution and in melt is lower than that of the linear polymers. Surprisingly, the viscosity decreases with increase in molecular weight *i.e.* higher dendrimers are less viscous [66]. This behaviour is attributed to the transition from an extended structure for lower generation to globular shapes at increased generations. The glass transition temperature (T_g) depends on the number of end groups and number of branch points [67, 68]. The increase in number of end groups lowers the T_g, while T_g is increased with increasing number of branch points and the polarity of the end groups. The other physical and chemical properties of dendrimers are determined by the shape and multiplicity of the core and building blocks and by the size and shape of the end groups, in addition to their chemical composition. Dendrimers can be prepared with highly reactive surface groups and controllable surface-functionalization of dendrimers provides segregated properties between surface and core. Numerous modifications of reactive groups like amines, alcohols, or halides have enhanced the scope for the application of dendrimers. The binding groups on the interior are called endo-receptors and those on the periphery are called exo-receptors. The functionality of a dendrimer can be enhanced by the judicious choice of the core, building block and terminal units according to the application. Due to their globular shape in solution, their cores are relatively loosely linked and have enough space to encapsulate guest molecules [69].

(e) General Applications

The surface functionalities, interior and core of the dendrimers can be tailored for a variety of applications including molecular electronics, molecular recognition, catalysis, sensors and electroluminescent devices [70-74]. Dendrimers containing photoactive or redox active components can serve as molecular antennas for light harvesting [33,75,76] and can be exploited in electrochemical sensors [77]. The dendritic boxes with encapsulated guest molecules can be opened and closed reversibly by means of an external stimulus and can be useful in controlled drug delivery applications [78-80]. The structural precision with high specificity along with the nanodimensions of the dendrimers has led to a variety of biomedical applications. Extensive interest in their use as protein mimics, genetic material transfer agents, targeted drug delivery agents, magnetic resonance imaging contrast agents, antiviral and antitoxin agents, angiogenesis inhibitors and artificial enzymes can be found in literature [81-84].

III. Electroactive Dendrimers

Electroactive dendrimers are defined as those that contain functional groups capable of undergoing fast electron transfer reactions [85]. The combination of specific electron transfer properties of redox active probes with the unique structural properties of dendrimers offers attractive prospects of their exploitation in electrocatalytic processes of biological and industrial importance [86]. Further, the interest in dendrimers containing electroactive units also relies on the fact that electrochemistry is a powerful technique to elucidate the structure and purity of dendrimers, to evaluate the degree of electronic interaction of their chemically and/or topologically equivalent or non- equivalent moieties, and also to study their endo- and exo-receptor capabilities [87].

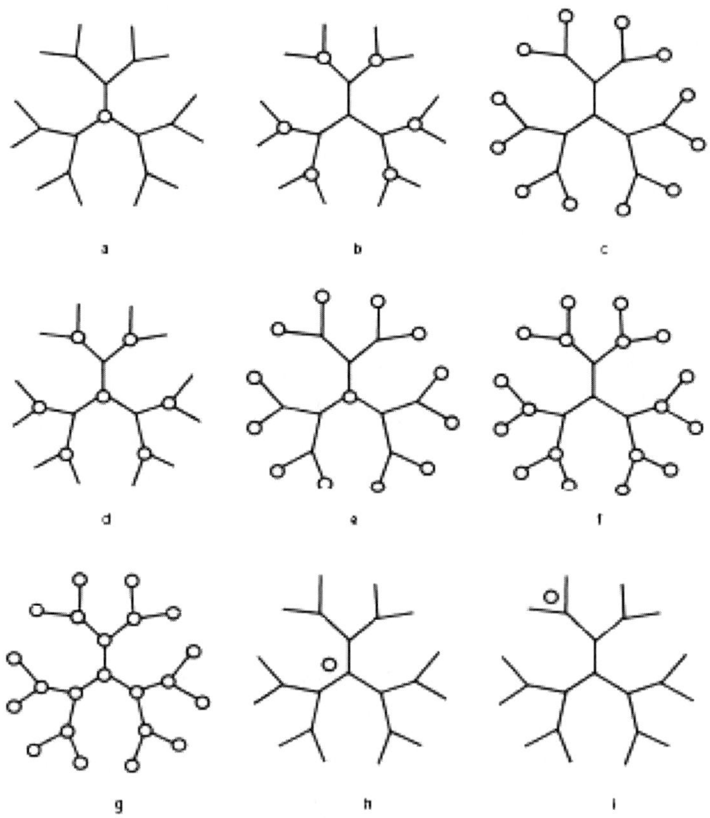

Figure 6. Schematic representation of dendrimers with positions where electroactive units (circles) can be located (Adapted from Ref.[87]).

Redox moieties can be buried in the central core, or incorporated in the branches or appended at the surface or located in topologically equivalent or non-equivalent sites of the dendrimer (Fig. 6). Since the first synthesis of an electroactive dendrimer containing 12 tetrathiafulvalene units in the periphery by Bryce et al in 1994 [88], several groups including those of Balzani, Kaifer, Casado and Cuadrado, Astruc, Newkome, Diederich and Gorman have made very valuable and interesting contributions on both the synthesis and applications of many different classes of dendrimers containing redox probes [89-95]. In general, the electrochemical behavior of an electroactive dendrimer with several redox centres resembles that of the redox group itself but the magnitude of current is enhanced in proportion to the total number of such redox centres. The redox potential may depend on the generation number and also the medium used. In many instances, the cyclic voltammetric data reveal that the redox process is thermodynamically hindered and kinetically slowed down as the dendrimer generation increases.

Redox-active metal core dendrimers are considered to be protein mimics [96]. Metal porphyrin complexes are particularly suitable for electroactive core dendrimers and can be regarded as models for proteins like cyctochrome c [85,90]. The electroactive properties of zinc and iron porphyrin core dendrimers have been investigated in detail [97,98]. Gorman et al developed novel dendrimers containing redox active iron-sulfur core [99]. Another notable example is that of the ferrocene core dendrimer with hemicarcerands as the encapsulating hosts [90,100]. Their voltammetric behaviour was investigated in CH_2Cl_2. The heterogeneous electron transfer rate constant was found to decrease as the dendrimer generation number increased. The decrease in the rate constant has been reasonably attributed to the increasing distance between the electroactive core and the electrode surface as the dendrimer generation increased.

Newkome's group developed a series of dendrimers containing a metal complex as the central core. The dendrimer assembly consists of terpyridine-derivatized macromolecular wedges wrapping around a Ru(II) metal centre. The terpyridines act as ligands to the metal ion [101,102]. Balzani's group [87] also made use of the transition metal coordination in the design of several novel dendrimers. The decanuclear Ru(II) dendrimer with bipyridyl ligands, is a typical example of dendrimers with an organized assembly of coordinated metal centres. It contains three kinds of metal centres: one in the central core, three internal ones and six peripheral ones (Fig.5B). The differential pulse voltammogram of this dendrimer showed only one anodic peak involving a transfer of six electrons. This anodic peak was assigned to the six peripheral metal centres. The oxidations of the four internal metal centres were not observed [87].

Ferrocene is the most widely used electroactive species for peripheral functionalization of dendrimers. Several reviews are available on the ferrocenyl dendrimers [86,91,103]. Casado's group [86,91] has synthesized silicon-based ferrocenyl dendrimers possessing 4, 8 and 16 peripheral ferrocenyl units. The ferrocenyl units are linked to the organosilicon dendritic framework through spaces of different nature and length. The same group also prepared five generations of organometallic dendrimers by surface functionalization of a series of diaminobutane-based dendrimers with 4, 8, 16, 32 and 64 ferrocenyl units. The electrochemical behaviour of these ferrocenyl dendrimers has been studied by cyclic voltammetry, differential pulse voltammetry and bulk coulometry. Irrespective of the number of ferrocenyl units, only a single reversible oxidation process corresponding to a multielectron transfer of 4, 8 or 16 electrons has been observed indicating the non-interacting nature of the topologically equilvalent ferrocenyl units. Another interesting example is the different generations of poly(propyleneimine) dendrimers containing varying numbers of peripheral ferrocenyl-urea groups [104]. The same class of dendrimers with alternative peripheral ferrocene and cobaltocenium species has also been reported [105]. There are examples of dendrimers functionalized with redox-active metal units or ferrocenyl groups in the branches [87]. Several other redox-active dendrimers have been well documented in the literature [106].

IV. DENDRIMERS IN BIOSENSORS

The application of dendrimers in electrochemical biosensors is an emerging area of research. The structural homogeneity, biocompatibility, internal porosity, high surface area and ease of functionalization of dendrimers make them very desirable for biosensor applications. In the past ten years, there has been a steady and gradual development in the evaluation of the bionanocomposites of dendrimers for electrochemical sensors. The expanding interest in the development of novel electroactive dendrimers has enabled their viability for this application.

(a) Preparation of Dendrimer Biocomposite-Modified Electrodes

The preparation of dendrimer biocomposite-modified electrode is the primary step in the development of biosensors. Appropriate strategies have been formulated to prepare stable and highly reproducible dendrimer-modified surfaces. Immobilization of biomolecules like enzymes, proteins and other suitable ligands on the dendrimer-modified electrode with extended lifetime is very important. Some general procedures adopted for the preparation of dendrimer biocomposite-modified surfaces for electrochemical biosensing are described below. Some of the unique procedures developed by various authors are elaborated later during the discussion of the performance of biosensors.

i) Direct Deposition

Dendrimers containing polymerizable groups can be electrodeposited onto suitable electrode surfaces (Pt or ITO) either by controlled potential electrolysis or by repeated cycling between the appropriate anodic and cathodic potential limits. The amount of electroactive material electrodeposited can be controlled with the electrolysis time or number of scans [86,107]. Enzymes or other biomolecules can be dissolved in the electrolyte of appropriate pH and the biocatalytic role of the dendrimer can be studied.

ii) Mixing/Blending

An appropriate amount of dendrimer dissolved in a suitable solvent can be mixed with a sufficient quantity of graphite powder. After evaporation of the solvent, the required quantity of the enzyme along with a small amount of paraffin oil are added and the mixture is blended into a paste. The modified carbon paste can be placed in an electrode holder and used [108].

iii) Drop-Casting

Some studies have made use of the traditional drop-casting method for preparing the dendrimer-modified electrodes [109]. Platinum, gold, glassy carbon and ITO electrodes can be modified by the dendrimer layers.Known quantities of the electroactive dendrimers can be dissolved in a solvent (often CH_2Cl_2 is used) and an appropriate quantity of the dendrimer solution is cast on the cleaned electrode surface and careful evaporation of the solvent leaves the dendrimer-modified surface. The surface coverage of the dendrimer is determined from the integrated charge of the cyclic voltammograms. Enzymes like glucose oxidase (GOx) can be immobilized onto the dendrimer-modified surface by drop-casting followed by cross-linking with glutaraldehyde and bovine serum albumin (BSA). Glutaraldehyde is a bifunctional cross-linking reagent which reacts with lysine residues on the exterior of the proteins and addition of BSA accelerates the cross-linking process due to the lysine groups present in its structure [110]. Biomolecules like DNA can be directly immobilized onto the dendrimer layer by simple drop-casting allowing sufficient time for the binding to take place.

iv) Layer-by-Layer Assembly

Layer-by-layer (LbL) assembly is a unique technique for the fabrication of composite films with precise thickness control at the nanometer scale [111, 112]. The method is based on the alternate adsorption of oppositely charged species from their solutions. The attractive feature of this approach is its ability to assemble complex structures from modular components, and integrate them into self-assembling constructions for a wide range of applications. The LbL method has been successfully exploited in the construction of dendrimer biosensors [113,114]. The LbL films provide a favorable environment for the intimate contact between the dendrimer and biomolecule (enzymes or proteins), promoting a direct electron transfer between them and the underlying electrodes.

v) Self-Assembly

In self-assembled systems, the basic construction units spontaneously associate to form a particular structure, the architecture of which is determined by the bonding properties of the individual components [115-117]. The formation of a self-assembled monolayer (SAM) proceeds towards a state of lower free energy and greater structural stability. Another feature of self-assembly is hierarchy, where primary building blocks associate into more complex secondary structures that are integrated into the next size-level in the hierarchy. These hierarchical constructions may exhibit unique properties that are not found in the individual components. SAM is widely used to modify a solid surface. Especially, the SAM of a long-chain alkanethiol on a gold support is very popular due to its strong chemisorption and high degree of thermal and chemical stability. A very simple method to prepare a SAM of the dendrimer involves the immersion of the gold electrode in an ethanolic solution containing suitable concentrations of a long chain alkanethiol and dendrimer for sufficiently long time (~ 20 h) to form a stable alkanethiol/dendrimer layer. A known quantity of the enzyme can then be immobilized by drop-casting on the SAM modified electrode.

(b) Dendrimer-Based Glucose Biosensors

Among the various dendrimers, the ferrocenyl dendrimers and the polyamidoamine (PAMAM) denrimers are the most frequently studied for biosensor applications. There are also some investigations based on poly(propyl imine) (PPI) dendrimers.

One of the first reports related to the application of dendrimers in biosensors demonstrated the use of ferrocenyl dendrimers containing organosilicon cores in glucose biosensing [118]. The main advantage is that the ferrocenyl moieties in the dendrimer act as redox mediator while the dendrimer provides a favorable environment for the immobilization of the biomolecule. The close proximity among the enzyme, mediator and sensing sites helps to achieve a rapid current response to glucose. Further, in conventional biosensors using monomeric ferrocene as the mediator, often there is a problem of sensor instability due to the solubility of the oxidized ferricinium ions causing their rapid diffusion away from the electrode surface. The anchoring of the ferrocene moieties to the high molecular weight dendrimer helps to accomplish better operational stabilities of the biosensors because their oxidized forms are less soluble than the ferricinium ions.

The cyclic voltammogram of ferrocenyl dendrimer/glucose oxidase (GOx)/carbon paste electrodes (CPE) showed a redox couple in the potential range 0 to 0.45 V *vs* SCE in sodium phosphate buffer containing 0.1 M KCl solution [118]. The addition of glucose led to the enhancement of the oxidation current, whereas the cathodic current decreased. The cyclic voltammogram obtained with electrodes containing only GOx without the dendrimer relay system did not display this behaviour. Based on the steady-state current response and the calculated values of the apparent Michaelis-Menten constants (K'_M), it was inferred that ferrocenyl dendrimers possessing the larger organosilicon branches and closer ferrocenyl neighbours are the most efficient electron transfer mediators. The ferrocenyl dendrimer-based glucose biosensors have been found to be better than the ferrocene-modified polymer mediated electrodes in terms of better operational stability and higher current sensitivity.

A fourth-generation PAMAM dendrimer partially functionalized with redox-active ferrocenyls was used by Yoon et al [119] to construct a reagentless enzyme electrode for glucose biosensing. Functionalization levels of dendrimers, determined by UV-visible absorption studies, ranged from 4 to 80 % depending on the molar ratio between ferrocenyls and amino groups from dendrimers. A 32 % dendrimer modification level of surface amines to ferrocenyls was found to be optimum in terms of enzyme-dendrimer network formation, electrochemical interconnectivity of ferrocenyls and electrode sensitivity. The multilayered GOx /ferrocenyl dendrimer electrode assembly was constructed on an aminated gold surface *via* a LbL deposition procedure (Fig.7). Figure 8A shows the cyclic voltammograms from one (E1D1), three (E3D3) and five (E5D5) GOx/ferrocenyl dendrimer bilayers assembled on a gold electrode in 0.1 M phosphate buffer. The cyclic voltammograms were typical of surface-immobilized redox species but the redox peaks were slightly more separated with increasing numbers of bilayers. Also, the surface concentration of the ferrocenyls increased linearly with respect to the number of bilayers. The cyclic voltammograms of the multilayered electrodes in 20 mM glucose solution were typical for the enzyme-catalyzed and mediated voltammograms and the anodic currents were significantly enhanced (Fig. 8B). Amperometry calibration helped to obtain a detection limit as low as 1×10^{-6} M range with a S/N ratio of 3 for a E5D5 electrode. The stability of the electrode was ascertained by the maintenance over 80 % of the initial response even after 20 days under daily calibrations. The same group has reported earlier the bioelectrocatalytic characteristics of multilayered assemblies of GOx/PAMAM dendrimer for glucose biosensing with ferrocene methanol as the solution mediator [120].

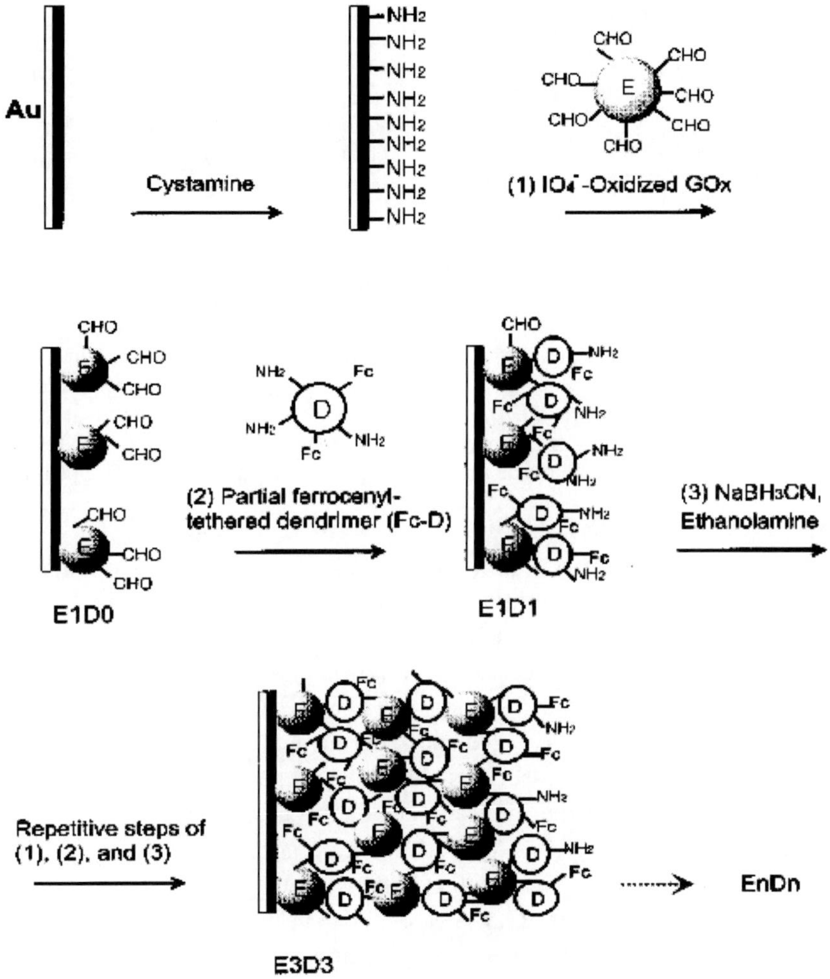

Figure 7. Organization of the multilayered GOx/ferrocenyl-tethered PAMAM dendrimer network on the Au electrode surface; EnDn – n-enzyme n-dendrimer layer (Adapted from Ref.[119]).

Cuadrado's group used a simple method to prepare dendrimer / enzyme electrodes for sensing hydrogen peroxide and glucose [121]. Three PPI dendrimers functionalized with 4, 8 and 32 octamethylferrocenyl moieties were used in the study. The dendrimer-modified platinum electrode was prepared by drop-casting technique. Then, GOx enzyme was immobilized by cross-linking using BSA and glutaraldehyde into the organometallic dendrimer film. The dendrimer/enzyme electrodes were found to show very good electrocatalytic effect for glucose. As expected, the higher generation dendrimer showed a better catalytic response of the biosensors. The linear range for calibration, sensitivity and detection limit for the amperometric determination of glucose were found to be very sensitive to the applied potential. The detection potential was lower at the octamethylferrocenyl dendrimer-modified electrodes compared to that at non-methylferrocenyl compounds.

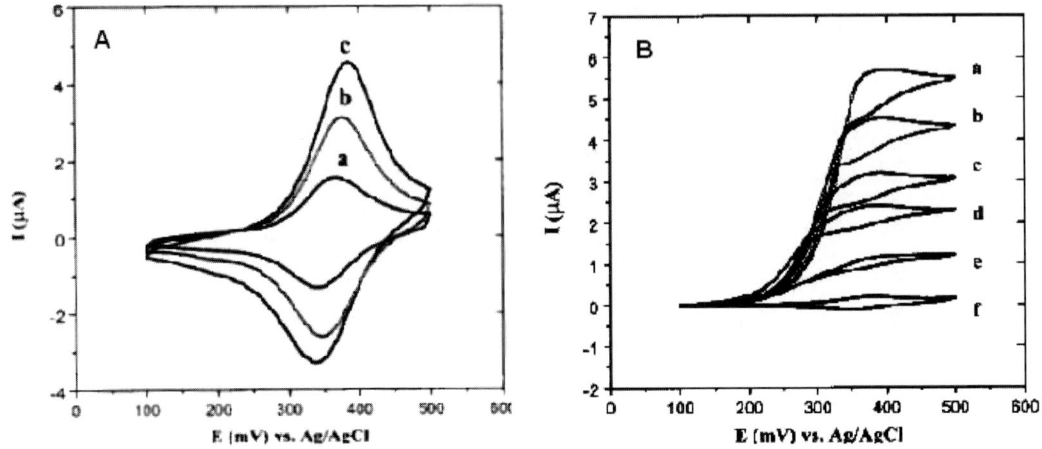

Figure 8. A. Cyclic voltammogram of GOx/ferrocenyl-tethered (32%) PAMAM dendrimer electrodes as a function of the number of bilayers in 0.1 M phosphate buffer (pH 7.0) at 50 mV/s (a) E1D1- (b) E3D3- and (c) E5D5- associated Au electrodes and B. Cyclic voltammograms at 5 mV/s for the bioelectrocatalytic glucose oxidation in the presence of 20 mM glucose as analyte (a) E5D5 (b) E4D4 (c) E3D3 (d) E2D2 (e) E1D1 (f) E1D1 in the absence of glucose (Adapted from Ref. [119]).

The same research group has also developed a bi-enzyme electrode based on GOx and horseradish peroxidase (HRP) co-immobilized on Pt electrodes modified with the octamethylferrocenyl poly(propyleneimine) dendrimer for the determination of glucose under aerobic conditions [122]. In conventional glucose sensors, hydrogen peroxide obtained by glucose oxidation is directly oxidized at the electrode. The direct oxidation of hydrogen peroxide requires sensor operation at +0.1 to +0.4 V *vs* SCE which is liable for interferences by other electroactive species like uric acid and ascorbic acid. The bi-enzyme electrode with a combination of the HRP and GOx permits the detection of glucose at substantially lower potentials (-0.3 V) and therefore the interferences due to the coexisting electroactive species can be avoided.

Another recent study also employed the bi-enzyme electrode for the determination of glucose using a fourth generation PAMAM dendrimer in the presence of hydroquinone mediator in the solution [123]. A looped nanocomposite with high enzyme loading was synthesized by tethering periodate-oxidized GOx and HRP bi-enzymes on the dendrimer in dark at 10°C for 3 days. A sol-gel modified glassy carbon electrode (GCE) was used as the sensing electrode. The best sensitivity was obtained for a 2:1 ratio of GOx to HRP in the bi-enzymatic mixture.

Instead of the bi-enzyme approach, a different strategy involving three components *viz.* a membrane-substrate with high capability for hydrogen peroxide diffusion, an efficient redox mediator for the exclusive electrocatalytic reduction of hydrogen peroxide and a hybrid membrane mediator suitable for enzyme immobilization was adopted [124]. First, Au nanoparticles were grown inside PAMAM dendrimer molecules in aqueous solution using formic acid as the reducing agent. The PAMAM-Au nanohybrid was used as cationic polyelectrolyte to assemble a 3-bilayer poly(vinylsulfonic acid) (PVS)/PAMAM-Au film onto the ITO electrode, where PVS was used as the anionic polyelectrolyte by the LbL technique (Fig. 9). This was followed by the electrodeposition of cobalt hexacyanoferrate (CoHCF) around the Au nanoparticles [125]. GOx was immobilized on the PVS/PAMAM-

Au@CoHCF electrocatalytic membrane by cross-linking with a mixture of BSA and glutaraldehyde. To optimize the biosensor construction, three different electrodes were assembled : i) applying PVS/PAMAM-Au nanoparticles three times, then depositing mediator followed by enzyme (PVS/PAMAM-Au)$_3$@CoHCF-GOx ii) applying PVS/PAMAM-Au nanoparticles and depositing mediator three times followed by the enzyme (PVS/PAMAM-Au @CoHCF)$_3$-GOx and iii) applying PVS/PAMAM-Au nanoparticle bilayer, mediator and enzyme layer three times (PVS/PAMAM-Au@CoHCF-GOx)$_3$. Among the three electrode configurations, the best response to glucose was obtained for the first one giving a sensitivity of 33.6 nA mmol L^{-1} cm^{-2} and a detection limit of 17 μmol L^{-1}. The selectivity of the biosensor was assessed by checking the influence of interferents like fructose, ethanol, acetic acid, ascorbic acid, citric acid , lactic acid, malic acid, oxalic acid and tartaric acid which are normally present in wines [126]. Among the interferents studied, only ascorbic acid was detected at 0.0 V vs SCE and at a glucose detection potential of -0.18 V, the interference due to ascorbic acid could be avoided.

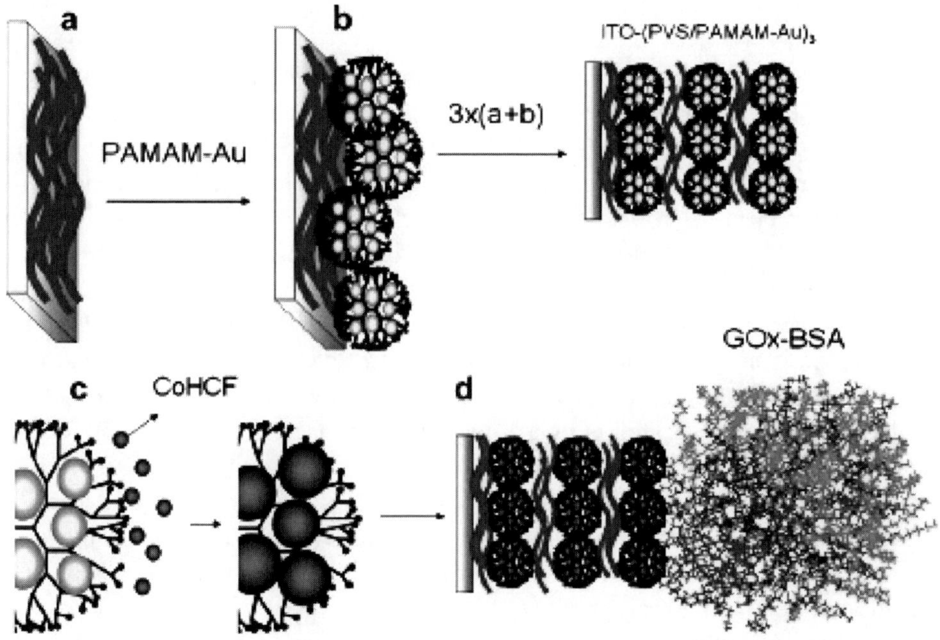

Figure 9. Schematic fabrication of LbL films comprising poly(vinylsulfonic acid) (PVS)and PAMAM-Au. The sequential deposition of LbL multilayers was carried out by immersing the substrate alternately into (a) PVS and (b) PAMAM-Au solutions for 5 min per step (c) After deposition of 3 bilayers, an ITO-PVS/PAMAM-Au)3 @ CoHCF electrode was prepared by potential cycling (d) The enzyme immobilization to produce ITO-PVS/PAMAM-Au)3@CoHCF-GOx was carried out in a solution containing BSA, glutaraldehyde and GOx (Adapted from Ref.[124])

An interesting investigation concerns the use of PPI dendrimers functionalized with both ferrocene and cobaltocenium moieties for glucose biosensor [105, 127]. Such dendrimers can exhibit a double function : while the ferrocene units act as mediators in enzymatic processes under anaerobic conditions, the cobaltocenium moieties take part in the electrocatalysis in the presence of oxygen. Another major advantage cited of these electrodes is that a large amount of enzyme can be immobilized due to electrostatic interactions between the positive ferrocenium and cobaltocenium moieties and the negatively charged enzyme. The dendrimer-modified electrode was prepared by electrodeposition onto Pt or GCE by cyclic voltammetry in the potential range between 0 and -1.1 V vs SCE in deaerated acetonitrile containing the dendrimer. The heteromultinuclear modified electrode in aqueous solution containing 0.1 M $LiClO_4$ shows two well-defined reversible systems with formal potentials at + 0.47 V and - 0.83 V corresponding to the ferrocene/ferrocenium and cobaltocenium/cobaltocene respectively. The GOx enzyme was immobilized by immersing the electrode in acetate buffer containing 0.1 % enzyme and 0.1 M $NaClO_4$ and holding the potential at +0.6 V for 30 minutes. Glucose was detected by measuring the amperometric response at + 0.5 V due to the mediation of the enzymatic reaction by the electrochemical oxidation of ferrocene. The catalytic activity of the cobaltocenium centres was proved by holding the potential at -0.65 V when a decrease in current due to oxygen reduction was detected as the concentration of glucose increased. The presence of cobaltocenium units prevents loss of GOx due to the reduction of ferrocenium groups and this increases the long-term stability of the sensor.

Hianik's group has made significant contributions on the development of stable glucose biosensors based on SAMs of PAMAM dendrimers of different generations [128-131]. The SAMs were formed by taking advantage of strong physical adsorption of dendrimers onto a gold support followed by chemisorption of hexylmercaptan [128] or hexadecane thiol [129] to impart stability to the dendrimer layer on the gold support. The enzyme GOx was immobilized into the SAM by cross-linking with glutaraldehyde. Quartz crystal microbalance technique was used to estimate the number of GOx molecules immobilized on the electrode surface. Amperometric determination of glucose at + 0.67 V *vs* SCE in 0.1 M KCl and 0.1 M Tris buffer at pH 7.1 indicated that the sensitivity of the biosensor increased with increasing dendrimer generation number. Two reasons *viz.* increased interior volume of the dendrimer and more number of binding sites for enzyme with increasing dendrimer content were attributed to the increase in current sensitivity [128]. Scanning electrochemical microscopy studies revealed that the electrodes with higher dendrimer content contained no visible defects or pinholes [130]. Atomic force microscopy studies ascertained that application of the potential to these layers caused substantial changes in the layer topography and increased the layer roughness [131]. These studies have helped to know that the method of preparation of dendrimer layers as well as the method of immobilization of the enzyme on the surface play crucial roles in determining the sensitivity, response time, detection limit, enzyme turnover and stability of the glucose biosensor.

A new type of biosensor based on PAMAM dendrimer encapsulated Pt nanoparticles (Pt-DENs)/GOx multilayered assembly has been reported by Zhu's group [132]. The encapsulated Pt nanoparticles act as efficient conduits for electrons facilitating their transfer in the enzyme layer. Platinum nanoparticles of size 3 nm were formed in situ within the dendrimer by a simple chemical reduction procedure. The Pt-DENs/GOx multilayer was assembled on a Pt electrode by the LbL procedure (Fig.10). AFM characterization confirmed the formation of a densely packed and structurally stable architecture attributable to a strong electrostatic interaction and covalent bonding between the charged amine terminated dendrimer and the periodate oxidized GOx. The amperometric response of a 5-bilayer electrode at -0.2 V in a buffer solution at pH 6.8 showed a linear range for the concentration of glucose from 5 μmol L^{-1} to 1.0 mmol L^{-1}. A low detection limit of 0.1 μmol L^{-1} was obtained. The biosensor sensitivity was 30.33 μA mM^{-1} cm^{-2} which was higher than the sensitivity value of 7.38 μA mM^{-1} cm^{-2} reported for the ferrocenyl-tethered PAMAM dendrimer [119]. These results led to the development of an enzyme-linked field effect transistor (ENFET) glucose biosensor device with three alternatively adsorbed layers of GOx and the Pt-DENs on the Si_3N_4 gate surface [133]. The ENFET (Fig.11) was first immersed in a blank solution for a few minutes to get a stable baseline and then known concentrations of the glucose solutions were injected into the measuring cell to monitor the change in the open circuit potential. The response time of 200 s was smaller than the normal 300 s and also the sensitivity of the device was about 12.5 mV/mM which is higher than the typical sensitivity of about 10 mV/mM observed for the ENFET devices doped with oxide nanoparticles [134].

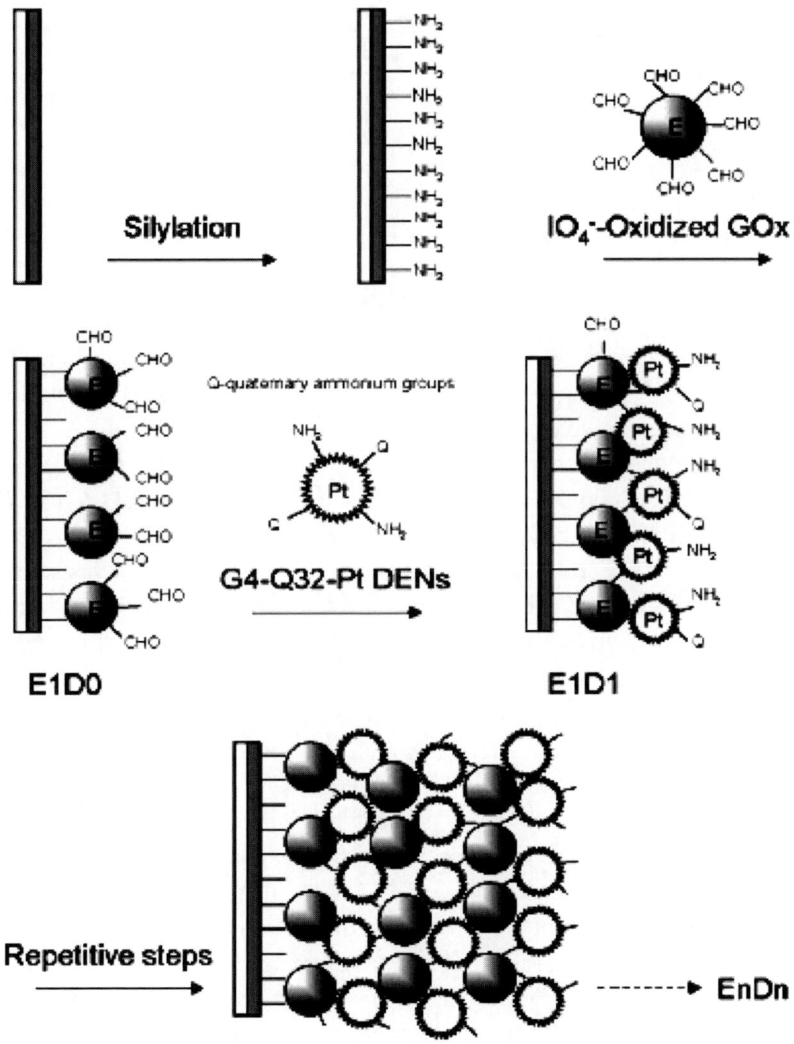

Figure 10. Schematic representation of the multilayered Pt-DENs/GOx network construction on the electrode using LbL approach (Adapted from Ref. [132]).

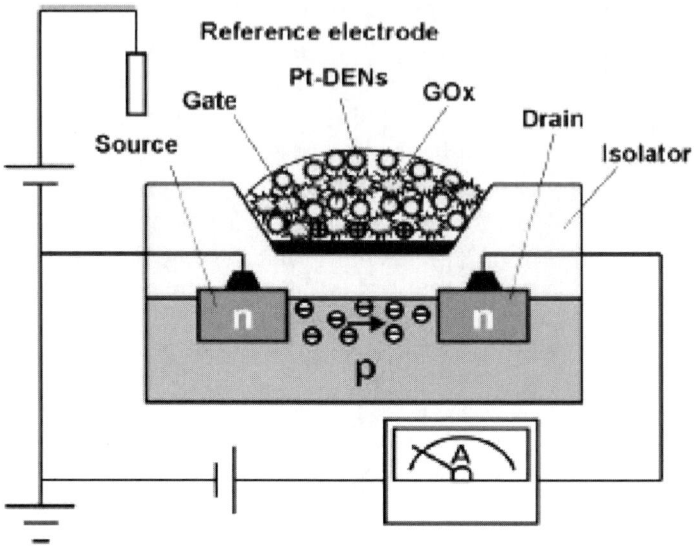

Figure 11. Schematic of ENFET assembled with Pt-DENs/GOx using LbL technique (Adapted from Ref. [133]).

The Pt-DENs have been exploited as dopant for a conjugated polymer *viz.* polypyrrole and the resulting nanocomposite has been found to give a very high sensitivity for glucose [135]. Polypyrrole itself is a good electrocatalyst for hydrogen peroxide and glucose [136, 137] and therefore one can expect a synergistic performance by the nanocomposite for glucose sensing. The nanocomposite was prepared by electropolymerization on a GCE from a solution consisting of 0.1 M pyrrole in phosphate buffer solution of pH 6.8 with the addition of Pt-PAMAM and GOx in the solution. The nanocomposite electrode had to be stored in phosphate buffer of pH 7.4 at 4 ^{o}C to prevent enzyme denaturation. Characterization of the nanocomposite by electrochemical impedance spectra showed a much lower charge transfer resistance compared to polypyrrole. The nanocomposite showed a short response time of 3 s with a high sensitivity of 164 μA mM^{-1} cm^{-2}. The detection limit for glucose was 10 nM. The selectivity of the glucose sensor in the presence of other interferents like uric acid, ascorbic acid and acetaminophen was also demonstrated. Zhu's group extended the study to the composites of Pt-DENs with carbon nanotube [138] polyaniline [139] and with both polyaniline and carbon nanotube [140] for glucose biosensing.

A mediator-free glucose sensor has been made possible by grafting PAMAM on carboxylated carbon nanotubes as shown in Fig.12 [141]. Acid-oxidized multi-walled carbon nanotube was treated with a methanolic solution of PAMAM in the presence of 1-(3-dimethylaminopropyl)-3-ethylcarbodiimide hydrochloride (EDC) and N-hydroxysuccinimide (NHS) to obtain the CNT-PAMMM composite. A bi-enzymatic matrix was prepared by treating the oxidized forms of GOx and HRP with the nanocomposite. The Schiff base formed was reduced by $NaBH_3CN$. In addition, the free carboaldehyde groups on the periphery of the enzymes were blocked with ethanolamine to avoid self-polymerization. A sol-gel film of the nanobiocomposite was drop-coated on a GCE. The sensor exhibited good current sensitivity to both hydrogen peroxide and glucose without any redox mediator. The mechanism of the sensor has been described as below [141] :

$GO_x(ox) + \beta\text{-D}(+)\text{-glucose} \longrightarrow GO_x(red) + \text{gluconic acid}$

$GO_x\,(red) + O_2 \longrightarrow GO_x\,(ox) + H_2O_2$

$H_2O_2 + HRP\,(red) \longrightarrow H_2O + HRP(ox)$

$HRP(ox) + e^-\,(CNT) \longrightarrow HRP(red)$

It is interesting to note that, without CNT, the oxidized form of HRP cannot get electrons from the electrode directly and in such case no current response to glucose will be observed. Another advantage of the sensor is the lower detection potential of -0.34 V which helps to avoid the interference of other biomolecules.

Table I provides a comparison of the performance of the dendrimer-based electrochemical glucose biosensors. It is found that many of the dendrimer electrode assemblies show reasonable linear range and detection limit. Their stability assessment and high sensitivity values indicate good scope for commercialization. The bi-enzyme model is better than the conventional mono-enzyme model in terms of lower detection potential which can help to circumvent the interferences due to other biomolecules during the measurements.

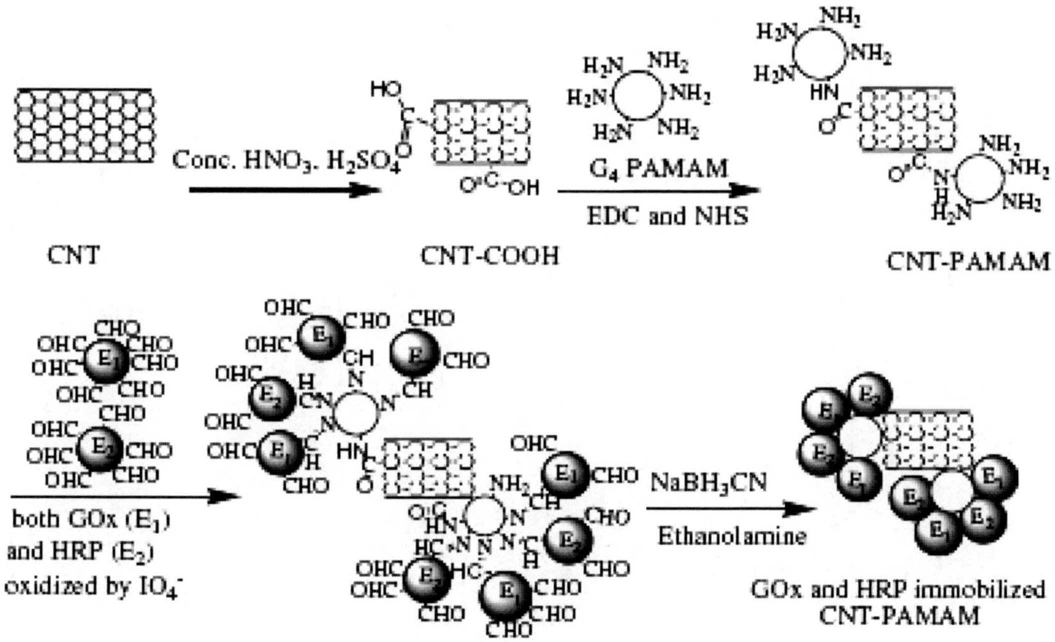

Figure 12. Procedure for the preparation of CNT-PAMAM and GOx-HRP immobilized CNT-PAMAM (Adapted from Ref.[141]).

Table I.Performance of dendrimer-based electrochemical glucose biosensors

No.	Enzyme(s) /electrode	Dendrimer or its composite	Immobilization method	Detection Technique	Electrolyte	Analytical Characteristics	Sensitivity*	Ref.
1.	GOx / CPE	Silicon dendrimers with 8 ferrocenyl peripheral groups	Blending	Steady-state polarization at +0.35 V *vs* SCE	0.1 M Phosphate buffer with 0.1M KCl, pH 7	Linear range – upto 1.5 mM; K'_M = 35.3 ±3.8; Stable response for 20 first measurements; Storage stability at 0°C in air for 120 h	57 mA mM^{-1}	[118]
2.	GOx / Au	Partial ferrocenyl-tethered PAMAM (G4)	LbL (one and five enzyme-dendrimer layers - E1D1 and E5D5)	Steady-state polarization at +0.37 V vs Ag/AgCl	0.1 M Phosphate buffer, pH 7	E5D5 : Linear range - upto 20 mM; Detection limit – 1 μM ; Response time =6s Storage stability in buffer for 20 days	-	[119]
3.	GOx / Au	PAMAM (G4)	LbL (one, three and five enzyme-dendrimer layers- E1D1, E3D3, E5D5)	Cyclic voltammetry, + 0.275 V *vs* Ag/AgCl	0.1 M Phosphate buffer, pH 8; 0.1 M ferrocene methanol as solution mediator	Storage stability in buffer for 20 days	E1D1-3.2; E3D3-8.3 E5D5-14.7 μA mM^{-1} cm^{-2}	[120]
4.	GOx/Pt	PPI functionalized with 4, 8 and 32 octamethyl ferrocenyl groups (Dend-1, Dend-2 and Dend-3)	Drop-coating	Steady-state polarization at +0.1 V vs SCE	0.1 M Phosphate buffer with 0.1 M $NaClO_4$, pH 7	Detection limit (μM); Dend-1: 43 Dend-2: 39 Dend-3: 15 K'_M(mM) : Dend-1: 2.0 Dend-2: 1.8 Dend-3: 3.0; Stable response for intermittent measurements during 6 days; Storage stability in air for 7 weeks	Dend-1: 0.17 Dend-2: 0.20 Dend-3: 0.32 μA mM^{-1}	[121]
5.	GOx/HRP/Pt	PPI functionalized with 4,8 and 32 octamethyl ferrocenyl groups (Dend-1, Dend-2 and Dend-3)	Drop-coating	Steady-state polarization at +100 mV vs SCE	0.1 M Phosphate buffer with 0.1 M $NaClO_4$, pH 7	Linear range (mmol L^{-1}) Dend 1: 4 Dend 2: 4 Dend 3: 4.5; Detection limit (μM) Dend 1: 12.8 Dend 2: 25.0 Dend 3: 22.1 ; K'_M (mM) Dend 1: 4.3 Dend 2: 4.8 Dend 3: 5.4	Dend 1: 5.51 Dend 2: 7.29 Dend 3: 7.43 μA mM^{-1} L cm^{-2}	[122]

Table I. (continued)

No.	Enzyme(s) /electrode	Dendrimer or its composite	Immobilization method	Detection Technique	Electrolyte	Analytical Characteristics	Sensitivity*	Ref.
6.	GOx/HRP/GCE	PAMAM (G4)	Silica sol-gel film	Chronoamperometry at - 0.3 V vs SCE	0.1 M phosphate buffer, pH 6.8 with 2mM hydroquinone as mediator	Linear range-H_2O_2: 3.1μM - 2 mM; Glucose : 3 μM-1.5 mM; Detection limit -H_2O_2::0.8 μM ; Glucose:1.2 μM ;Stability ~ 10 weeks	H_2O_2 – 360 μA L mol^{-1} cm^{-2} Glucose – 170 μA L mol^{-1} cm^{-2}	[123]
7.	GOx/ITO	PAMAM (G4)-Au-CoHCF	LbL	Amperometry at 0.0 V vs SCE	0.1 M phosphate buffer, pH 7	Linear range upto 1.5 mM; K'_M =2.03 mM;Detection limit 17 μM	33.6±0.2 nA mmol $L^{-1}cm^{-2}$	[124]
8.	GOx/GCE or Pt	Ferrocene -cobaltocenium PPI dendrimer With 4,8,16,32 metallic species(dend-1 to dend-4)	Potentiostatic deposition at -1.0 V vs SCE ; Enzyme immobilization in acetate buffer at +0.6 V	Steady state polarization +0.55 V (anaerobic) and -0.7 V (aerobic) vs SCE	0.1 M Phosphate buffer, pH 7	Anaerobic condn: K'_M, mM Dend 1:219 Dend 2:220 Dend 3:194 Dend 4:153 Response time = 5 to 10 s; Repeatability for 50 measurements; Storage stability-7 weeks	Anaerobic condn: Dend 1:15 Dend 2:22 Dend 3:38 Dend 4:53 nA mM^{-1} cm^{-2} Aerobic condn: Dend 1:0.28 Dend 2:0.33 Dend 3:0.42 Dend 4:0.68 μA $mM^{-1}cm^{-2}$	[127]
9.	GOx/Au	PAMAM (G0, G1 and G4)	SAM	Amperometry at + 0.67 V vs SCE	0.1 M KCl + 0.1 M Tris, pH 7.1	K'_M, mM, G0: 5.1±1.2, G1: 6.0±0.4 G4: 5.2 ED0E1D1:4.5;Stability highest for G0, 15 days	G0: 2.0, G1: 8.6 G4: 28 ED0ED1:95.1 nA mM^{-1} cm^{-2}	[128]
11.	GOx/Au	PAMAM (G1) SAM- Four types of electrodes prepared.Step-wise casting of dendrimer and hexadecanethiol A(G1); Simultaneous casting B(G1). Enzyme immobilization in vacuum A(GOx) and in solution B(GOx) ; E1 to E4 are A(G1)-A(GOx); B(G1)-A(GOx) A(G1)-B(GOx) ; B(G1)-B(GOx)		Amperometry at + 0.67 V vs SCE	0.1 M Tris-HCl mixed with 0.1 M KCl, 1:1v/v, pH 7.5,4 mM $K_4Fe(CN)_6$ as solution mediator	E1,E2,E3,E4 :K'_M (mM) - 2.7,1.1,5.8,1.7 ; Response time (min) = 1.2, 1.3,4.5,1.3 ; Linear range (mM)- 2,1,3.9.3.9 ; Detection limit (mM) – 0.025, 0.025, 1.03, 0.025 ; Stabilty (weeks)-2,8,1,1 respectively.	E1,E2,D3,E4 : 994.2±58.6 615.4±6.2 7.7±1.3 52.4±1.4 nA mM^{-1} cm^{-2}	[129]
12.	GOx/Au	PAMAM(G1) SAM Five types of electrodes with different hexadecanethiol /dendrimer ratio, E1 to E5 are 1:0.43; 1:0.82; 1:1.5; 1:3; 1:9		Amperometry at +0.67 V vs SCE	0.1 M Phosphate pH 7.6 $K_4Fe(CN)_6$ as solution mediator	E1,E2,E3,E4,E5: K'_M (mM)- 1.51±0.27, 1.64±0.08 1.01±0.27, 0.52±0.14, 0.75±0.22	E1,E2,E3,E4, E5: 52.2±14.4 164.9±23.6 531.9±50.9 243.3±16.0 558.2±112.1 nA mM^{-1} cm^{-2}	[130]

Table I. (continued)

No.	Enzyme(s) /electrode	Dendrimer or its composite	Immobilization method	Detection Technique	Electrolyte	Analytical Characteristics	Sensitivity*	Ref.
13.	GOx/Pt	PAMAM (G4)-Pt	LbL	Amperometry at -0.2 V vs SCE	0.1 M Phosphate buffer pH 6.8	Linear range 5 μM to 1 mM; Detection limit 0.1 μmol L^{-1}; Response time=5 s; Repeatability for 100 measurements; storage stability measured for 30 days	30.33 μA mM^{-1} cm^{-2}	[132]
14.	GOx Enzyme-linked field effect transistor (ENFET)	PAMAM(G4)-Pt	LbL	Potentiometry vs SCE	10 mM Phosphate buffer and 100 mM NaCl at pH 7.4	Linear range – 0.25-2.0 mM; Detection limit : 0.15 mM; Response time = 200s; Repetability for 5 measurements; storage stability measured for 30 days	12.5 mM/mV	[133]
15.	GOx/GCE	PAMAM(G4)-Pt-polypyrrole	Electrochemical codeposition	Amperometry at +0.3 Vvs SCE	0.1 M Phosphate buffer, pH 6.8	Linear range : 0.2 to 600 μM; Detection limit: 10 nM; Response time:<3 s; Storage stability measured for 4 weeks	164 μA mM^{-1} cm^{-1}	[135]
16.	GOx/GCE	PAMAM(G4)-Pt-Nanofibrous polyaniline	LbL	Amperometry at +0.6 V vs Ag/AgCl	0.05 M Phosphate buffer, pH 6	Linear range: 10 μM to 4.5 mM; Detection limit : 0.5 μM; Response time < 5 s; Storage Stability measured for 20 days	39.63 μA mM^{-1} cm^{-1}	[139]
17.	GOx/Pt	PAMAM (G4)-Pt-carbon nanotube	LbL	Amperometry at +0.60 V vs Ag/AgCl	0.05 M Phosphate buffer pH 6.8	Linear range : 5 μM-0.65 mM; Detection limit : 2.5 μM; response time < 5 s; Storage stability measured for 30 days	30.64 μA mM^{-1} cm^{-1}	[138]
18.	GOx/GCE	PAMAM (G4)-Pt-Polyaniline-carbon nanotube	LbL	Amperometry at +0.6 V vs Ag/AgCl	0.05 M Phosphate buffer pH 6	Linear range : 1 μM-12 mM; Detection limit: 0.5 μM; Response time = 5 s ; Storage stability measured for 3 weeks	42 μA mM^{-1} cm^{-1}	[140]
19.	GOx/HRP/GCE	PAMAM(G4)-CNT	Silica sol-gel film	Amperometry at -0.34V *vs* SCE	0.1 M Phosphate buffer, pH 6.8	Linear range: 4 μM to 1.2 mM; Detection limit – 2.5 mM; Response time =1 s	2.2 μA mM^{-1}	[141]

* The unit for sensitivity is as given in the respective references

Abbreviations : GOx-glucose oxidase; HRP-horse radish peroxidase ; PAMAM-poly(amidoamine) ; G_n – generation number; CPE-carbon paste electrode ; GCE-glassy carbon electrode; ITO-indium-tin oxide ; CoHCF-cobalt hexacyanoferrate ; K'_M - apparent Michaelis-Menten constant ; LbL-layer-by-layer ; SAM-self-assembled monolayer

(c) Biosensors for the Detection of other Analytes

Novel biointerfaces of dendrimers with heme proteins have been reported. Such studies have helped to accomplish direct electron transfer between the biomolecule and electrode. Several attempts have been made to widen the scope of the dendrimer-based electrochemical biosensors for environmental monitoring. Analytes like glutamate, ethanol and several pesticides have been detected. Exclusive studies to detect hydrogen peroxide at dendrimer-modified electrodes have also been made.

Hu's group has developed LbL assemblies of heme proteins with PAMAM [142] and PPI [143] dendrimers. At pH 7.0, protonated PAMAM possesses positive surface charges, whereas the proteins have net negative surface charges at pH above their isoelectric points. Thus, LbL (PAMAM/protein)$_n$ films were assembled with alternate adsorption of oppositely charged PAMAM and proteins from their aqueous solutions mainly by electrostatic interaction on pyrolytic graphite surface [142]. In the case of PPI dendrimer, the negatively charged hemoglobin protein at pH 9 not only alternately adsorbed with positively charged PPI by electrostatic attraction between them, but the positively charged hemoglobin protein at pH 5 was also successfully assembled with positively charged PPI into LbL films due to a possible localized electrostatic interaction or the charge reversal of proteins on PPI surface [143]. In another study, a LbL assembly of myoglobin with PPI dendrimer-stabilized gold core-shell nanoparticles has been reported [144]. All the three electrode assemblies have been evaluated for the electrocatalysis of hydrogen peroxide based on the direct electrochemistry of the proteins at the respective dendrimer-modified surfaces.

The nano-Au/PAMAM dendrimer/HRP assembly on a cystamine-modified gold electrode was found to show good sensitivity and stability in the detection of hydrogen peroxide [145].

Tang et al have reported the application of the dendrimer-encapsulated platinum nanoparticles in the detection of the glutamate neurotransmitter. Two types of sensing layers have been used : a self-assembled film comprising glutamate dehydrogenase and dendrimer-encapsulated platinum nanoparticles onto a carbon nanotubes-modified GCE and then a hybrid film of the above constituents with polypyrrole [146]. The film preparations were similar to those used by the authors for glucose biosensors [147]. Cyclic voltammetry and amperometry were used to follow the oxidation of glutamate in phosphate buffer solution at pH 7.4, containing 0.1 M β-nicotinamide adenine dinucleotide (NAD^+). Both the sensors showed a lower detection limit of 10 nM with a rapid response, low level of interference from ascorbic acid, uric acid and acetaminophen, good reproducibility and stability.

The detection of ethanol at concentrations of 1 ppm by volume, by electrical capacitance measurement using a PAMAM/alcohol dehydrogenase LbL film deposited onto Au-interdigitated electrode has been assembled [148]. The film growth and adsorption kinetics were followed nanogravimetrically with the help of a quartz crystal microbalance. The same group also developed a biosensor for the detection of catechol, using PAMAM/Cl-catechol 1,2-dioxygenase LbL film [149]. Catechol could be detected at concentrations as low as 10^{-10} M.

The effect of irreversible inhibition of acetylcholinesterase has been used in dendrimer-based electrochemical biosensors for environmental applications. Acetylcholinesterase is a very efficient protein catalyst for the hydrolysis of its physiological substrate acetylcholine. Organophosphorus and carbamic pesticides, heavy metals and detergents exert strong specific inhibition of this enzyme action which can be detected by electrochemical techniques [150]. Hianik's group investigated the response of the SAM-based PAMAM-enzyme biosensor for the detection of trichlorfon, carbofuran and eserine due to the inhibitory effect by adopting a bi-enzyme approach [151, 152]. Acetylcholinesterase and choline oxidase were the two enzymes used. Acetylcholine is hydrolyzed by acetylcholinesterase to form choline which is then oxidized by the second enzyme choline oxidase forming hydrogen peroxide. The electrochemical current in the hydrogen peroxide oxidation can be used as a measure of the acetylcholinesterase activity and hence as a response of the bi-enzyme sensor. Amperometric measurements in 0.1 M phosphate buffer solution at pH 7.5 revealed very low detection limits of dimethyl-2,2-dichlorovinylphosphate (1.3 pmol L^{-1}) [151], trichlorfon (0.03 nmol L^{-1}), carbofuran (0.04 nmol L^{-1}), and eserine (0.1 nmol L^{-1}) [152].

(d) Dendrimers in DNA Detection

DNA biosensors are useful to detect specific sequences of a target DNA. The development of DNA biosensors has been a very important area of research, especially after the realization of the potentialities of nanomaterials in bio applications [153]. Several materials and methods have been identified towards the goal of making cost- effective DNA chips or arrays for simultaneous determination of various gene sequences [154]. Tremendous progress has been made into the development of electrochemical DNA biosensors but there are still many challenges to be overcome [155]. The principle is based on the affinity of a single-strand DNA(ss-DNA) for a complementary strand of ss-DNA. DNA hybridization occurs between a DNA of known sequence (probe) and an unknown counterpart (target). The hybridization occurs due to the supramolecular phenomenon of bases paring in which the purine bases (Adenine and Guanine) are hydrogen-bonded to complementary pyrimidine bases (Cytosine and Thymine), creating A-T pairs and G-C pairs [156]. There have been two main approaches in the development of DNA biosensors: labeled method and label-free method. The labeled method involves the use of a redox probe that binds to DNA. The label-free method depends on the changes in the electroactivity of DNA due to hybridization.

The biocompatibility of dendrimers along with their enhanced surface area allow an increase in the immobilized DNA probe on the dendrimer-modified electrode which can result in a higher sensitivity in the detection of the target DNA [157]. PAMAM and PPI dendrimers possessing amine end groups are highly suitable for the DNA biosensors. Besides these dendrimers, DNA dendrimers have also been used for the DNA biosensors. These DNA dendrimers are nucleic acid dendrimers, built from dendritic monomers composed of single-stranded nucleic acid molecules partially hybridized, which can in turn be sequentially hybridized with a controlled exponential growth governed by supramolecular interactions [158].

There have been only very limited studies in literature on the exploitation of dendrimers in electrochemical DNA biosensors. The earliest report was by Wang et al on the chronopotentiometric detection of a 27-mer ss-DNA oligonucleotide of 2-layer and 4-layer dendrimers by adsorptive accumulation on carbon paste electrodes. The detection limits were found to be 3 and 12 pM for the 2- and 4- layers nucleic dendrimers respectively [159].

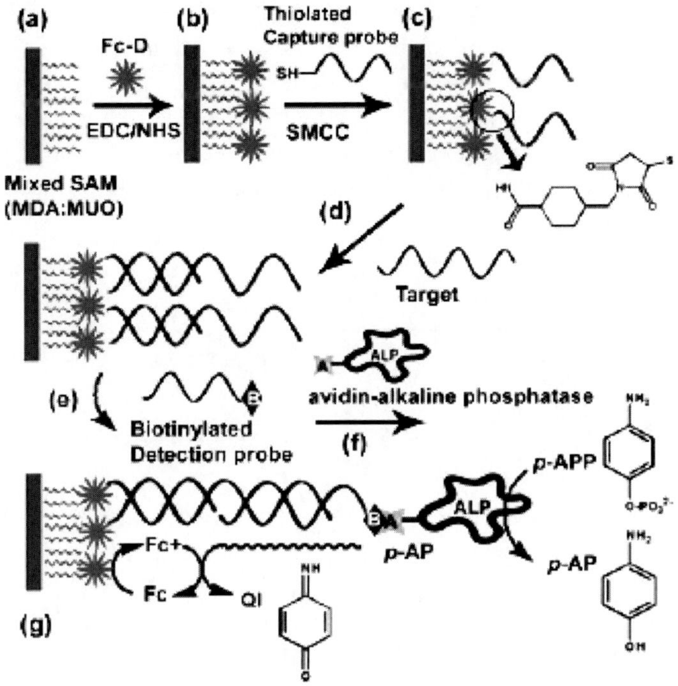

Figure 13. (a) Formation of mixed SAM on Au electrode, (b) immobilization of Fc-D, (c) immobilization of thiolated capture probe with bifunctional linker (succinimidyl 4-(*N*-maleimidomethyl)cyclohexane-1-carboxylate (SMCC)), (d) hybridization with target, (e) hybridization with biotinylated detection probe, (f) association with avidin-alkaline phosphatase, (g) description of the process of the electrocatalytic reaction of *p*-aminophenol (*p*-AP) via electronic mediation of ferrocenyl dendrimer (Adapted from Ref.[160])

A sandwich-type enzyme-linked DNA sensor based on a partially ferrocenyl-tethered PAMAM dendrimer has been reported [160]. The principle behind the sensor fabrication and operation is shown in Fig.13. A mixed SAM is formed on a clean gold electrode using a 1:4 mixture of mercaptododecanoic acid (MDA) and mercaptoundecanol (MDU). The SAM electrode is then immersed in a 2:1 mixed solution of EDC and NHS for activation of the carboxylic groups and then the ferrocenyl dendrimer is immobilized by covalent coupling of unreacted amine in the dendrimer to the acid groups. The probe DNA is modified with 5' thiol-terminated 6 carbon spacers. An ethylene glycol linker group is appended on the thiol modified probe DNA to improve hybridization efficiency and prevent nonspecific binding of proteins. The probe is 3'-labeled with a biotin group and a 5-T (thymine) spacer is inserted between the probe and the biotin. Three types of targets *viz.* complementary, non-complementary and single-base mismatched oligonucleotides are used for the sandwich hybridization. The hybridization step between the target and detection probe is carried out by incubation for 2 h at room temperature. If the target is complementary to the immobilized probe, it can then be hybridized with a biotinylated detection probe. Avidin-conjugated alkanline phosphate (Av-ALP) bound to the detection probe can generate the electroactive label *p*-aminophenol, from *p*-aminophenyl phosphate (*p*-APP) enzymatically. The *p*-aminophenol diffuses to near the ferrocene-tethered dendrimer layer which electrocatalyzes its oxidation. The magnitude of the electrocatalytic current indicates the extent of hybridization of the target DNA. The cyclic voltammograms showed strikingly different signals between the complementary (T1) and non-complementary target DNA (T2) (Fig. 14). For the hybridization with T_1, a sharp increase in the oxidation peak current was observed upon addition of *p*-APP, which was not the case with T_2. An oxidation current was also observed for the single-base mismatched target DNA (T_3) in which a single mismatched base was located in the middle of the section that was bound to the probe DNA. The hybridization signal for T1 increased with the target concentration in the range of 0.1 nM to 10 μM with a detection limit of 0.1 nM for a S/N =3.

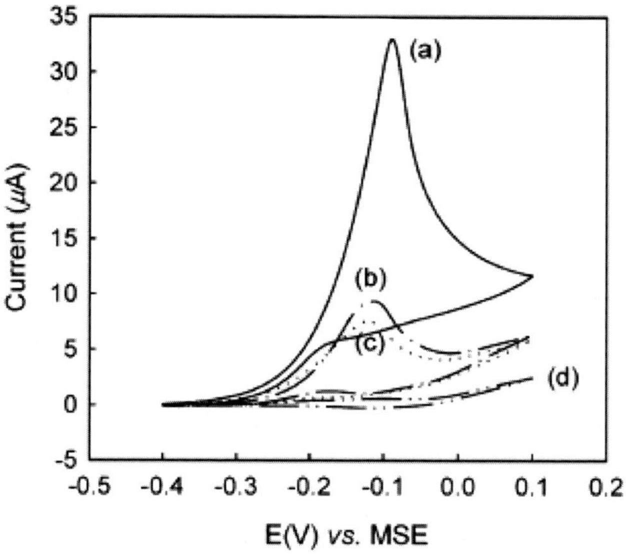

Figure 14. Cyclic voltammogram of enzyme-linked electrodes in a solution of 0.5 mM p-aminophenyl phosphate (p-APP) ; scan rate of 50 mV/s in the case of hybridization with (a) 1 μM complementary target (T1), (b) 1 μM single base- mismatched target (T3), (c) 1 μM non-complementary target (T2),and (d) without hybridization with target and detection probe (Adapted from Ref.[160]).

The SAM and covalent immobilization method have also been employed in the DNA hybridization detection based on PAMAM-modified gold electrode, using differential pulse voltammetry and daunomycin as the electroactive hybridization indicator [161]. Chemical modification of the gold electrode was carried out by treatment with mercaptoacetic acid for 2 h at room temperature. The electrode was then immersed in a solution containing appropriate quantities of dendrimer and EDC. The presence of EDC is very essential for firm anchoring of the dendrimer to the electrode surface. In the presence of EDC, peptide bond formation takes place, between the PAMAM dendrimer molecules and the surface attached thiol species. The immobilization of the ss-DNA probe was also performed by immersing the electrode in the oligonucleotide solution containing EDC in acetate buffer at pH 5.2 for 10 h. Hybridization reaction was carried out by immersing the ss-DNA probe captured electrode into a stirred solution containing different concentration of DNA target for 30 mins. The hybridized electrode was then placed in the stirred daunomycin solution containing 0.1% SDS phosphate buffer solution at pH 7.3 for 5 min in open circuit conditions. The differential pulse voltammetry (DPV) measurements were conducted from -0.1V to +0.5 V *vs* SCE in phosphate buffer solution. The peak current at + 0.23 V corresponding to the oxidation of daunomycin was taken as the electrochemical measurement signal. The daunomycin intercalated DNA duplex electrode gave an increased electrochemical response compared to ss-DNA in the concentration range between 1.1 x 10^{-10} and 1.1 x 10^{-11} mol L^{-1} with an estimated detection limit of 8 x 10^{-12} mol L^{-1}.

Recently, a DNA biosensor using a first generation PAMAM dendrimer and methylene blue as the electroactive indicator has been reported [162]. In this study, instead of the gold electrode, a pre-oxidized glassy carbon electrode was used to form the dendrimer modified electrode using the NHC and EDC as the coupling agents. The electroactive indicator, methylene blue, was also immobilized during the hybridization. The accumulated methylene blue was measured using cyclic voltammetry.

Electrochemical impedance technique has been used in the detection of DNA hybridization based on a fourth-generation PAMAM electrode [163]. The dendrimer was covalently attached to a 2-aminoethanethiol modified gold electrode through glutaraldehyde coupling. The aldehyde group of the glutaraldehyde reacts with the primary amino group of the aminoethanethiol and dendrimer to form a covalent bond, resulting in the Schiff base formation. The Schiff bases were reduced by $NaBH_4$ to get a dendrimer-modified electrode. The probe DNA was then attached to the modified electrode again through activation with glutaraldehyde in phosphate buffer solution at pH 7.4. followed by the reduction of the Schiff base. Hybridization was effected by immersing the probe DNA functionalized gold electrode in a solution of the target DNA. The impedance measurements have been done in a phosphate buffer solution containing 5 mM $[Fe(CN)_6]^{3-/4-}$ redox probe. The charge transfer resistance increased with increasing concentrations of the target DNA used for the hybridization. The increase in the charge transfer resistance is due to the charge repulsion between the negatively charged phosphate backbone of DNA and the $[Fe(CN)_6]^{3-/4-}$ redox probe. The DNA hybridization assay responded well in the concentration range from 10^{-11} to 10^{-8} M with a detection limit of 3.8 x 10^{-12} M.

In another study also, electrochemical impedance technique has been shown to be a useful method for a DNA biosensor using a multinuclear nickel(II) salicylaldimine metallodendrimer platform [164]. Both the preparation of the dendrimer-modified GCE surface and the immobilization of DNA have been effectively done by simple drop-coating procedures. The metallodendrimer is electroactive exhibiting two redox couples in phosphate buffer solution. The impedance study demonstrated that the DNA biosensor responded well to 5 nM of target DNA by displaying a decrease in charge transfer resistance in phosphate buffer solution and increase in charge transfer resistance in the presence of the $[Fe(CN)_6]^{3-/4-}$ redox probe.

(e) Dendrimers in Affinity Biosensors

Affinity sensors are based on selective binding of the biomolecules toward specific target species [165]. The binding interactions can be between protein-protein, receptor-ligand, antigen-antibody or enzyme-substrate. Immunosensors are based on immunological reactions involving the shape recognition of the antigen by the antibody binding site to form the antibody-antigen complex [166,167] The basic requirement to obtain good sensitivity from an electrochemical affinity sensor is the efficient immobilization of the biomolecule on the electrode surface with a favourable orientation for bio-specific interactions.

Dendrimers are molecularly controllable nanomaterials possessing multiple conjugation sites and are amenable for functionalization for specific applications. Especially PAMAM dendrimers with a large number of functional end groups are highly suitable for synthetic modifications of molecularly oriented nanostructures. Already several methodologies including SAM, LbL and micropatterning techniques have been developed for the construction of stable multilayered assemblies of biocomposites of dendrimers on electrode surfaces [117, 157, 168-171]. These characteristics enable dendrimers to be used in affinity biosensors.

Yoon's group has made significant contributions in the development of dendrimer-based electrochemical affinity biosensors [172-179] and highlights of their research work have been appraised recently [77].

The initial report was on the development of an affinity biosensor for avidin [172]. Avidin, an egg-white protein forms a very stable complex with biotin (vitamin H). The affinity biosensing surface is a SAM of ferrocenyl-tethered and biotinylated dendrimer on a gold electrode. An amine-reactive SAM was prepared by chemisorption of 3,3'-dithiopropionic acid bis-*N*-hydroxysuccinimide ester on gold surfaces. The activated ester groups were then reacted with the amino groups of ferrocenyl-tethered dendrimers. An aqueous solution of biotinyl-ε-amidocaproic acid *N*-hydroxysulfosuccinimide ester was added to the electrode for biotinylation of the amino groups of the ferrocenyl-tethered dendrimer monolayer. The principle of operation of the affinity biosensor is shown in Fig. 15. The SAM of the double-functionalized dendrimer plays the role of a molecular gate for free diffusing and signaling molecules in the electrolyte. The GOx enzyme in the electrolyte acts as a diffusional tracer and generates an electrochemical signal, depending on the degree of coverage of the sensing surface with avidin. The sensor signal (current) decreased with increasing avidin concentration and reached a minimum when the sensing surface was fully covered (Fig. 16). The sensor signal is affected by the amount of free GOx present in electrolyte and in order to avoid non-specific adsorption of GOx, a very low concentration is preferred. The sensor calibration showed good linearity in the range between 1.5 pM and 10 nM avidin with a detection limit of 4.5 pM. In a subsequent study, the authors reported an effective method for developing a renewable affinity surface by dissociation of the bound avidin molecules *via* a displacement reaction with free biotin in solution [173]. As another proof of the methodology developed, the reversible bio-specific recognition of the bifunctionalized dendrimer for the monoclonal anti-biotin immunoglobulin (I_gG) has also been reported [174].

Recently, the immunosensing of target antibody and antigen in a competition assay has been reported for the dinitrophenyl antigen/anti-dinitrophenyl antibody couple [175]. GOx-tagged anti-dinitrophenyl antibody was used as the signaling molecule. For competitive immunosensing, target anti-dinitrophenyl antibody and GOx-tagged anti-dinitrophenyl antibody were treated on the dinitrophenyl-functionalized electrode surface at the same time and the electrochemical current from GOx bioelectrocatalysis of GOx-tagged anti-dinitrophenyl antibody was monitored. The method was also applied for the detection of antigen as the target molecule. Free dinitrophenyl antigen was pre-mixed with GOx-tagged anti-dinitrophenyl antibody and the mixture was treated on the dinitrophenyl-modified electrode surface. The electrochemical signal decreased as the dinitrophenyl antigen concentration increased. Calibration plots could be made for both the target molecules.

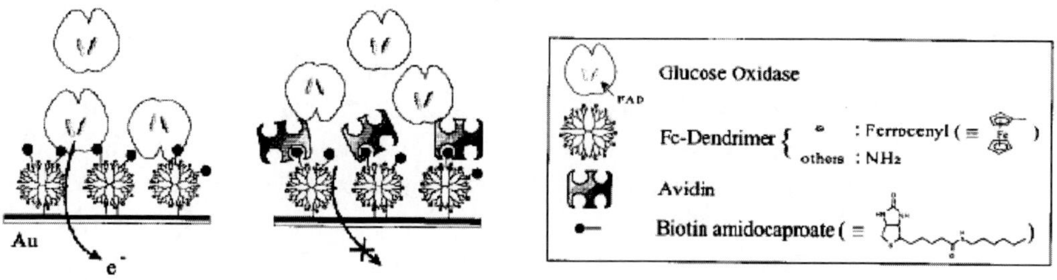

Figure 15. Construction and proposed operational principle for the affinity biosensor based on the avidin–biotin interaction on a gold electrode surface. (Right) Molecular models of the chemicals used for electrode construction and affinity biosensing. (Adapted from Ref. [172]).

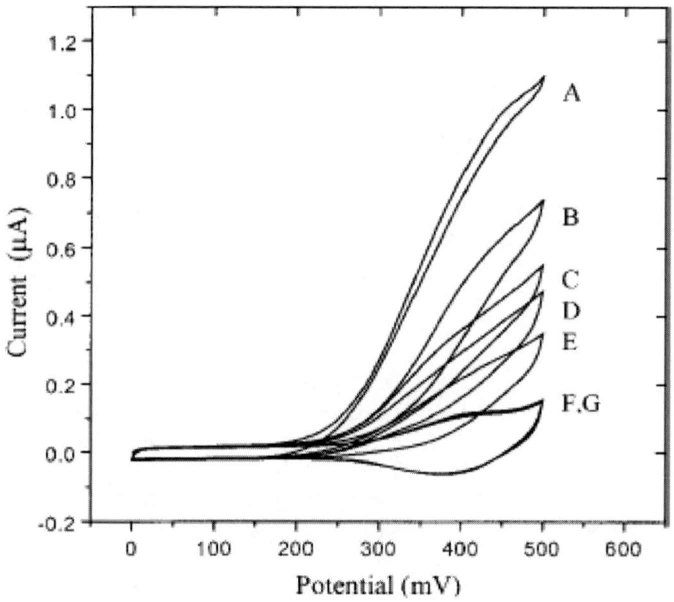

Figure 16. Cyclic voltammograms of the affinity biosensors as a function of reacted avidin concentration: (A) 0, (B) 1 ng/mL, (C) 10 ng/mL, (D) 100 ng/mL, (E) 1 μg/mL, and (F) 10 μg/mL. Cyclic voltammograms were obtained in the presence of 30 μg/mL of GOx as a signal generator and 10 mM glucose as a substrate; (G) background voltammogram in the absence of enzyme and substrate. All curves were registered in deoxygenated 0.1 M phosphate buffer (pH 7.2) solution under argon atmosphere. Potential scan rate was 5 mV/s. (Adapted from Ref. [172]).

Yoon's group further developed two impressive strategies for efficient electrochemical signaling from the affinity recognition reactions *viz.* immunoprecipitation-mediated signaling [176-178] and the enzymatic back-filling immunoassay [179].

For the biocatalytic precipitation, the sensing layer was the denrimer-activated SAM on a thin gold film surface deposited by electron-beam evaporation onto titanium-primed silicon wafers [176]. HRP was the enzyme label used. The analyte samples, containing the target proteins, antibiotin IgG–HRP or (strept)avidin–HRP conjugates, were then incubated with the biotinyl group functionalized surfaces. For the precipitate formation reaction, a mixture of H_2O_2 and 4-chloro-1-naphthol (4-CN) was used. HRP-mediated conversion of 4-CN to benzo-

4-chlorocyclohexadienone with H_2O_2 yielded insoluble precipitates on the sensor surface on which the biocatalyzed reaction took place. A film with a distinct color change was formed on the exposed and protein-associated region of the electrode surface confirming the efficient occurrence of the biocatalyzed reaction (Fig.17). A cyclic voltammetric signaling method, tracking the decrement in the active electrode area from the precipitation of the insolubles onto the electrode surfaces, was employed for signal registration. The sensor surface after the precipitation reaction can be renewed by the dissolution of the precipitate with an ethanolic phosphate buffer solution followed by the displacement of the bound antibody-enzyme conjugate with free biotin treatment [177].

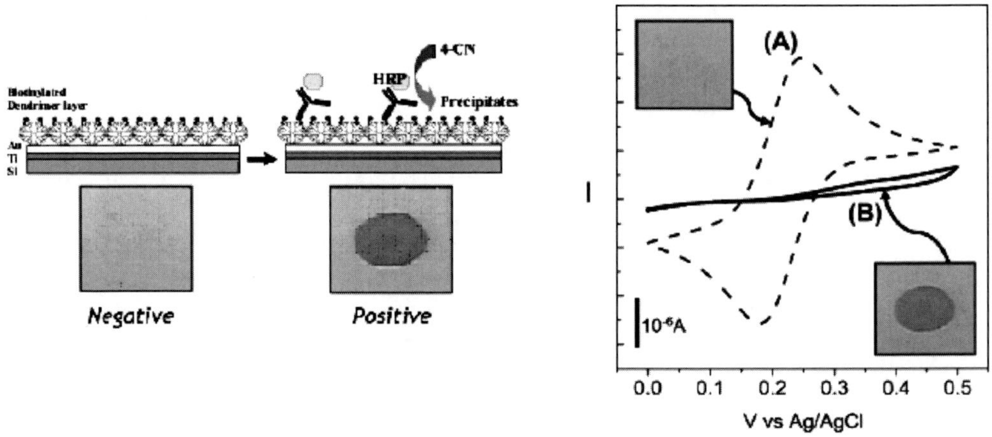

Figure 17. Schematic representation of the affinity biosensor construction and the proposed operational principle and voltammetric traces for affinity sensor signalling: a biotin-functionalized surface before (A) and after (B) target protein (antibiotin IgG–HRP) association and precipitation reaction steps. Voltammetric measurements were performed in 0.1 M phosphate buffer (pH 7.0),containing 0.1 mM ferrocene methanol as a signal tracer. Inset: charge coupled device (CCD) camera images of a sensor surface upon signalling reactions (Adapted from Refs. [176] & [177]).

The applicability of the method was further ascertained by the analysis of real samples such as blood serum using an array-type micropatterned gold electrodes of rectangular and circular geometries, exhibiting voltammetric characteristics of bulk and microelectrodes [178]. Ferritin was used as the recognition antigen which was functionalized on the immunosensing surface and anti-ferritin antibody was the target protein in applied antiserum samples. For signal generation, a HRP-catalyzed precipitate formation reaction was performed with either 4-CN or 3-amino-9-ethylcarbazole. Although, both rectangular and circular types of microfabricated immunosensors exhibited cyclic voltammograms with diminishing peak heights in correlation with the concentration of applied target protein in serum samples, the circular electrode was found to be advantageous for sensor operation since the current could be sampled at a fixed potential.

The enzymatic back-filling immunoassay model has been demonstrated with the dinitrophenyl antigen-functionalized surface and anti-dinitrophenyl antibody as target analyte [179]. The method is based on the covalent immobilization of enzyme onto the immunosensor surface, circumventing the use of enzyme-tagged antibody and alleviating the signal instability from low-affinity binding. The electrochemical signal can be maintained even if the analyte has a low affinity to the binding ligand because the signal generating enzyme is separated from the analyte.

V. CONCLUSION

The rapid advancements in nanoscience and nanotechnology have yielded a number of new materials such as gold nanoparticles, nanostructured metal oxides and carbon nanotubes for exploitation in electrochemical biosensors [180-182]. Among the nanostructured materials, dendrimers stand unique owing to their high biocompatibility and internal porosity which make them extremely suitable for the immobilization of biomolecules in their matrices. The intensive studies reported so far in literature using some novel dendrimer-modified bioelectrode platforms have already shown promising trends in terms of short response time, improved sensitivity, high stability and least interferences due to the presence of other analytes. However, the elaborate synthetic procedures required to prepare designer dendrimers in a pure form along with the intricate steps that need to be followed for making the sensing layer are presently the impediments in the exploration of many other dendrimers for the biosensor applications.

ACKNOWLEDGMENT

RS is grateful for a visiting scientist fellowship under the Exchange Program in Research, Education and Training between Taiwan and India and also for the financial assistance under the University with Potential for Excellence scheme from the University Grants Commission, New Delhi, India.

VI. REFERENCES

[1] Buhleier, E.; Wehner, W.; Vogtle, F. *Synthesis* 1978, 155-158.
[2] Newkome, G.R.; Moorefield, C.N.; Vogtle, F. *Dendritic Macromolecules : Concepts, Synthesis, Perspectives* ; Wiley-VCH : Weinheim, 1996.
[3] Newkome, G.R. Ed.; *Advances in Dendritic Macromolecules* ; JAI Press: Greenwich, CT, 1996; Vol. 3.
[4] Tomalia, A.; Frechet, J.M.J. Ed.; *Dendrimers and Other Dendritic Polymers* ; John Wiley : NY, 2002.
[5] Newkone, G.R.; Moorefield, C.N.; Vogtle, F. *Dendrimers and Dendrons : Concepts, Syntheses, Applications* ; John Wiley: NY, 2002.
[6] Vogtle, F. Ed.; *Dendrimers, Topics in Current Chemistry* ; Springer: Berlin, 1998; Vol. 197.
[7] Vogtle,F. Ed.; *Dendrimers – II Architecture, Nanostructure and Supramolecular Chemistry, Topics in Current Chemistry* ; Springer: Berlin, 2000; Vol. 210.
[8] Vogtle,F. Ed.; *Dendrimers – III Design, Dimension, Function* ; *Topics in Current Chemistry* ; Springer: Berlin, 2001; Vol. 212.

[9] Vögtle, F.; Schalley, C.A. Ed.; *Dendrimers – IV Metal Coordination, Self Assembly, Catalysis* ; *Topics in Current Chemistry* ; Springer: Berlin, 2001; Vol. 217.
[10] Schalley, C.A.; Vögtle, F. Ed.; *Dendrimers – V Functional and Hyperbranched Building Blocks, Photophysical Properties, Applications in Materials and Life Sciences*; *Topics in Current Chemistry* ; Springer: Berlin, 2003; Vol. 228.
[11] Boas, U.; Christensen, J. B.; Heegaard, P. M. H. *Dendrimers in Medicine and Biotechnology: New Molecular Tools* ; RSC: London, 2006.
[12] Gade, L.H. Ed.; *Dendrimer Catalysis*, *Topics in Organometallic Chemistry*; Springer: Berlin, 2006; Vol. 20.
[13] Zeng, F.; Zimmerman, S.C. *Chem. Rev.* 1997, *97*, 1681-1712.
[14] Constable, E.C. *Chem. Commun.* 1997, 1073-1080.
[15] Mathews, O.A.; Shipway, A.N.; Stoddart, J.F. *Prog. Polym. Sci.* 1998, *23*, 1-56.
[16] Newkome,G.R. *Pure Appl. Chem.* 1998, *70*, 2337-2343.
[17] Roovers, J.; Comanita, B. *Adv. Polym. Sci.* 1999, *142*, 179-228.
[18] Fischer, M.; Vögtle, F. *Angew.Chem. Int. Edn.* 1999, *38*, 884-905.
[19] Hearshaw, M.A.; Moss, J.R. *Chem. Commun.* 1999, 1-8.
[20] Caminade, A.-M.; Majoral, I.-P. *Prog. Polym. Sci.* 2005, *30*, 491-505.
[21] Smith, D.K. *Chem. Commun* 2006, 34-44.
[22] Boas,U.; Christensen, J.B.; Heegaard, M.H. *J. Mater. Chem.* 2006, *16*, 3785-3798.
[23] Caminade, A.-M.; Wei,Y.; Majoral, J.-P. *C. R. Chim.* 2008, 1-16.
[24] Tomalia, D.A.; Baker, H.; Dewald, J.; Hall, M.; Kallos, G.; Martin, S.; Roeck, J.; Ryder, J.; Smith, P. *Polym. J.* 1985, *17*, 117-132.
[25] Tomalia, D.A.; Baker, H.; Dewald, J.; Hall, M.; Kallos, G.; Martin, S.; Roeck, J.; Ryder, J.; Smith, P. *Macromolecules* 1986, *19*, 2466-2468.
[26] Tomalia, D.A.; Hall, M.; Hedstrand, D.J. *J. Am. Chem. Soc.* 1987, *109*, 1601-1603.
[27] Hawker, C.J.; Frechet, J.M. *J. Am. Chem. Soc.* 1990, *112*, 7638-7647.
[28] Wooley, K.L.; Hawker, C.J.; Frechet, J.M. *J. Am. Chem. Soc.* 1991, *113*, 4252-4261.
[29] Kawaguchi,T.; Walker, K.L.; Wilkins, C.L.; Moore, J.S. *J. Am. Chem. Soc.* 1995, *117*, 2159-2165.
[30] Nagasaki, T.; Ukon, M.; Arimori, S.; Shinkai. S. *J. Chem. Soc. Chem. Commun* 1992, 608-610.
[31] Scott, R.W.J.; Wilson, O.M.; Crooks, R.M. *J. Phys. Chem. B* 2005, *109*, 692-704.
[32] Mery, D; Astruc, D. *Coord. Chem. Rev.* 2006, *250*, 1965-1979.
[33] Balzani,V.; Campagna, S.; Denti,G.; Juris, A.; Serroni, S.; Venturi, M. *Acc. Chem. Res.* 1998, *31*, 26-34 ; Balzani,V.; Credi, A.; Venturi, M. *ChemSusChem* 2008, 1, 26-58.
[34] Jiang, D.-L.; Aida, T. *Prog. Polym. Sci.* 2005, *30*, 403-422.
[35] Cuadrado, I.; Moran, M.; Casado, C.M.; Alonso, B.; Losado, J. *Coord. Chem. Rev.* 1999, *193*, 395-445.
[36] Ceroni, P.; Vicinelli,V.; Maestri, M; Balzani,V.; Lee, S.-K.; Heyst, J.V.; Gorka, M.; Vogtle, F. *J. Organomet. Chem.* 2004, *689*, 4375-4383.
[37] Balzani,V.; Vogtle, F. *C.R.Chim.* 2003, *6*, 867-872.
[38] Serroni, S.; Canapagna, S.; Puntoriero, F.; Pietro, C.D.; Mc Clenaghan, N.D.; Loiseau. F, *Chem. Soc. Rev.* 2001, *30*, 367-375.
[39] Smith, D.K.; Hirst, A.R.; Love, C.S.; Hardy, J.G.; Brignell, S.V.; Huang, B. *Prog. Polym. Sci.* 2005, *30*, 220-293.

[40] Inoue, K. *Prog. Polym. Sci.* 2000, *25*, 453-571.

[41] Vogtle, F.; Gestermann, S.; Hesse, R.; Schwierz, H.; Windisch, B. *Prog. Polym. Sci.*2000, *25*, 987-1041.

[42] Caminade, A.-M,; Laurent, R.; Majoral, J.-P. *Adv. Drug Delivery Rev.* 2005, *57*, 2130-2146.

[43] Balzani, V.; Bergamini, G.; Ceroni, P.; Vogtle, F. *Coord. Chem. Rev.* 2007, *251*, 525-535.

[44] Chow, H.F.; Mong, T.K.K.; Wan, C.W.; Wang, Z.Y. *Adv. Dendritic Macromol.* 1999, *4*, 107-133.

[45] Hummelen, J.C.; Van Dongen, J.L.J.; Meijer, E.W. *Chem. Eur. J.* 1997, *3*, 1489-1493.

[46] Kallos, G.J.; Tomalia, D.A.; Hedstrand, D.M.; Lewis, S.; Zhou, J. *Rapid Commun. Mass Spectrom.* 1991, *5*, 383-386.

[47] Sahota, H.; Lloyd, P.M.; Yeates, S.G.; Derrick, P.J.; Taylor, P.C.; Haddleton, D.M. *J. Chem. Soc. Chem. Commun.* 1994, 2445-2446.

[48] Prosa, T.J.; Bauer, B.J.; Amis, E.J. *Macromolecules* 2001, *34*, 4897-4906.

[49] Potschke, D.; Ballauff, M.; Lindner, P.; Fischer, M.; Vogtle, F. *Macromolecules*1999, *32*, 4079-4087.

[50] Li, X.; He, X.; Ng, A.C.H.; Wu, C.; Ng. D.K.P. *Macromolecules* 2000, 33, 2119-2123.

[51] Jackson, C.L.; Chanzy, H.D.; Booy, F.P.; Drake, B.J.; Tomalia, D.A.; Bauer, B.J.; Amis, E.J. *Macromolecules* 1998, *31*, 6259-6265.

[52] Li, J.; Piehler, L.T.; Qin, D.; Baker Jr., J.R.; Tomalia, D.A.; Meier, D.J. *Langmuir* 2000, *16*, 5613-5616.

[53] Cardona, C.M.; Kaifer, A.E. *J. Am. Chem. Soc.* 1998, *120*, 4023-4024.

[54] Pollak, K.W.; Leon, J.W.; Frechet, J.M.J.; Maskus, M.; Abruna, H.D. *Chem. Mater.* 1998, *10*, 30-38.

[55] Kukowska-Latallo, J.F.; Bielinska, A.U.; Johnson, R.; Splindler, D.A.; Tomalia, D.A.; Baker Jr., J.R. *Proc. Natl. Acad. Sci. U.S.A.* 1996, *93*, 4897-4902.

[56] Jansen, J.F.G.A..; de Brabander van den Berg, E.M.M.; Meijer, E.W. *Science* 1994, *266*, 1226-1229.

[57] Hawker, C.J.; Wooley, K.L.; Frechet, J.M.J. *J.Am.Chem.Soc.* 1993, *115*, 4375-4376.

[58] Klajnert, B.; Bryszewska, M. *Acta Biochim. Pol.* 2001, *48*, 199-208.

[59] Tomalia, D.A.; Mardel, K.; Henderson, S.A.; Holan, G.; Esfand, R. in *Handbook of Nanoscience Engineering and Technology*, Goddard.W.A.III.; Brenner.D.W.; Lyshevski, S.E.; Jafrate, G.J. Ed.; CRC Press: NY, 2003, Chapter 20, pp 1-34.

[60] Imae, T. in *Encyclopedia of Nanoscience and Nanotechnology*; Nalwa.H.S. Ed.; American Scientific Publishers: NY, 2004, Vol. 3, pp 685-701.

[61] Hawker, C.J.; Malmstrom, E.E.; Frank, C.W.; Kampf, J.P. *J.Am.Chem.Soc.* 1997, *119*, 9903-9904.

[62] Tomalia, D.A.; Naylor, A.D.; Goddard III ,W.A. *Angew. Chem. Int. Ed. Engl.* 1990, *29*,138-175.

[63] Gupta, U.; Agashe,H.B.; Asthana, A.; Jain, N.K. *Biomacromolecules* 2006, *7*, 649-658.

[64] Newkome, G.R; Moorefield, C.N.; Baker, G.R.; Saunders, M.J.; Grossman, S.H. *Angew. Chem. Int. Ed. Engl.* 1991, *30*, 1178-1180.

[65] Kofoed, J.; Reymond, J.-L. *Curr. Opin. Chem. Biol.* 2005, *9*, 656-664.

[66] Mourey, T.H.; Turner, S.R.; Rubinstein, M.; Frechet, J.M.J.; Hawker, C.J.; Wooley, K.I. *Macromolecules* 1992, *25*, 2401-2406.

[67] Wooley, K.L.; Hawker, C.J.; Pochan, J.M.; Frechet, J.M.J. *Macromolecules* 1993, *26*, 1514-1519.

[68] Tande, B.M.; Wagner, N.J.; Kim, Y.H. *Macromolecules* 2003, *36*, 4619-4623.

[69] Cameron. C.S.;Gorman, C.B.in *Encyclopedia of Nanoscience and Nanotechnology*;Nalwa. H.S. Ed. American Scientific Publishers: 2004, Vol. 2, 327-335.

[70] Astruc,D.; Ornelas,C.; Aranzaes, R. *J. Inorg. Organomet. Polym. Mater.* 2008, *18*, 4-17.

[71] Astruc, D. *Pure. Appl. Chem.* 2003, *75*, 461-481.

[72] Credi, A.; Ribera, B.F.; Venturi. M. *Electrochim. Acta* 2004, *49*, 3865-3872.

[73] Reek, J.N.H.; Arevalo, S.; van Heerbeek, R.; Kamer, P.C.J.; van Lecuwen, P.W.N.M. *Adv. Cat.* 2006, *49*, 71-151.

[74] Lo, S.-C.; Burn, P.I. *Chem. Rev.* 2007, *107*, 1097-1116.

[75] Kaifer, A.E. *Acc. Chem. Res.* 1999, *32*, 62-71.

[76] Nantalaksakul, A.; Reddy, D.R.; Bardeen, C.J.; Thayumanavan, S. *Photosyn. Res.* 2006, 87, 133-150.

[77] Kim, H.-S.; Yoon, H.C. in *Nanomaterials for Biosensors, Nanotechnologies for Life Sciences*; Challa.S.S.R.Kumar Ed.; Wiley-VCH: Weinheim, 2007; Vol.8, pp 240-258.

[78] Svenson, S.; Tomalia, D.A. *Adv. Drug Delivery Rev.* 2005, *57*, 2106-2129.

[79] Jain, N.K.; Asthana, A. *Exp. Opin. Drug Delivery* 2007, *4*, 495-512.

[80] Boas,U.; Heegaard, P.M.H. *Chem. Soc. Rev.* 2004, *33*, 43-63.

[81] Cloninger, M.J. *Curr. Opin. Chem. Biol.* 2002, *6*, 742-748.

[82] Yang, H.; Kao, W.J. *J. Biomater. Sci., Polym. Ed.* 2006, *7*, 3-19.

[83] Parekh, H.S. *Curr. Pharm. Design* 2007, 13, 2837-2850.

[84] Takada, K.; Goldsmith, J.I.; Bernhard, S.; Abruna, H.D. in *Encyclopedia of Electrochemistry*, Fujihira, M.; Rubinstein, I.; Rusling, J.F. Ed.; Wiley-VCH: Weinheim, 2007; Vol.10, pp 729-754.

[85] Kaifer, A.; Kaifer, M.-G, *Supramolecular Electrochemistry* ; Wiley-VCH: NY, 1999; pp 207-221.

[86] Casado, C.M.; Cuadrado, I.; Moran,M.; Alonso, B.; Garcia, B.; Gonzalez, B.; Losada, J. *Coord. Chem. Rev.* 1999, *185-186*, 53-80.

[87] Juris, A.; Venturi. M.; Paola,C.; Balzani.V.; Campagna.S.; Serroni.S. *Collect. Czech. Chem. Commun.* 2001, *66*, 1-32.

[88] Bryce, M.R.; Devonport,W.; Moore, A.J. *Angew. Chem. Int. Ed. Engl.* 1994, *33*, 1761-1763.

[89] Venturi, M.; Credi, A. Balzani, V. *Coord. Chem. Rev.* 1999, *185*, 233-256.

[90] Cardona, C.M.; Mendoza, A.; Kaifer, A.E. *Chem. Soc. Rev.* 2000, *29*, 37-42.

[91] Cuadrado, I.; Moran, M.; Casado, C.M.; Alonso, B.; Losada, J. *Coord. Chem. Rev.* 1999, *193-195*, 395-445.

[92] Valério, C.; Alonso, E.; Ruiz, J.; Fillaut, J.-L.; Guittard. J.; Blais, J.-C.; Astruc, D. *Pure Appl. Chem.* 1998, *70*, 809-818.

[93] Hwang, S.-H.; Newkome, G. R. in *Frontiers in Transition Metal-Containing Polymers* ; Abd-El-Aziz, A. S.; Manners, I. Ed.; John Wiley & Sons Inc.: NY,2007; Chapter 10, pp 399-438.

[94] . Dandilker, P.J.; Diederich, F.; Gisselbrecht, J,-P.; Louati, A.; Gros, M. *Angew. Chem. Int. Ed. Engl.* 1996, *34*, 2725-2728.

[95] Gorman, C.B. *C. R. Chim.* 2003, *6*, 911-918.
[96] Cardona, C.M., Kaifer, A.E. *J. Am. Chem. Soc*. 1998, *120*, 4023-4024.
[97] Dandilker, P.J.; Diederich, F.; Gross, M.; Knobler, C.B.; Louati, A.; Sanford, E.M. *Angew. Chem. Int. Ed. Engl.* 1994, *33*, 1739-1742.
[98] Dandilker, P.J.; Diederich, F.; Zingg, A.; Gisselbrecht, J.-P, ; Gross, M.; Louati, A.; Sanford, E.M. *Helv. Chim. Acta* 1997, *80*, 1773-1801.
[99] Gorman, G.B.; Parkhurst, B.L.; Su, W.Y,; Chen, K.-Y. *J. Am. Chem. Soc*. 1997, *119*, 1141-1142.
[100] Mendoza, S.; Davidov, P.D.; Kaifer, A.E. *Chem. Eur. J.* 1998, *4*, 864-870.
[101] Newkome, G.R.; Guther, R.; Moorefield, C.N.; Cardullo, F.; Echegoyen, L.; Cordero, E.-P,; Luftmann, H. Angew. *Chem. Int. Ed. Engl.* 1995, *34*, 2023-2026.
[102] Newkome, G.R.; Cardullo, F.; Constable, E.C.; Moorefield, C.N.; Thompson, A.M.W.C. *Chem. Soc. Chem. Commun* 1993, 925-927.
[103] Peris, E. *Coord. Chem. Rev.* 2004, *248*, 279-297.
[104] Valero, C.; Fillaut, J.-L.; Ruiz. J, ; Guittard, J.; Blais, J.-C.; Astruc. D. *J. Am. Chem. Soc*. 1997, *119*, 2588-2589.
[105] Casado, C.M.; Gonzalez, B.; Cuadrado, I.; Alonso, B.; Moran. M.; Losada, J. *Angew. Chem. Int. Ed.* 2000, *39*, 2135-2138.
[106] Juris.A *Annu. Rep. Prog. Chem. Sect. C*. 2003, *99*, 177-241.
[107] Chen, S.-M.; Chuang,G.-H. *J. Electroanal. Chem*. 2005, *575*, 125-137.
[108] Losada, J.; Cuadrado, I.; Moran, M.; Casado, C.M.; Alonso, B.; Barranco, M.*Anal. Chim. Acta* 1997, *338*, 191-198.
[109] Armada, M.P.G.; Losada, J.; Zamora, M. ; Alonso, B.; Cuadrado, I.; Casado, C.M. *Bioelectrochemistry* 2006, *69*, 65-73.
[110] Silva, C.J.S.M.; Sousa, F.;Gubitz, G.; Cavaco-Paulo, A. *Food Technol.Biotechnol.* 2004, *42*, 51-56.
[111] Decher, G. *Science* 1997, 277, 1232-1237.
[112] Salditt, T.; Schubert, U.S. *Rev. Mol. Biotech.* 2002, *90*, 55-70.
[113] Lojou, E.; Bianco, P. *Bioelectrochemistry* 2006, *69*, 237-247.
[114] Paez, J.I.; Froimowicz, P.; Baruzzi, A.M.; Strumia, M.C.; Brunetti, V. *Electrochem. Commun.* 2008, *10*, 541-545.
[115] Gooding, J.J.; Mearns, F.;Yang, W.R.; Liu, J.Q. *Electroanal.* 2003, *15,* 81-96.
[116] Schreiber, F. *Prog. Surf. Sci*. 2000, *65*, 151-257.
[117] Zhang,S.; Marini, D.M.; Hwang, W; Santoso, S. *Curr. Opin. Chem. Biol.* 2002, *6*, 865-871.
[118] Losada, J.; Cuadrado, I.; Moran, M; Casado, C.M.; Alonso, B.; Barranco, M. *Anal. Chim. Acta* 1997, 338, 191-198.
[119] Yoon, H.C.; Hong, M.-H,; Kim,H.-S. *Anal. Chem.*, 2000, *72*, 4420.
[120] Yoon, H.C.; Kim, H.-S. *Anal.Chem*. 2000, *72*, 922-926.
[121] Armada, M.P.G.; Losada, J.; Zamora, M.; Alonso, B.; Cuadrado, I.; Casado, C.M. *Bioelectrochemistry* 2006, *69*, 65-73.
[122] Losada, J.; Zamora, M.; Armada, P.G.; Cuadrado, L.; Alonso, B.;Casado, C.M. *Anal. Bioanal. Chem*. 2006, *385*, 1209-1217.
[123] Zeng,Y.-L,; Huang, H.-W,; Jiang, J.-H.; Tian, M.-N,; Li, C.-X, ; Tang, C.-R,; Shen, G.-L,; Yu, R.-Q. *Anal. Chim. Acta* 2007, *604*, 170-176.

[124] Crespilho, F.N.; Emilia Ghica, M; Florescu, M.; Nart, F.C.; Oliveira Jr.,O.V.; Brett, C.M.A. *Electrochem. Commun.* 2006, *8,* 1665-1670.

[125] Crespilho, F.N.; Emilia Ghica, M; Zucolono,V.; Nart, F.C.; Oliveira Jr.,O.V.; Brett, C.M.A. *Electroanal.* 2007, *19*, 805-812.

[126] Crespilho, F.N.; Emilia Ghica,; Carla,G.-C, Oliveira Jr.,O.V.; Brett, C.M.A. *Talanta,* 2008, *76*, 922-928.

[127] Alonso, B.; Armada, P.G.; Losada, J.; Cuadrado, I.; Gonzalez, B.; Casado, C.M. *Biosens. Bioelectron.* 2004, *19*, 1617-1625.

[128] Snejdarkova, M.; Svobodova, L.; Gajdos,V.; Hianik,T. *J. Mater.Sci. Mater. Med.* 2001, *12*, 1079-1082.

[129] Svobodova, L.; Snejdarkova, M.; Hianik, T. *Anal. Bioanal. Chem.* 2002, *373*, 735-741.

[130] Svobodova, L.; Snejdarkova, M.; Toth, K.; Gyurcsanyi, R.E.; Hianik, T. *Bioelectrochem*istry 2004, *63*, 285-289.

[131] Polohova,V.; Snejdarkova, M.; Podskocova, J.; Svobodova,L.; Chorvat Jr.D.; Hianik,T. *Electroanal.* 2007, *19*, 324-330.

[132] Zhu,Y.; Zhu, H.; Yang, X.; Xu, L.; Li, C. *Electroanal.* 2007, *19*, 698-703.

[133] Yao, K.; Zhu,Y.; Yang, X.; Li, C. *Mater.Sci. Engg: C* 2008, *28*, 1236-1241.

[134] Luo, X.-L,; Xu. J.-J.; Zhao,W.; Chen, H.-Y. *Sens. Actuators, B* 2004, *97*, 249-255.

[135] Tang, L.; Zhu, L.; Yihua,; Xu, L.; Yang, X.; Li, C. *Electroanal.* 2007, *19*, 1677- 1682.

[136] Malinauskas, A. *Synth. Met.* 1999, *107*, 75-83.

[137] Ramanavicius, A.; Kansaite,A.; Ramanaviciene, A. *Sens. Actuators B* 2005, 111-112, 532-539.

[138] Xu, L.; Zhu, L.; Tang, L.; Yang, X.; Li, C. *Electroanal*, 2007, 19, 717-722.

[139] Xu, L.; Zhu, L.; Tang, L.; Yang, X.; Li,C. *J. Appl. Polym. Sci.* 2008, 109, 1802

[140] Xu, L.; Zhu, L.; Tang, L.; Yang, X.; Li, C. *Mater. Sci. Eng. C* doi: 10.1016/j.msec.2008.10.031

[141] Zeng, Y.-L.; Huang, Y.-F.; Jiang, J.-H.; Zhang, X.-B,; Tang, C.-R, ; Shen, G.-L, Yu, R.-Q. *Electrochem. Commun.* 2007, *9*, 185-190.

[142] Shen, L.; Hu, N. *Biomacromolecules* 2005, *6*, 1475-1483.

[143] He, P.; Li, M.; Hu, N. *Biopolymers* 2005, *79*, 310-323.

[144] Zhang, H.; Hu, N. *Biosens. Bioelectron.* 2007, *23*, 393-399.

[145] Liu, Z.-M,; Yang, Y.; Wang, H.; Liu,Y.-L,; Shen,G.-L,; Yu, R.-Q. *Sens. Actuators, B* 2005, *106*, 394-400.

[146] Tang, L.; Zhu,Y.; Xu, L.; Yang, X.; Li,C. *Talanta* 2007, *73*, 438-443.

[147] Tang, L.; Zhu,Y.; Xu, L.; Yang, X.; Li,C. *Anal. Chim. Acta* 2007, *597*, 145-150.

[148] Perinotto, A.C.; Caseli, L.; Hayasaka,C.O.; Riul Jr. A.; Oliveira Jr, O.N.; Zucolotto,V. *Thin Solid Films* 2008, *516*, 9002-9005.

[149] Zucolotto,V.; Pinto, A.P.A.; Tumolo, T.; Moraes, M.L.; Baptista, M.S.; Riul Jr. A.; Araujo, A.P.U.; Oliveira Jr., O.N. *Biosens. Bioelectron.* 2006, *21*, 1320-1326.

[150] Nicole, J.-R. *Sensors* 2001, 1, 60-74.

[151] Snejdarkova, M.; Svobodova, L.; Nikolelis, D.P.; Wang, J.; Hianik, T. *Electroanal*. 2003, *15*, 1185-1191.

[152] Snejdarkova, M.; Svobodova, L.; Evtugyn, G.; Budnikov,H.; Karyakin, A.; Nikolelis, E.P.; Hianik, T. *Anal. Chim. Acta* 2004, *514*, 79-88.

[153] Merkoci, A.; Aldavert, M.; Martin, S.; Alegret, S. *Trends Anal. Chem.* 2005, *24*, 341-349.

[154] Teles, F.R.R.; Fonseca, L.P. *Talanta* 2008, *77*, 606-623.
[155] Odenthal, K.J.; Gooding, J.J. The *Analyst* 2007, *132*, 603-610.
[156] Watson, J.D.; Crick, F.H.C. *Nature* 1953, *171*, 737-738.
[157] Caminade, A.-M,; Padie, C.; Laurent, R.; Maravel, A.; Majoral, J.-M. *Sensors* 2006, *6*, 901-914.
[158] Nilsen, T.W.; Grayzel, J.; Prensky, W. *J. Theor. Biol.* 1997, *187*, 273-284.
[159] Wang, J.; Rivas, G.; Fernandes, J.R.; Jiang, M.; Lopez Paz, J.L.; Waymire, R.; Nielsen, T.W.; Getts, C. *Electroanal.* 1998, *10*, 553-556.
[160] Kim, E; Kim, K.; Yang, H.; Kim,Y.T.; Kwak, J. *Anal. Chem.* 2003, *75*, 5665-5672.
[161] Zhu, N.; Gu,Y.; Chang,Z.; He, P.; Fang,Y. *Electroanal.* 2006, *18*, 2107-2114.
[162] Shi. W.-J.; Ai. S,-Y.; Li, J.-H,; Zhu, L.-S. *Chinese J. Anal. Chem.* 2008, *36*, 335-338.
[163] Li, A.; Yang, F.; Ma,Y.; Yang, X. *Biosen. Bioelectron.* 2007, *22*, 1716-1722.
[164] Arotiba, O.; Ignaszak, A.; Malgas, R.; Amir, A.-A,; Baker, P.C.L.; Mapolie, S.F.; Iwuoha, E.I. *Electrochim. Acta* 2007, *53*, 1689-1696.
[165] Wang, J. *Analytical Electrochemistry*; VCH: NY,1994, Chapter 5, pp133-160.
[166] Aizawa, M. *Phil. Trans. R. Soc. Lond. B* 1987, *316*, 121-134.
[167] Liu,G.; Lin, Y. *Talanta* 2007, *74*, 308-317.
[168] Shen, L.; Hu, N. *Biomacromol*ecules 2005, 6, 1475-1483.
[169] Lojou, E.; Bianco, P. *Bioelectrochem*istry 2006, 69, 237-247.
[170] Zhang, H.; Hu, N. *Biosens. Bioelectron.* 2007, *23*, 393-399.
[171] Liu, Z.; Amiridis, M.D. *Colloids Surf. B* 2004, *35*, 197-203.
[172] Yoon, H.C.; Hong, M.Y.; Kim, H.S., *Anal. Biochem.* 2000, 282, 121-128.
[173] Yoon, H.C.; Hong, M.Y.; Kim, H.S. *Langmuir* 2001, *17*, 1234-1239.
[174] Yoon, H.C.; Lee,D.; Kim, H.S. *Anal. Chim. Acta* 2002, *456*, 209-218.
[175] Lee, J.W.; Yang, S.S., Kim, B.W.; Sim, S.J.; Chae, H.; Yoon, H.C. *Colloids Surf. A* 2008, *313*, 509-514.
[176] Yoon, H.C.; Yang, H.; Kim,Y.T. *The Analyst* 2002, *127*, 1082-1087.
[177] Yoon, H.C.; Ko, J.S.; Yang, H.; Kim, Y.T. *The Analyst* 2002, *127*, 1576-1579.
[178] Yoon, H.C.; Yang, H.; Byun, S.Y. *Anal. Sci.* 2004, *20*, 1249-1254.
[179] Won, B.Y.; Choi,H.G.; Kim, K.H.; Byun, S.Y.; Kim, H.S.; Yoon, H.C.; Kim, H.S.*Biotechnol. Bioeng.* 2005, *89*, 815-821.
[180] Pingarro, J.M.; Paloma, Y.-S.; Araceli, G.-C. *Electrochim. Acta.* 2008, *53*, 5848-5866.
[181] Liu, A. *Biosens. Bioelectron.* 2008, *24*, 167-177.
[182] Wang, J.; Lin, Y. *TrA, Trends Anal. Chem.* 2008, *27*, 619-626.

In: Nanostructured Materials for Electrochemical Biosensors ISBN: 978-1-60741-706-4
Editors: U. Yogeswaran; S. Kumar; S. Chen ©2009 Nova Science Publishers, Inc.

Chapter 2

FUNCTIONALISATION OF POLYANILINE NANOMATERIALS FOR AMPEROMETRIC BIOSENSING

Tesfaye T. Waryo, Everlyne A. Songa, Mangaka C. Matoetoe, Rachel F. Ngece, Peter M. Ndangili, Amir Al-Ahmed, Nazeem M. Jahed, Priscilla G.L. Baker, Emmanuel I. Iwuoha*

SensorLab, Department of Chemistry,
University of the Western Cape Western Cape, Republic of South Africa.

ABSTRACT

This chapter summarizes some procedures for intrinsic functionalization, doping and preparation, analysis and biosensor applications of polyaniline nano-composite materials. Details of the synthesis of four novel nanostructured polymeric composites formed with pristine or substituted polyanilines and sulfonated polyanion, as well as their microscopy, spectroscopy, electrochemistry and multifunctional properties in enzyme electrodes, are presented. In the case of the pristine polyaniline (PANI) and poly(dimethoxy aniline) (PDMA), the polyelectrolyte dopants used were polyvinyl sulfonate (PVS) and polystyrene sulfonic acid (PSS). No dopant was used in conjunction with poly(8-anilino naphthalene sulfonic acid) (PANSA) – a self-doping conducting polymer. A final section deals with the application of the resulting nanocomposites as enzyme-immobilization and conducting platforms in amperometric biosensors involving two oxidoreductase enzymes (horseradish peroxidase and cytochrome P450-2D6). The analytical performances of the resulting biosensors in batch operation mode with regard to their responses to standard samples of selected clinical and environmental analytes, including drugs (e.g. sertraline and fluoxetine), hydrogen peroxide (a strategic biomedical analyte) and some pesticides (e.g., glufosinate and glyphosate) are described. The chapter also demonstrates the application of cyclic voltammetry, scanning electron microscopy, uv-visible spectroscopy and infrared spectroscopy in the development and analysis of biosensors based on functionalized polyaniline nanomaterials.

* Correspondence, email: eiwuoha@uwc.ac.za, Tel: +27-21-9593054, Fax: +27-21-959-1562

Keywords: polyaniline; hydrogen peroxide, nanomaterials; glufosinate ; glyphosate; sertraline; fluoxetine; pesticide; anti-depressant; horseradish peroxidase; Cytochrome P450-2D6.

1. Introduction

Polyaniline is a conducting polymer that has been found to be suitable for application in the development of amperometric chemical sensors due to its air-moisture stability, aqueous phase preparation, and simple doping-dedoping chemistry [1, 2]. Over the years there has been intensive research work on the preparation, characterisation and application of polyaniline [3-20]. It is widely agreed that polyaniline's electroactivity and conductivity is restricted to acidic media. The retention of polyaniline's electroactivity in physiological pH's for biosensor applications has been achieved by various strategies including the incorporation of anionic dopants – usually anionic polyelectrolytes [21-23]. Polymerization of dopant-functionalized aniline or post-synthesis functionalization of PANI[1] or copolymerization of aniline with a variety of its substituted derivatives as co-monomers are widely followed strategies [21, 24]. The literature shows that properties of PANI can easily be tailored, via functionalization and composite formation, to suit specific technological needs such as anticorrosion coating, batteries, electrochromic displays, sensors and separation membranes [17, 23, 25-32]. It has also been used in manufacturing of interference shielding materials as well as in broadband microwave adsorbing materials [33]. In contrast to its traditional micro/macro bulk forms, nanostructured polyanilines exhibit interesting physic-chemical properties [1]. For example, while microstructured polyaniline has been known to possess poor dispersibility in appropriate solvents, a property that is highly desired for easy fabrication and study of biosensors, nano-fibrillar PANI has been reported to be easily dispersible in water. Other general advantages of nanomaterials in electrode modification are their high effective surface area, better mass transport, better catalysis and higher sensitivity.

The conventional methods for the synthesis of PANI produce insoluble, irregularly shaped and integrally macro- and micro-particulate products that are difficult to process, due to extensive secondary growth the follow the formation of the initial polymer. Conductivity of these PANIs critically depends on the degree of hydration – the hydrated polymers exhibit the lowest conductivity. Traditional PANI is not only infusible but also hardly soluble in most common (organic) solvents except strong acids and N-methylpyrollidone (NMP) [34]. The insolubility of PANI in most solvents has been ascribed to its chemical structure (see Figure 1) that consists of aromatic rings, inter-chain hydrogen bonding and effective charge delocalisation. As a result the exploitation of the outstanding electrical characteristics of this pristine form of PANI has been limited. PANI's infusibility and insolubility in water and

1 Abbreviations: AAO: anodic aluminium oxides; ANSA: 5-aminonaphthalene-2-sulfonic acid; APS— Ammonium persulphate; ASA — Anthracene Sulfonic acids; CB — conduction band; CPs — conducting polymers; CSA — Camphor sulfonic acid; CV: cyclic voltammogram; CYP2D6 — cytochrome P450-2D6; DBSA: dodecyl benzenesulfonic acid; EAQ — Eastman AQ polymersTM; FTIR — Fourier Transform infrared spectroscopy; HRP — Horseradish peroxidase; NMP: N-methylpyrollidone; PTM: particle track-etched membrane; PANIs — Polyanilines; NSA: naphthalenesulfonic acid; PANI – Polyaniline; PDMA-PSS — Poly (-dimethoxyaniline-poly (4-styrene sulfonic acid); PANSA — 8-anilino-1-napthalene sulfonic acid; PPY: polypyrrol; PESA: polyester sulfonic acid; PVS - polyvinyl sulfonate; SEM — Scanning electron Microscopy; PVA: poly(vinyl alcohol)

other common organic solvents has led to an emphasis on the development of functionalized and nanostructured polyanilines. While "polymer functionalization" may be defined in general as the "introduction of desired chemical groups into polymer molecules to create specific chemical, physical, biological, pharmacological, or other properties" [35], functionalization and doping of PANI have been carried out in order to increase the electroactivity of the polymer and to obtain materials for specific tasks. Introduction of the functional groups into PANI is usually done through co-polymerization or post-polymerization [36]. Nano-structuring of conducting polymers in general and of the polyaniline in particular, has been shown to improve their dispersibility in liquids, thermoplasticity, biocompatibility, optical and electrical characteristics [1, 37-43].

Several procedures have been developed for intrinsic functionalization, doping and formation of composite of polyaniline. These are summarized in Section 2. The development of nanostructured polyanilines with appropriate physico-chemical retractability will have a lot of impact on sensor research and technology. Sections 3 of this chapter will deal with some electrochemical and a purely chemical technique for the preparation of novel nanostructured composites of pristine or substituted polyanilines. Also contained in the section is the use of sulfonated polyanion as multifunctional components of amperometric biosensors. In the case of the pristine polyaniline (PANI) and poly(dimethoxy aniline) (PDMA), the polyelectrolyte dopants used were polyvinyl sulfonate (PVS) and polystyrene sulfonic acid (PSS). No dopant was used in conjunction with poly(8-anilino naphthalene sulfonic acid) (PANSA). Section 4 will deal with the application of PANI nanocomposites as enzyme-immobilization and conducting platforms in amperometric biosensor technology involving two important oxidoreductase enzymes (horseradish peroxidase and cytochrome P450-2D6). The analytical performances of these biosensors in batch operational mode are reported for selected clinical and environmental analytes, including drugs (sertraline and fluoxetine), hydrogen peroxide (a strategic biochemical analyte) and some pesticides (glufosinate and glyphosate).

2. General Methods for Preparation of Nanostructured Polyanilines

The common synthetic routes for PANI production are either chemical or electrochemical. The c*hemical synthesis methods* involve the oxidation of aniline using strong oxidising agents (potassium persulphate, potassium dichromate, ferric ions or hydrogen peroxide) in an acid medium. Radical chain polymerization techniques such as cationic, anionic and Ziegler-Natta as well as the co-ordination step–growth polymerization have also been reported [44-46]. Chemical synthesis routes are simple, inexpensive, and suitable for bulk production of polyanilines. Preparation of polyaniline via e*lectrochemical polymerization* is generally accomplished by galvanostatic, potentiostatic or potential scanning voltammetry [18, 47, 48]. It involves the electrooxidation of the monomer atop the surface of an anodically polarized working electrode, and it is a technique of choice in the fabrication of biosensors as it allows easy control of film thickness and polymer properties. A typical potentiodynamic electropolymerization processes is shown in the cyclic voltammogram of Figure 3(a) for pristine polyaniline. To perform electropolymerization, the working electrode (together with the necessary accessories such as the reference and counter electrodes) is placed in the solution of the monomer in an appropriate medium, and then the electrode potential is scanned oxidatively within the potential window of interest. A successful formation of conducting polymer on the electrode surface is principally indicated by increase of current with successive scan as shown in Figure 3(a) by the two arrows. The thickness of the polyaniline film could be monitored, tailored, and set to the desired magnitude based on the number of cycles (for potentio-dynamic) or the polymerization time (for potentiostatic) the electro-oxidation is allowed to proceed.

Polymerization mechanisms for polyaniline have been proposed in the literature [45, 46]. Figure 2 illustrates some of the basic steps occurring during polymerization of aniline. The oxidation states of PANI, and of polyanilines in general, are indicated by an index for the degree of oxidation (Y). It is in its completely reduced form (leucoemeraldine) when Y = 1, and its completely oxidised form (pernigraniline) is dominant when Y = 0. At Y = 0.5, the 50% intrinsically oxidized polymer (emeraldine) is ambient [49, 50]. The molecular structures of the different forms (oxidation states) of PANI are illustrated in Figure 1.

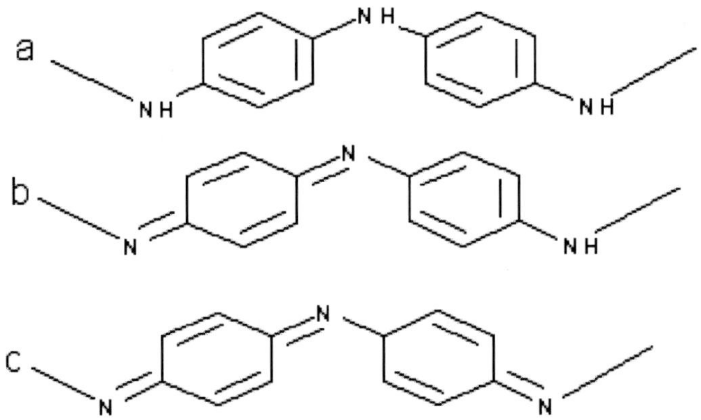

Figure 1. Structures of PANI oxidation states: (a) leucoemeraldine, (b) emeraldine salt and (c) pernigraniline.

The synthesis of polyaniline and its derivatives has been found to be generally influenced by the conditions under which the polymerization is carried out including the type of supporting electrolyte (electropolymerization), monomer concentration, applied potential, the type of solvent and pH of the electrolyte [51, 52]. It has also been shown that the nature of the anion present in the reactant solution determines the morphology and properties of the generated polyaniline [3, 51, 53-55]. As already mentioned, the processibility and applicability of PANI have been mostly hampered by its infusibility or insolubility in organic solvents due to its rigid π-π conjugation system. Several strategies have therefore been employed to improve the solubility of PANI in organic solvents. Accordingly, synthesis of nanostructured PANI has become the key step in preparing highly dispersed blends of PANI with other processable polymers. Apart from the physical routes like electrospinning, mechanical stretching and the doping–induced solution route, the chemical approaches adopted for production of one-dimensional nanostructured PANI can generally be categorized as chemical and electrochemical polymerization, as is the case for the synthesis of the conventional PANI powders [56].

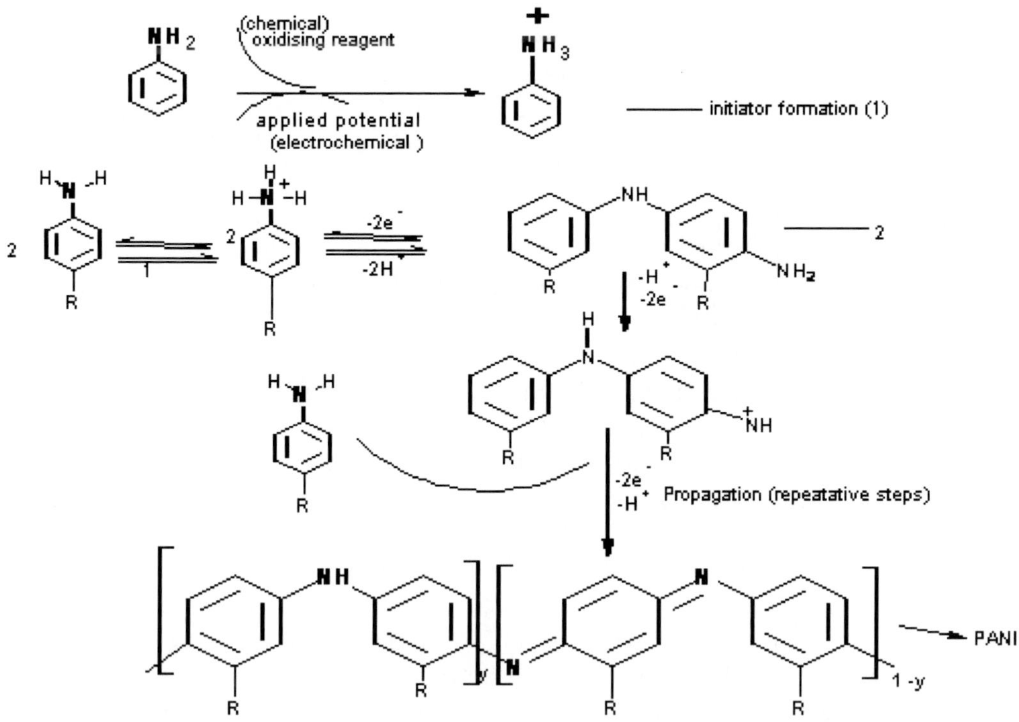

Figure 2. Proposed aniline polymerization mechanism; R = H for PANI otherwise a derivative when substituted monomers are used. The allowed Y values are 0, 0.5 and 1.

Substituted PANIs (polymers of functionalize aniline molecules), on the other hand, have also become an alternative choice to obtaining the desired properties of processability and solubility. For example, the polymerization of a derivatised aniline such as 2-methoxyaniline, results in a soluble conducting polymer. In general, substituent groups present in the units of the polymer chain cause decrease in the stiffness of the polymer chain to result in better solubility. Unfortunately such improvements by substitution of groups in the phenyl ring or *N*-position of polyaniline units are also accompanied by decrease of conductivity. Nevertheless, aniline substituted with two methoxy groups, 2,5-dimethoxyaniline, has been reported to contrarily produce a soluble polymer, poly(2,5-dimethoxyaniline), PDMA, with a conductivity similar to PANI [57].

The chemical methods for the preparation of nanomaterial could be categorized as either template-directed or template-free. The template synthesis methods commonly used for the production of one-dimensional nanostructured PANI are further subdivided into hard template (physical template) synthesis and soft template (chemical template) synthesis approach according to the solubility of the templates in the reaction media. Non-template routes for the synthesis of one-dimensional nanostructured PANI such as rapid–mixing reaction method, radiolytic synthesis, interfacial polymerization, and sonochemical synthesis have also been reported [56]. Other approaches like combined soft and hard template synthesis are also known. An overview of hard-template, soft-template, and template-free procedures are presented in the following paragraphs.

Hard Template Synthesis

Nanomaterials of intrinsically conducting polymers such as PANI, PPY as well as other materials including metals, carbon can be obtained by chemically derivatizing the pore walls, by providing molecular anchors or channels to hard templates such as membranes, zeolites, anodic aluminium oxides (AAO) and track-etched membranes, so that the electrodeposited material preferentially directed into the pore walls [56, 58]. The technique is simple and nanostructures with extraordinary low dimensions (a few nm) have been reported to be produced. For example, PANI filaments with diameters of 3 nm have been achieved in the hexagonal channels of mesoporous aluminosilicate [59]. However, the disadvantage of this method is that a tedious post-synthesis process is required in order to remove the templates and the nanostructured polymers may be destroyed or form undesirable aggregated structures after being released from the templates [56]. The requirement of 'molecular anchors' to maintain the nanostructured shapes is in itself a challenge.

For example, in a typical application of the hard template method to the chemical synthesis of PANI, the hard templates were first immersed in a pre-cooled acidic solution of aniline monomer, and then the oxidant solution at the same temperature was added to start the polymerization. During the procedure, PANI was produced and deposited within the pores or channels of the templates. With the templates eliminated partly or completely, one-dimensional nanostructured PANI was isolated. If the templates were not removed, one-dimensional nanostructured PANI-filled composite materials were produced. In some cases, aniline was adsorbed from vapor phase into the channels of the templates, and polymerization was then carried out in an identical fashion as mentioned above. PANI nanotubules were also synthesized by placing solutions of aniline and ammonium peroxydisulfate (APS), the oxidant, in a two-compartment cell with the particle track-etched membrane (PTM) as the dividing wall, which serves as the hard template. The monomer and the oxidant diffused toward each other through the membrane and reacted, yielding the PANI nanotubules in the pores of the membrane [56]. PANI nanofibers, nanotubules and nanoribbons were also prepared by electrochemical oxidative polymerization with hard templates such as PTM, AAO and enclosed nanochannels. Polymers generated using electrochemical oxidative polymerization within PTM templates are associated with increased electric conductivity because the polymerization is confined to the pore spaces and electrostatic interactions between the ionic species allow alignment on the walls of the pores [17]. While using electrochemical method, one surface of the membrane is coated with a metal film which acts as an anode and the polymer is grown within the pores. Using a polycarbonate membrane, the polymer was shown to preferentially nucleate and grow on the pore walls, producing polymeric tubules whose wall thickness controlled through the polymerization time. In some polymers like PPY, the tubules close up to form solid fibrils, while in PANI the tubules do not close up even after long polymerization time [58]. Mazur *et al.* [12] prepared PANI and poly-*o*-methoxyaniline nanotubes in polycarbonate membranes through the chemical *in situ* deposition method.

Soft Template Synthesis

Due to the limitations presented by hard template method, new approaches towards PANI dispersibility through nanostructurization are now focused on the use of soft templates. The soft template synthesis method referred to as the "template-free" method (in that no hard template is used) involves the synthesis of PANI or its derivatives in the presence of structure-directing molecules such as surfactants, polyelectrolytes, deoxyribonucleic acid (DNA), thiolated cyclodextrins, sulfonated porphyrins, liquid crystals and ethanol, which act as templates for the production of one-dimensional nanomaterials [56]. The surfactants are often complex acids with bulky side groups, such as the naphthalenesulfonic acid (NSA) [60], camphorsulfonic acid (CSA) [61], dodecyl benzenesulfonic acid (DBSA) [62], 5-aminonaphthalene-2-sulfonic acid (ANSA) [63], etc. In solution the surfactant molecules exist in micelles leaving nanoscopic spaces available for monomer polymerization. In this way surfactants act as soft templates for nanostructurization. The polyelectrolytes include poly(acrylic acid), poly(styrenesulfonic acid), poly(vinylsulfonic acid), etc. The "template-free" method is simple and cheap in comparison with the hard template method because it does not require post synthesis processing. It results nanostructured materials with improved processability, conductivity and morphology. Also, through the "template-free" method, various dispersible one-dimensional structures are formed, the final structure depending on the nature of template. The formation of dispersible one-dimensional nanostructured PANI depends on the polymerization conditions, such as the concentration of aniline, the molar ratio of aniline to oxidant or the soft template, reaction temperature and time. Generally low concentrations of aniline favor the formation of nanotubes or nanofibers, while high concentrations favor the formation of granular PANI [56]. Although the control of the diameters of the nanostructures is not easily achieved through this method, it has been described as an elegant method for the fabrication of new smart materials (composites) by simply varying the contents of the polymerization solution.

In a typical surfactant-based procedure, aniline and surfactants such as CSA, NSA, ANSA, *o*-aminobenzenesulfonic acid, etc. with different molar ratios are added to predetermined amount of distilled water. A transparent solution of the aniline/surfactant salt formed is brought to a specified temperature, and then an aqueous solution of the oxidant, usually ammonium peroxydisulfate (pre-cooled to the same temperature) added to initiate the polymerization. After a predetermined reaction time, the mixture is filtered, washed and dried to obtain the one-dimensional nanostructured PANI [56]. For instance, Huang and Wan [64] synthesized microtubes of PANI by this method, using $(NH_4)_2S_2O_8$ as an oxidant in the presence of β-naphthalene sulfonic acid (NSA) as a dopant. It was proposed that the formation of these PANI microtubes can be attributed to self-assembling of β-NSA molecules and/or their aniline salts into microstructural intermediate [65] which acts as both a super molecular template [66] and a self-doping agent. The reliability and practicability of this method have been proven through changing polymer chains [64, 67-71], dopants [66, 72, 73] and using different polymerization methods [74]. At the same time, the size of the tubes, from micrometer to nanometer (100-300 nm), could be controlled through changing the synthesis conditions [66, 73]. Furthermore, it was discovered that the diameter and length of the tubes strongly depended on the polymerization conditions [70, 73]. Zhang and Wan [75] reported the formation of composite nanostructures (e.g. nanotubes or nanorods of 60-80 nm) of PANI blended with water-soluble poly(vinyl alcohol) (PVA) as a matrix. The PANI nanostructures were synthesized by a "template-free" method in the presence of β-NSA as a dopant. Yang et al. synthesized chiral PANI nanotubes with inner diameter of 50–130 nm, outer diameter of 80–220 nm and aspect ratio of 6–10, with chiral 2-pyrrolidone-5-carboxylic acid (PCA) as the template [56]. Nickels *et al.* and Ma *et al.* synthesized nanowires of PANI with DNA as the template, and the nanowires were immobilized on silicon surface with pre-stretched strand DNA as the template [56]. Iwuoha and co-workers [76] synthesized nanofibrils of PANI with diameters less than 200 nm using anthracenesulfonic acid (ASA) as the structure-directing molecule. It was proposed that the resultant ASA–micelles guided the formation of the fibrillar morphology. Similar structures were reported for CSA–doped PANI [77, 78]. Elsewhere, the chemical oxidative polymerization of aniline was performed in a micellar solution of DBSA to obtain nanoparticles with enhanced thermal stability and processability [62]. The average size of the PANI particles was between 20-30 nm.

In a typical polyelectrolyte–template procedure, the polyelectrolyte is first dissolved in an organic solvent such as tetrahydrofuran and then aniline is added to the solution to form a gel composed of a molecular complex of aniline and the polyelectrolyte. After washing with tetrahydrofuran in order to eliminate the excess aniline, the gel complex is re-dissolved in an acidic aqueous solution. Polymerization is then initiated by adding the oxidant solution which results in the formation of PANI nanofibers that are collected by filtration after a specied period of reaction. As far as the mechanism is concerned, Liu and Yang, Hwang and Yang in independent studies suggested that aniline molecules were first bound onto the polyelectrolytes, followed by polymerization of aniline attached to the polyelectrolyte templates. Therefore, PANI nanofibers with diameters of 50 nm are produced when the template molecule is an extended linear chain of poly(acrylic acid), while globular morphology is obtained when the random coil conformation of poly(styrenesulfonic acid) is used as the template [56].

Polyaniline and its derivatives exhibit redox properties only in acidic media of $pH < 4$ [51], a feature that limits their application in combination with biomolecules which normally require a neutral pH environment for their activity and stability. It was, however, reported that the doping of PANI or its derivatives with anionic species or the formation of composite polymer blends between PANI and negatively charged polymers (anionic polyelectrolytes) such as poly(styrenesulfonate), poly(vinylsulfonic acid) or poly(acrylic acid) switches the redox activity of PANI to neutral pH values and also leads to the increase in its structural stability and conductivity at a broader range of pH values in aqueous media [51, 52, 79]. This is attributed to the effective doping of PANI by the trapped polyelectrolytes in a broad pH range. Employing a polyelectrolyte to bind to and preferentially align the aniline monomers prior to polymerization has also shown promise in facilitating the desired head-to-tail coupling of the aniline substrates. During polymerization, the anionic polyelectrolytes such as poly(styrenesulfonate) and poly(acrylate) also provide the required counter ions for charge compensation in the doped PANI products. This can lead to water-soluble or water-dispersed emeraldine salt products [51]. PANI can be deposited onto electrode surfaces through chemical or electrochemical polymerization. Electrosynthesis by galvanostatic, potentiostatic or potentiodynamic procedures allows the incorporation of a wide range of dopant ions since the reaction only requires the presence of an appropriate electrolyte rather than a chemical oxidant. Electrochemical oxidation also gives better control over film properties, such as thickness and morphology [79].

3. Preparation of Electrodes-Modified with Sulfonate-Functionalized Polyanilines

This section discusses the reactivities and biosensor applications of functionalized electrosynthetic polyanilines prepared by (i) electropolymerization and (ii) chemical polymerization of aniline on the surfaces of Au, glassy carbon or Pt disk electrodes. Four such polyaniline or substituted composite polyaniline films developed by our research group are: (a) nanofibrillar polyaniline-polyvinyl sulfonate (PANI-PVS), (b) poly(2,5-dimethoxyaniline)-polystyrene sulfonate (PDMA-PSS), (c) poly(anilinonaphthalene sulfonic acid) (PANSA), and (d) polyaniline/polyester sulfonic acid/polystyrene sulfonate (PANI-PESA-PSS). The electrochemical cells used for carrying out electrochemical measurements consisted of a working electrode modified by PANI film or PANI composite film, Pt wire auxiliary electrode and Ag/AgCl reference electrode. Before each electrode modification experiment, the bare Pt, glassy carbon or Au disk electrode is polished successively with aqueous slurries of 1.0, 0.3 and 0.05 μm alumina, rinsed with de-ionized water after each polishing step, and finally sonicated in water for 5 min. A good way of cleaning a counter electrode after an electropolymerization experiment is by flaming the Pt wire until all impurities are removed. This procedure was followed before using the counter electrode in subsequent electroanalytical measurements. Dissolved oxygen is removed from electrochemical cell solution by purging it with ultra high purity argon and maintaining a head-space of the gas above the solution until the experiment is completed.

Characterisation of an amperometric biosensor may be considered as the evaluation of quantitative and qualitative physiochemical observables based on input-output behaviour of the biosensor, and trying to understand the underlying structural, chemical, and dynamic principles based on the measurements. Biosensor characterization is critical in ensuring that the biomolecule is successfully immobilised on, and electrochemically communicating with, the electrode. These assessments are usually performed by electrochemical and spectroscopic techniques. In broad terms, the analyses of senors are based on the determination of changes in physico-chemical properties which may be linked to the functional groups or molecular structure or morphology of the biosensing layer. Structural changes are checked using FTIR and UV-Visible spectroscopy. Morphology is assessed using SEM and TEM techniques. Electrochemical techniques are used to assess redox and electrocatalytic activities and their corresponding kinetic and thermodynamic parameters.

Electrosynthetic and Electroless Modification

Recently we found that keeping $FcPF_6$ in an aniline/PVS electropolymerization solution promoted the formation of a film of nanofibral PANI a carbon electrode in contrast to the cauliflower-morphology of PANI which resulted in the absence of $FcPF_6$. The polymerization solution contained 0.05 M $FcPF_6$, 0.2 M aniline, and 1 mL of the stock PVS sodium salt (18%) all dissolved in 1 M HCl. Figure 3(c) shows a typical PANI/PVS composite electropolymerization CV (20-cycles, 100 mV s^{-1}). The resulting modified electrode will be referred to as GCE|PANI-PVS. The PDMA/PSS [80] and PANSA [81] films can be prepared by electrochemical polymerization of the respective monomers on Au electrode surfaces in acidic medium (1.0 M HCl or 0.5 M H_2SO_4). In a typical experiment, the DMA to PSS dopant ratio was 2:1 and the anilino naphthalene sulfonic (0.1 M) was polymerized alone. Six and 10 polymerization cycles (at CV scan rate of 40 or 50 mV s^{-1}) were used for the electrosynthesis of PDMA-PSS and PANSA, respectively on Au disk electrodes (see Figure 3(b)). The resulting modified electrodes will be referred to as Au|PDMA/PSS and Au|PANSA. A PANI-PESA-PVS composite film can be prepared via purely chemical oxidative initiation as follows. 5 μL of a mixture of polyester sulfonic acid (PESA) and aniline (7:100 w/w) is placed on the surface of a Pt disk electrode which is then dipped (with the droplet side down) in 1 M HCl containing 0.1 M APS (oxidant) and 0.5% w/v PVS. The ensuing electroless chemical polymerization of PANI on the Pt electrode surface is allowed to proceed for 12 h in an ice bath. The resulting modified electrode will be referred to as Pt|PANI-PESA-PVS.

The electropolymerization voltammograms in Figure 3 (a) to (d) show that the peak current increases with the number of voltammetric cycles, which is characteristic of layer-by-layer deposition and growth of a conducting polymer on the surface an electrode [82, 83]. Electropolymerization of PANI has been known to show two pairs of prominent peaks belonging to the intrinsic electrochemical property of the polymer itself and in the middle of the CV is a pair of less prominent peaks arising from intermediate PANI structures or trapped molecular species [83]. The peaks are observed in Figure 3 (a) for polyaniline and in Figure 3 (b) for PDMA-PSS. The origin and interpretation of the PANI peaks are well documented in the literature [83,84]. The redox couple represented by peak pair a/a′ arises from leucoemeraldine/emeraldine transitions and the peak pair d/d′ is due to emeraldine/pernigraniline transition [84]. In contrast, during the electropolymerization of PANI in the presence of $FcPF_6$, four redox peaks were observed, three of which were similar to PANI peaks in terms of peak potentials and other CV characteristics. The redox couple that was and not found in PANI is represented by the peak pair b/b′ (see Figure 3 (c)). This peak pair was formed in the first polymerization cycle and there was no change in peak characteristics with successive cycles. The anodic peak is wide and centered at about 350 mV while the cathodic wave is significantly sharper and situated at about 200 mV. Both peaks appear to originate from surface adsorbed $FcPF_6$, and their heights increased with increasing concentration of $FcPF_6$ in the polymerization solution. The anodic peak was wider in accordance with the stronger adsorption of ferrocene than the ferrocenium ion [85]. The fact that the peak currents of the three redox couples attributed to PANI (a/a′, c/c′ and d/d′) in Figure 3(c) were not affected by changes in the concentration of $FcPF_6$ in the polymerization solution strongly confirmed the assignment of peaks b/b′ to $FcPF_6$. It was further observed that the peak potentials of the characteristic PANI peaks remained invariant regardless of the absence or presence of $FcPF_6$. Also, the absence or presence of $FcPF_6$ in the polymerization solution did not make any significant difference in the peak currents of peaks a/a′, c/c′ or d/d′. This observation indicated that similar amounts of PANI were electrosynthesized in the absence or presence of $FcPF_6$.

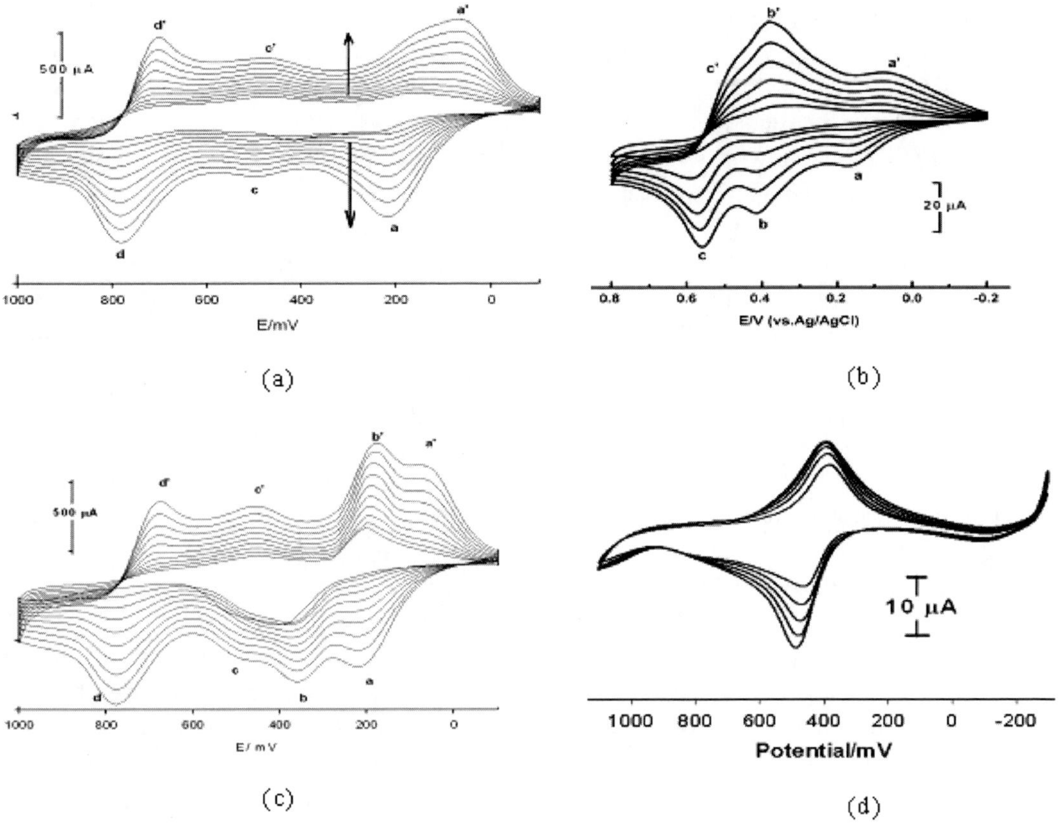

Figure 3. Polymerization cyclic voltammograms for (a) PANI (at GCE); (b) PDMA-PSS (at Au); (c) PANI-PVS-PFcPF$_6$ (at GCE); and (d) PANSA, in 0.5 M H_2SO_4 or HCl.

Anilino naphthalene sulfonic acid's (ANSA) polymerization CV (Figure 3 (d)) depicts only one pair of redox couple at about 0.5 V. The presence of a substituent on aniline also altered the CVs of PDMA-PSS in comparison with that of the pristine PANI. The successful polymerization of ANSA was confirmed by the voltammogram shown in Figure 4 (d) which exhibited similar cyclic voltammetric peaks as established for polyaniline.

Characterization of the Modified Electrodes: Electrochemical, Surface Morphology and Spectroscopic

The electrochemical behaviour (cyclic voltammetry) of the PANI derivatives and composites were studied in acid media (1 M HCl or 0.5 H_2SO_4) after rinsing the freshly modified electrodes with water. In the case of the nanofibral PANI-PVS which was formed in the presence of FcPF$_6$, the peaks associated with FcPF$_6$ oxidation/reduction in the polymerization voltammogram, disappeared altogether in the characterization CVs shown in Figure 4 (a), and only peaks with qualitative characteristics of a PANI were observed [82]. Both leucoemeraldine ↔ emeraldine (a/a′) and emeraldine ↔ pernigraniline (b/b′) transformations are evident. However, a broad anodic peak is observed between 300 mV and 500 mV. Therefore, there was a strong possibility that the FcPF$_6$ was not incorporated within the polymer matrix. Actually, $FcPF_6$ is not only appreciably soluble but also tends to be unstable in aqueous media as indicated in the literature [85]. The effect of the presence of the $FcPF_6$ was rather seen in the morphology of the PANI film formed on the surface of the electrode as shown in Figure 5 (a) in contrast to the SEM image of PANI formed in the absence of $FcPF_6$ (not shown). According to the image, the PANI-composite formed as nano-fibres with average cross-sectional diameters measuring about 100 nm, in contrast to the film formed in the absence of $FcPF_6$ that exhibited cauliflower-like morphology with image diameters of about 500 to 1000 nm. Thus ferrocenium hexafluorophosphate inhibited secondary growth over the PANI nanofibers.

The SEM image of PDMA-PSS film depicted in Figure 5 (b) showed globular particles with cross-sectional diameters of about 200 nm. The globules appeared clustered together with signs of inter-particle fusions either forming or disappearing. The voltammogram of PDMA-PSS (Figure 4 (b)) exhibits two redox couples centered at +0.20 V (a/a′) and +0.56 V (c/c′). It is clear that PANI composite retained some PANI characteristics as indicated by the existence of leucoemeraldine ↔ emeraldine (a/a′) and emeraldine ↔ pernigraniline (c/c′) transitions. The results confirm that PDMA-PSS film was successfully attached onto the gold electrode surface. PDMA being a polyaniline derivative shows features characteristic of polyaniline.

As shown in Figure 4 (c), the CV of the PANSA films in acid medium exhibited the two redox peaks characteristic of PANI voltammograms in the literature [7] confirming that aniline in anilinonapthalene sulfonic acid could be polymerized. The redox couples A/B and C/D are attributed to intrinsic redox processes of the polymer. The redox couple A/B observed at approximately +350 mV is as a result of the transformation of aniline in anilinonapthalene sulfonic acid from the reduced leucoemeraldine state to the partly oxidized emeraldine state. The redox couple C/D in the region 600 mV is due to the transition of leucoemeraldine state to the pernigraniline state which is accompanied by oxidation of aniline-1-napthalene sulfonic acid monomer. Scanning electron microscopy of PANSA shown in Figure 5 (c)), revealed nanorod constituents with cross-sections of approximately 100 nm.

The SEM image of the PANI/PVS/PESA composite film which was formed by chemical oxidative initiation of polymerization is shown in Figure 5 (d). This composite appears to be characterized by long and multi-folded nano-ropes with cross-sectional diameters of about 100 nm. A closer examination of the digitally zoomed-in section of the image shows that each nano rope appears to be either decorated with clusters of about 20 nm particles or it is a loose template-guided trace of these particles. Multi-scan voltamograms of the PANI/PVS/PESA composite film in 1 M HCl are shown in Figure 4 (d). This film exhibited two broad but distinct anodic peaks around 300 mV and 600 mV which were accompanied by two broad reverse cathodic peaks at about 500 mV and 200 mV. These peaks get wider and overlap as the scan rate increases to 20 mV s^{-1}, but without any shift in the respective peak potentials.

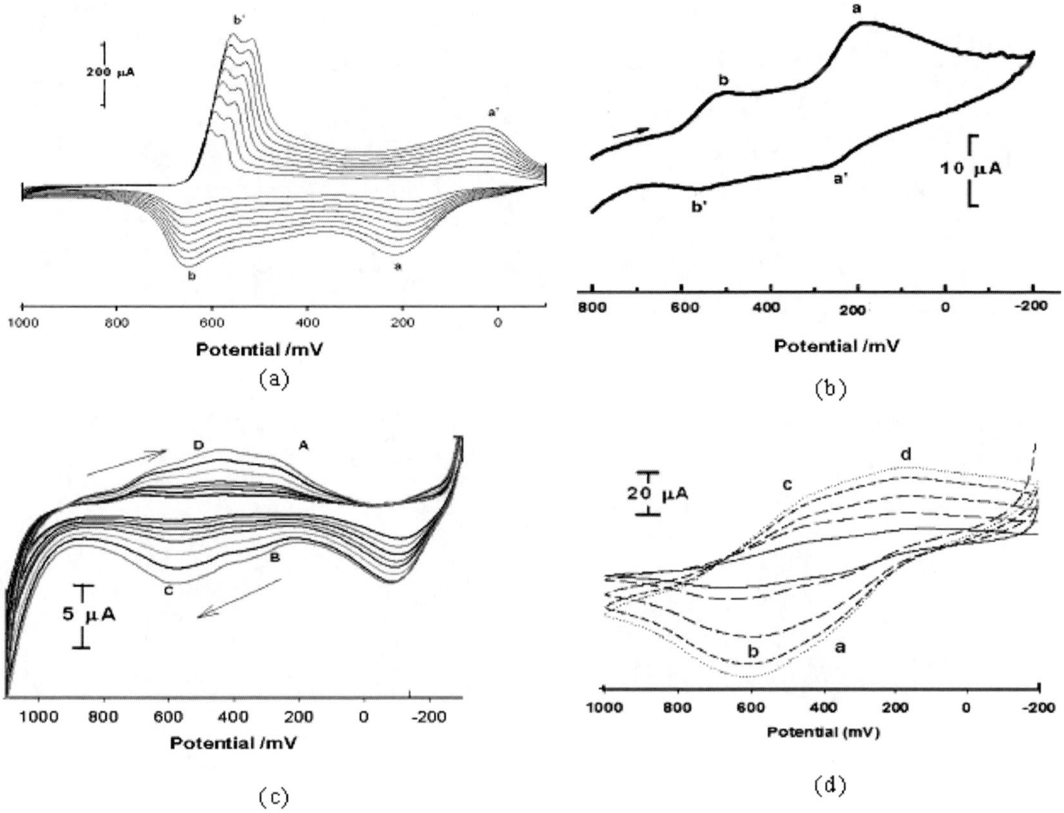

Figure 4. Cyclic voltammograms of nanostructured polyaniline composite films in strong acid solutions (aq. HCl or H_2SO_4): (a) GCE|PANI/PVS; (b) Au|PDMA-PSS; (c) Au|PANSA; and (d) Pt|PANI-PVS-PESA.

FTIR spectroscopy has been used to monitor the conducting states of a conducting polymer as well as to know if a doping experiment is successful [86, 87]. The FTIR and UV-Vis spectra of unsubstituted PANI is similar to that of substituted PANI though with slight band shifts. Doped PANI and its derivatives exist in the emeraldine salt forms which are essentially delocalized polysemiquinone radical cations whose stability is maintained by the presence of dopant anions. The degree of electron delocalization in the polysemiquinone forms of the doped PANI manifests itself in the form of an 'electronic-like band' at ca. 1100 cm^{-1} associated with polarons [86]. The structures of emeraldine base and emeraldine salt form of PANI are presented in Figure 6.

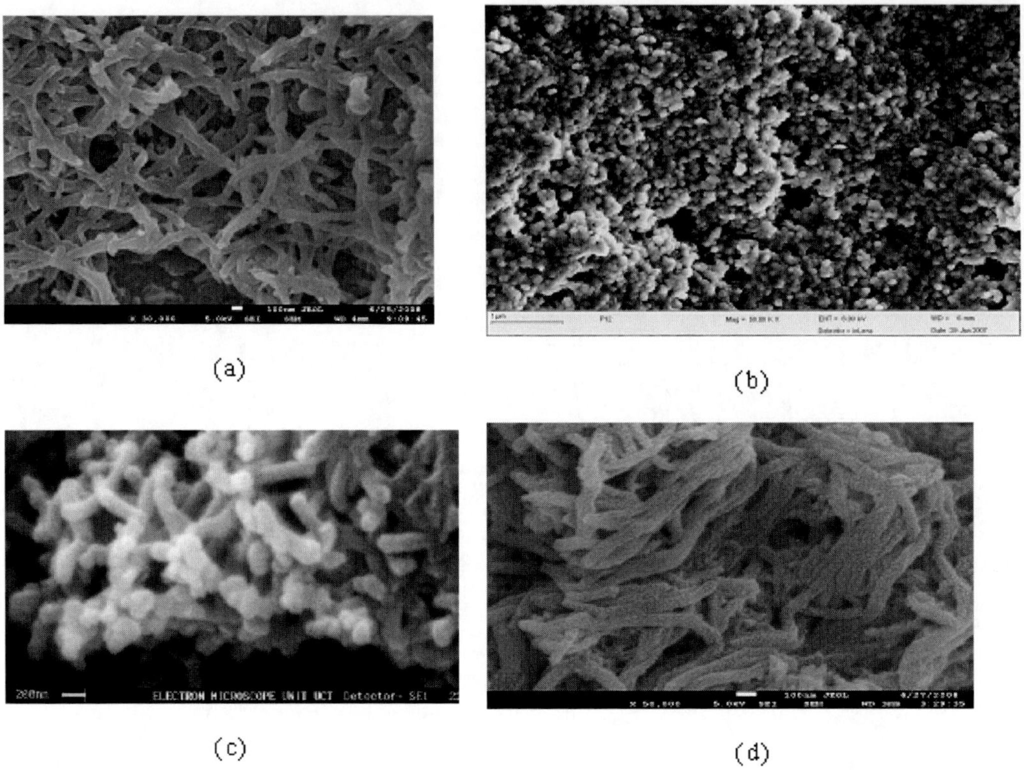

Figure 5. Scanning electron micrograph of (a) PANI-PVS [from ref. 111 by permission]; (b) PDMA-PSS; (c) PANSA [83]); (d) PANI-PES-PVS. Scale bars: (a) 100 nm; (b) 1000 nm; (c) 220 nm; and, (d) 100 nm.

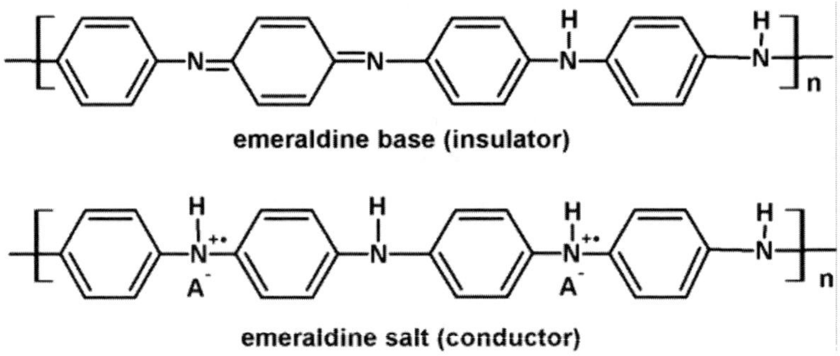

Figure 6. The structures of emeraldine base and emeraldine salt forms of PANI. A^- represents the dopant anion.

As revealed by FTIR and UV-Vis spectra in other studies, all PANI nanotubes, nanofibers, nanowires, nanorods, as well as microtubes, have backbone structures similar to that of the conventionally prepared granular PANI. In some cases, the Einstein shifts observed in the FTIR and UV-Vis spectra were ascribed to the interaction between the PANI chains and some small molecules, such as ethanol rather than to the chemical structures.

Furthermore, conductivity measurements on hard-template synthesized PANI nanotubules showed that the conductivities decreased as tube diameter increases and often reaching the conductivity of the conventional PANI powder [56].

In our own studies as well, the FTIR and UV-Vis results obtained for the nanostructured PANI/ or PANI derivatives (nanofibers, nanotubes and nanoparticles) showed characteristics similar to those of the conventional PANI/ or PANI derivatives confirming that they have backbone structures similar to that of the conventional granular PANI. Figure 7 shows typical FTIR and UV-Vis spectra of the nanostructured PDMA and PDMA-PSS films synthesized by electrochemical soft template method as described above. Incorporation of PSS into the PDMA film during electrosynthesis was confirmed by comparing the FTIR spectrum of PDMA with that of PDMA-PSS. PDMA-PSS spectrum shows the introduction of PSS bands at 1170 cm^{-1} and 1050 cm^{-1} as a result of the asymmetric and symmetric stretching modes of the $-SO_2$-OH group respectively [87]. The PDMA-PSS spectrum also shows a strong band at 1500 cm^{-1} due to the *para*-linked polymerization and confirms the presence of 1,4-amino (-NH-) substituted aromatic compound (1525-1485 cm^{-1}). This confirms that the anionic polyelectrolyte PSS present in the electrolyte solution, played the critical role of preferentially aligning the dimethoxyaniline monomers prior to polymerization promoting a more ordered *para*-linked (head-to-tail) coupling of the dimethoxyaniline substrates. The PDMA-PSS spectrum shows the double bond character of C=N stretching frequency at 1663 cm^{-1} suggesting that PSS played a role in doping the synthesized PDMA to the highly conducting emeraldine salt form. The presence of sharp duplex peaks at 1321 and 1251 cm^{-1} for PDMA-PSS is characteristic of C-O groups. The C-O duplex peaks for PDMA appear at 1330 and 1298 cm^{-1} but with lower intensity than that of PDMA-PSS.

The UV-Vis spectrum of nanostructured PDMA-PSS film shows a strong peak in the region around 800 nm due to the polaron → π* band transition for emeraldine salt form of PANI. This polaron band is a diagnostic test for the conformation of the PANI chains and it appears in the region 750-850 nm [88]. This confirms that the nanostructured polyanilines possess backbone structures similar to that of doped conventionally prepared granular PANI. The undoped nanostructured PDMA displays a strong band at ca. 600 nm that is characteristic of emeraldine base. This can be attributed to a local charge transfer between a quinoid ring and the adjacent imine-phenyl-amine units giving rise to an intramolecular charge transfer exciton [51].

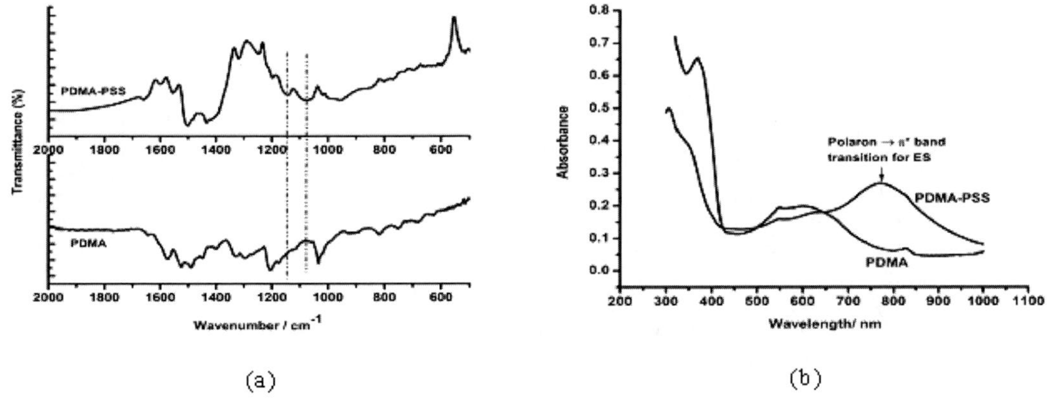

Figure 7. (a) FTIR spectra and (b) UV-Vis spectra of nanostructured PDMA and PDMA-PSS films.

4. Amperometric Biosensors with Enzymes Electrohemically Communicated Via Sulfonate-Functionalized Polyanilines

Polyanilines have attracted much interest as suitable conducting matrices for the immobilization of functional proteins, especially enzymes. As a transducer in biosensors, PANI has been effectively to enhance biosensor response time, sensitivity and versatility for clinical diagnostics, industrial and environmental monitoring [89]. Several reviews on the use of conducting polymers in the fabrication of biosensors have been published [16, 78, 89, 90]. Biological recognition agents such as purified enzymes, enzyme-rich tissues, antibody (antigens), microbes such as bacteria and yeast, liposomes and organelles have been used for developing specific and sensitive biosensors [91, 92]. The methods for immobilizing these bio-recognition agents include adsorption [93, 94], entrapment [95], cross-linking and covalent bonding [56, 92, 96-99]. In the case of amperometric enzyme biosensors, which are of particular focus in this book chapter, molecules to be detected are let to diffuse and partition between the enzyme layer of the biosensor and the sample solution. Signals are generated by electrochemical interrogation of the enzyme itself or the product of the enzymatic reaction. The direct or indirect electrochemical communication of an enzyme's redox center with the electrode so that the enzyme could be regenerated electrochemically rather than by its reaction with a co-factor or a co-substrate has been the focus of many studies. An amperometric biosensor working on this transduction principle would exploit the ultimate selectivity that could be offered by the biological reaction towards the analyte of interest. Advantages of polyaniline as a matrix for the immobilization and electrochemical interrogation of biomolecules, especially enzymes, can be summarised below.

- *Flexibility of the chemical structure which can be easily modified* as required by the formation of blends or composites as demonstrated in pesticides and glucose sensors [100-102].
- *Post-polymerization incorporation of the biomolecules* into the electrodeposited PANI permits localisation of biomolecules on electrodes of any size or geometry and it is useful in multi-analyte micro amperometric biosensors [52, 103, 104].
- *Polyanilines have been shown to be compatible with biomolecules* in neutral and near neutral aqueous solutions – a medium of preference for most biomolecules [97, 105].
- *Electrochemical synthesis of PANI allows the direct deposition* of the polymer on the electrode surface, while simultaneously trapping the biomolecules [16, 90].

Figure 8 is a possible redox cycle occurring in an amperometric sensor for hydrogen peroxide involving enzyme-wiring of a typical enzyme (*Horseradish peroxidase,* HRP) with polyaniline. HRP immobilized on the electrode surface can be oxidized by H_2O_2 to compound I that contains an oxyferryl centre with the iron in the ferryl state ($Fe^{IV} = O$), and a porphyrin π cation radical, followed by further direct (mediatorless) electroreduction of compound I at the electrode surface to the initial HRP state [106]. The electrode is considered as an electron donor.

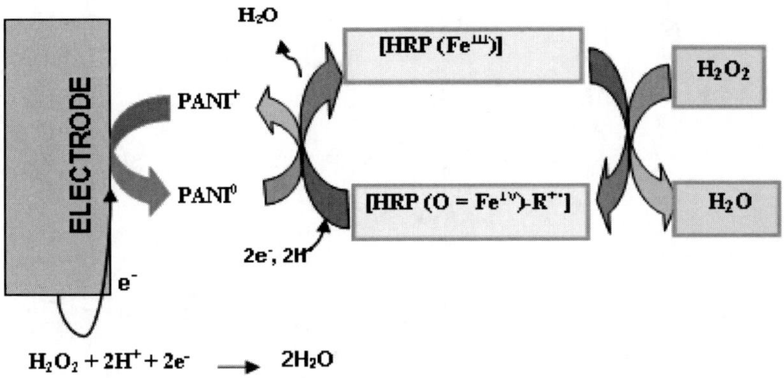

Figure 8. Reaction scheme for PANI-HRP based peroxide biosensor.

Immobilization of Enzymes: Biosensors for Hydrogen Peroxide, Glufosinate, Glyphosate, Fluoxetine and Setraline

Two typical enzyme immobilization methods, electrostatic and cross-linking, were followed in developing biosensors with polyaniline nanocomposites discussed in the previous sections. In the electrostatic method of enzyme incorporation into the conducting polymer platform, the modified-electrode is transferred to a pH 7 phosphate buffer solution and subjected to a constant reductive potential (-0.5 V) in order to convert the polymer film into its completely reduced state. Then it is transferred into a solution containing HRP or CYP2D6 (0.1 mg/mL in PBS) and re-oxidized for 20 min at +0.65 V. During the oxidation process, the heme protein HRP became electrostatically attached onto the PDMA-PSS film. In the case of the biosensor developed by immobilizing the enzyme via the combination of drop-coating and cross-linking, the enzyme layer casting solution which was prepared just before use in phosphate buffer (pH 7.0, 0.1 M) contained the enzyme (~ 15 mg/mL), bovine serum albumin (BSA, ~30 mg/mL) and glutaraldehyde (Glu, ~1%). 5 µL of the enzyme layer casting solution was pipetted out onto the PANI-modified GCE surface and allowed to dry. We shall assume that the enzyme/BSA/glutaraldehyde mixture sipped into the porous PANI layer. This strategy was used for the HRP biosensor developed on the PANI-$FcPF_6$ nanofibre platform. While the biosensors thus fabricated could be stored wet in PBS or dry at 4 °C when not in use, in these studies the biosensors were kept in the working buffer at 4° C when not in use, and rinsed with deionised water between experiments.

Verification of the Occurrence of Electrochemical Enzyme–Interrogation

Figure 9 shows the electrocatalytic responses of biosensors for H_2O_2 (a, b, and d) and fluoxetine (c) demonstrating the occurrence of electrochemical communications between the electrode and the enzymes (HRP and CYP2D6). For the nanofibral PANI, the electrocatalytic half wave of the amperometric signal occurred at about -400 mV. For PDMA-PSS, it was -200 mV; and +100 mV for PANI-PVS-PESA when they were tested in the presence of H_2O_2.

The biosensors were applied in the analysis of herbicides and clinical drugs. Concentration dependence of the responses of the biosensors is displayed in Figure 10.

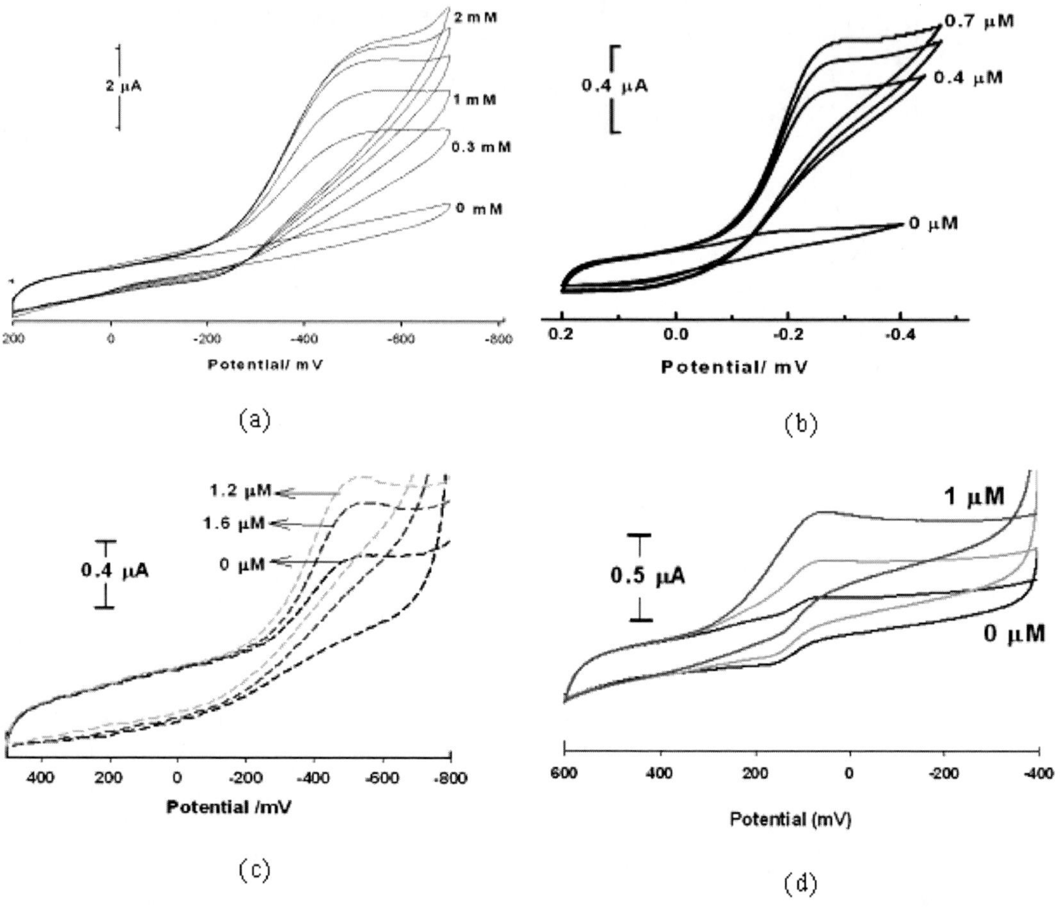

Figure 9. Biosensor CV responses (in phosphate buffer) of: (a) GCE|PANI-PVS/HRP to H_2O_2 [from ref. 111 by permission]; (b) Au|PDMA-PSS/HRP to H_2O_2; (c) Au|PANSA/CYP2D6 to sertraline; and (d) Pt|PANI-PVS-PESA/HRP to H_2O_2. The respective buffer pH values are 7, 6.1, 7.4 and 6.5.

Analytical Responses

HRP Biosensors for hydrogen peroxide (H_2O_2) – a strategic biomedical analyte. Both GCE|PANI-PVS/HRP and Pt|PANI-PVS-PESA/HRP biosensors were successfully demonstrated for applications in the detection of hydrogen peroxide. Linear responses were observed as shown by Figures 10 (a) and (b). The analytical figures of merits of these biosensors and those discussed below are summarized in Table 1.

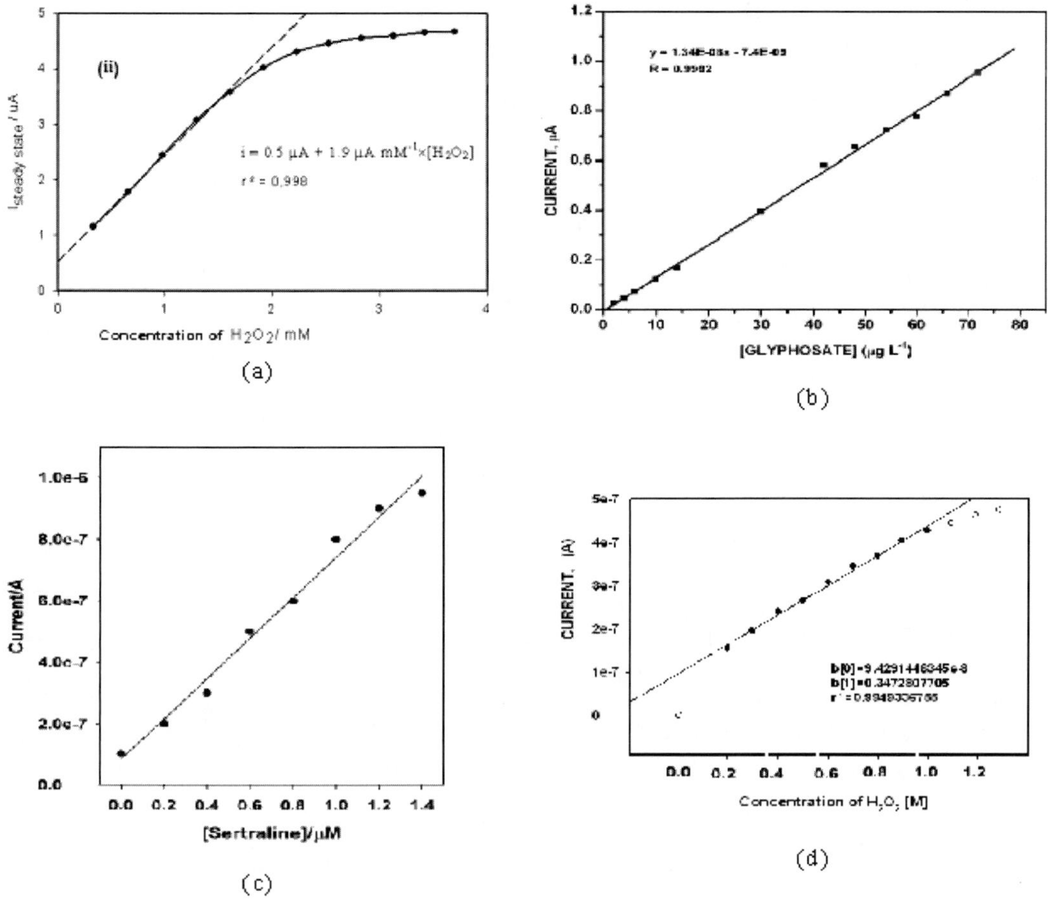

Figure 10. Biosensor calibration curves for data obtained with phosphate buffer: (a) GCE/PANI-PVS/HRP for H_2O_2 (-400 mV; steady state amperometry, 300 rpm stirring, pH 7); (b) Au|PDMA-PSS/HRP for glyphosate (-100 mV, steady state amperometry, 400 rpm stirring, pH 6.1); (c) Au|PANSA/CYP2D6 (-250 mV, DPV, pH 7.4); and (d) Pt|PANI-PVS-PESA/HRP to H_2O_2 (-100 mV, CV, pH 6.5).

HRP-inhibition biosensor for herbicides. The detection of H_2O_2, glyphosate and glufosinate herbicides was achieved using the Au|PDMA-PSS/HRP biosensor. Herbicides are known to suppress the photosynthetic reactions as well as the activity of tyrosinase or peroxidase enzymes [107]. The transduction of the herbicides's (glyphosate and glufosinate) concentrations was based on signal–attenuation caused by the inhibition of the HRP by the herbicides [107] and hence the decrease in the amperometric signals from the biosensor in the presence of constant background concentration of H_2O_2. Inhibition of an enzyme can be easily and directly observed with enzyme sensors without having to resort to techniques that require long extractions, such as dialysis or gel filtration, which are normally used to separate an inhibitor from a soluble enzyme. This is illustrated in Figure 11 for the amperometric response of the biosensor to H_2O_2, glyphosate and glufosinate standard solutions.

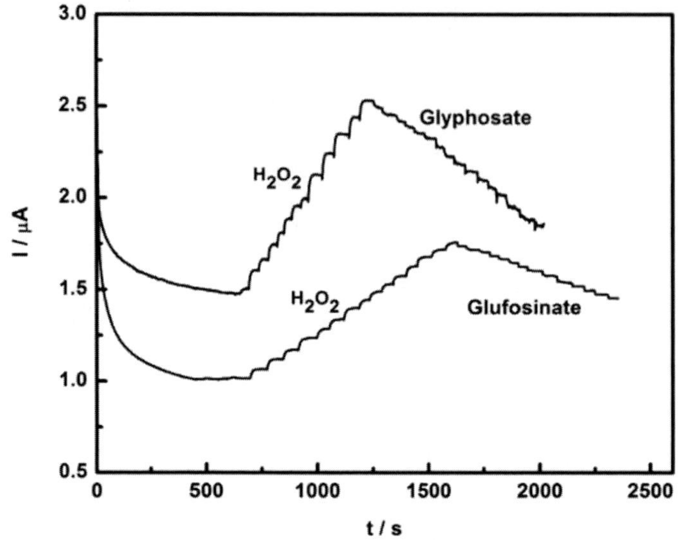

Figure 11. Amperometric responses of Au|PDMA-PSS/HRP to H_2O_2, glyphosate and glufosinate standards in pH 6.1 phosphate buffer; applied potential: -100 mV; Stirring: 400 rpm.

The response of the Au|PDMA-PSS/HRP biosensor to H_2O_2 would serve as a measure of the activity of the immobilized enzyme, whether or not its inhibitor is present in the sample. The relative change in activity of the enzyme HRP could thus be estimated from signal measured before and after the addition of herbicide in the presence of a constant concentration of H_2O_2. It is observed from Figure 11 that the response of the biosensor to H_2O_2 reduced in the presence of the inhibitors glyphosate and glufosinate. The magnitude of the decrease in signal could also be related to the concentrations of glyphosate and glufosinate in the test solutions. Glyphosate and glufosinate could be classified as reversible inhibitors because the biosensor could be reactivated simply by rinsing off with phosphate buffer. The sensor-to-sensor (fabrication) reproducibility was generally within 5% (standard deviation, N = 3) and a typical biosensor was operational for days.

Table 1. Performance parameters of the biosensors

Analyte	Biosensor	Detection Limit	Upper Linear Range	Sensitivity	Operating Potential (and Mode)	Ref.
H_2O_2	GCE|PANI–PVS/HRP	30 µM	2 mM	1.9 µA/mM	-400 mV (stir)	[111]
Glyphosate	Au|PDMA–PSS/HRP	5.0 nM	400 nM	1.6 nA/nM	-100 mV (stir)	[80]
Glufosinate	Au|PDMA–PSS/HRP	6.0 nM	350 nM	1.0 nA/nM	-100 mV (stir)	[80]
H_2O_2	Pt|PANI–PVS–PESA/HRP	0.2 µM	10 µM	1.4 µA/µM	-100 mV (CV)	This report
Fluoxetine	Au|PANSA/CYP2D6	0.09 µM	1.0 µM	0.6 nA/nM	-250 mV (DPV)	This report
Sertraline	Au|PANSA/CYP2D6	0.13 µM	1.4 µM	0.3 µA/µM	-250 mV (DPV)	[81]

CYP2D6 biosensor for antidepressants (sertraline and fluxetine). Previous studies on PANI– and polythiophene–based CYP–biosensors for fluoxetine showed that the uncompetitive inhibition kinetics between the CYP enzyme and fluoxetine is based on the mono-oxygenation reaction of the enzyme [13]. The response of the Au|PANSA/CYP2D6 biosensor in the presence of sertraline was studied using CV and DPV under aerobic conditions. A linear calibration curve was obtained for the DPV response of the biosensor to sertraline as shown in Figure 10c, and the corresponding analytical parameters are summarised in Table 1. The detection limits of fluoxetine and sertraline are higher than those reported in the literature. This is especially true for the fluoxetine biosensor whose intra-hepatic concentration is reported in the range from 2 to 7 μmol/L [13].

Although not all the biosensors presented in this chapter have detection limits lower than values reported in the literature [76], biosensor technology is still preferable to chromatographic detection techniques which involve labourious derivatisation procedures [108-111]. Electrochemical biosensors based on nanostructured material as sensor platforms have been reviewed recently by Wang (2005) [19]. A more recent review on organic conjugated polymer–based electrochemical sensors by Rahman et.al (2008) [19,109,110] highlighted that in combination with nanotechnology, novel functional nanomaterials, nanobiostructures and nanobiotechnologies, chemical sensors are exerting a profound influence on the quality of services in various sectors of real life.

ACKNOWLEDGMENTS

The authors gratefully acknowledge financial assistances from the Department of Labour (DST, South Africa), the National Research Foundation (NRF, South Africa), the Claude Leon Foundation (CLF, South Africa), the Third World Organization for Women in Science (TWOWS, Italy), and the African Network of Scientific and Technological Institutions (ANSTI, Kenya). We thank Dr Gerald Malgas of the National Centre for Nano-Structured Materials, Council for Scientific and Industrial Research (CSIR), Pretoria - South Africa, for the permission to use CSIR's scanning electron microscopy facility.

REFERENCES

[1] Huang, J. *Pure Appl. Chem.* 2006, *78*, 15-27.
[2] Virji, S.; Kaner, R. B.; Weiller, B. H. *ACS Symp. Ser.* 2007, *980*, 101-115.
[3] Zotti, G.; Cattarin, S.; Comisso, N. *J. Electroanal. Chem.* 1988, *239*, 387-396.
[4] Kalaji, M.; Peter, L. M.; Abrantes, L. M.; Mesquita, J. C. *J. Electroanal. Chem.* 1989, *274*, 289-295.
[5] Inzelt, G. *J. Electroanal. Chem.* 1990, *279*, 169-178.
[6] Kalaji, M.; Nyholm, L.; Peter, L. M.; Rudge, A. J. *J. Electroanal. Chem.* 1991, *310*, 113-126.
[7] MacDiarmid, A. G.; Manohar, S. K.; Masters, J. G.; Sun, Y.; Weiss, H.; Epstein, A. J. *Proc. Int. Conf. Sci. Tech. Synth. Met.* 1991, *41*, 621-626.
[8] Karyakin, A. A.; Bobrova, O. A.; Lukachova, L. V.; Karyakina, E. E. *Eurosensors IX* 1996, *33*, 34-38.
[9] Cosnier, S.; Gondran, C. *Biosensors: Analusis* 1997, *27*-.
[10] Wan, M. X.; Li, J. C. *Synth. Met.* 1999, *101*, 844-845.
[11] Tian, F. M.; Xu, B.; Zhu, G. Y. *Chinese Chemical Letters* 2001, 12, 625-628

[12] Mazur, M.; Tagowska, M.; Palys, B.; Jackowska, K. *Electrochem. Commun.* 2003, *5*, 403-407.

[13] Iwuoha, E. I.; Wilson, A.; Howel, M.; Mathebe, N. G. R.; Montane-Jaime, K.; Narinesingh, D.; Guiseppi-Elie, A. *Anal. Lett.* 2004, *37*, 929-941.

[14] Ali, M. A.; Saion, E.; Yahya, N.; Kassim, A.; Dahlan, K. M.; Hashim, S. *J. Eng. Sci. Technol.* 2007, *2*, 111-118.

[15] Syed, A. A.; Dinesan, M. K. *Talanta* 1991, *38*, 815-837.

[16] Cosnier, S. *Biosens. Bioelectron.* 1999, *14*, 443-456.

[17] Malinauskas, A.; Malinauskiene, J.; Ramanavicius, A. *Nanotechnology* 2005, *16*, R51-R62.

[18] Tahir, Z. M.; Alocilja, E. C.; Grooms, D. L. *Selected Papers from the Eighth World Congress on Biosensors, Part I* 2005, *20*, 1690-1695.

[19] Wang, J. *Analyst* 2005, *130*, 421-426.

[20] Gospodinova, N.; Terlemezyan, L. *Prog. Polym. Sci.* 1998, *23*, 1443-1484.

[21] Zheng, L.; Xiong, L.; Liu, C.; Jin, L. *Eur. Polym. J.* 2006, *42*, 2328-2333.

[22] Lee, H. -Y.; Rwei, S. -P.; Wang, L.; Chen, P. -H. *Mater. Chem. Phys.* 2008, 112, 805-809.

[23] Prakash, S.; Rao, C. R. K.; Vijayan, M. *Electrochim. Acta* 2008, *53*, 5704-5710.

[24] Shah, A. -A. -H. A.; Holze, R. *Electrochim. Acta* 2008, *53*, 4642 - 4653.

[25] Genies, E. M.; Lapkowski, M.; Santier, C.; Vieil, E. *Synth. Met.* 1987, *18*, 631-636.

[26] Goto, F.; Abe, K.; Ikabayashi, K.; Yoshida, T.; Morimoto, H. *J. Power Sources* 1987, *20*, 243-248.

[27] Ryu, K. S.; Kim, K. M. *J. Power Sources* 2007, *165*, 420-426.

[28] Bartlett, P. N.; Ling-Chung, S. K. *Sens. Actuators* 1989, *20*, 287-292.

[29] Karyakin, A. A.; Bobrova, O. A.; Lukachova, L. V.; Karyakina, E. E. *Sens. Actuators, B* 1996, *33*, 34-38.

[30] Jin, Z.; Su, Y.; Duan, Y. *Sens. Actuators, B 2000*, *71*, 118-122.

[31] Syed, A. A.; Dinesan, M. K. *React. Polym.* 1992, *17*, 145-157.

[32] Illing, G.; Hellgardt, K.; Wakeman, R. J.; Jungbauer, A. *J. Membr. Sci.* 2001, *184*, 69-78.

[33] Kim, B.; Koncar, V.; Devaux, E.; Dufour, C.; Viallier, P. *Synth. Met.* 2004, *146*, 167-174.

[34] Barbero, C.; Salavagione, H. J.; Acevedo, D. F.; Grumelli, D. E.; Garay, F.; Planes, G. A.; Morales, G. M.; Miras, M. C. *Electrochim. Acta* 2004, *49*, 3671-3686.

[35] IUPAC. In *Compendium of Chemical Terminology;* McNaught, A. D.; Wilkinson, A.; Eds.; 2nd ed. (the "Gold Book"); Blackwell Scientific Publications: Oxford, 1997.

[36] Morales, G. M.; Salavagione, H. J.; Grumelli, D. E.; Miras, M. C.; Barbero, C. A. *Polymer* 2006, *47*, 8272-8280.

[37] Li, D.; Xia, Y. *Nat. Mater.* 2004, *3*, 753-754.

[38] Hopkins, A. R.; Lipeles, R. A.; Kao, W. H. *Thin Solid Films* 2004, *447-448*, 474-480.

[39] Hopkins, A. R.; Sawall, D. D.; Villahermosa, R. M.; Lipeles, R. A. *Thin Solid Films* 2004, *469-470*, 304-308.

[40] Chronakis, I. S.; Grapenson, S.; Jakob, A. *Polymer* 2006, *47*, 1597-1603.

[41] Guimard, N. K.; Gomez, N.; Schmidt, C. E. *Prog. Polym. Sci.* 2007, *32*, 876-921.

[42] Karim, M. R.; Lim, K. T.; Lee, C. J.; Lee, M. S. *Synth. Met.* 2007, *157*, 1008-1012.

[43] Al-Mashat, L.; Tran, H. D.; Wlodarski, W.; Kaner, R. B.; Kalantar-zadeh, K. *Sens. Actuators, B* 2008, *134*, 826-831.

[44] Akinyeye, R.; Sekota, M.; Baker, P.; Iwuoha, E. *Fullerenes, Nanotubes, Carbon Nanostruct.* 2006, *14*, 49-55.

[45] Jang, J.; Bae, J.; Lee, K. *Polymer* 2005, *46*, 3677-3684.

[46] Jiaxing, H. *Pure Appl. Chem.* 2006, *78*, 15-27.

[47] Lei, T. *Trans. Nonferrous Met. Soc. China* 2007, *17*, 1343-1346.

[48] Eftekhari, A. *Synth. Met.* 2004, *145*, 211-216.

[49] Masters, J. G.; Sun, Y.; MacDiarmid, A. G.; Epstein, A. J. *Proc. Int. Conf. Sci. Tech. Synth. Met.* 1991, *41*, 715-718.

[50] Matveeva, E. S.; Gimenez, C. F.; Tejera, M. J. G. *Synth. Met.* 2001, *123*, 117-123.

[51] Wallace, G. G.; Spinks, G. M.; Kane-Maguire, L. A.; Teasdale, P. R. *Conductive electroactive polymers: Intelligent materials systems*; 2nd ed.; Taylor & Francis Group: United States of America, 2003, 121-177.

[52] Iwuoha, E. I.; de Villaverde, D. S.; Garcia, N. P.; Smyth, M. R.; Pingarron, J. M. *Biosens. Bioelectron.* 1997, *12*, 749-761.

[53] Tang, H.; Kitani, A.; Shiotani, M. *Electrochim. Acta* 1996, *41*, 1561-1567.

[54] Kalaji, M.; Nyholm, L.; Peter, L. M. *J. Electroanal. Chem.* 1991, *313*, 271-289.

[55] Inzelt, G.; Horányi, G. *Electrochim. Acta* 1990, *35*, 27-34.

[56] Zhang, D.; Wang, Y. *Mater. Sci. Eng., B* 2006, *134*, 9-19.

[57] Chen, S.-S.; Wen, T.-C.; Gopalan, A. *Synth. Met.* 2003, *132*, 133-143.

[58] Chakarvarti, S. K.; Vetter, J. *Radiat. Meas.* 1998, *29*, 149-159.

[59] Wu, C. G.; Bein, T. *Science (Washington, DC)* 1994, *264*, 1757-1759.

[60] [Wei, Z.; Zhang, Z.; Wan, M. *Langmuir* 2002, *18*, 917-921.

[61] Zhang, Z.; Wei, Z.; Zhang, L.; Wan, M. *Acta Mater.* 2005, *53*, 1373-1379.

[62] Han, M. G.; Cho, S. K.; Oh, S. G.; Im, S. S. *Synth. Met.* 2002, *126*, 53-60.

[63] Wei, Z.; Wan, M. *J. Appl. Polym. Sci.* 2003, *87*, 1297-1301.

[64] [Huang, J.; Wan, M. *J. Polym. Sci., Part A: Polym. Chem.* 1999, *37*, 151-157.

[65] Wan, M.; Li, J. *J. Polym. Sci., Part A: Polym. Chem.* 2000, *38*, 2359-2364.

[66] Qiu, H.; Wan, M.; Matthews, B.; Dai, L. *Macromolecules* 2001, *34*, 675-677.

[67] Liu, J.; Wan, M. *J. Polym. Sci., Part A: Polym. Chem.* 2001, *39*, 997-1004.

[68] Liu, J.; Wan, M. *J. Mater. Chem.* 2001, *11*, 404-407.

[69] Wan, M.; Huang, J.; Shen, Y. *Synth. Met.* 1999, *101*, 708-711.

[70] Shen, Y.; Wan, M. *J. Polym. Sci., Part A: Polym. Chem.* 1999, *37*, 1443-1449.

[71] Wan, M.; Li, J. *J. Polym. Sci., Part A: Polym. Chem.* 1999, *37*, 4605-4609.

[72] Wan, M.; Liu, J.; Qiu, H.; Li, J.; Li, S. *Synth. Met.* 2001, *119*, 71-72.

[73] Qiu, H.; Wan, M. *J. Polym. Sci., Part A: Polym. Chem.* 2001, *39*, 3485-3497.

[74] Yang, Y.; Wan, M. *J. Mater. Chem.* 2002, *12*, 897-901.

[75] Zhang, Z.; Wan, M. *Synth. Met.* 2002, *128*, 83-89.

[76] Michira, I. N.; Klink, M.; R.O. Akinyeye; Somerset, V.; M. Sekota; Al-Ahmed, A.; P.G.L. Baker; Iwuoha, E. I. In *Recent advances in analytical electrochemistry: Anthracene sulfonic acid-doped polyanilines: electrodynamics and application as amperometric peroxide biosensor;* Kenneth, O.; Ed.; *Chapter 5;* Transworld Research Network: Karala India, 2007; Vol., pp. 137.

[77] Zhang, X.; Manohar, S. K. *Chem. Commun.* (Cambridge, United Kingdom) 2004, 2360-2361.

[78] Kim, B. -K.; Kim, Y. H.; Won, K.; Chang, H.; Choi, Y.; Kong, K. -J.; Rhyu, B. W.; Kim, J. -J.; Lee, J. -O. *Nanotechnology* 2005, *16*, 1177-1181.
[79] Grennan, K.; Killard, A. J.; Hanson, C. J.; Cafolla, A. A.; Smyth, M. R. *Talanta* 2006, *68*, 1591-1600.
[80] Songa, E. A.; Somerset, V. S.; Waryo, T.; Baker, P. G. L.; Iwuoha, E. I. *Pure Appl. Chem.* 2009, *81,* 39-55.
[81] Iwuoha, E.; Ngece, R.; Klink, M.; Baker, P. *IET Nanobiotechnol.* 2007, *1*, 62-67.
[82] Mathebe, N. G. R.; Morrin, A.; Iwuoha, E. I. *Talanta* 2004, *64*, 115-120.
[83] Rajendra Prasad, K.; Munichandraiah, N. *Synth. Met.* 2001, *123*, 459-468.
[84] Iwuoha, E. I.; Mavundla, S. E.; Somerset, V. S.; Petrik, L. F.; Klink, M. J.; Sekota, M.; Baker, P. G. *Microchim. Acta* 2006, *155*, 453-458.
[85] Sanchis, C.; Salavagione, H. J.; Morallón, E. *J. Electroanal. Chem.* 2008, *618*, 67-73.
[86] Patil, V.; Sainkar, S. R.; Patil, P. P. *Synth. Met.* 2004, *140*, 57-63.
[87] Cataldo, F.; Maltese, P. *Eur. Polym. J.* 2002 *38*, 1791-1803.
[88] Kim, S. -C.; Huh, P.; Kumar, J.; Kim, B.; Lee, J. -O.; Bruno, F. F. *Green Chem.* 2007 *9*, 44-48.
[89] Ahuja, T.; Mir, I. A.; Kumar, D.; Rajesh *Biomaterials* 2007, *28*, 791-805.
[90] Wei, D.; Ivaska, A. *Chem. Anal. (Warsaw)* 2006, *51*, 839-852.
[91] Piras, L.; Adami, M.; Fenu, S.; Dovis, M.; Nicolini, C. *Anal. Chim. Acta* 1996, *335*, 127-135.
[92] Gerard, M.; Malhotra, B. D. *Curr. Appl. Phys.* 2005, *5*, 174-177.
[93] Pan, X.; Kan, J.; Yuan, L. *Sens. Actuators, B* 2004, *102*, 325-330.
[94] Garjonyte, R.; Malinauskas, A. *Biosens. Bioelectron.* 2000, *15*, 445-451.
[95] Luo, Y. -C.; Do, J. -S. *Microsens. Microsyst. 2003* 2004, *20*, 15-23.
[96] Ivanov, A. N.; Evtugyn, G. A.; Lukachova, L. V.; Karyakina, E. E.; Budnikov, H. C.; Kiseleva, S. G.; Orlov, A. V.; Karpacheva, G. P.; Karyakin, A. A. *Sensors* 2003, *3*, 333-340.
[97] Gerard, M.; Chaubey, A.; Malhotra, B. D. *Biosens. Bioelectron.* 2002, *17*, 345-359.
[98] Teles, F. R. R.; Fonseca, L. P. *Mater. Sci. Eng., C In Press, Corrected Proof.*
[99] Snejdarkova, M.; Svobodova, L.; Evtugyn, G.; Budnikov, H.; Karyakin, A.; Nikolelis, D. P.; Hianik, T. *Anal. Chim. Acta* 2004, *514*, 79-88.
[100] Zhou, H.; Chen, H.; Luo, S.; Chen, J.; Wei, W.; Kuang, Y. *Biosens. Bioelectron.* 2005, *20*, 1305-1311.
[101] Ma, Y.; Ali, S. R.; Dodoo, A. S.; He, H. *J. Phys. Chem. B 2006, 110, 16359-16365.*
[102] Zhang, M.; Yamaguchi, A.; Morita, K.; Teramae, N. *Electrochem. Commun.* 2008, *10*, 1090-1093.
[103] Qu, F.; Yang, M.; Jiang, J.; Shen, G.; Yu, R. *Anal. Biochem.* 2005, *344*, 108-114.
[104] Ruan, C.; Li, Y. *Talanta* 2001, *54*, 1095-1103.
[105] Akinyeye, R.; Michira, I.; Botha, S.; Baker, P.; Iwuoha, E. In *Recent advances in analytical electrochemistry: Electrocatalytic sensor applications of Nanostructured polypyrroles and polythiopenes;* Kenneth, O.; Ed.; Chapter 4; Transworld Research Network: Karala India, 2007, Vol., pp. 99.
[106] Ferapontova, E.; Schmengler, K.; Börchers, T.; Ruzgas, T.; Gorton, L. *Biosens. Bioelectron.* 2002, *17*, 953-963.
[107] Evtugyn, G. A.; Budnikov, H. C.; Nikolskaya, E. B. *Talanta* 1998 *46*, 465-484.

[108] Sato, K.; Jin, J. Y.; Takeuchi, T.; Miwa, T.; Suenami, K.; Takekoshi, Y.; Kanno, S. *J. Chromatogr. A* 2001, *919*, 313-320.
[109] Rahaman, M. A.; Kumar, P.; Park, D. -S.; Shim, Y. -B. *Sensors* 2008, *8*, 118-141.
[110] Khanna, V. K. *Sensors* 2008, *28*, 39-45.
[111] Ndangili, P.M.; Waryo, T.T.; Muchindu, M.; Baker, P.G.L.; Ngila, C.J.; Iwuoha, E.I. *Electrochimica Acta* DOI 10.1016

In: Nanostructured Materials for Electrochemical Biosensors ISBN: 978-1-60741-706-4
Editors: U. Yogeswaran; S. Kumar; S. Chen ©2009 Nova Science Publishers, Inc.

Chaper 3

METAL NANOPARTICLES EMBEDDED POLYMER MATRIX MODIFIED ELECTRODES FOR DIRECT ELECTROCATALYSIS AND ELECTROCHEMICAL SENSOR

Ramasamy Ramaraj* and Govindhan Maduraiveeran
Centre for Photoelectrochemistry, School of Chemistry,
Madurai Kamaraj University Madurai, INDIA

ABSTRACT

Recent electrochemical research interest in nanomaterials modified electrodes is focused on the fabrication of new direct electrocatalytic and electrochemical sensing devices using potentially useful metal nanoparticles embedded in suitable support matrices. In recent times, the simple fabrication of direct electrocatalytic and electrochemical sensor devices by employing metal (platinum (Pt) and gold (Au)) nanoparticles (Pt_{nano}, and Au_{nano}) embedded in matrices such as Nafion (Nf) and functionalized silicate sol-gel (SG) network (Nf/Pt_{nano} and SG-Au_{nano}) for the detection and determination of biomolecules such as dopamine (DA), ascorbic acid (AA), serotonin (5-HT), uric acid (UA) and toxic chemicals such as hydrazine, sulfite and nitrite was reported from our laboratory. In direct electrocatalysis and electrochemical detection systems, metal nanoparticles at the modified electrodes play a major role as mediator and catalyst for the direct oxidation/reduction of substrates. The mediators, such as enzymes or similar molecules, free modified electrodes prepared using metal nanoparticles are a reagentless electrochemical sensor and exhibit low operating potential for substrates reaction at the modified electrode. These electrodes are simple to design, cost-effective, and require no external modification to metal nanoparticles or layer by layer modification. The embedded metal nanoparticles in matrix improve the transducer property of the sensor by providing the necessary electronic conduction pathway and facilitating the electron transfer events between the analyte and electrode surface in the absence of any other external electron transfer mediator. The metal nanoparticles embedded matrix networks are characterized by scanning electron micrograph (SEM),

* Corresponding author. Phone: +91-452-2459084; E-mail: ramarajr@yahoo.com.

atomic force micrographs (AFM), X-ray photoelectron spectroscopy (XPS), X-ray diffraction (XRD), optical and electrochemical techniques. The simultaneous and selective detection and determination of chemically and biologically important molecules are achieved at the metal nanoparticles based electrochemical sensors. Such simple sensor devices designed from Nf/Pt_{nano} and SG-Au_{nano} are expected to play an important role in clinical diagnostics and environmental monitoring and in ensuring our food safety. Such protocols may be used to design simple sensor devices for routine diagnostic applications, which is only a matter of time.

1. INTRODUCTION

The combination of nanotechnology and information processing helps to create new devices that promise to open the door to solving numerous analytical problems in areas such as healthcare, food and drink, industries, environmental monitoring, defense and security [1]. The chemistry of metal nanoparticles leads to interesting applications in the fields of catalysis, sensing, electronics and optics [2]. The physical (electromagnetic, mechanical, thermal and optical) and chemical (chemiluminescence, surface funtionalization, etc.) properties of metal nanoparticles can be tailored by altering the particle size, morphology and composition. These properties have been purposefully engineered to enhance and tailor the performance of sensors developed with the help of new nanomaterials. Such features make nanomaterials very attractive for unique sensing applications [3]. Metal nanoparticles embedded in matrices network are attracting much attention in recent times and they pave the way for construction of new generation direct electrocatalytic systems and sensor devices, since the network matrices exhibit tunable porosity, high thermal stability and chemical inertness [4].

The direct electrocatalytic and electrochemical sensing devices were fabricated by using metal nanoparticles embedded in matrix system. They could be utilized in the fabrication of transducer structures. Some of the micro-/nano-fabrication technologies are very mature and used widely [5]. The main focus on the electrochemical sensing platforms which are fabricated and integrated with nanostructured materials is that it will enhance their performance and consequently lead to increased sensitivity towards measurands. The two main effects, (i) Volta effect (voltammetry) and (ii) Galvanic effect (amperometry), are utilized in electrochemical sensors. The performance of both types of sensors can be enhanced by utilizing the nanomaterials [6,7]. Thin films consisting of nanomaterials can increase the surface area to volume ratio at the sensitive regions of the electrode and enhance the performance of sensors (electrochemical and optical). The fabrication of direct electrocatalytic and electrochemical sensor devices using metal nanoparticles (Pt_{nano} and Au_{nano}) embedded in matrices such as Nafion (Nf) and functionalized silicate sol-gel (SG) network (Nf/Pt_{nano} and SG-Au_{nano}) for detection and determination of chemically and biologically important molecules has recently been introduced from our laboratory. Such sensing systems (Nf/Pt_{nano} and SG-Au_{nano}) also exhibited selective and simultaneous detection and determination molecules. This chapter mostly summarizes the work carried out in our laboratory on these systems.

1.1. Synthetic Strategies

Extensive research works have been published in nanoscience and nanotechnology on gaining the control of metal nanoparticles size, shape and composition under mild conditions. Generally, the synthesis of nanoscale particles grouped into two broad categories: "bottom-up" (starting with a molecular system and expanding its size) and "top-down" (starting from a solid and confining it to a limited size). The interatomic interaction causes the performance of a solid, or a cluster of atoms and the adjustment of the relative number of under-coordinated surface atoms provides an additional freedom that allows one to tune the properties of a nanosolid with respect to that of its bulk counterpart. Particularly, the "bottom-up" route is very interesting due to the possibilities of controlling the size, shape, stoichiometry and surface area and that can easily be utilized for sensor applications [8].

1.2. General Methods for Synthesis of Metal Nanoparticles

Nano-dimensional metal particles are synthesized from their corresponding metal salts. For sensor applications, the sensing system may be suspended in liquid or gas phase (e.g. colloidal suspensions) or ordered arrays formed on the surface of the transducer/substrate. The organization of metal nanoparticles on substrates plays a major role in the development of sensor devices [9]. Numerous methods are available for synthesizing metal nanoparticles with different structures such as nanospheres [10], nanowires [11], nonorods [12], nanodisks [13], nanorings [14], nanocube [15] and branched nanocrystals [16] using the solution-phase bottom-up approach. Depending on the nanoparticle type, its functional medium and the surface to which it is attached, the method of synthesis has to be designed. Enormous amount of research work has been carried out to synthesize a variety of metal nanoparticles, especially noble metals such as gold, silver and platinum, for novel applications in a wide variety of applications, such as in medicine, electronics, optics, sensors, etc. [17]. In sensor type applications, metal nanoparticles could be used as catalyst, biomaterial tags, optical resonators and in the fabrication of many other functional devices [18]. The inert nature of noble metals is generally attractive in biosensing and biotechnology. Metal nanoparticles are very stable, and their size can easily be controlled by choosing the synthetic methods. Especially, colloidal gold nanoparticles are most stable among other stable metal nanoparticles and they show many fascinating properties and applications [19]. The most conventional method for the synthesis of colloidal nanoparticles using Au(III) salt is schematically shown in Figure 1. To prepare gold nanoparticles, Turkevitch *et al.* [20] in 1951 used citrate as reducing agent for $HAuCl_4$ in an aqueous environment. Later, Frens *et al.* [21] showed the preparation of predetermined dimensions of gold nanoparticles by controlling the ratio of the reducing and stabilizing agents (citrate to gold ratio). These methods still remains very popular and useful from the application point of view. Template methods also play a major role for the synthesis of a variety of nanostructures and researchers have reported the use of dendrimers as templates for the synthesis of gold [22], platinum [23] and other metals [24]. Metal nanoparticles were prepared within supramolecular organic assembly using the corresponding metal ions followed by chemical reduction of metal ions to yield the corresponding metal nanoparticles. The dendrimers played a major role during the synthesis of nanoparticles as both template and stabilizer.

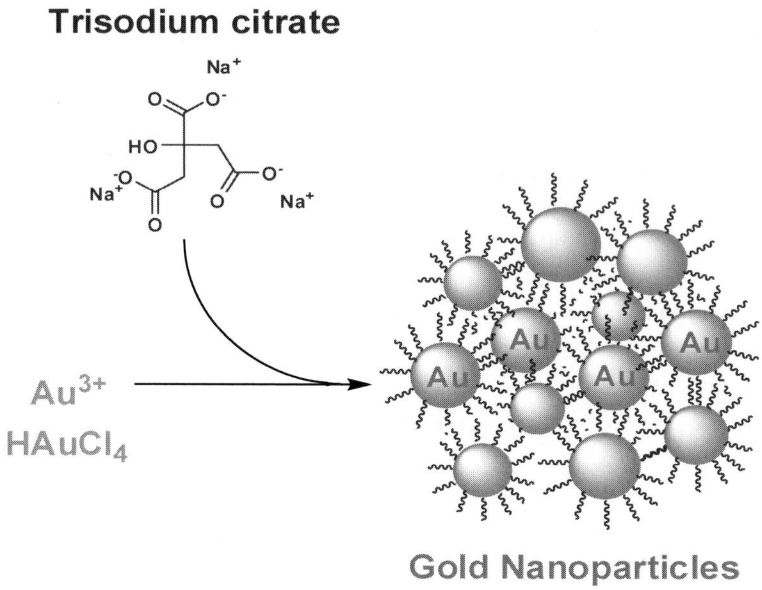

Figure 1. Schematic representation of synthesis of colloidal gold nanoparticles.

The formation of a thin film of metallic nanoparticles on electrode surface is very important in designing sensor devices. The uniform growth of thin film of nanoparticles may be achieved by the adsorption attachment of nanoparticles on the surface and the desorption of by-products. In layer-by-layer deposition of metal nanoparticles, the thickness of the monolayer depends on the molecular length, orientation, rigidity and the type of packing. The electroless deposition (ED) method produced a thin film of nanoparticles without the use of a connection to an external electrical power source [25]. A Langmuir-Blodgett (LB) film is deposited from the surface of a liquid onto a solid, at the air-water interface or by immersing the solid substrate into (or from) the liquid. With each immersion or emersion step a monolayer is added to the surface, and thus the film with very accurate thickness can be formed. Electroplating and electrodeposition methods are typically limited to electrically conductive materials. The electrodeposition process is well suited for making thin films of metals such as gold [26], platinum, etc. [27]. The thickness of the metal film in the range from a few nm to well in excess of 100 μm can easily be formed. The electrodeposition of nanomaterials can be formed without the assistance of template. Electrodeposition is quite a versatile and inexpensive technique to fabricate nanoscaled arrays with systematically reproducible properties [28a,b]. The deposition of nanomaterials on substrates by spin coating, drop casting, dip coating and spray coating are also reported [28c]. In these methods, the solvent is allowed to evaporate leaving behind a thin film of nanomaterials on the substrate (Figure 2). The nanomaterials so formed on the substrate are used for chemical and biosensing applications [29]. Metal nanoparticles have been successfully applied to modify the substrate surface with the help of a self-assembled monolayer formation of alkanethiol molecules and silane-functionalized molecules using -S-Au, -S-Ag and -S-Pt or -NH_2-Ag bond. The metal nanoparticles modified substrates enhance the performance of an electrochemical sensor [30].

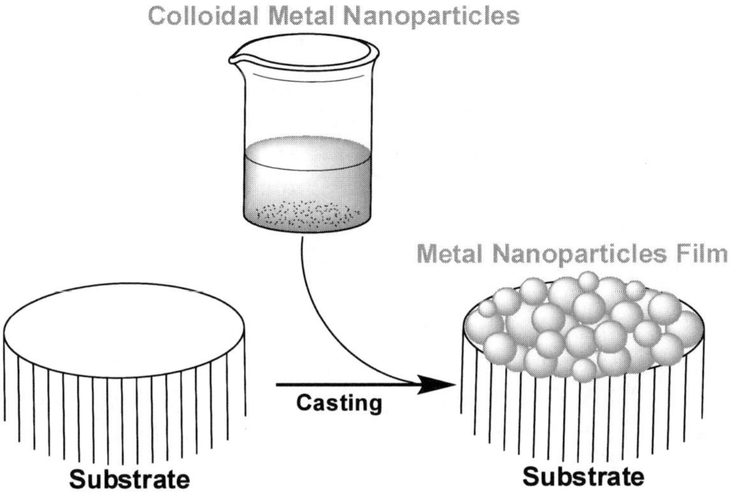

Figure 2. Schematic representation of metal nanoparticles film fabrication by casting and solvent evaporation technique.

2. Electrochemical Preparation of Platinum Nanoparticles

Nanostructured materials in electrochemistry are unique and the main focus in electrochemical sensing ranges from the electrochemical fabrication of nanostructures to the behavior of the nanostructured electrodes to the applications of nanostructured electrodes in chemical analysis [31]. The electrochemical deposition of metal nanoparticles on the surface of a conductive substrate is a very convenient approach [1a,32]. The electrodeposition of metal nanoparticles involves the reduction of the appropriate metal salt (Au(III), Ag(I), Pt(II) or Pt(IV) precursor) in the presence and absence of stabilizers such as polymers, surfactants or special ligands [33a]. Researchers are interested in platinum nanoparticles because platinum nanoparticles have been utilized in various applications due to their extraordinary physical and chemical properties [33]. Efforts were made to synthesize various shapes of platinum nanoparticles in order to investigate their influence on the catalytic activity [34]. Recently, several reports have appeared on the fabrication of platinum nanoparticles by electrodeposition onto substrates and their applications in electrochemical sensing [35]. Our group has designed an electrochemical sensor with high efficiency and good stability using electrodeposited nanostructured platinum particles on polymer coated electrode surface [36].

2.1. Platinum Nanoparticles in Nafion Matrix

The greatest interest in Nafion (Nf), a perfluorinated polymer with sulfonate groups, derives from its consideration as a proton conducting membrane in fuel cells to many sensor applications [37]. The use of Nf and other polyanions to control ion-transport during electrode reaction is a recurring theme [38]. The electrodeposition of platinum nanoparticles at the Nafion (Nf) modified glassy carbon (GC) electrode (GC/Nf/Pt_{nano}) by the two-step method was reported [36]. The GC electrode was polished using an aqueous suspension of alumina and then rinsed with doubly distilled water and sonicated in a water bath for 3 min. The cleaned electrode was pretreated [39] by cycling the potential between -0.2 and 1.2 V at a scan rate of 100 mV s^{-1} in 0.1 M phosphate buffer solution (pH 7.4) until a stable voltammogram was obtained and the potential was stepped to 1.2 V for 2 min. The first step for the fabrication of a sensor was the Nf film formation on the GC electrode. A known amount of Nf solution was casted on the GC electrode surface (0.07 cm^2 area) and the solvent was allowed to evaporate at room temperature [40]. The so formed Nf film thickness was calculated as 0.9 μm [41]. The Nf film deposited GC electrode was dipped into doubly distilled water for 30 min. The second step for the fabrication of the sensor was the electrodeposition of nanostructured platinum particles at the Nf film (GC/Nf/Pt_{nano}) [36,42] as shown in Figure 3. The electrochemically deposited nanostructured platinum particles on the GC/Nf electrode were accomplished with 25 cycles of scanning between 1.0 and -0.2 V(SCE) at a scan rate of 10 mV s^{-1} by dipping the GC/Nf electrode in a fresh solution containing 10 mM H_2PtCl_6 in 0.1 M H_2SO_4. The electrochemically deposited nanostructured platinum particles modified electrode (GC/Nf/Pt_{nano}) was washed with doubly distilled water.

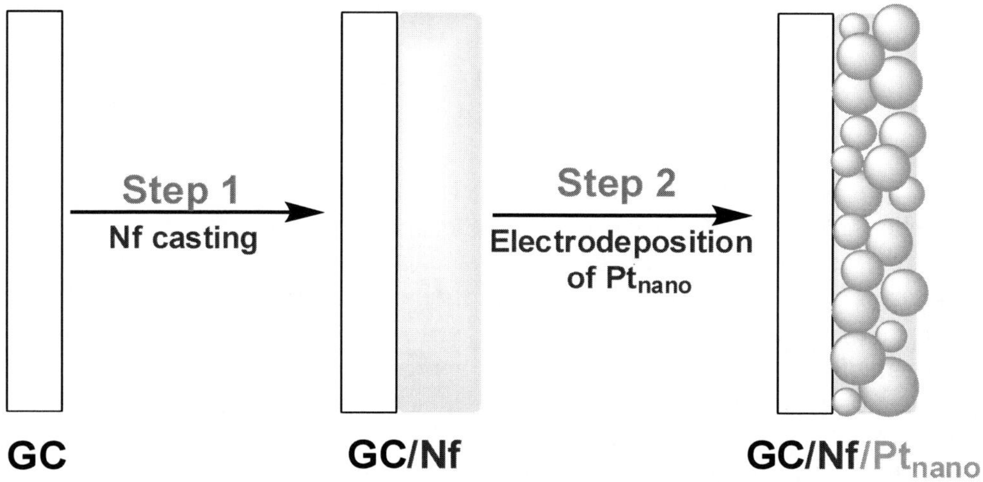

Figure 3. Schematic representation of step wise fabrication of nanostructured Pt particles modified electrode (GC/Nf/Pt_{nano}).

The continuous cyclic voltammograms recorded during the electrodeposition of platinum nanoparticles on the GC/Nf electrode by dipping it in a mixture of 10 mM H_2PtCl_6 and 0.1 M H_2SO_4 at a scan rate of 10 mV s^{-1} are shown in Figure 4. The main characteristic peaks due to Pt formation appeared in the negative potential range (0 to -0.2 V) and in the positive potential region (0.4 to 1.0 V). These peaks correspond to the electrochemical characteristics of the Pt electrode showing the typical regions of the adsorption of hydrogen and oxygen [43] on Pt_{nano} at GC/Nf/Pt_{nano} electrode. The reduction of H_2PtCl_6 at the appropriate potential leads to the formation of the Pt_{nano} at the GC/Nf electrode (Eq. (1)) [44].

$$[PtCl_6]^{2-} + 6\ H_30^{+} + 4\ e^{-} \longrightarrow Pt^{0} + 6\ HCl + 6\ H_2O \qquad (1)$$

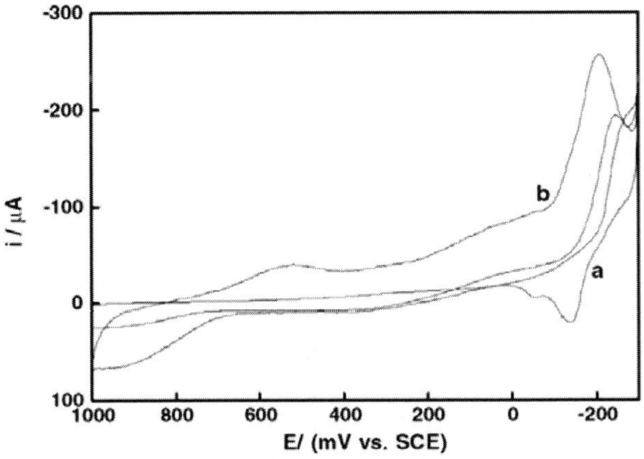

Figure 4. Continuous cyclic voltammograms recorded during electrodeposition of platinum nanoparticles on GC/Nf electrode in 0.1 M H_2SO_4 and 0.01 M H_2PtCl_6. Scan rate = 10 mV s^{-1}. (a) 1st cycle and (b) 25th cycle. (Reprinted from Ref. 36 with permission from Elsevier)

2.2. Characterization of Platinum Nanoparticles in Nafion Matrix

AFM Measurements

The surface morphology and homogeneity of Pt_{nano} at the Nf modified electrode was studied by recording the AFM and the 3D image is shown in Figure 5. The AFM image provides detailed information about the formation of Pt_{nano} on the Nf film and the surface morphology and homogeneity of the same (Figure 5). The Pt_{nano} deposited electrode shows a smooth surface with a wide range of grain size [36]. The Pt_{nano} are densely packed in the film and each particle is in contact with adjacent ones (Figure 5). The AFM image in Figure 5 shows a three dimensional network and it also shows the uniform dispersion of Pt_{nano} on the Nf coated electrode.

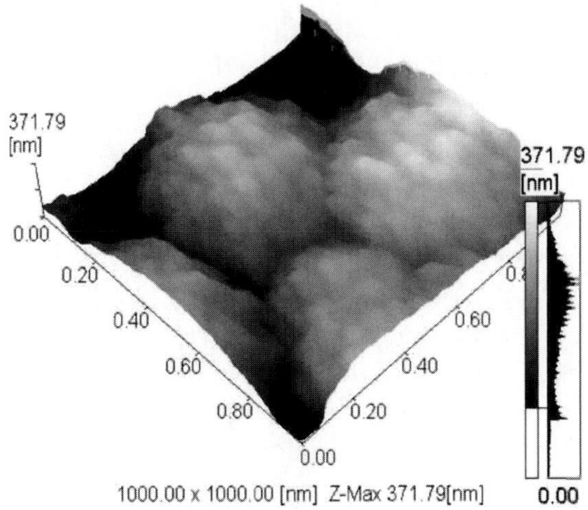

Figure 5. Tapping-mode 3D image of ITO/Nf/Pt_{nano} electrode surface. (Reprinted from Ref. 36 with permission from Elsevier)

XPS Measurements

The valance of the platinum formed at the Nf coated electrode was investigated by XPS. Figure 6 shows the XPS observed for the Pt_{nano} in the Nf film. The observed emission of 4f photoelectrons from Pt is identified in two peaks of the XPS spectra; one is assigned to Pt(0) (71.2 eV) and the other one to Pt(IV) (74.8 eV). The XPS measurement confirms the complete reduction of $PtCl_2^{6-}$ and the formation of Pt(0) on Nf film. The observed Pt(4f) BEs indicate the presence of Pt(0) and Pt(IV) species (74.7 and 74.3 eV, respectively) [44].

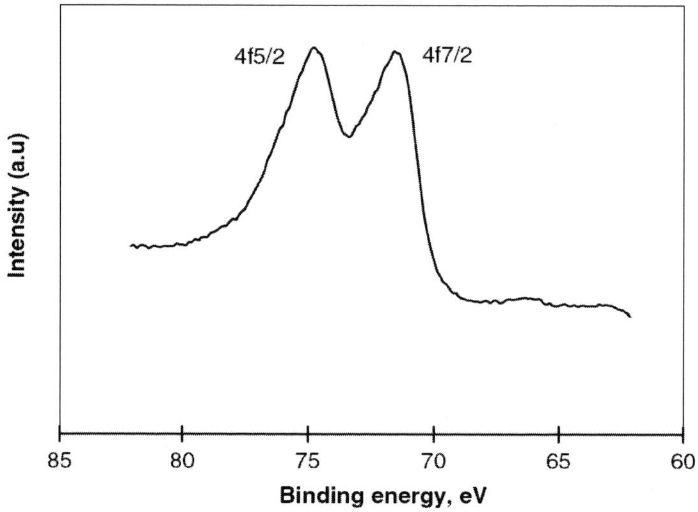

Figure 6. High-resolution XPS of Pt(4f7/2-5/2) core-level spectra of electrodeposited metallic Pt on Nf coated electrode. (Reprinted from Ref. 36 with permission from Elsevier)

XRD Measurements

The crystallographic nature of platinum nanoparticles at the Nf coated electrode was determined by XRD measurements. The presence of metallic Pt was clearly revealed by the characteristic diffraction peaks of Pt. The main diffraction peak of Pt (111) ($2\theta = 39.8°$, JCPDS 04-802) and other diffraction peaks of Pt ((200) and (220) planes) at 2θ values of 46.2° and 67.4° were clearly revealed by the characteristic diffraction peaks of the metallic Pt.

Electrochemical Measurements

The electrochemical behavior of $GC/Nf/Pt_{nano}$ electrode was studied by cyclic voltammetry. Figure 7 shows the cyclic voltammograms recorded for $GC/Nf/Pt_{nano}$ electrode in 0.1 M H_2SO_4 and it shows two peaks observed between 0 and -0.1 V (Figure 7(A)) and platinum oxide peak at 0.4 V (Figure 7(B)). It is well known that the hydrogen adsorption/desorption process and PtO reduction are very sensitive to the Pt electrode [43]. The nanostructured platinum particles modified electrode clearly exhibited the characteristics of reversible hydrogen adsorption/desorption process (Figure 7(A)) and the PtO reduction peak (Figure 7(B)). This means that the electrochemical characteristics of Pt_{nano} modified electrode are very similar to the bulk Pt electrode. It is possible to quantitatively characterize the Pt_{nano} electrode using voltammetric data.

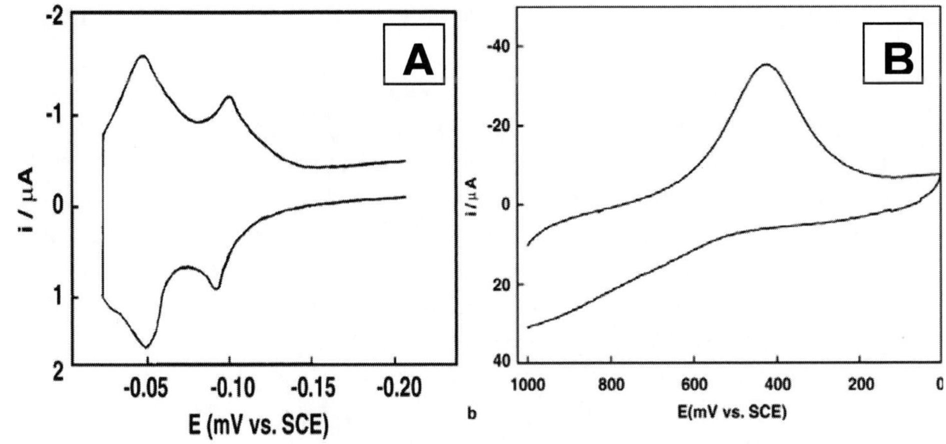

Figure 7. (A). Cyclic voltammetric profile of the hydrogen adsorption/desorption and (B). the reduction peak of platinum oxide observed at GC/Nf/Pt_{nano} electrode in 0.1 M H_2SO_4. Scan rate = 10 mV s^{-1}. (Reprinted from Ref. 36 with permission from Elsevier)

The influence of pH on the electrochemical characteristics of Pt_{nano} was studied at different pHs 1-7. The PtO reduction peak potential observed for the electrochemically deposited Pt_{nano} was found to be dependent on the solution pH. Differential pulse voltammograms (DPV) recorded for GC/Nf/Pt_{nano} electrode at different pHs are shown in Figure 8. The irreversible reduction peak potential shifts to more negative potentials when the pH is lowered. The peak potential fits well to a straight line in the pH range 1-7 as shown in Figure 8(inset) and the slope of the straight line was found to be 59 mV/pH. According to the Nernst equation, this system indicates that the electrode potential varies with the pH and the variance of the formal potential with respect to pH has been attributed to proton-coupled reaction (Eq. (2)).

$$PtO + 2\,e^- + 2H^+ \longrightarrow Pt + H_2O \tag{2}$$

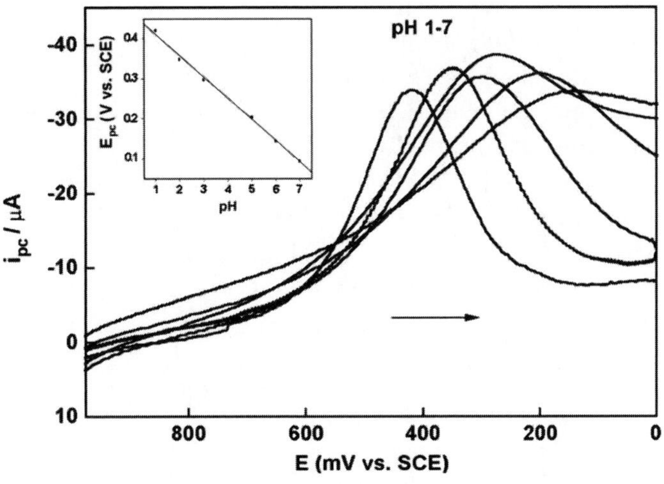

Figure 8. Cathodic DPV recorded at different pHs for GC/Nf/Pt_{nano} electrode. Inset: Plot of cathodic peak potential (E_{pc}) against pH for GC/Nf/Pt_{nano} electrode. (Reprinted from Ref. 36 with permission from Elsevier)

3. Gold Nanoparticles in Silicate Sol-Gel Matrix

The combination of inorganic and organic moieties in a single-phase material provides unique possibilities to tailor the mechanical, electrical and optical properties with respect to numerous applications [46]. The silicate sol-gel based hybrid materials combine the most important properties of their constituents, like high transparency (glasslike), low processing temperatures (polymer-like), sufficient thermal stability (silicone-like) and are easily accessible because of an unique availability of the respective precursors [47]. The number of possible compositions, synthetic routes and potential applications are most attractive features in this research field. This technique offers versatile methods to synthesize new and advanced multi-functional materials and tailor their properties and their industrial applications [48]. The sol-gel process allows mild chemical conditions and provides a versatile access to electrochemical devices in electroanalysis associated with electrocatalysis, voltammetry and amperometry detection, permselective coatings and electrochemical sensors [49]. The dispersion of nanomaterials in silicate sol-gel matrix showed various morphologies (xerogels, aerogels, thin and thick films, uniform particles and monoliths), properties (chemical, mechanical, optical, and electrical) and applications in various fields, including electrocatalysis, electroanalysis, polymer science, protective coatings, surface analysis, electrosynthesis, molecular electronics and some others [50]. Particularly, the encapsulation of gold nanoparticles in functionalized silicate sol-gel matrix help to avoid aggregation and improve stabilization of metal nanoparticles in silicate based sol-gel matrix and provides a way to derive benefits of homogeneously dispersed metal nanoparticles for optical, catalytic and electrochemical sensor applications with the convenience of solid handling [51]. Recently, we have designed electrochemical sensors based on gold nanoparticles embedded in three-dimensional silicate sol-gel matrix [52]. The so-designed sensors showed long term stability and high sensitivity performance [52]. As a first step for designing a sensor, gold nanoparticles were prepared using reported procedure [21,22,53]. The 20 nm size spherical gold nanoparticles were often prepared by using citrate as reducing agent and as stabilizing agent. The 20 nm size gold nanoparticles solution so-prepared was characterized by its characteristics surface plasmon band (SPB) at 520 nm. The homogeneous methyltrimethoxysilane (MTMOS) silicate sol-gel matrix was prepared by adopting reported procedure [54] and the dispersion of gold nanoparticles in the silicate sol-gel matrix was prepared (Figure 9). Known amounts of MTMOS silicate sol-gel matrix (MTMOS(SG) and gold nanoparticles solutions were mixed (MTMOS(SG):Au_{nano} (Si:Au = 55:1 molar ratio)) under vigorous stirring for 5 min. The color of the solution mixture (dispersion of gold nanoparticles in silicate sol-gel matrix) turned wine red to purple in color. As a result of the dispersion of gold nanoparticles in the silicate sol-gel matrix (represented as MTMOS(SG)-Au_{nano}), the absorption spectrum of the MTMOS(SG)-Au_{nano} solution showed the surface plasmon band at 524 nm. As a general procedure, the gold nanoparticles embedded in silicate sol-gel matrices were prepared by an easy approach. The reduction of Au(III) to Au(0) and the formation of MTMOS or APS (3-(aminoproppyl) triethoxysilane) silicate sol-gel matrix occurs simultaneously when the corresponding precursors were mixed at appropriate experimental conditions [51]. The gold nanoparticles so prepared are spherical in shape and of 4-6 nm size [51]. We have successfully prepared the gold nanoparticles embedded in functionalized silicate sol-gel matrices and used them to design electrochemical sensor devices.

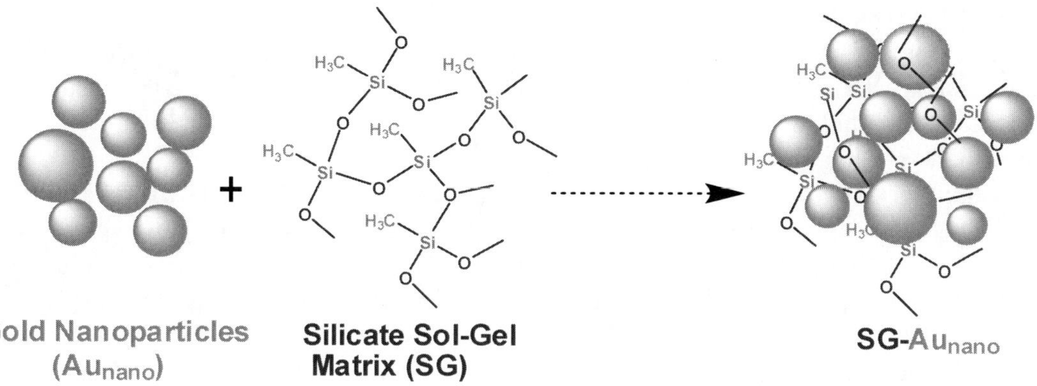

Figure 9. Schematic representation of dispersion of Au_{nano} in MTMOS silicate sol-gel matrix (SG-Au_{nano}).

The fabrication of thin film of SG-Au_{nano} on the electrode surface (represented as GC/MTMOS(SG)-Au_{nano} and GC/APS(SG)-Au_{nano}) was done by casting a known volume of gold nanoparticles embedded silicate sol-gel matrix onto the cleaned and pretreated GC electrode. The solvent was allowed to evaporate in air at room temperature for 2 hours. The SG-Au_{nano} film coated electrode was dipped in water for 1 hour. The sol-gel film thickness was calculated as 3 μm using the reported procedure [54,52a]. The modified electrode so designed was used to construct sensors for the direct electrochemical reduction/oxidation and the detection of molecules without immobilizing any other mediator/enzymes (Figure 10).

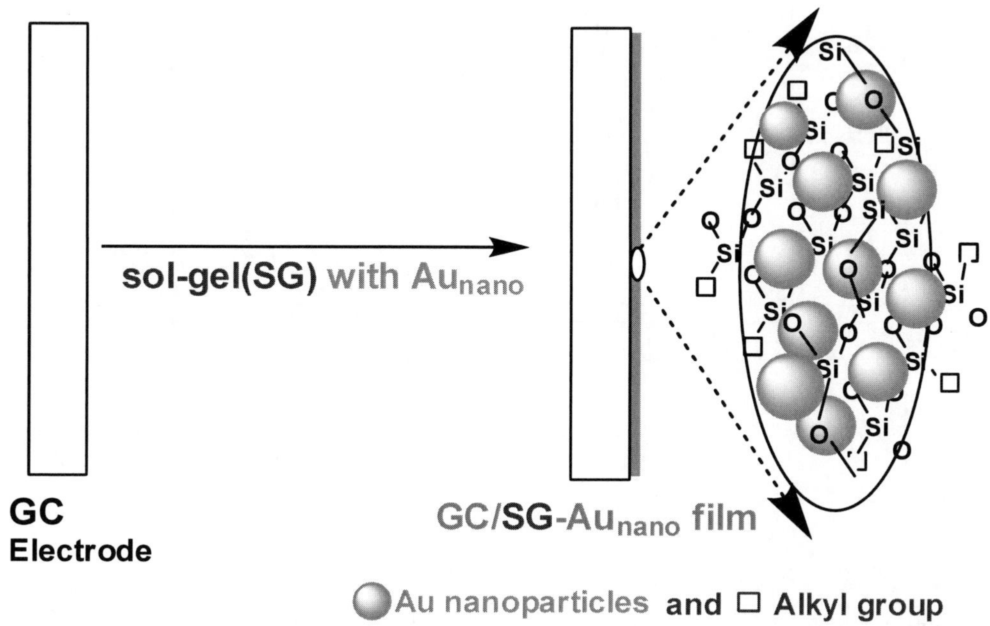

Figure 10. Schematic representation of Au_{nano} dispersed in silicate matrix (MTMOS(SG)-Au_{nano}).

3.1. Characterization of Gold Nanoparticles Embedded Silicate Sol-Gel Matrix

Optical Measurements

The spectral characterization of gold nanoparticles was carried by recording the absorption spectra of the gold nanoparticles. The collective excitation of the free electrons of the gold nanoparticles (Au_{nano}) shows the SPR band at 520 nm as shown in Figure 11(a). The absorption spectrum for gold nanoparticles dispersed in MTMOS silicate matrix (MTMOS(SG)-Au_{nano}) solution showed the SPR band at 524 nm (Figure 11(b)). The observed red shift (4 nm) was due to the interaction of gold nanoparticles with the silicate sol-gel matrix [51]. For the gold nanoparticles embedded in amine functionalized (APS) silicate sol-gel (APS(SG)-Au_{nano}) solution, the surface plasmon band was observed at 516 nm [51]. The gold nanoparticles embedded MTMOS silicate sol-gel matrix (MTMOS(SG)-Au_{nano}) was coated onto a clean glass plate and the absorption spectrum recorded on glass plates showed the SPR band at 520 nm (Figure 11(inset)). The SPR band was observed at 520 nm for the MTMOS(SG)-Au_{nano} film. In the case of the APS(SG)-Au_{nano} film the SPR band was observed at 524 nm for gold nanoparticles embedded in APS silicate. The observation of SPR band for the gold nanoparticles in silicate sol-gel matrices clearly shows that the gold nanoparticles are more stable and the particle size was not changed in the film state. The observed small red shift in the surface plasmon resonance band was due to the formation of the thin film of polymer on the gold nanoparticles [51].

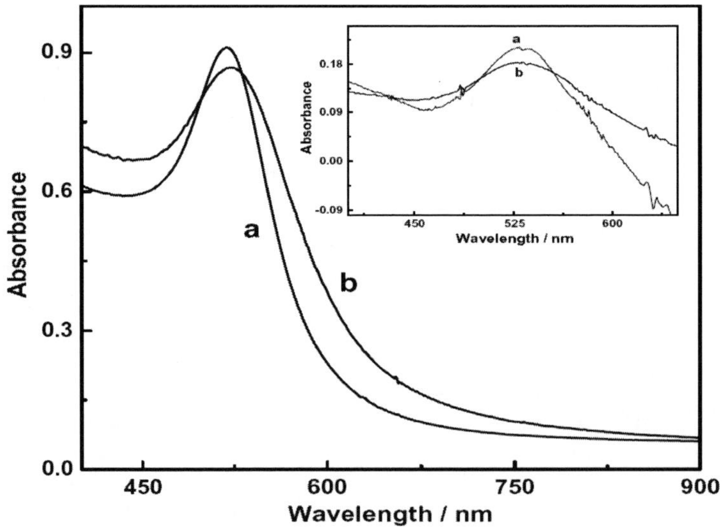

Figure 11. Absorption spectra of Au_{nano} (a) and SG-Au_{nano} (b). Inset: Absorption spectra of Au_{nano} (a) and MTMOS(SG)-Au_{nano} (b) coated on glass plates. (Reprinted from Ref. 52a with permission from Elsevier)

SEM Measurements

The SEM provides the surface morphology of gold nanoparticles embedded in silicate sol-gel matrix. Figure 12 displays the SEM images of the APS sol-gel film (APS(SG)) and the gold nanoparticles embedded in the APS sol-gel network (APS(SG)-Au_{nano}). Figure 12(A) shows a clear SEM image of the plain APS sol-gel matrix film and Figure 12(B) shows the uniform distribution of gold nanoparticles in the APS silicate matrix. A blurred image of the gold nanoparticles was also visible due to the buried nanoparticles inside the APS sol-gel film. In the case of the MTMOS sol-gel film (MTMOS(SG)), some agglomerates heterogeneity was observed due to the heterogeneous nature of the MTMOS film in the absence of gold nanoparticles. When the gold nanoparticles were embedded into the MTMOS silicate matrix, the particles interacted strongly at the edge of the agglomerated heterogeneous spots and the uniform distribution of the gold nanoparticles was observed [52a].

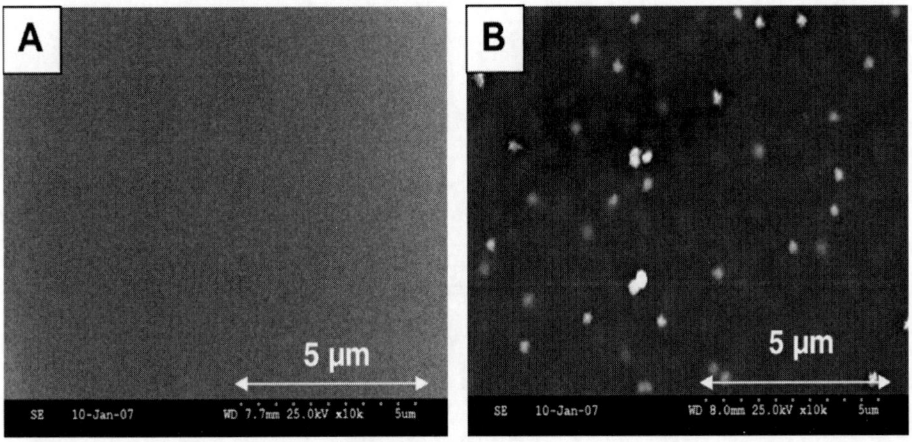

Figure 12. SEM images observed for APS(SG) sol-gel film (A) and gold nanoparticles embedded in APS sol–gel matrix (APS(SG)-Au_{nano}) (B). (Reprinted from Ref. 52b with permission from Elsevier)

Electrochemical Measurements

The electrochemical characteristics of the gold nanoparticles embedded in silicate matrix (GC/MTMOS(SG)-Au_{nano}) was studied by cyclic voltammetry. Figure 13 shows the cyclic voltammograms obtained for the sol-gel coated GC electrode in the presence and absence of Au_{nano}. In the absence of the gold nanoparticle the characteristic electrochemical response due to Au was not observed (Figure 13(a-b) at the plain GC and GC/SG electrodes. The gold nanoparticles dispersed sol-gel film modified electrode showed an anodic peak at 1.0 V and a cathodic peak around 0.43 V as shown in Figure 13(c) [55,52a]. The gold nanoparticles embedded amine functionalized silicate sol-gel matrix (APS(SG)-Au_{nano}) showed an anodic peak at 0.9 V and a cathodic peak at 0.5 V showing the presence of Au_{nano} at the APS sol-gel film at the modified electrode (GC/APS(SG)-Au_{nano}) [52b]. This electrochemical response corresponds to the formation of gold oxide and its reduction at the MTMOS(SG)-Au_{nano} and APS(SG)-Au_{nano} electrodes [52]. This electrochemical behavior confirms that the gold nanoparticles are dispersed in the silicate sol-gel matrix and the gold nanoparticles are in electrical contact with each other in the silicate sol-gel film.

The kinetic barrier of the interface for electron-transfer between the species in solution and electrode was tested using the electroactive species such as the $[Fe(CN)_6]^{3-/4-}$ couple [56]. As expected, the $[Fe(CN)_6]^{3-/4-}$ couple exhibits reversible behavior at the plain GC electrode. A quasi-reversible voltammetric response with very low peak currents and large peak-to-peak separation was observed when the plain GC electrode was modified with silicate sol-gel (MTMOS(SG)) [52a]. The introduction of gold nanoparticles in the MTMOS silicate sol-gel lead brought about reversible voltammetric response with a decreased peak-to-peak separation (ΔE_p) and a small increase in the peak currents when compared to bare GC electrode [52a]. This observation clearly reveals that the gold nanoparticles embedded silicate sol-gel matrix (MTMOS(SG)-Au_{nano} and the acts as a new electrode surface with increased electrode area. The designed network achieves good electrical communication with the underlying electrode surface [57].

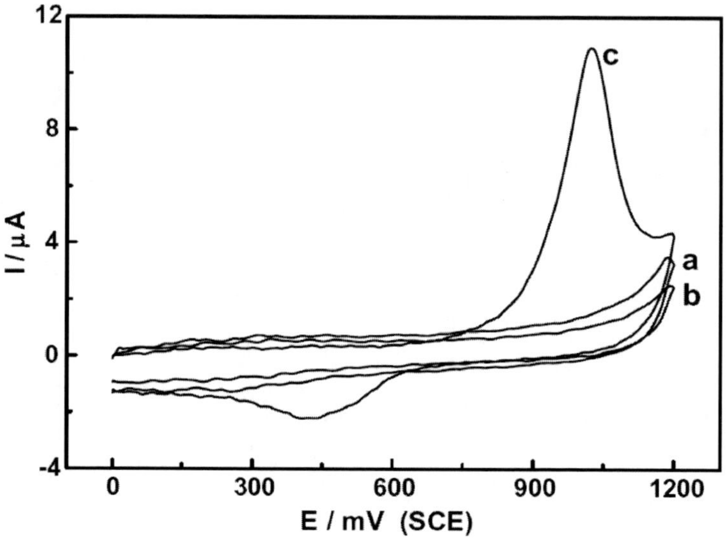

Figure 13. Cyclic voltammograms of bare GC (a), GC/MTMOS(SG) (b) and GC/MTMOS(SG)-Au_{nano} (c) electrodes in 0.5M of H_2SO_4, Scan rate = 50 mV s^{-1}. (Reprinted from Ref. 52a with permission from Elsevier)

4. Applications of Metal Nanoparticles in Sensors

Sensor is a device that responds to some stimulus by generating a functionally related output. The word "sensor" in Latin means "sentire" (perceive) [58]. In recent times, sensor technology has been flourishing as the need for physical, chemical and biological recognition systems is growing [59]. A modern chemical sensor consists of a "transducer" and a chemically selective material. Different strategies can be employed to extract maximum information about the sample. The label "chemical sensor" is used to describe an analytical procedure that should be more appropriately called an "analytical assay" or "sensing system" [60]. The development of new sensing materials is essential for the advancement of modern chemical sensors [60]. Nanomaterials based development of small, inexpensive and efficient sensors has broad applications with greater sensitivity and selectivity, lower production costs, reduced power consumption as well as improved stability. The unique properties of nanoscale materials make them ideal for sensor applications and could be used to form new generation sensing devices [61]. The electroanalytical detection limit at a micro-/nano-electrode ensemble can be much lower than that of an analogous macro-sized electrode because the ratio of faradaic to capacitive current is very high [62]. The development of electrochemical sensors based on micro-/nano-electrode ensembles have been widely used due to the advantages over conventional macro-electrodes such as increased mass transport, decreased influence of solution resistance, low detection limits, and better signal-to-noise ratios [63]. The metal nanoparticles such as Pt, Au, Cu, etc., find novel applications in electrocatalysis, electrochemical sensors and analytical chemistry [64,65]. In our laboratory, research work on a metal nanoparticles embedded silicate matrix system was carried out to explore the applications in the field of electrochemical sensors.

4.1. Detection of Biomolecules at Nanostructured Platinum Particles Modified Electrode

The biologically active small molecules (DA and its metabolites, AA, UA, etc.) are attributed importance in neuroscience, owing to the diversity of model systems for many neuronal processes and neurodegenerative diseases [66]. The requirement of detection methods for these important biomolecules attracted much attention in the past decades [67,68]. The catalytic transformation systems involving nanomaterials, which act as sensors, could be simple to design and to operate but they cover a limited number of biomolecules. The interaction between such biomolecules and nanomaterials should induce significant changes in the electrical properties of nanostructured interfaces. A variety of metal nanoparticles, nanotubes, nanowires, etc., prepared from metals, semiconductors, carbon and polymeric species were used to fabricate functional interfaces to enhance the sensitivity and selectivity of the electrochemical sensors towards biomolecules [69]. Platinum nanoparticles were used in the design of nanostructured interfaces for biological sensing applications. Thiagarajan *et al.* fabricated an electrochemical sensor device using the electrochemically deposited platinum and gold nanoparticles on a glassy carbon electrode and used it for the simultaneous determination of DA, AA and UA [70]. Cao *et al.* designed an amperometric glucose sensor based on ultrafine platinum nanoparticles [71]. Many research groups have developed electrochemical detection methods for detection of biomolecules [72]. For the first time, our research group designed [36] a direct electrochemical device based on the electrochemically deposited platinum nanoparticles in Nf membrane for the simultaneous determination of dopamine and serotonin in the presence of interfering molecules such as AA and UA with practical applications to real samples.

4.2. Electrocatalytic Oxidation of Dopamine

Electrocatalysis is a process in which the electrochemical reaction rate is increased by introducing a mediator, known as an electrocatalyst, to the electrode surface [1a]. The metal nanoparticles, the well known electrocatalysts, can be prepared using metals and alloys [74]. The electrode can be modified by attaching the metal nanoparticles on the electrode surface to facilitate the flow of electrons between the electrode surface and the substrates due to its larger active surface area [1b]. Recently, a number of research groups have studied the electrocatalytic oxidation of dopamine at a nanomaterials modified electrode [73]. The intrinsic electrocatalytic activity of platinum nanoparticles depends on the particle size, shape and composition [74]. The role of electrocatalytic activity of platinum nanoparticles has been widely investigated by many groups [75]. Our group has designed nanostructured platinum particles deposited Nf membrane modified electrodes for the direct electrocatalytic oxidation of DA in 0.1 M PBS (pH 7.4) [36]. The electrocatalytic oxidation of DA at the nanostructured platinum particles incorporated Nf membrane (GC/Nf/Pt_{nano}) showed better performance towards DA when compared to GC/Pt_{nano}. The nanostructured platinum particles provide the necessary conduction pathway and facilitate the electron transfer process between DA and electrode interface. Figure 14 shows the DPV response of the electrocatalytic oxidation of DA at different electrodes. The GC/Nf/Pt_{nano} electrode showed the anodic peak potential at 0.13 V due to the oxidation of dopamine. A negative potential shift of 60 mV was observed for the oxidation of DA at the GC/Nf/Pt_{nano} electrode when compared to bare GC electrode and a 11.6 fold enhancement in the anodic peak current was also observed (Figure 14(a) and (c)). The positively charged DA molecule was expected to occupy the ionic cluster region (–SO^{3-} groups) and the interfacial regions of the Nf film due to the electrostatic interaction. Figure 14 displays the efficient electrocatalytic oxidation of DA at the GC/Nf/Pt_{nano} electrode whereas the GC/Pt_{nano} electrode exhibits a lower peak current when compared to the GC/Nf/Pt_{nano} electrode. The oxidation of 100 μM DA at the bulk Pt plate electrode was observed with a very small current (Figure 14(inset)) when compared to GC/Pt_{nano} and GC/Nf/Pt_{nano} electrodes. The direct electrocatalytic oxidation of DA observed at the GC/Nf/Pt_{nano} electrode suggests that the Pt_{nano} promote the electron transfer process at the modified electrode. The anodic peak current was measured as a function of DA concentration ranging from 3×10^{-6} to 60×10^{-6} M DA. The DPV peaks are well defined and the peak current was proportional to the DA concentration. The lowest detection limit was calculated as 10 nM [36]. The designed electrochemical sensor was stable for 2 weeks when stored in PBS at room temperature with a decrease of 5% anodic peak current. The platinum nanoparticles based electrochemical sensing system may find applications in DA release *in vitro* and *in vivo* applications.

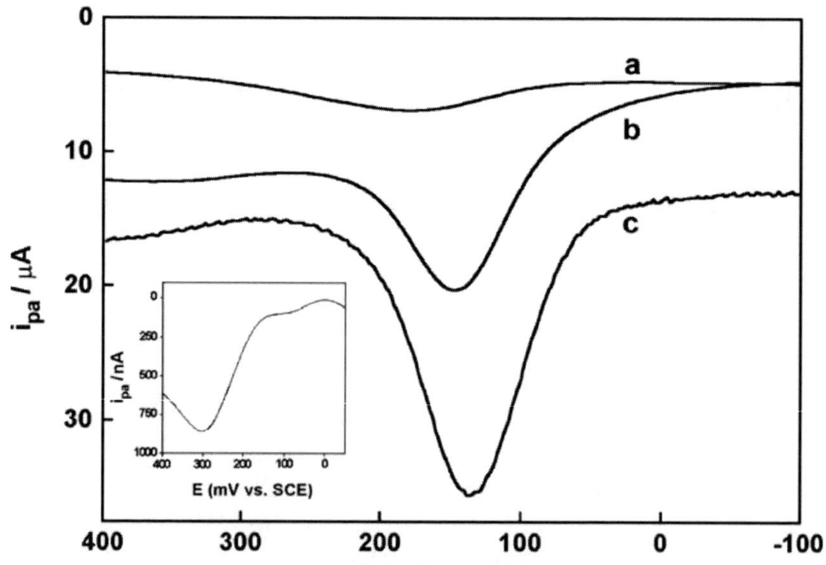

Figure 14. Anodic DPVs recorded for 100 μM DA at (a), plain GC electrode (b), GC/Pt_{nano} electrode and (c). GC/Nf/Pt_{nano} electrode in 0.1 M PBS. Inset: Anodic DPV for 100 μM DA at bulk Pt electrode. (Reprinted from Ref. 36 with permission from Elsevier)

4.2.1. Simultaneous Detection of Dopamine and Serotonin

Simultaneous detection of DA and 5-HT was achieved at the nanostructured platinum particles embedded Nf modified electrode [36]. The development of sensors for the selective detection of biomolecules such as DA, AA, UA, etc. is attracting attention [76]. The designed sensing substrate involves the preconcnetration of electrostatic binding of cationic analytes at the electrodes coated with permselective Nf membrane. It has been demonstrated that the Nf film is a sufficient barrier for several anionic interfering analytes [77]. The modified electrode used for the detection of DA and its metabolites should be free from interferences of other anionic electroactive substances co-existing in biological fluids, such as AA, UA, nitrite, nitrate, etc. Among these compounds, AA and UA are important interfering species owing to their higher concentrations in biological systems. The oxidation potentials of AA and UA are very close to that of DA. Hence it is very important to eliminate the interference of the co-existing substances. Figure 15 shows the schematic representation of the nanostrucured platinum particles embedded Nf modified electrode for the selective detection of DA and its metabolites in the presence of interferences such as AA and UA.

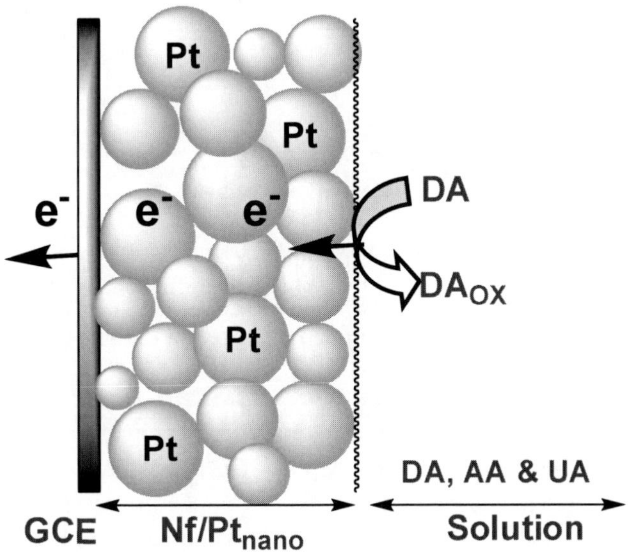

Figure 15. Schematic representation of electrocatalytic oxidation of DA and 5-HT at GC/Nf/Pt_{nano} in the presence of interferences such as AA and UA.

The Nf polymer coated GC electrode (GC/Nf) acts as a very effective barrier for anions such as AA and UA. A better peak separation for DA and 5-HT in a mixture was observed (Figure 16(a)) in the presence of higher concentrations of interferences such as AA and UA where the bare GC electrode was not able to distinguish the four species in a mixture containing 50 μM DA, 500 μM 5-HT, 1 mM AA and 0.1 mM UA and all the four species showed a single peak at the same potential as shown in Figure 16(inset). The two anodic peaks corresponding to the oxidation of DA and 5-HT were observed at the GC/Nf/Pt_{nano} modified electrode (Figure 16(b)). The cyclic voltammetric response observed for the DA and 5-HT at the GC/Nf/Pt_{nano} electrode with physiological concentrations was increased dramatically. A large anodic peak current with a decrease in overpotential (Figure 16(b)) was observed when compared to the GC/Nf electrode (Figure 16(a)). The electrocatalytic oxidation potential of metallic platinum was less positive when compared to substrate oxidation potential indicating a significant interaction (i.e., chemical catalysis) of DA and 5-HT with the platinum nanoparticles. In this regard, the published work shows that, among neurotransmitters, DA and 5-HT are easily accommodated by the distal site of carbon nanotubes, as well as in nano-goldself-assembled layer and ε-mercaptocarboxylic acid monolayer carbon disk electrode [78]. Therefore, a similar type of interaction could be achieved at the $GC/Nf/Pt_{nano}$ electrode.

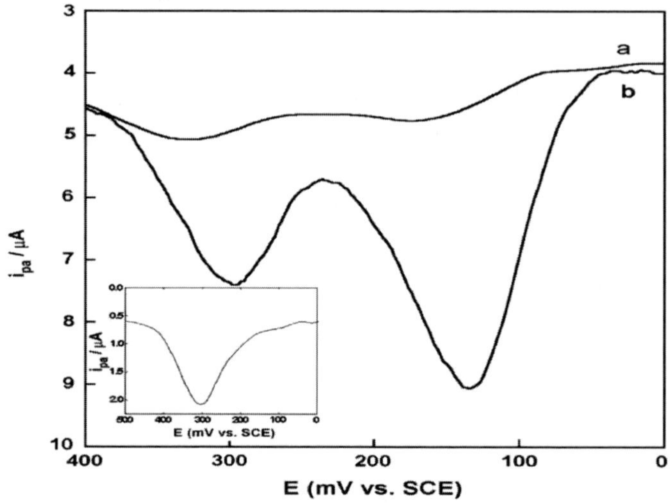

Figure 16. Anodic DPVs recorded for a mixture of 50 μM DA and 500 μM 5-HT in presence of 1.0 mM AA and 0.1 mM UA at GC/Nf (a) and at $GC/Nf/Pt_{nano}$ electrode (b) in 0.1M PBS. Inset: Anodic DPV for a mixture of 50 μM DA and 500 μM 5-HT in presence of 1.0 mM AA and 0.1 mM UA at plain GC electrode. (Reprinted from Ref. 36 with permission from Elsevier)

4.2.2. Detection and Determination of Dopamine in Real Samples

The $GC/Nf/Pt_{nano}$ electrode was utilized in analytical applications using practical samples such as the DA injection solution blood plasma [36]. Both the CV and DPV anodic peak currents were linearly related as a function of the DA concentration in the range from 1.0×10^{-8} to 1.4×10^{-6} M. The lowest detection limit was calculated as 8 nM and it could be estimated at a signal-to-noise ratio of 3. The CV and DPV techniques were used to determine the DA concentration in the DA injection solution at the $GC/Nf/Pt_{nano}$. The determination of the DA in dopamine hydrochloride injection solution was studied by the standard DA addition method using the $GC/Nf/Pt_{nano}$ electrode and the results are listed in Table 1. DA was repeatedly determined with duplicate samples and the relative standard deviation was found to be 4.5%. Interference studies were carried out with species such as AA and UA and no interference was observed when AA and UA (100-200 times higher concentrations than DA) were added to the DA injection solution. The $GC/Nf/Pt_{nano}$ electrode was also used to sense DA in blood plasma sample. The recovery was calculated for blood plasma spiked (50-fold) with varying amounts of DA. A reproducible result was observed with five determinations of each sample. Acceptable recovery and reproducible data were obtained as shown in Table 2. The designed electrochemical sensing device, $GC/Nf/Pt_{nano}$, was found to be very effective for the construction of selective, sensitive and stable sensors. In addition, the estimation of biologically important molecules in real samples was also demonstrated.

Table 1. Estimation of DA in dopamine hydrochloride injection solution using GC/Nf/Pt_{nano} electrode[a].

Sample	Found[b] (mg)	Quoted value	Spike (mg)	Found[b] (mg)	Mean recovery (%) ±
Injection 1	9.5	10	10	9.7	97.0 ± 3.1
Injection 2	10.5	10	10	9.8	99.8 ± 1.8
Injection 3	10	10	10	10.3	103.0 ± 4.0

[a] Potential scan rate: 5 mV s^{-1} in DPV and 50 mV s^{-1} in CV and other conditions as given in Figure 16.
[b] Average values of five determinations.

Table 2. Recovery of DA in diluted (50-fold) blood plasma spiked with different DA concentrations using GC/Nf/Pt_{nano} electrode[a].

Sample	Spiked concentration (nmol DA per 0.2 ml)	Mean recovery (%) ± SD (n = 5)
Plasma	10	102.2 ± 3.
	50	103.5 ± 2.4
	200	97.3 ± 4.8

[a] Potential scan rate: 5 mV s^{-1} in DPV and 50 mV s^{-1} in CV and other conditions as given in Figure 16.

5. Detection and Determination of Hydrogen Peroxide at Gold Nanoparticles Modified Electrode

The requirement of rapid, accurate, reliable and reagentless detection and determination of hydrogen peroxide (H_2O_2) is very important in the fields of food, industry, environmental protection, clinical control and so on [79]. H_2O_2 is not only a by-product of several highly selective oxidases, but also an essential mediator in biology, medicine, industry and many other fields [80]. Among the many techniques developed for this purpose, amperometric biosensors based on direct electron transfer reaction between an electrode and immobilized peroxidase, which catalyzes the reduction of H_2O_2, is especially promising [81]. The determination of H_2O_2 reported utilizing the gold nanoparticles [82]. Recently, a modified electrode was developed using gold nanoparticles embedded in a functionalized silicate sol-gel matrix without immobilizing any other mediator/enzyme for electrochemical sensing of H_2O_2 [52a].

5.1. Electrocatalytic Reduction of Hydrogen Peroxide

The direct electrocatalytic activity of gold nanoparticles embedded in MTMOS silicate sol-gel matrix modified electrode was demonstrated towards H_2O_2 reduction (Figure 17) [52a]. Cyclic voltammograms were recorded in the presence of H_2O_2 at plain GC, GC/MTMOS(SG) and GC/MTMOS(SG)-Au_{nano} electrodes in 0.1 M phosphate buffer (pH 7.0). In the absence of gold nanoparticles at the GC electrode, no obvious cathodic current occurred due to H_2O_2 reduction. The dispersion of gold nanoparticles in MTMOS silicate matrix exhibited good electrocatalytic activity towards the reduction of H_2O_2. Gold nanoparticles mediate the electrochemical reduction of H_2O_2 and a large cathodic current was observed starting around 0 V. This observation clearly shows that the catalytic current was mainly due to the direct electron-transfer between dispersed gold nanoparticles and H_2O_2. A polycrystalline Au electrode was also used for H_2O_2 reduction under similar experimental condition; but noticeable H_2O_2 reduction current was not observed in the potential window. Gold nanoparticles distributed in the MTMOS silicate network (GC/MTMOS(SG)-Au_{nano}) are in electrical contact with each other and an efficient electron-transfer process is occurring at the gold nanoparticles modified electrode without immobilizing any other mediator/enzyme in the MTMOS silicate sol-gel film. Gold nanoparticles provide a large surface area with specific interaction towards substrate [19] resulting in an improved electron-transfer kinetics and enhancement in the reduction of H_2O_2. The direct electrocatalytic activity of dispersed gold nanoparticles in MTMOS silicate matrix at the modified electrode depends on the amount of nanoparticles dispersed in the silicate film. When the amount of dispersed gold nanoparticles was increased in constant amounts of MTMOS silicate sol-gel, the electrocatalytic performance towards H_2O_2 reduction also increased [52a]. The maximum catalytic current was observed for the molar ratio of Si:Au = 55:1 in the silicate film and no further increase in the catalytic current upon increasing the amount of gold nanoparticles was observed. The designed sensor using homogeneously distributed gold nanoparticles in a silicate sol-gel film modified electrode without immobilizing any redox mediator/enzyme was found to be electrocatalytically active for H_2O_2 reduction.

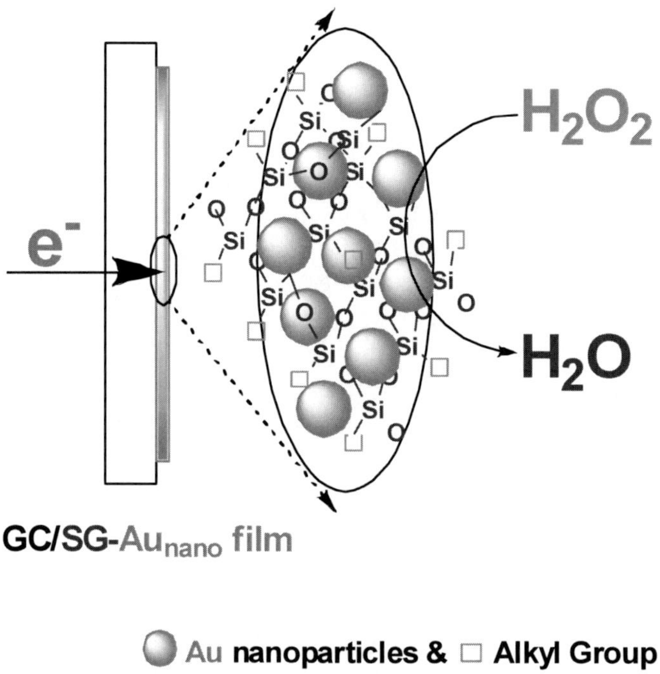

Figure 17. Schematic representation of electrocatalytic reduction of H_2O_2 at gold nanoparticles (Au_{nano}) embedded in MTMOS silicate sol-gel modified electrode.

5.2. Amperometric Detection of Hydrogen Peroxide

The electrochemical sensing device so designed was utilized to detect H_2O_2 by the amperometry technique [52a]. Figure 18 displays the schematic representation of amperometric detection of H_2O_2 at the GC/MTMOS(SG)-Au_{nano} electrode. The foot of the direct electrocatalytic reduction of H_2O_2 was observed around 0 V and the steady-state current was increased when the applied potential was more and more negative (-0.5 to -0.8 V) at the GC/MTMOS(SG)-Au_{nano} electrode. The preferred applied potential for the detection of H_2O_2 was chosen as -0.5 V since the sensor showed higher sensitivity at -0.5 V. The H_2O_2 reduction current was recorded using the GC/MTMOS(SG)-Au_{nano} electrode at an applied potential of -0.5 V with subsequent spiking of 2.5 μM H_2O_2. The calibration curve was plotted based on the steady-state H_2O_2 reduction current-time response curve in the concentration range from 2.5 to 45 μM with a correlation coefficient of 0.998 (n = 17) at a signal to noise ratio of 3. The lowest detection limit at the gold nanoparticles modified electrode was estimated to be 3.15 nM. The amperometric response time was ca. 3 s, which indicates a fast electron-transfer process at this electrode. The electrode was stable for at least one week when stored at room temperature and the reproducibility of the GC/MTMOS(SG)-Au_{nano} was also demonstrated.

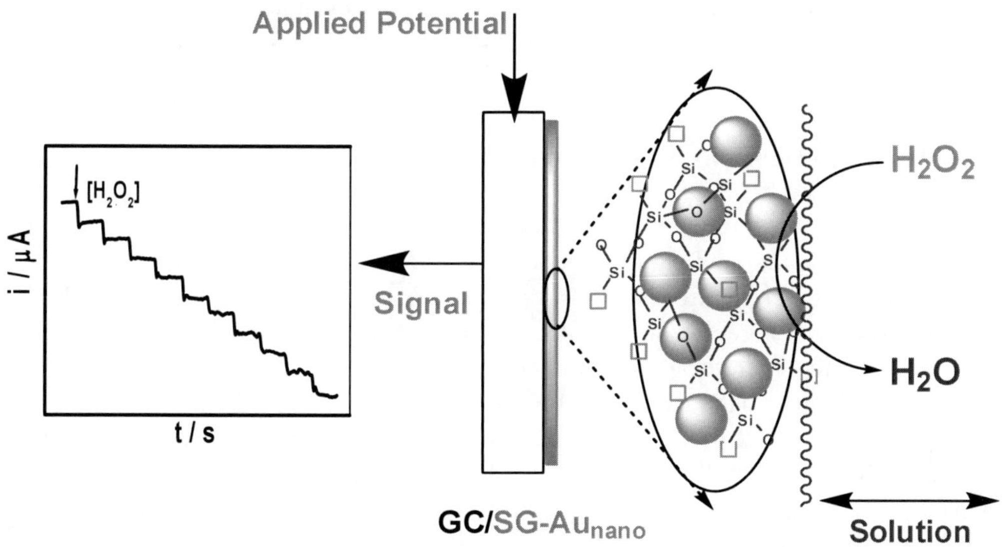

Figure 18. Schematic illustration of gold nanoparticles embedded in MTMOS silicate sol-gel matrix (MTMOS(SG)-Au_{nano}) sensor for amperometric sensing of H_2O_2.

6. Simultaneous Detection of Hydrazine, Sulfite and Nitrite at Gold Nanoparticles Modified Electrode

Hydrazine is a neurotoxin and produces carcinogenic and mutagenic effects and has low threshold limit values of 10 ppb [83]. It is widely used as high-energy propellants in rockets and spacecraft by the military and aerospace industries and fuel for zero-emission fuel cells

[84]. Hydrazine has been implicated in a terrorist incident reported in 2003 [85]. Due to its importance in industry and its toxicity, the developement of sensitive methods for the detection of hydrazine is essential. Other than gold nanoparticles, Pt, Pd and Cu-Pd nanoparticles have been utilized for the electrocatalytic oxidation of hydrazine [86]. The metal nanoparticles show high catalytic activity and oxidation of substrates occurs at more positive potential at these modified electrodes, and the detection limit is well above the threshold level of hydrazine [87]. The sulfite is used as a preservative in view of the fact that it is an antioxidant and an inhibitor of enzymatic or microbial activity in beverage, food and pharmaceutical products [88]. The food and drug administration (FDA) (in 1958) considered sulfites as a recognized safe preservative, but reports from consumers and the medical community show the adverse health reactions [89]. In 1982, the FDA concluded that sulfite additives are safe for the majority of people, but can result in the aggravation of asthmatic conditions, hypotension and gastrointestinal problems [90]. The FDA has recommended labeling of all foods, non-alcoholic beverages and wine products with sulfite agents in concentrations at least >10 ppm (1.25×10^{-4} M) from 1986 [91]. The environmentally and biologically important nitrite ion is an important precursor in the formation of nitrosamines, many of which have been shown as potent carcinogens in human bodies. It exists widely in the environment, beverages, and food products as a preservative [92]. Therefore, the importance of improved analytical methods for nitrite detection in food, water and biological fluids has received considerable attention. Olga *et al.* [93] published the determination of sulfite using gold ultra microelectrode arrays with 6 μM of detection limit.

6.1. Electrocatalytic Oxidation of Hydrazine, Sulfite and Nitrite

Gold nanoparticles embedded amine functionalized silicate sol-gel network (APS(SG)-Au_{nano}) have been used in the field of direct electrocatalysis and electrochemical sensor [52b]. The detection and determination of hydrazine (N_2H_4), sulfite (SO_3^{2-}) and nitrite (NO_2^-) in aqueous solution have attracted attention in chemical, pharmaceutical, agricultural and food industries in order to develop electrochemical sensors [94]. The gold nanoparticles embedded in amine functionalized silicate (APS) sol-gel matrix were coated on the GC electrode (GC/APS(SG)-Au_{nano}) and used for the electrocatalytic oxidation of hydrazine, sulfite and nitrite [52b]. The electrocatalytic oxidation peaks were observed at 0.05, 0.2 and 0.55 V for hydrazine, sulfite and nitrite, respectively at GC/APS(SG)-Au_{nano} electrode (Figure 19). Such voltammetric peaks were not observed at bare GC and GC/APS(SG) coated electrodes for these analytes. The electrooxidation of these analytes at >0.8 V with ill-defined voltammograms with electrode fouling was noticed at unmodified electrodes. It requires a high overpotential when compared to a gold nanoparticles modified electrode. The designed electrochemical sensor using gold nanoparticles modified electrode could effectively catalyze the electrooxidation of hydrazine, sulfite and nitrite at lower overpotentials (Figure 19). Gold nanoparticles facilitate the electron transfer process and decrease the overpotential to a large extent of ~750 mV, ~600 mV and ~250 mV, respectively for the oxidation of hydrazine, sulfite and nitrite (Figure 20).

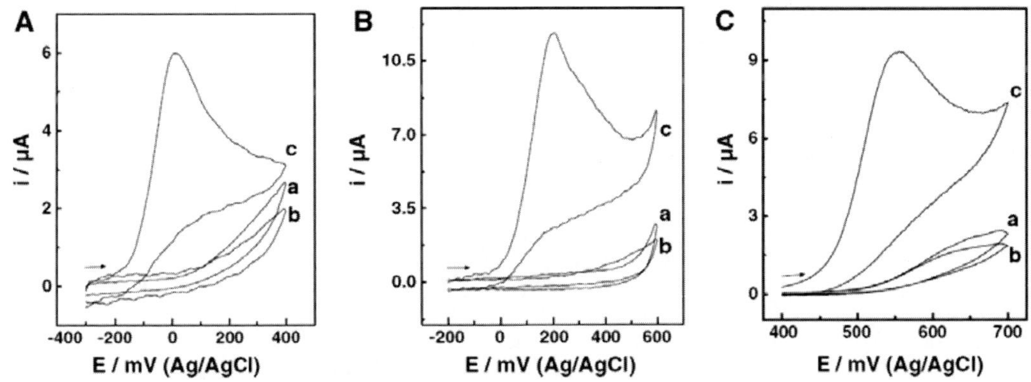

Figure 19. Cyclic voltammograms recorded at GC (a), GC/APS(SG) (b) and GC/APS(SG)-Au_{nano} (c) electrodes for 250 μM hydrazine (N_2H_4) (A), sulfite (SO_3^{2-}) (B) and nitrite (NO_2^-) (C) in 0.1 M PBS (pH 7.2). Scan rate = 50 mV s^{-1}. (Reprinted from Ref. 52b with permission from Elsevier)

6.2. Simultaneous Electrochemical Detection of Hydrazine, Sulfite and Nitrite

The importance of detection and determination of hydrazine, sulfite and nitrite has lead to designing the electrochemical sensor for the detection and determination of these molecules, both individual and simultaneous [52b,94]. This is the first report that appeared in the literature for the simultaneous detection and determination of these toxic chemicals [52b]. The cyclic voltammograms were recorded for the mixture of analytes (each 250 μM of N_2H_4, SO_3^{2-} and NO_2^-) at bare GC, GC/APS(SG) and GC/APS(SG)-Au_{nano} electrodes in 0.1 M PBS (pH 7.2). The schematic illustration of simultaneous detection of a mixture of analytes at the gold nanoparticles embedded in APS silicate matrix sol-gel modified electrode (GC/APS(SG)-Au_{nano}) is shown in Figure 20. The bare GC and GC/APS(SG) electrodes could not show individual oxidation peak for N_2H_4, SO_3^{2-} and NO_2^-. The GC/APS(SG)-Au_{nano} electrode could resolve the voltammetric signal into three well-defined voltammetric peaks with maxima at -0.08, 0.17 and 0.52 V corresponding to the oxidations of N_2H_4, SO_3^{2-} and NO_2^-. The plotted anodic peak currents against the square root of the scan rates showed a linear response for all three analytes, N_2H_4, SO_3^{2-} and NO_2^-, indicating the diffusion controlled electron transfer processes of the analytes at the modified electrode. The gold nanoparticles embedded in the three dimensional APS silicate sol-gel network (GC/APS(SG)-Au_{nano}) act as a nanoscale electrode and provide the conduction pathway and the catalytically active sites of APS(SG)-Au_{nano} efficiently partake the electrocatalytic oxidation process.

Linear sweep voltammetric (LSV) responses were obtained for the mixture of N_2H_4, SO_3^{2-} and NO_2^- at the GC/APS(SG)-Au_{nano} electrode with successive additions of their concentrations (Figure 21A). The observed anodic peak currents for the analytes increased linearly with the concentrations of analytes (Figure 21B). The sensitivity of this system was found to be 0.0241 ± 0.0007, 0.0098 ± 0.0007 and 0.2577 ± 0.0012 μA/μM towards the electrooxidation of N_2H_4, SO_3^{2-} and NO_2^-, respectively. The designed sensor was stable for 25 days at room temperature as the results were found to be reproducible within ±10% difference in the peak current. Gold nanoparticles embedded in APS silicate sol-gel matrix system efficiently electrocatalyze the oxidation and concurrent detection of N_2H_4, SO_3^{2-} and NO_2^- in the absence of any other immobilized redox mediator/enzyme in the APS sol-gel film with a large decrease in the over potentials. The constructed electrochemical sensing device could be applied for direct electrochemical sensing of other chemically and biologically important analytes which is a challenging task in the design of nanoscale building blocks for electrochemical sensing.

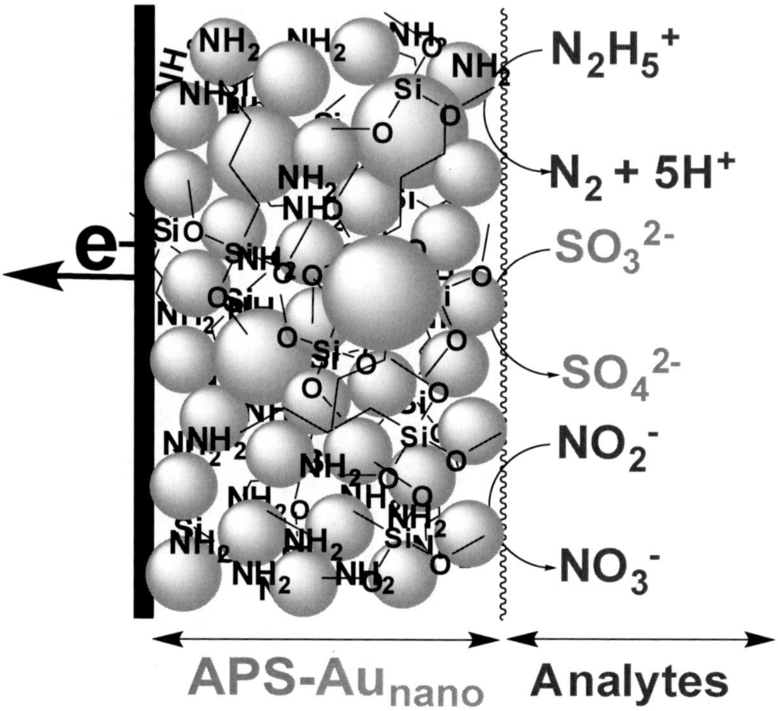

Figure 20. Schematic representation of gold nanoparticles embedded in APS silicate sol-gel matrix (APS(SG)-Au_{nano}) modified GC electrode and simultaneous electrocatalytic oxidation of hydrazine, sulfite and nitrite.

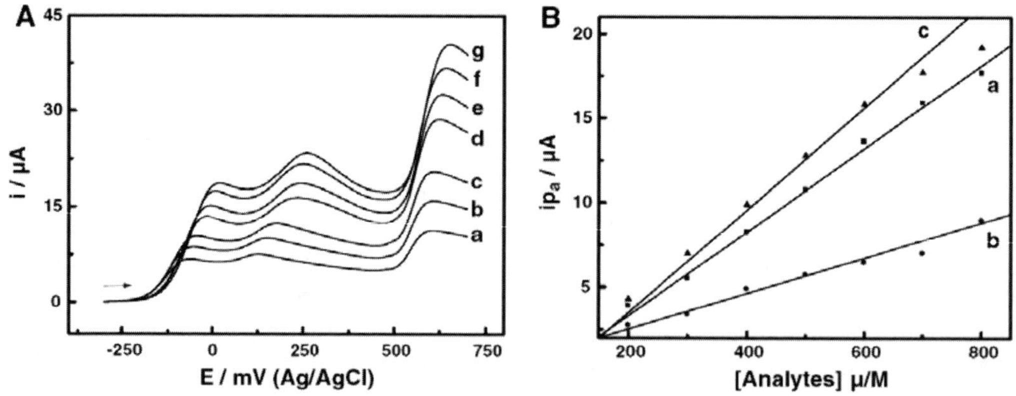

Figure 21. (A) LSV recorded at GC/APS(SG)-Au_{nano} electrode for the mixture of N_2H_4, SO_3^{2-} and NO_2^- with successive addition of their concentrations in 200 µM (a), 300 µM (c), 400 µM (d), 500 µM (e), 600 µM(f), 700 µM (g) and 800 µM (h) in 0.1 M PBS (pH 7.2). (B). Corresponding calibration plots for N_2H_4 (a), SO_3^{2-} (b) and NO_2^- (c). (Reprinted from Ref. 52b with permission from Elsevier)

CONCLUSION

The chemical inertness and resistance to surface oxidation make gold an important material for use in nanoscale devices. This property is crucial when the particle's size approaches the nanoscale and the dominance of surface atoms results in an enhanced chemical reactivity. Other metals that share similar corrosion resistance as gold are platinum and silver. The surface modification of electrodes has been directed toward several goals, often involving electrode kinetics. The surface bound functional groups on the electrode can affect the selectivity or can serve as a catalyst for certain electrochemical reaction. The deliberate modification of the electrode surface with a selected reagent embedded in a suitable matrix that governs its electrochemical properties is advantageous for designing powerful catalytic and sensing devices. The judicious choice of the catalyst that has to be attached to the modified electrode using suitable support material is a major challenge. Nanoparticles-on-electrodes comprise a fundamentally interesting class of materials, in part because of an apparent dichotomy which exists between their sizes and many of their physical and chemical properties. There is no doubt that the importance of nanoscience and nanotechnology based fabrication of electrochemical sensing devices will continue to grow over the coming years for sensor applications.

In this chapter, we presented the facile fabrication of new generation electrochemical sensors using the metal nanoparticles embedded in Nafion and silicate matrices modified electrodes without incorporating any other enzyme or mediator. Indeed, these metal nanoparticles embedded in various matrices act as very good transducers in sensing devices through direct electrocatalysis. The metal nanoparticles show very high selectivity and sensitivity to the sensing molecules when compared to their bulk metal counterparts and the detection limit is also found to be above the threshold level. The present work paves the way for the construction of metal nanoparticles embedded in a suitable matrix modified electrode and for exploring its applications in mediator free concurrent electrochemical sensing of other analytes which is a challenging task in the new generation of nanoscale building blocks for electrochemical sensing.

REFERENCES

[1] (a)Kerman, K.; Saito, M.; Yamamura, S.; Takamura, Y.; Tamiya, E. *Trends in Anal. Chem.* 2008, *27*, 585-592. (b) Sharpe, M. *J. Environ. Monit.* 2003, *5*, 109N-113N.

[2] Moores, A.; Goettmann, F. *New J. Chem.* 2006, *30*, 1121-1132.

[3] Angulo, A. M.; Noguez, C. *J. Phys. Chem. A* 2008, *112*, 5834-5838.

[4] Walcarius, A.; Mandler, D.; Cox, J. A.; Collinson, M.; Lev, O. *J. Mater. Chem.* 2005, *15*, 3663-3389.

[5] Kalantar-zadeh, K.; Fry, B. *Nanotechnology-Enabled Sensors*; ISBN 978-0-387-32473-9; Springer Science+Business Media: New York, USA, 2008, *1*, 135.

[6] Kalantar-zadeh, K.; Fry, B. *Nanotechnology-Enabled Sensors;* ISBN 978-0-387-32473-9; Springer Science+Business Media: New York, USA, 2008, *1*, 79.

[7] Kalantar-zadeh, K.; Fry, B. *Nanotechnology-Enabled Sensors;* ISBN 978-0-387-32473-9; Springer Science+Business Media: New York, USA, 2008, *1*, 8.

[8] (a)D'souza, L.; Richards, R. In *Synthesis, Properties, and Applications of Oxide Nanoparticles;* Rodríguez, J. A.; Fernández-García, M. ISBN 978-0-471-72405-6, JohnWiley & Sons, Inc., CA, 3, 83, (b) Egerton, T. A.; Tooley, I. R. *J. Phys. Chem. B* 2004, *108*, 5066-5072. (c) Fox, M.A.; Dulay, M. T. *Chem. Rev.* 1993, *93*, 341-357.

[9] Alivisatos, A. P. *Science* 1996, *271*, 933-937.

[10] (a)Huang, C. -C.; Yang, Z.; Lee, K-H.; Chang, H-T. *Angew. Chem. Int. Ed.* 2007, *46*, 6824-6828. (b) Chen, Z.; Zu, Y. *Langmuir* 2007, *23*, 11387-11390.

[11] (a)Lin, B.; Gelves, G. A.; Haber, J. A.; Sundararaj, U. *Ind. Eng. Chem. Res.* 2007, *46*, 2481-2487. (b) Wang, D.; Jakobson, H. P.; Kou, R.; Tang, J.; Fineman, R. Z.; Yu, D.; Lu, Y. *Chem. Mater.* 2006, *18*, 4231-4237.

[12] (a)Lu, X.; Au, L.; McLellan, J.; Li, Z. -Y.; Marquez, M.; Xia, Y. *Nano Lett.* 2007, *7*, 1764-1769. (b) Hu, M.; Petrova, H.; Sekkinen, A. R.; Chen, J.; McLellan, J. M.; Li, Z. -Y.; Marquez, M.; Li, X.; Xia, Y.; Hartland, G. V. *J. Phys. Chem. B* 2006, *110*, 19923-19928.

[13] (a)Reeja-Jayan, B.; Rosa, D. E.; Sepulveda-Guzman, S.; Rodriguez, R. A.; Yacaman, M. *J. J. Phys. Chem. C* 2008, *112*, 240-246. (b) Wolcott, A.; Kuykendall, T. R.; Chen, W.; Chen, S.; Zhang, J. Z. *J. Phys. Chem. B* 2006, *110*, 25288-25296.

[14] (a)Wang, X.; Xi, G.; Xiong, S.; Liu, Y.; Xi, B.; Yu, W.; Qian, Y. *Cryst. Growth Des.* 2007, *7*, 930-934. (b) Shen, G.; Chen, D. *J. Am. Chem. Soc.* 2006, *128*, 11762-11763.

[15] (a)Wang, C.; Daimon, H.; Lee, Y.; Kim, J.; Sun, S. *J. Am. Chem. Soc.* 2007, *129*, 6974-6975. (b) Guo, Q.; Zhao, Y.; Mao, W. L.; Wang, Z.; Xiong, Y.; Xia, Y. *Nano Lett.* 2008, *8*, 972-975.

[16] (a)Wu, H.-Y.; Liu, M.; Huang, M. H. *J. Phys. Chem. B* 2006, *110*, 19291-19294. (b) Xie, J.; Lee, J. Y.; Wang, D. I. C. *Chem. Mater.* 2007, *19*, 2823-2830.

[17] (a)Wen, F.; Zhang, W.; Wei, G.; Wang, Y.; Zhang, J.; Zhang, M.; Shi, L. *Chem. Mater.* 2008, *20*, 2144-2150. (b) Baker, G. A. *J. Am. Chem. Soc.* 2004, *126*, 15632-15633. (c) Jain, P. K.; Huang, X.; El-Sayed, I. H.; El-Sayed, M. A. *Acc. Chem. Res.* 2008, *41*, 69-77.

[18] (a)Zhang, J.; Liu, J.; Peng, Q.; Wang, X.; Li, Y. *Chem. Mater.* 2006, *18*, 867-871. (b) Pantano, P. J. *Am. Chem. Soc.* 2007, *129*, 10963-10963. (c) Li, Z.; Cai, W.; Yang, S.; Duan, G.; Ang, R. *J. Phys. Chem. C* 2008, *112*, 1837-1841.

[19] Daniel, M-C.; Astruc, D. *Chem. Rev.* 2004, *104*, 293-346.

[20] Turkevich, J.; Stevenson, P. C.; Hillier, J. *Discuss. of the Faraday Soc.* 1951, *11*, 55-75.

[21] Frens, G. *Nature* 1973, *241*, 20-22.

[22] (a)Kim, J. -H.; Lee, T. R. *Langmuir* 2007, *23*, 6504-6509. (b) Satti, A.; Aherne, D.; Fitzmaurice, D. *Chem. Mater.* 2007, *19*, 1543-1545.

[23] (a)Surendran, G.; Ramos, L.; Pansu, B.; Prouzet, E.; Beaunier, P.; Audonnet, F.; Remita, H. *Chem. Mater.* 2007, *19*, 5045-5048. (b) Ma, Z.; Liu, Q.; Cui, Z. -M.; Bian, S. -W.; Song, W. -G. *J. Phys. Chem. C* 2008, *112*, 8875-8880.

[24] (a)Berti, L.; Alessandrini, A.; Bellesia, M.; Facci, P. *Langmuir* 2007, *23*, 10891-10892. (b) Yang, L.; Shen, Y.; Xie, A.; Zhang, B. *J. Phys. Chem. C* 2007, *111*, 5300-5308. (c) Chowdhury, D.; Maoz, R.; Sagiv, J. *Nano Lett.* 2007, 7, 1770-1778.

[25] Niesen T. P.; De Guire, M. R. *J. Electroceram.* 2001, *6*, 169-207.

[26] (a)Wang, L.; Mao, W.; Ni, D.; Di, J.; Wu, Y.; Tu, Y. *Electrochem. Commun.* 2008, *10*, 673-676. (b) Wang, H.; Tian, T.; Zhang, Y.; Pan, Z.; Wang, Y.; Xiao, Z. *Langmuir*

2008, *24*, 8918-8922. (c) Umeda, R.; Awaji, H.; Nakahodo, T.; Fujihara, H. *J. Am. Chem. Soc.* 2008, *130*, 3240-3241.

[27] (a)Chou, J.; Jayaraman, S.; Ranasinghe, A. D.; McFarland, E. W.; Buratto, S. K.; Metiu, H. *J. Phys. Chem. B* 2006, *110*, 7119-7121. (b) Chen, G.; Xia, D.; Nie, Z.; Wang, Z.; Wang, L.; Zhang, L.; Zhang, *J. Chem. Mater.* 2007, *19*, 1840-1844.

[28] (a)Zach, M. P.; Ng, K. H.; Penner, R. M. *Science* 2000, *290*, 2120-2123. (b) Gimeno, Y.; Creus, A. H.; Carro, P. Gonzalez, S.; Salvarezza, R. C.; Arvia, A. J. *J. Phys. Chem. B* 2002, *106*, 232-4244. (c) Kalantar-zadeh, K.; Fry, B. *Nanotechnology-Enabled Sensors;* ISBN 978-0-387-32473-9; Springer Science+Business Media: New York, USA, 2008, *3*, 182-184.

[29] (a)Hansen, J. A.; Mukhopadhyay, R.; Hansen, J. O.; Gothelf, K. V. *J. Am. Chem. Soc.* 2006, *128*, 3860-3861. (b) Hansen, J. A.; Sumbayev, V. V.; Gothelf, K. V. *Nano Lett.* 2007, *7*, 2831-2834.

[30] (a)Badia, A.; Lennox, R. B.; Reven, L. *Acc. Chem. Res.* 2000, *33*, 475-481. (b) Fendler, J. H. *Chem. Mater.* 1996, *8*, 1616-1624. (c) Yang, T.; Li, Z.; Wang, L.; Guo, C.; Sun, Y. *Langmuir* 2007, *23*, 10533-10538.

[31] Díaz, D. J. *J. Am. Chem. Soc.* 2008, *130*, 10033-10034.

[32] (a)Herricks, T.; Chen J.; Xia, Y. *Nano Lett.* 2004, *4*, 2367-2371. (b) Kijima, T.; Yoshimura, T.; Uota, M.; Ikeda, T.; Fujikawa, D.; Mouri, S.; Uoyama, S. *Angew. Chem., Int. Ed.* 2004, *43*, 228-232. (c) Song, Y.; Yang, Y.; Medforth, C. J.; Pereira, E.; Singh, A. K.; Xu, H.; Jiang, Y.; Brinker, C. J.; van Swol, F.; Shelnutt, J. A.; *J. Am. Chem. Soc.* 2004, *126*, 635-639.

[33] (a)Huab, X.; Dong, S. *J. Mater. Chem.* 2008, *18*, 1279-1295. (b) Kim, D. W.; Lee, J. S.; Lee, G. S.; Overzet, L.; Kozlov, M.; Aliev, A. E.; Park, Y. W,; Yang, D. J. *J. Nanosci. and Nanotech.* 2006, *6*, 3608-3613. (c) Chow, K. -F.; Mavre, F.; Crooks, R. M. *J. Am. Chem. Soc.* 2008, *130*, 7544-7545.

[34] Chen, D.; Wang, G.; Li, J. *J. Phys. Chem. C* 2007, *111*, 2351-2367.

[35] (a)Du, X.; Wang, M.; Liu, L.; Gong, W.; Wang, B. *Sensor Letters* 2008, *6*, 226-230. (b) Chow, K-F.; Mavre, F.; Crooks, R. M. *J. Am. Chem. Soc.* 2008, *130*, 7544-7545. (c) Thiagarajan, S.; Chen, S-M. *Talanta* 2007, *74*, 212-222. (d) Kang, X.; Mai, Z.; Zou, X.; Cai, P.; Mo, J. *Anal. Biochem.* 2007, *369*, 71-79. (e) Wang, A.; Ye, X.; He, P.; Fang, Y. *Electroanalysis* 2007, *19*, 1603-1608.

[36] Selvaraju, T.; Ramaraj, R. *J. Electroanal. Chem.* 2005, *585*, 290-300.

[37] Mauritz, K. A.; Moore, R. B. *Chem. Rev.* 2004, *104*, 4535-4586. (b) Choi, H. N.; Cho, S.-H.; Lee, W.-Y. *Anal. Chem.* 2003, *75*, 4250-4256.

[38] (a) Yeager, H. L.; Kipling, B.; Dotson, R. L. J. *Electrochem. Soc.* 1980, *127*, 303-310. (b) Covitch, M. J.; Lowry, S. R.; Gray, C. L.; Blackford, B. *In Polymeric Separation Media*; Cooper, A. R., Ed.; Plenum: New York, 1982; p 257. (c) Eisenberg, A.; Yeager, H. L. *Perflourinated Ionomer Membranes, ACS Symposium series 180*, American Chemical Society, Washington, 1982. (d) Mao, L.; Zhang, D.; Sotomura, T.; Nakatsu, K.; Koshiba, N.; Ohsaka, T. *Electrochim. Acta* 2003, *48*, 1015-1021. (e) Yasuzawa, M.; Kunugi, A. *Electrochem. Commun.* 1999, *1*, 459-464.

[39] Hrapovic, S.; Liu, Y.; Male, E. B.; Luong, J. H. T. *Anal. Chem.* 2004, *76*, 1083-1088.

[40] John, S. A.; Ramaraj, R. *Langmuir* 1996, *12*, 5689-5695.

[41] Martin, C. R.; Dollard, K. A. *J. Electroanal. Chem.* 1983, *159*, 127-135.

[42] (a)Mikhaylova, A. A.; Khazova, O. A.; Bagotzky, V. S. *J. Electroanal. Chem.* 2000, *480*, 225-232. (b) Premkumar, J.; Ramaraj, R. *J. Solid State Electrochem.* 1997, *1*, 172-179.
[43] (a)Ross, P. N. *J. Electrochem. Soc.* 1979, *126*, 67-. (b) Clavilier, J.; Faure, R.; Guinet, G.; Durand, R. *J. Electroanal. Chem.* 1980, *107*, 205-209. (c) Clavier, J. in *Electrochemical Surface Sciences: Molecular Phenomena at Electrode Surfaces*, M. Soriaga, Ed., ACS Books, Washington, D. C., 1988, p. 205. (c) Bard, A. J.; Faulkner, L. R. *Electrochemical Methods Fundamentals and Applications*, Wiley, New York, 2004, *13*, 570.
[44] (a)Vetter, K. J.; Schultze, J. W. *J. Electroanal. Chem.* 1972, *34*, 131-141. (b) Dong, S.; Qiu, Q. *J. Electroanal. Chem.* 1991, *314*, 223-229. (c) Jiang, J.; Kucernak, A. *J. Electroanal. Chem.* 2004, *567*, 123-137.
[45] (a)Wagner, D. In *Practical Surface Analysis;* Second Ed; Briggs, D.; Scah M. P. Wiley, Chichester, 1990, *1,* (Appendix 5). (b) Bard, A. J.; Faulkner, L. R. *Electrochemical Methods, Fundamentals and Applications*, Wiley, New York, 2001.
[46] Schottner, G. *Chem. Mater.* 2001, *13*, 3422-3435.
[47] (a)Schmidt, H. J. *Non-Cryst. Solids* 1985, *73*, 681-691. (b) Ravaine, D.; Seminel, A.; Charbouillot, Y.; Vincens, M. *J. Non-Cryst. Solids* 1986, *82*, 210-219.
[48] (a)Uhlmann, D. R.; Teowee, G. J. *Sol-Gel Sci. Technol.* 1998, *13*, 153-162. (b) Mackenzie, J. D.; Bescher, E. P. J. *Sol-Gel Sci. Technol.* 1998, *13*, 371-377.
[49] Walcarius, A. *Chem. Mater.* 2001, *13*, 3351-3372.
[50] (a)Walcarius, C. A.; Mandler, D.; Cox, J. A; Collinson, M.; Lev, O. *J. Mater. Chem.* 2005, *15*, 3663-3689. (b) Sanchez, L.; De G. J.; Soler-Illia, A. A.; Ribot, F.; Grosso, D. C. R. *Chimie* 2003, *6*, 1131-1151. (c) Caruso, R. A.; Antonietti, M. *Chem Mater.* 2001, *13*, 3272-3282.
[51] Bharathi, S.; Fishelson, N.; Lev O. *Langmuir* 1999, *15*, 1929-1937.
[52] (a)Maduraiveeran, G.; Ramaraj, R. *J. Electroanal. Chem.* 2007, *608*, 52-58. (b) Maduraiveeran, G.; Ramaraj, R. *Electrochem. Commun.* 2007, *9*, 2051-2055.
[53] (a)Grabar, K. C.; Freeman, R. G.; Hommer, M. B.; Natan, M. *J. Anal. Chem.* 1995, *67*, 735-743. (b) Lin, H.-Y.; Chen, C.-T.; Chen, Y.-C. *Anal. Chem.* 2006, *78*, 6873-6878. (c) Xie, F.; Baker, M. S.; Goldys, E. M. *Chem. Mater.* 2008, *20*, 1788-1797. (d) Tao, W.; Yao, S. *J. Electroanal. Chem.* 2004, *572*, 109-116.
[54] (a)Schmidt, C. *J. Sol-Gel Sci. Technol.* 1994, *1*, 217-22. (b) Hsueh, C. H.; Collinson, M. M. *J. Electroanal. Chem.* 1997, *420*, 243-249. (c) Khoo, S. B.; Chen, F. *Anal. Chem.* 2002, *74*, 5734-5741.
[55] (a)Rand, D. A.; Woods, R. *J. Electroanal. Chem.* 1971, *32*, 29-35. (b) Woods, R.; in Bard, A. J (Ed.), *Electroanalytical Chemistry; A series of Advances,* 1976, Marcel Dekker, Newyork, *9*, 1-162. (c) Bharathi, S.; Nogami, M.; Lev, O. *Langmuir* 2001, *17*, 2602-2609.
[56] Jia, J.; Wang, B.; Wu, A.; Cheng, G.; Li, Z.; Dong, S. *Anal. Chem.* 2002, *74*, 2217-2223.
[57] Raj, C. R.; Abdelrahman, A. I.; Ohsaka, T. *Electrochem. Commun.* 2005, *7*, 888-893.
[58] (a)Usher, M. J.; Keating, D. A. *Sensors and transducers: characteristics, applications, instrumentation, interfacing;* Macmillan, London, UK, 1996. (b) W. Göpel, J. Hesse, and J. N. Zemel, *Sensors: A Comprehensive Survey*; VCH, Weinheim, Germany, 1991.
[59] Sinclair, I. R. *Sensors and transducers*; Newnes, Oxford, UK, 2001.

[60] Janata, J. *Chem. Rev.* 2008, *108*, 327-328.

[61] Kalantar-zadeh, K.; Fry, B. *Nanotechnology-Enabled Sensors*; ISBN 978-0-387-32473-9; Springer Science+Business Media: New York, USA, 2008, *1*, 5-6.

[62] (a)Cassidy, J.; Ghoroghchian, J.; Sarfarazi, F.; Smith, J. J.; Pons, S. *Electrochim. Acta* 1986, *31*, 629-636. (b) Penner, R. M.; Martin, C. R. *Anal. Chem.* 1987, *59*, 2625-2630.

[63] (a)Reller, H.; Kirowa-Eisner, E.; Gileadi, E. *J. Electroanal. Chem.* 1984, *161*, 247-268. (b) Cassidy, J.; Ghoroghchian, J.; Sarfarazi, F.; Smith, J. J.; Pons, S. *Electrochim. Acta* 1986, *31*, 629-636.

[64] Huab, X.; Dong, S. *J. Mater. Chem.* 2008, *18*, 1279-1295.

[65] (a)Hansen, J. A.; Mukhopadhyay, R.; Hansen, J. O.; Gothelf, K. V. *J. Am. Chem. Soc.* 2006, *128*, 3860-3861. (b) Orozco, J.; Fernández-Sánchez, C.; Jiménez-Jorquera, C. *Environ. Sci. Technol.* 2008, *42*, 4877-4882. (c) Hansen, J. A.; Wang, J.; Kawde, A.-N.; Xiang, Y.; Gothelf, K. V.; Collins, G. *J. Am. Chem. Soc.* 2006, *128*, 2228-2229. (d) Hwang, S.; Kim, E.; Kwak, J. *Anal. Chem.* 2005, *77*, 579-584.

[66] Bauer, A. J.; Stockwell, B. R. *Chem. Rev.* 2008, *108*, 1774-1786.

[67] Wilson, G. S.; Johnson, M. A. *Chem. Rev.* 2008, *108*, 2462-2481.

[68] Sharpe, M. *J. Environ. Monit.* 2003, *5*, 109N-113N.

[69] Chen, D.; Wang, G. Li, J. *J. Phys. Chem. C* 2007, *111*, 2351-2367.

[70] Thiagarajan, S.; Chen, S-M. *Talanta* 2007, *74*, 212-222.

[71] Cao, Z.; Zou, Y.; Xiang, C.; Sun, Li-X.; Xu, Fen. *Anal. Lett.* 2007, *40*, 2116-2127.

[72] (a)Du, X.; Wang, M.; Liu, L.; Gong, W.; Wang, B. *Sensor Letters* 2008, *6*, 226-230. (b) Chow, K-F.; Mavre, F.; Crooks, R. M. *J. Am. Chem. Soc.* 2008, *130*, 7544-7545. (c) Yuan, L.; Yang, M.; Qu, F.; Shen, G.; Yu, R. *Electrochimica Acta* 2008, *53*, 3559-3565.

[73] (a)Ali, S. R.; Parajuli, R. R.; Ma, Y.; Balogun, Y.; He, H. *J. Phys. Chem. B* 2007, *111*, 12275-12281. (b) Siqueira, J. R., Jr.; Gasparotto, L. H. S.; Crespilho, F. N.; Carvalho, A. J. F.; Zucolotto, V.; Oliveira, O. N., Jr. *J. Phys. Chem. B* 2006, *110*, 22690-22694. (c) Ali, S. R.; Ma, Y.; Parajuli, R. R.; Balogun, Y.; Lai, W. Y.-C.; He, H. *Anal. Chem.* 2007, *79*, 2583-2587.

[74] (a)Kinoshita, K. *Electrochemical Oxygen Technology*; Wiley, New York, 1992. (b) Markovic, N. M., Gasteiger, H. A.; Ross, P. N. *J. Electrochem. Soc.* 1997, *144*, 1591-1597. (c) Stamenkovici, V. R.; Mun, B. S.; Arenza, M.; Mayrhofer, K. J. J.; Lucas, C. A.; Wang, G.; Ross, P. N.; Markovic, N. M. *Nature Mater.* 2007, *6*, 241-247.

[75] (a)Du, H. -Y.; Wang, C. -H.; Hsu, H. -C.; Chang, S. -T.; Chen, U. -S.; Yen, S. C.; Chen, L. C.; Shih, H. -C.; Chen, K. H. *Diamond and Related Materials* 2008, *17*, 535-541. (b) Sevilla, M.; Sanchis, C.; Valdes-Solis, T.; Morallon, E.; Fuertes, A. B. *Carbon* 2008, *46*, 931-939. (c) Abe, H.; Matsumoto, F.; Alden, L. R.; Warren, S. C.; Abruna, H. D.; DiSalvo, F. J. *J. Am. Chem. Soc.* 2008, *130*, 5452-5458.

[76] (a)Ali, S. R.; Ma, Y.; Parajuli, R. R.; Balogun, Y.; Lai, W. Y. -C.; He, H. *Anal. Chem.* 2007, *79*, 2583-2587. (b) Ali, S. R.; Parajuli, R. R.; Ma, Y.; Balogun, Y.; He, H. *J. Phys. Chem. B* 2007, *111*, 12275-12281. (c) Ciszewski, A.; Milczarek, G. *Anal. Chem.* 1999, *71*, 1055-1061.

[77] Karyakin, A. A.; Puganova, E. A.; Budashov, I. A.; Kurochkin, I. N.; Karyakina, E. E.; Levchenko, V. A.; Matveyenko, V. N.; Varfolomeyev, S. D. *Anal. Chem.* 2004, *76*, 474-478.

[78] (a)Poh, W. C.; Loh, K. P.; Zhang, W. D.; Triparthy, S. ; Ye, J. -S.; Sheu, F. -S. *Langmuir* 2004, *20*, 5484-5492. (b) Raj, C. R.; Okajima, T.; Ohsaka, T. *J. Electroanal. Chem.* 2003, *543*, 127-133. (c) F. Malem, D. Madler, *Anal. Chem.* 1993, *65*, 3204-3211.

[79] (a)Kulys, J.; Wang, L.; Maksimoviene, A. *Anal. Chim. Acta* 1993, *274*, 53-58. (b) Yanxia, X.; Chengguo, H.; Shengshui, H.; *Sensors and Actuators B* 2008, *130*, 816-822.

[80] Notsu, H.; Tatsuma, T.; Fujishima, A.; *J. Electroanal. Chem.* 2002, *523*, 86-92. (b) Hill, H. A. *Coord. Chem. Rev.* 1996, *151*, 89-15. (c) Shu, X.; Chen, Y.; Yuan, H.; Gao, S.; Xiao, D. *Anal. Chem.* 2007, *79*, 3695-3702. (d) Rubianes, M. D.; Rivas, G. A. *Electroanalysis* 2005, *17*, 73-78. (e) Rubianes, M. D.; Rivas G. A. *Electrochem. Commun.* 2003, *5*, 689-694. (f) Mark, V.; Maidan, R.; Heller A.; *Anal. Chem.* 1992, *64*, 3084-3090.

[81] (a)Ferapontova, E.; Schmengler, K.; Borchers, T.; Ruzgas, T.; Gorton, L. *Biosens. Bioelectron.* 2002, *17,* 953-963. (b) Wang, L.; Wang, E. *Electrochem. Commun.* 2004, *6*, 225-229. (c) Wang, B.; Zhang, J.; Cheng, G.; Dong, S. *Anal. Chim. Acta.* 2000, *407*, 111-118. (d) Di , J.; Shen, C.; Peng, S.; Tu, Y.; Li, S. *Anal. Chim. Acta* 2005, *553*, 196-200. (e) Zhao, J.; Henkens, R. W.; Stonehuerner, J.; O'Daly, J. P.; Crumbliss, A. L. *J. Electroanal. Chem.* 1992, *327*, 109-119. (f) Jia, J.; Wang, B.; Wu, A.; Cheng, G.; Li, Z.; Dong, S. *Anal. Chem.* 2002, *74*, 2217-2223.

[82] (a) Chen, S.; Yuan, R.; Chai, Y.; Zhang, L.; Wang, N.; Li, X.; Chongqing. *Biosens. Bioelectron.* 2007, *22*, 1268-1274. (b) Feng, J-J.; Xu, J-J.; Chen, H.-Y. *J. Electroanal. Chem.* 2005, *585*, 44-50. (c) Feng, J-J.; Zhao, G.; Xu, J-J.; Chen, H-Y. *Anal. Biochem.* 2005, *342*, 280-286. (d) Yang, W.; Li, Y.; Bai, Y.; Sun, C. *Sensors and Actuators B* 2006, *115*, 42-48. (e) Gao, F.; Yuan, R.; Chai, Y.; Tang, M.; Cao, S.; Chen, S. *Colloids and Surfaces, A: Physicochemical and Engineering Aspects* 2007, 295, 223-228.

[83] (a)Becker, R. A.; Barrows, L. R.; Shank, R. C. *Carcinogenesis* 1981, *2*, 1181-1188. (b) McAuley, C. B.; Banks, C. E.; Simm, A. O.; Jonesb, T. G. J.; Compton, R. G. *Analyst* 2006, *131*, 106-110 and references cited therein.

[84] Yamada, K.; Yasuda, K.; Fujiwara, N.; Siroma, Z.; Tanaka, H.; Miyazaki, Y.; Kobayashi, T. *Electrochem. Commun.* 2003, *5*, 892-896.

[85] Homeland Security Information Bulletin; U.S. Department of Homeland Security: Washington, DC, May 2003.

[86] (a)Gimeno, Y.; Hernandez Creus, A.; Gonzalez, S.; Salvarezza, R. C.; Arvia, A. J. *Chem. Mater.* 2001, *13*, 1857-1864. (b) Batchelor-McAuley, C.; Banks, C. E.; Simm, A. O.; Jones, T. G. J.; Compton, R. G. *Analyst* 2006, *131*, 106-110. (c) Yang, C. -C.; Kumar, A. S.; Kuo, M. -C.; Chien, S. -H.; Zen, J. -M. *Anal. Chim. Acta* 2005, *554*, 66-73.

[87] Jena B. K.; Raj, C. R. *J. Phys. Chem. C* 2007, *111*, 6228-6232.

[88] Dinc¸kaya, E.; Sezgintu¨rk, M. K.; Akyılmaz, E.; Erta, F. N. *Food Chem.* 2007, 101, 1540-1544 and references cited therein.

[89] Situmorang, M.; Brynn Hibbert, D.; Gooding, J. J.; Barnett, D. *Analyst* 1999, *124*, 1775-1779.

[90] (a)Vally, H.; Thompson, P. J. *Clin. Exp. Allergy* 2002, *32*, 186-191. (b) Vally, H.; Klerk, N.; Thompson, P. J. *J. Allergy Clin. Immun.* 2000, *105*, 462-467. (c) Vally, H.; Thompson, P. J. *Thorax* 2001, *56*, 763-769.

[91] In *Fed. Regist.* 1986, *51*, 25012-25020.

[92] Agboola, B. O.; Ozoemenab, K. I.; Nyokong, T. *Electrochim. Acta* 2006, *51*, 6470-6478 and references cited therein.

[93] Olga, O.; Craig E.; Banks, F.; Javier C.; Francesc, X. M.; Davis, J.; Compton, R. G. *Electroanalysis* 2006, *18*, 247-252.

[94] (a)Garrod, S.; Bollard, M. E.; Nicholls, A.W.; Connor, S. C.; Connelly, J.; Nicholson, J. K.; Holmes, E. *Chem. Res. Toxicol.* 2005, *18*, 115-122. (b) Mellor, R. B.; Ronnenberg, J.; Campbell, W. H.; Diekmann, S. *Nature* 1992, *355,* 717-722. (c) Almeida, P. J.; Rodrigues, J. A.; Guido, L. F.; Santos, J. R.; Barros, A. A. A.; Fogg, G. *Electroanalysis* 2003, *15*, 587-590. (d) Davis, J.; Compton, R. G. *Anal. Chim. Acta* 2000, *404*, 241-247.

In: Nanostructured Materials for Electrochemical Biosensors ISBN: 978-1-60741-706-4
Editors: U. Yogeswaran; S. Kumar; S. Chen ©2009 Nova Science Publishers, Inc.

Chapter 4

GOLD NANOPARTICLES MODIFIED ELECTRODES FOR BIOSENSORS

A. Sivanesan and S. Abraham John*
Gandhigram Rural University, Dindigul, India

OVERVIEW

Biomolecules are chemical compounds found in living organisms which are the building blocks of life and perform important functions. Fluctuation from the normal concentration of these biomolecules in living system leads to several disorders. Thus the exact determination of them in human fluids is essential in the clinical point of view. High performance liquid chromatography, flow injection analysis, capillary electrophoresis, fluorimetry, spectrophotometry, electrochemical and chemiluminescence techniques were usually used for the determination of biologically important molecules. Among these techniques, electrochemical determination of biomolecules has several advantages over other methods viz., simplicity, selectivity and sensitivity. In the past two decades, electrodes modified with polymer films, self-assembled monolayers containing different functional groups and carbon paste have been used as electrochemical sensors. But in recent years, nanomaterials based electrochemical sensors play an important role in the improvement of public health because of its rapid detection, high sensitivity and specificity in clinical diagnostics. To date gold nanoparticles (AuNPs) have received arousing attention mainly due to their fascinating electronic and optical properties as a consequence of their reduced dimensions. These unique properties of AuNPs make them as an ideal candidate for the immobilization of enzymes for biosensing. Further, the electrochemical properties of AuNPs reveal that they exhibit interesting properties by enhancing the electrode conductivity, facilitating electron transfer and improving the detection limit of biomolecules. In this chapter, we summarized the different strategies used for the attachment of AuNPs on electrode surfaces and highlighted the electrochemical determination of glucose, ascorbic acid (AA), uric acid (UA) and dopamine derivatives using the AuNPs modified electrodes.

---

* Corresponding author e-mail: abrajohn@yahoo.co.in; Tel.: 91-451-2452371; fax: 91-451-2453071. Department of Chemistry, Gandhigram Rural University,Gandhigram-624 302, Dindigul, India

1. INTRODUCTION

1.1. What are Biomolecules?

Biomolecules are chemical compounds that naturally occur in living organisms and are primarily composed of carbon, hydrogen, oxygen, nitrogen, sulfur and phosphorus. Other elements sometimes are incorporated but are much less common. These biomolecules are the fundamental building blocks of living cells which provide the foundation of life [1]. Even though one can subdivide an organism into substructures like tissues, cells, blood, bones etc., the biomolecules make their basic role felt across the entire hierarchy of biological order. They plays a vital role in all living organisms such as Pheromones which link male and female in disperse societies, drugs to treat diseases in individuals, cells which are guided in their development through hormones, and every process in cells is directly linked to biomolecules. Therefore naturally, the search for a theory of living systems starts with the fundamental building blocks, i.e., biomolecules [2]. Thus, the presence of an each and every biomolecules in a living system is very essential for the proper functioning of that organism. Further, the concentration of these biomolecules in an organism is as important as the presence of biomolecules in that particular organism. Generally, all living systems need an appropriate concentration of a particular biomolecule for its proper function. If there is any fluctuation in the concentration of that particular biomolecules, then the malfunctioning of the system starts. Therefore, to rectify a malfunctioning of a biological system we should adjust the concentration of a biomolecule by external source. To sum up, the exact measurement of the concentration of a biomolecules in a living system is very important both in the medicinal and clinical point of view.

1.2 Biosensor

In the history of determination of the concentration of biomolecule several methods were used such as high performance liquid chromatography [3], flow injection analysis [4,5], capillary electrophoresis [6,7], fluorimetry [8], spectrophotometry [9], chemiluminescence [10] and electrochemical method [11,12]. Among these methods recently exhaustive research effort has been focused in the field of analytical electrochemistry to design a biosensor because the biosensors based on electrochemical method are highly selective, sensitive and stable. Further, the fabrication and usage of electrodes are easy and affordable [11, 12]. Thus, electrochemical biosensors have been the subject of basic as well as applied research for more than 45 years. The history of electrochemical biosensor starts with Leland C. Clark, who introduced the principle of the first enzyme electrode with immobilized glucose oxidase at the New York Academy of Sciences Symposium in 1962 [13]. Springs Instruments (Yello Springs, OH, USA) in 1975 first commercialized the biosensor for glucose assay in blood samples from diabetic patients. From then to till date huge number of electrochemical biosensors have been commercialized for sensing various important biomolecules.

Now a question may arise what is a biosensor? Various definitions and terminologies are used depending on the field of application. A commonly used definition is "*a biosensor is a chemical sensing device in which a biologically derived recognition entity is coupled to a transducer that transforms the quantitative information of a biomolecule into an analytically useful signal*". Thus, biosensors usually contain two primary components connected in series i.e., a biomolecule recognition system otherwise known as receptor or bio-element and a physiochemical transducer or sensor element (Figure 1) [14-17].

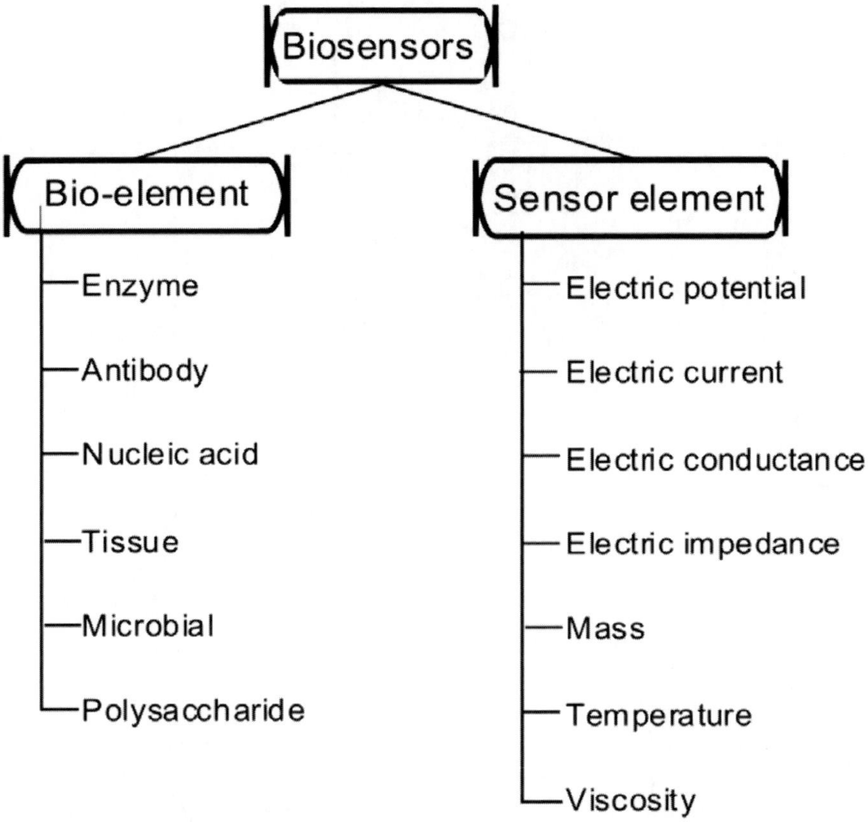

Figure 1. Elements of biosensors

Generally, the biological recognition system recognizes a specific biomolecule or analyte and translates information about the concentration of that biochemical domain into a specific output signal with a defined sensitivity. The biomolecule recognition system is very specific to the biomolecule to which it is sensitive. Mostly biomolecule recognition system does not recognize other analytes. The transducer is an electronic device which converts energy from one form to another form. Here the transducer part of the sensor serves to transfer the signal from the output domain of the recognition system to specific domain of the sensor used. Depending on the output signal of the transducer used, the biosensors are of many types such as: resonant biosensors, colorimetric biosensor, optical-detection biosensors, thermal-detection biosensors, ion-sensitive field-effect transistor (ISFET) biosensors and electrochemical biosensors. In electrochemical biosensors the transducer is an electrode which converts the chemical reaction into an electrical signal (Figure 2) [16, 17].

The electrochemical biosensors, based on the parameter measured, can be further classified into potentiometric, amperometric, conductometric, impedimetric and ion charge or field effect biosensor [18].

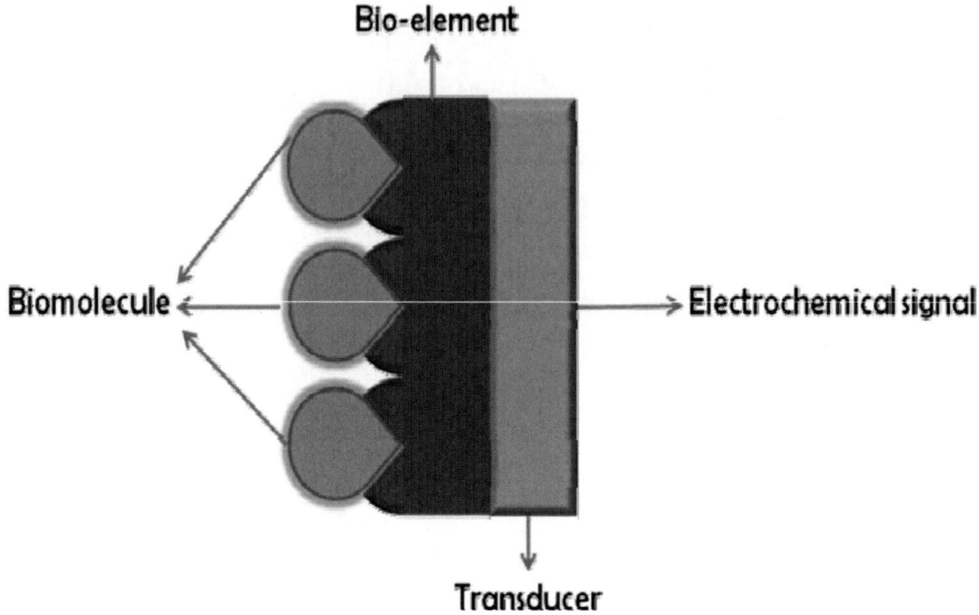

Figure 2. Pictorial representation of a biosensor.

1.3. Importance of Nanomaterials

It has been well established that the performance of a biosensor depends greatly on the material used for the immobilization of receptor molecule on the electrode surface. In this context, the use of nanomaterials for the construction of biosensing devices constitutes one of the most exciting approaches [19]. Nanomaterials have attracted particular interest owing to their ease in synthesis and functionalization, chemical stability, low inherent toxicity (biocompatibility), and tunable optical and electronic properties (absorption, fluorescence and conductivity) [20,21]. These unique properties of nanomaterials found its usage in the construction of novel and improved sensing devices, in particular electrochemical sensors and biosensors. Generally, the nanomaterials have excellent conductivity and catalytic properties, which make them suitable for acting as "electronic wires" to enhance the electron transfer between the bio-element and the electrode surface [22]. Further, the adsorption of biomolecules or bio-element directly onto the naked surfaces of bulk electrode materials may frequently result in the denaturation followed by the loss of bioactivity. However, the adsorption of such biomolecule onto the surfaces of nanomaterials can retain their bioactivity because of the biocompatibility of the nanomaterials [19,22].

Although different nanomaterials such as nanoparticles, nanowires and nanotubes are used for the construction of biosensor, this chapter is mainly devoted to the use of AuNPs for the construction of electrochemical biosensor and their analytical performances. Further, in this chapter we restrict ourselves in the electrochemical sensing of glucose, ascorbic acid, uric acid and dopamine derivatives using the AuNPs modified electrodes.

2. Synthesis of Gold Nanoparticles

2.1. Wet Chemical Methods

The very first method for the synthesis of gold nanoparticles (AuNPs) was reported by Faraday in 1857 [23]. He prepared deep red solutions of colloidal gold by reducing the aqueous solution of gold (III) chloride using phosphorus in carbon disulfide (CS_2). Later, in the 20th century numerous methods were reported and reviewed for the synthesis of colloidal gold [20,21]. In 1951, Turkevitch [24] reported the preparation of colloidal gold by citrate reduction method with an average diameter of 20 nm. The synthetic procedure is as follows: a solution of 100 mL 1mM hydrogentetrachloroaurate ($HAuCl_4$) in water is boiled in reflux conditions under vigorous stirring and secondly 10 mL of 38.8 mM aqueous sodium citrate is added all at once to the $HAuCl_4$ solution. The yellow color in the aqueous solution due to the presence of $AuCl_4^-$, turns clear over dark blue leaving a deep reddish color within a few minutes indicating the formation of AuNPs. This mixture is further stirred and boiled for 15 minutes, and is then removed form the heat while stirring is continued till room temperature is reached. In this reaction, the citrate ions reduce the $HAuCl_4$ according to the following equation (1).

$$3(H_2CCOOH)_2C(OH)COO^- + 2AuCl_4^- \rightleftharpoons 3(H_2CCOOH)_2\,C{=}O + 2Au + 8Cl^- + 3CO_2 + 3H^+ \quad (1)$$

Here the gold colloids are stabilized by negatively charged citrate ions and chloride ions that are still present in the solution.

In 1973, Frens [25,26] succeeded in the synthesis of colloidal gold with average sizes differing from 16 nm to 147 nm by changing the concentration of the added sodium citrate. When the concentration of sodium citrate addition is decreased, colloidal particles of greater size are formed. The gold sol produced by this method is less reproducible but it proves the importance of the citrate ions stabilizing the gold colloids. The larger particles are less monodisperse and the color of the solution is violet. A typical UV-Vis spectrum of gold colloids prepared according to the citrate reduction method described by Frens is shown in Figure 3. The absorption band around 520 nm is the surface plasmon resonance band which is responsible for the remarkable colors of the colloidal gold sols. The properties of colloids depend on the particle size and the surface plasmon band shifts to longer wavelengths when larger (less monodisperse) AuNPs are prepared. This method is very often used even now when a rather loose shell of ligands is required around the gold core in order to prepare a precursor to valuable AuNPs-based materials.

The stabilization of AuNPs with alkanethiols was first reported in 1993 by Mulvaney and Giersig [27]. The TEM image of the AuNPs is shown in Figure 4. They showed the possibility of using thiols of different chain lengths as stabilizing agents. In this method, the

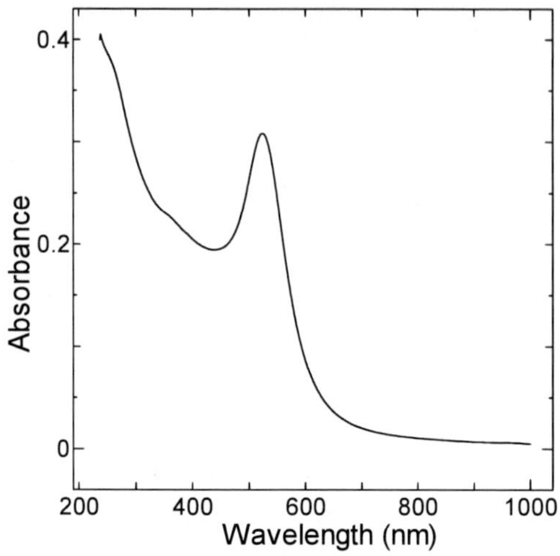

Figure 3. UV-visible spectrum of citrate stabilized AuNPs.

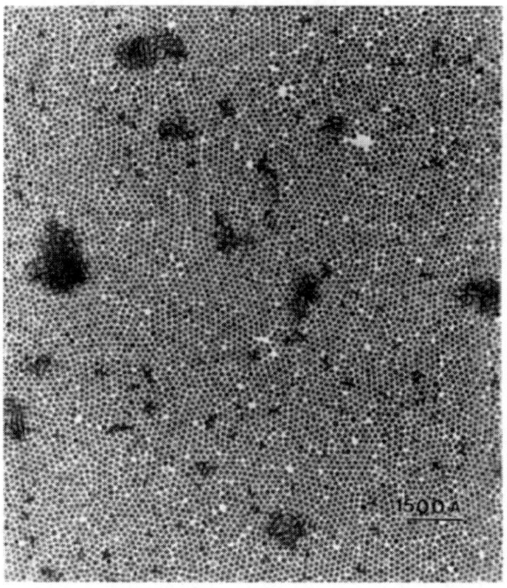

Figure 4. Electron micrograph of a 2D gold colloid monolayer prepared on carbon-coated copper grids (coating thickness 100 Å) by electrophoresis of a 0.5 mM citrate stabilized Au sol at an applied positive voltage of 50 mV. Reprinted with permission from ref 27. Copyright 1993 American Chemical Society.

citrate stabilized AuNPs were equilibrated with suitable water soluble thiolates for several hours. The entire citrate molecules were replaced from the particles surface and resulting new thiol stabilized AuNPs. The reason for gold binding specifically to sulfur atom of the thiol group is due to soft-soft interaction based on hard soft acid base concept.

One year later, Brust and Schiffrin [28,29] published a method for AuNPs synthesis which has a considerable impact on the overall field in less than a decade because it allowed the facile synthesis of thermally stable and air-stable AuNPs of reduced dispersity and controlled size for the first time. In this method, the gold colloids are sterically stabilized by organic molecules having thiol, amide or acid groups in contrast to the citrate reduction method where the gold colloids are kinetically stabilized in aqueous solutions by an electrical double layer [28,29]. The main advantage of the Brust method is that the gold particles behave in a way as chemical compounds. These AuNPs can be repeatedly isolated and redissolved in common organic solvents without irreversible aggregation or decomposition, and they can be easily handled and functionalized just as stable organic and molecular compounds. Further, several stabilization agents with thiol, amide or acid groups can be used to sterically stabilize the gold colloids. Therefore, interesting hybrid materials can be prepared by using this method. In 1994, they have reported the synthesis of AuNPs in a two-phase system as inspired by Faraday [28]. The two-phase redox reactions can be carried out by an appropriate choice of redox reagents present in the adjoining phases. In this case, $HAuCl_4$ was transferred from aqueous solution to toluene using tetraoctylammonium bromide (TOAB) as the phase-transfer reagent and reduced with aqueous $NaBH_4$ in the presence of dodecanethiol. The organic phase changes color from orange to deep brown within a few seconds upon addition of $NaBH_4$. The overall reaction is summarized in the below equations where the source of electrons are BH_4^-.

$$AuCl_4^-(aq) + N(C_8H_{17})_4^+(C_6H_5Me) \longrightarrow N(C_8H_{17})_4^+AuCl_4^-(C_6H_5Me) \quad (2)$$

$$mAuCl_4^-(C_6H_5Me) + nC_{12}H_{25}SH(C_6H_5Me) + 3me^- \longrightarrow$$

$$4mCl^-(aq) + (Au_m)(C_{12}H_{25}SH)_n(C_6H_5Me) \quad (3)$$

The preparation method was as follows: an aqueous solution of $HAuCl_4$ (30 ml, 30 mmol dm^{-3}) was mixed with a solution of TOAB in toluene (80 ml, 50 mmol dm^{-3}). The two-phase mixture was vigorously stirred until all the $HAuCl_4$ was transferred into the organic layer and dodecanethiol (170 mg) was then added to the organic layer. A freshly prepared aqueous solution of $NaBH_4$ (25 ml, 0.4 mol dm^{-3}) was slowly added with vigorous stirring. Further stirring for 3 h the organic phase was separated, evaporated to 10 ml in a rotary evaporator and mixed with 400 ml ethanol to remove excess thiol. The mixture was kept for 4 h at -18°C and the dark brown precipitate was filtered off and washed with ethanol. The crude product was dissolved in 10 ml toluene and again precipitated with 400 ml ethanol. The TEM images of the thiol derivatized AuNPs are shown in Figure 5. An unusual property of these thiol-derivatized AuNPs is that they can be handled and used as a simple chemical compound.

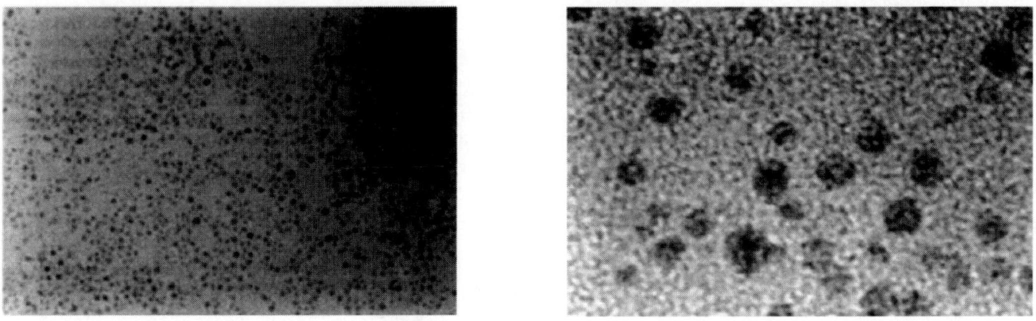

(a) (b)

Figure 5. TEM images of the thiol derivatised AuNPs at (a) low and (b) high magnification. Reprinted with permission from ref 28. Copyright 1994 Royal Society of Chemistry.

Later in 1995, the same group reported the single phase synthesis of AuNPs using a mercapto compound as a stabilizing agent [29]. $HAuCl_4$ (0.76 mmol) and p-mercaptophenol (1.8 mmol) were dissolved in methanol (150 ml). Acetic acid (3 ml) was added to the mixture to prevent the deprotonation of p-mercaptophenol and 30 ml of freshly prepared 0.4 mol dm^{-3} aqueous $NaBH_4$ were added carefully in small portions of 1 ml with vigorous stirring. The solution turned brown immediately indicating the formation of gold clusters with a size around 2~5 nm. Further stirring for 30 min the solvent was removed under reduced pressure without exceeding a temperature of 50°C, and the dark-brown residue was washed thoroughly with diethyl ether to remove excess p-mercaptophenol. After evaporation of diethyl ether the material was washed with water to remove borates and acetates and dissolved in propan-2-ol and then dried over anhydrous Na_2SO_4. The solvent was removed under reduced pressure to give 162 mg of the pure product as a dark-brown solid. The average particle diameter was found to be 5 nm.

The synthesis of colloidal AuNPs reported by both Turkevitch and Frens methods has several drawbacks. The particle concentration is low (typically pM), the particles are polydisperse, and the success in making a predetermined particle diameter is low compared to that of small particle syntheses. Moreover, it is extraordinarily difficult to produce particles with the same (mean) diameter for two syntheses carried out under presumably identical conditions. To overcome these difficulties Natan in 1998 [30,31], described a method for enlargement of colloidal Au nanoparticles called "seeding", based on the colloidal Au surface-catalyzed reduction of Au^{3+} by NH_2OH. Here NH_2OH is thermodynamically capable of reducing Au^{3+} to bulk metal and this reaction is dramatically accelerated by AuNP surfaces. As a result, no new particle nucleation occurs in solution, and all added Au^{3+} goes into production of larger particles (Figure 6). The seeding approach to the synthesis of larger colloidal Au nanoparticles is noteworthy in several respects:

i. it produces particles of improved monodispersity relative to the Frens method.
ii. it allows smaller particles to be grown into larger particles of a predetermined size.
iii. it can be applied successfully to surface-confined Au nanoparticles.

These interesting features make NH_2OH/Au^{3+} seeding as a useful tool in the fabrication of colloidal Au-based materials.

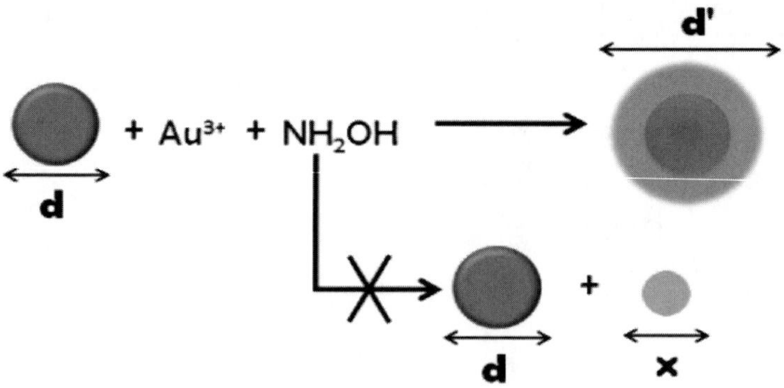

Figure 6. Hydroxylamine seeding of colloidal AuNPs

Other sulfur-containing ligands, such as xanthates, disulfides, di- and trithiols, and resorcinarene tetrathiols have been used to stabilize AuNPs. Apart from sulfur containing ligands, other ligands such as phosphine, phosphine oxide, amine and carboxylic acids.

2.2. Physical Methods

In addition to chemical methods variety of physical methods has been employed for the synthesis of AuNPs. UV irradiation is used to improve the quality of the AuNPs when it is used in synergy with micelles or seeds [32,33]. Near-IR laser irradiation provokes an enormous size growth of thiol-stabilized AuNPs [34]. The presence of an ultrasonic field (200 kHz) allowed the control of the rate of $AuCl_4^-$ reduction in an aqueous solution containing only a small amount of 2-propanol and the sizes of the formed AuNPs are controlled by varying the parameters such as the temperature of the solution, the intensity of the ultrasound, and the positioning of the reactor [35,36]. Sonochemistry was also used for the synthesis of AuNPs within the pores of silica and for the synthesis of Au/Pd bimetallic particles [37,38]. Radiolysis has been used to control the size of AuNPs [39]. Laser photolysis has been used to form AuNPs in block copolymer micelles. Laser ablation is another technique of AuNP synthesis that has been used under various conditions whereby size control can be induced by the laser [40,41].

3. Immobilization of AuNPs on Electrode Surface

This section deals with the ordered immobilization of AuNPs on the solid surface or electrodes. Attachment of AuNPs onto an electrode surface is very important task in developing an electrochemical biosensor. There are numerous approaches to fabricate nanomaterials on electrode surfaces, depending on the exact material and substrate. The modified electrodes usually exhibit different electrochemical and electrocatalytic characteristics even if there is a slight change in the modification procedure. Therefore, it is necessary to discover different electrode materials as well as novel attachment approaches for AuNPs [42]. Generally, AuNPs modified electrode surfaces can be prepared in three major ways:

(a) binding AuNPs with self-assembled monolayers (SAMs) containing different functional groups and sol-gel network
(b) binding AuNPs by layer-by-layer assembly method
(c) direct deposition of nanoparticles onto the bulk electrode surface by electrochemical and Langmuir Blodgett methods.
(d) incorporating colloidal gold onto the electrode surface by mixing the AuNPs with the other composite material.

3.1. Self-Assembly Method

Among the various methods, the simplest method of nanoparticles fabrication on electrode surface which gives some remarkable results is the so-called self-assembly method [44]. Since gold tends to covalently bind with thiol group, the self-assembled monolayer (SAM) of a mercapto functionalized molecule can be easily self-assembled on bulk Au surface by spontaneous adsorption form the solution medium. For fabricating AuNPs on electrode surface usually a bi-functional molecule (either a dithiol or a thiol and amine) is selected and resulting SAM will be in such a way that one thiol moiety will adsorb to the bulk Au surface and the other thiol, or amine moiety will protrude away from the surface. Then the modified electrode is immersed into a colloidal solution of AuNPs for an optimum time period. Since AuNPs have strong affinity towards mercapto or amine functionality, it can easily self-assemble on to the functionalized electrode by displacing the weak stabilizing or capping agents like citrate, TOAB and so on. The commonly used bifunctional molecules for covalently binding AuNPs on electrode surfaces are 1,6-hexanedithiol [44-46], benzenedimethanethiol [47], 4-aminothiophenol [48], 3-mercaptopropyltrimethoxy silane (MPTS) (Figure 7) [49-51], cysteine [52,53], cysteamine [54-56], cystamine [57,58], 1,9-nonanedithiol [59] etc. Similarly SAM prepared by silane molecules on glass surface [60,61], amine functionalized molecules on indium tin oxide (ITO) surface [62,63], carboxylic acid functionalized molecules on titanium dioxide surface were also used for the immobilization of AuNPs on solid electrode surface.

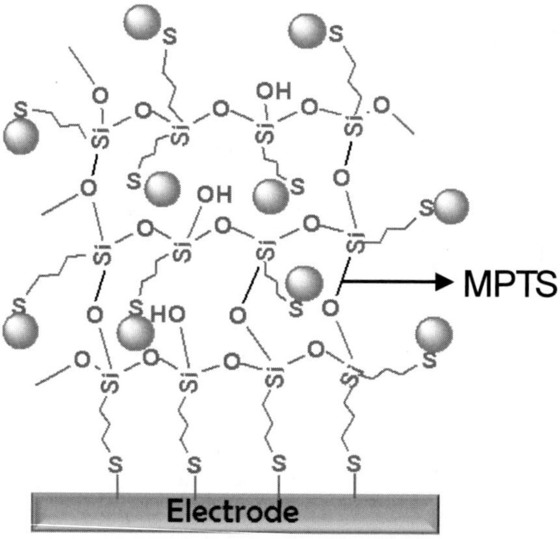

Figure 7. Schematic representation of AuNPs immobilized on sol-gel net work.

Similar to covalent interaction, AuNPs can also be self-assembled onto the electrode surface by electrostatic interaction (Figure 8). Nowadays, electrostatic self-assembly of nanomaterials on functionalized surfaces is a versatile approach for generating monodispersed 2D arrays [64-67]. Surface functionalization can be performed by self-assembly of ionic species of a particular charge onto the substrate. Onto this charged surface, species of the opposite charge can be adsorbed, such as the protecting shell of the nanostructures. An example for the self-assembly of AuNPs on electrode surface through electrostatic interaction is as follows [64]: first, the freshly evaporated gold film electrode was immersed into 11-mercaptoundecanoic acid (MUA) solution in ethanol for over 12 h. The excess of MUA was removed by rinsing with a large amount of absolute ethanol and MilliQ water. Subsequently, the modified gold electrode was immersed into poly-L-lysine (PYLS) (pH 6) for 20 min. The modified electrode was rinsed with copious amounts of MilliQ water and dried under a high-purity nitrogen flow. Then the above modified electrode was immersed in citrate stabilized AuNPs (Figure 8). Thus, adsorption of the negatively charged citrate-stabilized nanoparticles occurs by electrostatic interaction with the positively charged PLYS-terminated film. The number density of particles was controlled by the time of immersion of the modified electrode in colloidal solution.

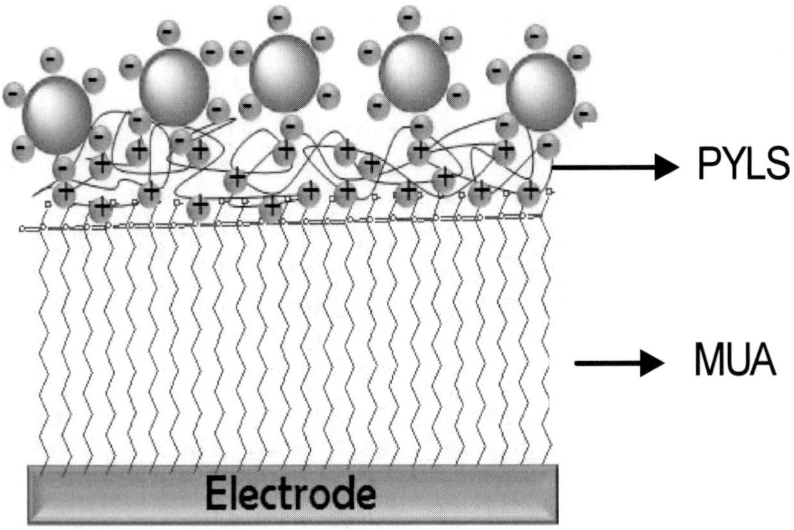

Figure 8. Schematic representation of AuNPs modified electrode prepared by electrostatic interactions.

Although linker molecules such as alkanethiols terminated with amino and thiol functional groups and polymers were successfully used to attach the AuNPs either covalently or electrostatically, the linker molecules often hinder the electron transfer reactions as a non-conductive component on the surface. Therefore, in order to overcome this, very recently direct self-assembly of AuNPs on gold electrode surface without the linker molecule has been reported [68]. In this work, either 2,5-dimercapto-1,3,4-thiadiazole (DMT) or 5-amino-2-mercapto-1,3,4-thiadiazole (AMT) were used as capping agents for the synthesis of AuNPs. The procedure is as follows: 0.5 ml of DMT (1 mM) was added to 44 ml ultrapure water in a round bottom flask with constant stirring under argon atmosphere. Then 5 ml of $NaBH_4$ (0.25%) was added to the stirred solution of DMT followed by the immediate addition of 0.5 ml of $HAuCl_4 \cdot 4H_2O$ (0.0317 M) and the stirring was continued for another 30 min. The color of the solution turns red immediately after the final addition, indicating the formation of AuNPs. For the preparation of AMT-AuNPs, 0.5 mM of the respective compound was used. The presence of free thiolate and amino groups on the surface of the DMT- and AMT-AuNPs, respectively was utilized to self-assemble AuNPs directly on Au surface [68].

3.2. Electrochemical Deposition

So far we have seen the attachment of AuNPs on the electrode surface through suitable functional groups. The other method of binder-free approach is electrodeposition. This is a novel electroless method to fabricate AuNPs on electrode surface without using peculiar binder molecules, which can exert the catalysis of AuNPs in electrochemical measurements and applications. AuNPs were deposited on the surface of a GCE by electrodeposition from a $HAuCl_4$ solution. The procedure involves applying a constant potential of -200 mV for 60 s in an acidic solution containing 1.2 μM $HAuCl_4$ [69]. The AuNPs were also electrochemically deposited along with a suitable stabilizing agent. A simple method for the fabrication of a chitosan film containing AuNPs on electrode surface has been reported [70, 71]. Here, $HAuCl_4$ solution is mixed with chitosan and electrochemically reduced to AuNPs directly, and the produced AuNPs were stabilized by chitosan and subsequently deposited onto the GCE under a certain voltage along with chitosan. Recently, a mesoporous material has been used as a template for the synthesis AuNPs on the electrode surface by electrodeposition method. These materials possess uniform void spaces and these voids served as templates for the formation of nanoparticles. Several kinds of mesoporous silica are commercially available, such as hexagonal mesoporous silica (HSM), mesoporous molecular sieve (MCM-41), and SBA-15. They have a two-dimensional pore structure with a channel diameter of less than 10 nm and a high surface area of up to 1,000 $m^2\ g^{-1}$ [72]. In such pore structure, metal particles can interact with each other only in the same pore and no interaction occurs between the neighboring pores [73]. Nanoparticles deposited on those materials are confined in the pores. Thus, they have controlled size and high dispersion. Initially the electrode material was modified with a mesoporous material. Then the modified electrode was immersed in the solution of $HAuCl_4$ for a period of time to allow $AuCl_4^-$ ion to diffuse into the pores. Subsequently, the potential was adjusted to 0.80 V, and stepwise decreased to 0.65 V for the electrodeposition of AuNPs into the pores [74].

3.3. Langmuir-Blodgett Method

Langmuir–Blodgett (LB) film contains one or more monolayers of an organic material, deposited from the surface of a liquid onto a solid by immersing the solid substrate into the liquid. A monolayer is added with each immersion or emersion step, thus films with very accurate thickness can be formed. The monolayers are usually composed of amphiphilic molecules with a hydrophilic head and a hydrophobic tail. Nowadays, AuNPs with suitable capping agent are attached to the electrode surface similar to that of organic molecule using LB film technique (Figure 9). Fendler and co-workers first demonstrated that surface-modified hydrophobic colloidal nanoparticles may also be organized on the surface of water and their films could be formed on suitable substrates by the LB technique [75]. A number of other groups have now used this method to form multilayer films of AuNPs [76-80], polymer-capped platinum colloidal particles [81], and fullerenes [82]. For the deposition of AuNPs, the key step consists of surface modification of the particles to render them hydrophobic and amenable to organization on the surface of water. In the Brust procedure [28] AuNPs are synthesized and capped with alkanethiols in a non-polar organic phase which continues to be the most popular means of obtaining hydrophobic AuNPs that are readily dispersible in different non-polar/weakly polar organic solvents [76]. Recently, hydrophobic AuNPs in water are also synthesized by electrostatic coupling with fatty amine molecules present in non-polar organic solvents [83].

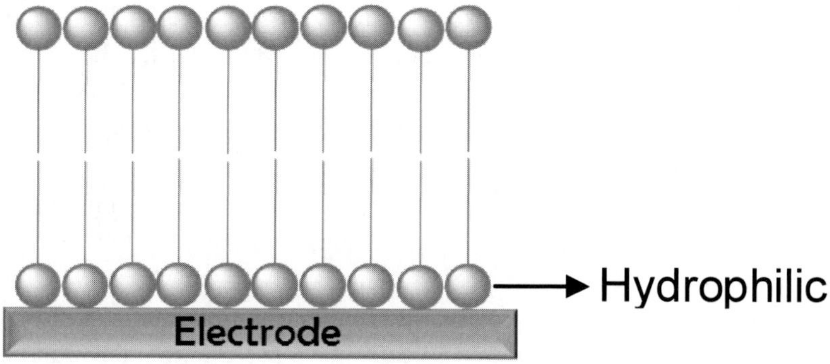

Figure 9. Schematic representation of AuNPs modified electrode prepared by L-B method.

3.4. Spin Coating and Casting

Previously, the immersion method was typically employed to fabricate AuNPs on the electrode surface. Generally, it will take a long time to get a structure with high packing density of nanoparticles by the immersion method. Additionally, large volume of AuNPs solution is required to immerse the substrate completely. It seems to be diametrically opposed to develop large-scale process with low cost. Conversely, the spin coating method is a standard process for applying uniform thin films on various substrates [84-86]. In this technique, initially 0.5 ml of AuNPs solution was placed on the electrode surface and spun out by a spin coater (spin speed of 1000 rpm). Then the substrate was washed with suitable solvent and dried well in N_2 atmosphere [85,86].

Another easy way of attaching AuNPs on electrode surface is by casting method. In this method a known quantity AuNPs dispersed in easily volatile solvent is placed on the electrode surface and allowed to dry [87] (Figure 10).

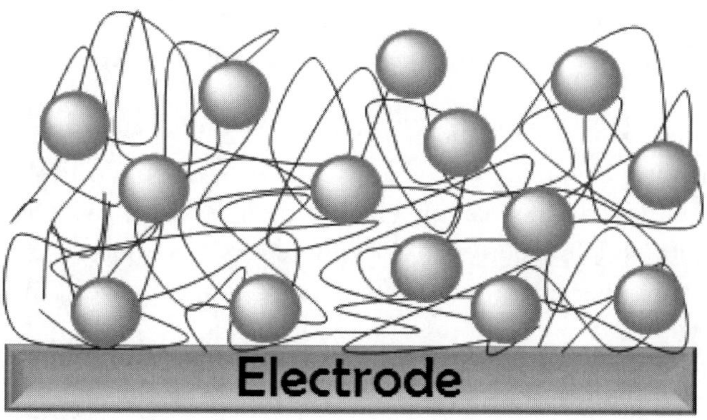

Figure 10. Schematic representation of AuNPs modified electrode prepared by cast method.

4. Conjugation of Bio-Element on AuNPs Surface

The success of the biosensing device mainly depends on the bio-element used. Sometimes bare electrode itself used as a biomolecule recognition element i.e., the transducer itself is acting as a recognition element [88]. But, it often undergoes fouling due to the oxidized product of the corresponding biomolecule. Further the selectivity and sensitivity of the bare electrode is very poor. Thus chemically modified electrodes were used as biomolecule recognition element. These electrodes have good reproducibility, stability, sensitivity, selectivity and no fouling effect [89, 90]. In recent years, AuNPs modified electrode is used as a biomolecule recognition element [12]. In this case the capping agent is playing a versatile role in the sensing of biomolecule. Although variety of electrodes was used as a biomolecule recognition element still there is a question regarding the selectivity? Since the biological fluid, for example blood contains numerous biomolecules, it is a tough job for the chemically modified electrode to selectively sense a particular biomolecule which we are interested. The only way to overcome this problem is using a biological receptor such as enzymes, antibodies, cells or tissues as a bio-element since it has very high bio-activity selectivity and specificity [16]. These molecules can be immobilized as a thin layer at the transducer surface either directly or through a chemical (coupling) or AuNPs which serves as an electronic communicator between the bio-element and the transducer. The conjugation of the biological receptor on the electrode surface is achieved by using the following procedures (Figure 11):

a) *Entrapment of biological receptor behind a membrane*: A thin film of a suitable membrane is formed on the electrode surface which should permit the diffusion of analyte or biomolecule. Before that the enzyme molecules or antibodies are entrapped inside that membrane [13,91].
b) *Entrapment within a polymer matrix*: The electrode surface modified with a thin film of polymer matrix inside which the bio-element is entrapped [11,92-97]. Some commonly used polymer matrix are polyacrylonitrile, polymethacrylate, polypyrrole, polythiophene, agar gel, poly(vinyl) alcohol, polyurethane, sol-gels, cellulose acetate and Nafion.
c) *Bulk modification of entire electrode*: The entire electrode material is modified with the bio-element [98,99]. For example, bio-element modified carbon paste electrode or graphite epoxy resin in which the bio-element is mixed well with the electrode material.
d) *Chemical binding of the bio-element with the SAMs on electrode surface*: First the electrode surface is modified with a suitable SAM molecule. After that the bio-element is either covalently or electrostatically bind with the SAM modified electrode [100,101]. Recently, AuNPs modified electrodes were used to conjugate the bio-element either through a strong chemical bond or weak interaction.

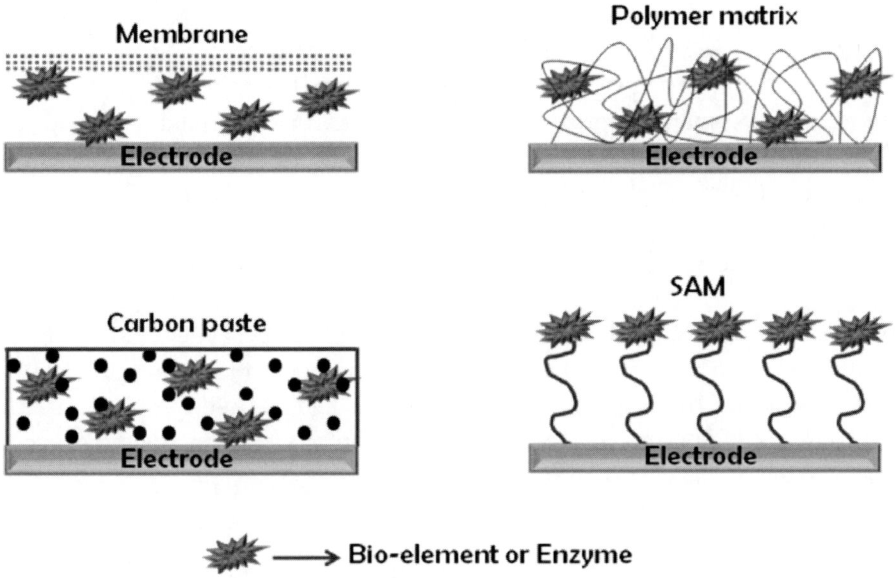

Figure 11. Different types of immobilization of the bio-element on the electrode

Nowadays, enzymatic biosensors utilizing nanomaterials, especially AuNPs, have attracted significant attention in the area of biosensors. Such biosensors use the biospecificity of the enzymatic reaction with the added advantage of AuNPs. Thus, the conjugation of bio-element on AuNPs surface is having lot of advantages when compared to other methods. One of the attracting salient features of AuNPs are the enzyme molecules immobilized on the AuNPs modified electrode could retain their bioactivity because AuNPs possess good biocompatibility. Thus no chemical modification is required prior to bioconjugation. Further, AuNPs itself used as a biomolecule recognition element without using any enzymes or antibodies for sensing variety of biomolecules.

4.1. Bioconjugation through Covalent Bond

Covalent binding of biomolecules via direct coupling to the surface of metal nanoparticles represents a simple conjugation strategy. Among the different metal nanoparticles, the conjugation strategy is best suited for AuNPs because of its high affinity towards the sulfur atom of the thiols and also the amine functionality to form a covalent bond. Generally, covalent conjugation of biomolecules at the surface of AuNPs can be mediated via a bi-functional cross-linker molecule. Monolayer protected AuNPs with bi-functional groups such as –SH at one end and –COOH or $-NH_2$ or even another –SH at the other end have been used in the direct coupling of biomolecules. Zhang et al. reported a feasible method to construct a covalently bound nanoparticle-enzyme biosensor [102]. Briefly, AuNPs were first self-assembled on gold electrode by dithiol (1,6-hexanedithiol) via Au–S bond. A cystamine monolayer was then chemisorbed onto those AuNPs through the thiol moiety and the amino groups are projecting away from the AuNPs surface. The exposed arrays of amino groups will then react with aldehyde groups of periodate oxidized *glucose oxidase* (GOx) via the well known Schiff base reaction. Oxidization of carbohydrate groups on the peripheral surface of the GOx into aldehydes with periodate is an established method [103-106], and proved to retain the activity of GOx [106].By this means, GOx could be covalently attached to the electrode surface, resulting in a stable biosensing interface. The same group just replaced 1,6-hexanedithiol with (3-mercaptopropyl)trimethoxysilane (MPTS) and repeated the same procedure to immobilize GOx [107]. In some reports, the enzyme molecule was covalently attached to the electrode surface through the Schiff base condensation reaction [108-111]. In another report, GOx is covalently bound to the electrode through 1-ethyl-3,3-dimethylaminopropyl carbodiimide (EDC) coupling [112]. The procedure is as follows: initially, a carboxylic acid terminated SAM was formed on Au electrode surface using DL-thiorphan. Covalent immobilization of GOx to the carboxylic acid terminated SAM was achieved in two steps. The SAM modified surface was treated first with EDC/NHS in DMF for 48 h at 4 °C, dried by evaporating DMF, and washed out with ethanol to remove the unreacted residues. Finally, the covalent immobilization of GOx was done by placing a few drops of the enzyme on the electrode surface.

4.2. Bioconjugation Via without Chemical Bond

Immobilization of enzyme molecule can also be done through several non covalent approaches. Casting was the widely used method to immobilize the enzyme molecule on the electrode surface. Zhao et al. used Nafion film to immobilize GOx and AuNPs on electrode surface [113]. Firstly, 10 μl of the solution containing GOx and AuNPs are placed on the electrode surface and allowed to dry. Secondly, 1 μL of Nafion was casted to stably hold the GOx and AuNPs on the electrode surface. Layer-by-layer deposition of chitosan, AuNPs and GOx on the poly(allylamine) (PAA) modified electrode was reported by Wu et al [114]. Hoshi et al. reported a method to prepare multilayer membranes via the layer-by-layer deposition of GOx and AuNPs on sensor substrates, such as a Pt electrode and a quartz glass plate, to prepare glucose sensors [115]. There are few reports in which electrochemical deposition of a biocomposite film consisting of chitosan, GOx and AuNPs [116-118]. Here a clean electrode was dipped into a solution containing suitable amount of chitosan, GOx and AuNPs and a constant potential of -1.5 V was applied for a particular time period. At this potential, H^+ was reduced to H_2 and as a result the pH near the electrode surface gradually increased. When the pH was higher than 6.3, chitosan became insoluble [119], and chitosan hydrogel incorporated with GOx and AuNPs was electrodeposited on the electrode surface. Li et al. reported a composite film coated glassy carbon electrode which comprises of GOx, DMF, AuNPs and ionic liquid 1-butyl-3-methylimidazolium hexafluophosphate ($BMIMPF_6$) [120]. GOx was also incorporated in carbon paste electrode for sensing glucose [121]. For the preparation of enzyme based carbon paste electrode, initially, a suitable amount of graphite powder, AuNPs, GOx, polyphenol oxidase and albumin were mixed and grounded well. A portion of the above paste was packed firmly into the cavity of a Teflon tube.

5. Sensing of Biomolecules

In this section we will discuss about the importance of some selective biomolecules and how the AuNPs modified electrodes can be used for the selective and stable determinations of these biomolecules.

5.1. Electrochemical Sensors for Glucose

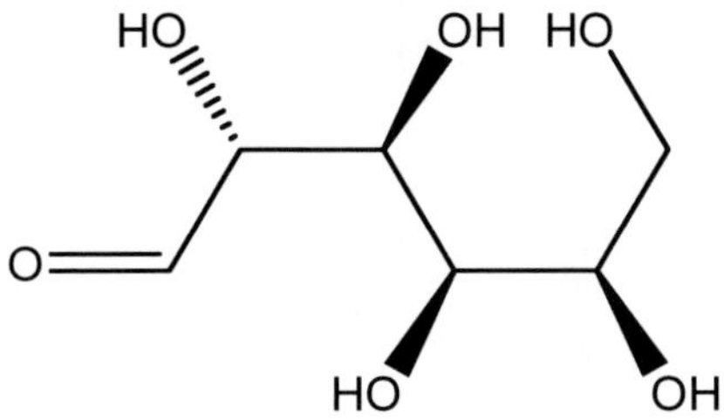

Glucose

Diabetes mellitus often simply referred as "diabetes", which is a major worldwide public health problem. In greek diabetes means "to pass through urine". This metabolic disorder develops due to a diminished production of insulin or resistance to its production which results in the increased blood glucose level. The normal range of blood glucose level is 80-120 mg/dl. As the blood glucose level exceeds this normal level it is known as hyperglycemia and it goes down below 80 mg/dl it is known as hypoglycemia. These effects lead to lot of complications in the body and are one of the leading causes of death and disability in the world. Hyperglycemia results in higher risks of heart disease, kidney failure and blindness. On the other hand, hypoglycemia leads to lethargy, impaired mental functioning, and loss of consciousness or coma stage and finally even death occurs. But the above severe complications can be greatly reduced through stringent personal control of blood glucose level. Thus the diagnosis and management of diabetes mellitus requires a tight monitoring of blood glucose levels. Every day millions of diabetes patient test their blood glucose level and making glucose as the most commonly tested analyte. To be sure, glucose biosensors account for about 85% of the entire biosensor market. Such huge market size makes diabetes a model disease for developing new biosensing concepts. Thus, the invention of new clinically and economically viable glucose biosensor still faces challenge and it leads to a considerable amount of fascinating research and innovative detection strategies [122,123]. Amperometric enzyme electrodes, based on GOx have played a leading role in simple and easy testing of blood glucose and are expected to play a similar role in the move towards continuous glucose monitoring.

In 1962, Clark and Lyons of the cincinnatti children's hospital first developed the enzyme based electrodes for glucose sensing [13,124]. In the design of the original biosensor by them, a solution of GOx was physically entrapped between the gas-permeable membrane of the oxygen measuring Pt electrode and an outer dialysis membrane. The dialysis membrane was of a low molecular weight cutoff such that it will allow glucose and oxygen to pass but not proteins and other macromolecules. The GOx catalyzed oxidation of glucose was the principle behind this measurement. Here GOx oxidizes glucose into gluconic acid by consuming oxygen.

$$\text{Glucose} + O_2 \xrightarrow{\text{Glucose oxidase}} \text{Gluconic acid} + H_2O_2 \qquad (4)$$

$$O_2 + 4H^+ + 4e^- \longrightarrow 2H_2O \qquad (5)$$

The rate of decrease in Po_2 (partial pressure of oxygen) depends on the glucose concentration and the former is monitored by the Po_2 electrode. The concentration of remaining oxygen was measured by applying a negative potential to the platinum electrode where oxygen is reduced to water. In contrary, if the polarizing voltage of the Po_2 is reversed i.e., making platinum electrode positive then it is possible to oxidize H_2O_2 produced in the above reaction to O_2.

$$H_2O_2 \longrightarrow 2H^+ + O_2 + 2e^- \qquad (6)$$

Clark's technology was subsequently transferred to Yellow Spring Instrument (YSI) Company, which launched in 1975 the first dedicated glucose analyzer (the Model 23 YSI analyzer) for direct measurement of glucose in 25 μL whole blood samples. The principle they used for detecting glucose concentration is based on the amperometric detection of H_2O_2. In 1973, Guilbault and Lubrano demonstrated an enzyme electrode for the measurement of blood glucose based on anodic amperometric measuring of H_2O_2 formed as product after the oxidation of glucose [125]. The resulting biosensor offered good accuracy and precision with 100 μL blood samples. A wide range of amperometric enzyme electrodes, differing in electrode design or material, immobilization approach, or membrane composition, has since been described. But there are some drawbacks associated with the measurement of O_2 or H_2O_2 concentration. The above glucose sensor devises rely on the use of oxygen as the physiological electron acceptor and they are subjected to errors resulting from fluctuations in oxygen pressure. In the case of H_2O_2 measurement, it needs large overpotential of +0.7 V or greater for the anodic oxidation of H_2O_2 to oxygen. At such a high potential, many compounds commonly coexisting in biological samples such as uric acid, ascorbic acid etc. can also be electrochemically oxidized, giving electrochemical signals overlapping with that of glucose, which certainly affect the selective and quantitative detection of glucose.

To avoid these difficulties, in 1980s researchers designed a new mediator based second generation glucose biosensor which is able to shuttle electrons from the redox center of the enzyme to the surface of the electrode [126-128]. In this case a mediator is required because GOx does not directly transfer electrons to conventional electrodes because a thick protein layer surrounds its flavin adenine dinucleotide (FAD) redox center. Such thick protein shell introduces a spatial separation of the electron donor-acceptor pair, and hence an intrinsic barrier to direct electron transfers between the enzyme and electrode surface [129]. The minimization of the electron-transfer distance between the immobilized GOx and the electrode surface is crucial for ensuring best performance of the biosensor. Thus, various innovative strategies have been reported for establishing and tailoring the electrical contact between the FAD redox center of GOx and electrode surfaces. The past two decades witnessed extensive research works directed toward the establishment of electrical communication between the redox center (FAD) of GOx and the electrode surface through a mediator. Hence different mediating materials including polymers [130-133], silica sol–gel film [134] and polyacrylamide microgel matrix, [135], paste electrode materials mixed with mediator and/or the enzyme [136,137], and the successive layering of positively charged mediator between the negatively charged enzyme and polyanionic polymer [138,139]. Recently, combination of nanosized materials and biomolecules is of interest in the field of biosensors since AuNPs are playing an important role in the immobilization of biomolecules due to their large specific surface area, excellent biocompatibility and good conductivity [20,21,140]. Generally AuNPs are not toxic to biological systems and also known to provide a microenvironment similar to that of redox proteins in native systems and give protein molecules more freedom in orientation [141]. Several reports have demonstrated that AuNPs can be used as a hopping bridge of electrons between the enzyme's catalytic redox center and electrode surface [142-146]. It has been suggested that the AuNPs placed adjacent to the redox-active center of enzyme could act as a nano collector of electrons and effectively relay them to the electrode [142]. The efficiency of electron taking or releasing of AuNPs in biosensors has been explained with quantum size effect [143] and biocompatibility to the attached protein structure [144].

Zhao et al. reported glucose oxidation based on the combination of GOx and AuNPs immobilized in Nafion film on glassy carbon electrode [113]. The immobilized GOx displayed a pair of well-defined and nearly reversible redox peaks with a formal potential ($E°'$) of -0.434 V in 0.1 M pH 7.0 phosphate buffer solution. The redox peak is due to surface confined electrode process which is confirmed by varying the scan rate. The experimental results were also demonstrated that the immobilized GOx retained its electrocatalytic activity for the oxidation of glucose. The modified electrode was used for stable sensing of glucose with a detection limit of 3.4×10^{-5} M at a signal to noise ratio of 3. There are several reports based on electrodes modified with AuNPs and GOx in which GOx is covalently attached by the well known Schiff base condensation reaction between the aldehyde group of GOx and amine group of the linker molecule [113, 147-151]. The multilayer film of cysteamine, GOx, and AuNPs was constructed by layer-by-layer covalent attachment approach [110]. The biosensors constructed after six bilayers of GOx and AuNPs showed a wide linear response to glucose in the range of 1×10^{-5} to 1.3×10^{-2} M, with a fast response less than 4 s, high sensitivity of 5.72 $\mu A\ mM^{-1}\ cm^{-2}$, as well as good stability and long-term life. A novel amperometric glucose biosensor based on the nine-layers of multilayer films composed of multi-wall carbon nanotubes (MWCNTs), AuNPs and GOx was reported [148]. The biosensor was prepared by first immersing a platinum electrode in poly(allylamine) (PAA), MWCNTs, cysteamine and AuNPs, respectively, followed by the adsorption of GOx. This leads to the one layer of multilayer films on the surface of Pt electrode. Repeating the above process could assemble different layers of multilayer films on the Pt electrode. The modified electrode showed a wide linear range of 0.1-10 mM for glucose, with a remarkable sensitivity of 2.527 $\mu A\ mM^{-1}\ cm^{-2}$ and a detection limit of 6.7 μM. The bienzymatic sensor was fabricated by covalent attachment of periodate-oxidized glucose oxidase (IO_4^--GOx) and horseradish peroxidase (HRP) on controlled multilayer films of sulfonate-capped AuNPs and thionine (SCAuNPs/TH) [149]. Using LBL deposition method, SCAuNPs and TH were deposited alternately on gold electrode through the electrostatic and covalent interactions. The biosensor constructed with six bilayers of SCAuNPs/TH showed a good performance of glucose detection with a response time of less than 20 s, acceptable sensitivity of 3.8 μA mM^{-1} cm^{-2} and the detection limit of 3.5×10^{-5} M. A good method to fabricate glucose biosensor was developed by immobilizing GOx on AuNPs, which was self-assembled on Au electrode modified with a three-dimensional network of (3-mercaptopropyl)trimethoxysilane (MPTS) [107]. This sensor exhibited fast amperometric response (3 s) to the mediated electrocatalyzed oxidation of glucose, and the catalytic current is proportional to the concentration of glucose up to 6 mM with a sensitivity of 8.3 μA mM^{-1} cm^{-2}. The detection limit of the sensor was estimated to be 23 μM. In addition, the sensor has good reproducibility, and can remain stable over 60 days.

Recently, composite film comprising of electrodeposited chitosan (CS) along with AuNPs and GOx has showed promising glucose sensor with high sensitivity and practical utility [116, 151-153]. A new strategy for fabricating glucose biosensor was presented by layer-by-layer assembled (CS)/AuNPs/GOx multilayer film modified Pt electrode [152]. The amperometric biosensor formed by six layers showed best response towards glucose oxidation. It showed a wide linear range of 0.5-16 mM, with a detection limit of 7.0 μM estimated at a signal-to-noise ratio of 3 and fast response time (within 8 s). Moreover, it exhibited good reproducibility, long-term stability and interference free. An improved amperometric glucose biosensor was constructed in situ by incorporating GOx within the electrodeposited chitosan–AuNPs hybrid film on a Prussian Blue modified electrode [150]. The method is simple and controllable. It combined the merits of in situ immobilizing biomolecules in the chitosan–AuNPs hybrid film by electrochemical method and the synergic catalysis effects of PB and GOx molecule. The biosensor prepared under optimal conditions showed fast response time (3 s), high sensitivity (69.26 μA mM^{-1} cm^{-2}), long-term operational stability, good suppression of interference and low detection limit (6.9×10^{-7} M). This biosensor was also successfully applied to determine the glucose concentration in human serum samples.

5.2. Electrochemical Sensors for Ascorbic Acid

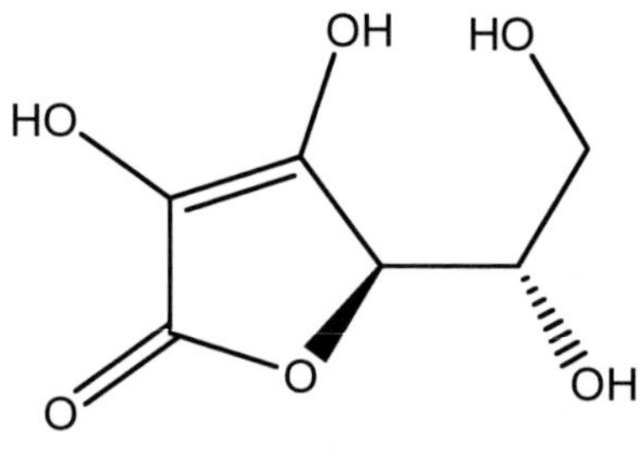

Ascorbic acid

Ascorbic acid (AA) acts as a powerful antioxidant because it can donate a hydrogen atom and form a relatively stable ascorbyl free radical. Many reactive oxygen and nitrogen oxide species are superoxide radical ion, hydrogen peroxide, the hydroxyl radical, singlet oxygen and nitric oxide. Since these species contain an unpaired electron they are highly reactive and creates damages to humans at the molecular level. This is due to their interaction with *nucleic acid*, proteins, and lipids. Reactive oxygen species oxidize (take electrons from) ascorbate first to monodehydroascorbate and then dehydroascorbate. The reactive oxygen species are reduced to water, while the oxidized forms of ascorbate are relatively stable and unreactive and do not cause cellular damage. AA enhances the non-heme iron absorption. A study by Hallberg (1987) showed that iron absorption from non-heme food sources can be increased significantly with a daily AA intake of at least 25 mg for each meal. This water-soluble vitamin is important in forming collagen, a protein that gives structure to bones, cartilage, muscle, and blood vessels. AA is a reducing agent which is necessary to maintain the enzyme prolyl hydroxylase in an active form, most likely by keeping its iron atom in a reduced state. It protects folic acid reductase, which converts folic acid to folinic acid, and may help release free folic acid from its conjugates in food [1,2].

Severe deficiency of AA causes scurvy. Symptoms appear when the concentration of AA in serum level falls below 0.2 mg/dl. Otherwise when the amount of AA falls less than 300 mg in the total body fluid then the symptoms of scurvy arises while the maximum body concentration allowed is 2 g. Several recognized symptoms of AA deficiency includes follicular hyperkeratosis, swollen and inflamed gums, loosening of teeth, dryness of the mouth and eyes, loss of hair, anemia and dry itchy skin. These symptoms reflect the role of AA in the maintenance of collagen and blood vessel integrity. The psychological manifestations of scurvy include depression and hysteria. The above disorders can be prevented with at least 10 mg of AA per day, an amount easily obtained through consumption of fresh fruits and vegetables. AA is widely distributed in fresh fruits and leafy vegetables such as guava, mango, papaya, cabbage, mustard leaves and spinach [154]. It is the least stable of all vitamins and is easily destroyed during processing and storage. Exposure to oxygen, prolonged heating in the presence of oxygen, contact with minerals (iron and copper) and exposure to light will destruct the AA content of foods.

While scanning the literature we can find huge number of papers published in the electrochemical sensing of AA for the past several decades. Besides this huge number of papers published for sensing of AA still it is gaining interest because of its importance. Recently, AuNPs modified electrodes have been exploited for the selective and stable sensing of AA.

Sivanesan et al. describes a method for the electrocatalytic oxidation of AA in phosphate buffer solution by the immobilized citrate capped AuNPs on 1,6-hexanedithiol (HDT) modified Au electrode [46]. The AuNPs fabricated electrode exhibits excellent electrocatalytic activity towards the oxidation of AA by enhancing the oxidation peak current to more than two times with a 210 mV negative shift in the oxidation potential when compared to a bare Au electrode. The oxidation peak of AA at AuNPs electrode was highly stable upon repeated potential cycling and the lowest detection limit achieved was 1 μM using differential pulse voltammetry (DPV). The common physiological interferents such as glucose, oxalate ions and urea do not show any interference within the detection limit of AA. The selectivity of the AuNPs modified electrode was illustrated by the determination of AA in the presence of uric acid. Zhang et al. reported a method for attaching AuNPs on GC electrode surface through a thiol terminated monolayer and it has been applied to the electrocatalytic oxidation of AA which reduces the overpotential by about 200 mV with obviously increased current when compared to bare GC electrode [155]. Further the AuNPs modified electrode resolved the overlapped voltammetric waves of AA and dopamine into two well-defined peaks with peak-to-peak separation of about 300 mV. Thus this electrode can be used for the selective determination of AA in the presence of dopamine. The catalytic current obtained from DPV is linearly dependent on AA concentration over the range of 6.5 x 10^{-6} to 1.45 x 10^{-4} M with correlation coefficient of 0.998 in the presence of dopamine. The detection limit for AA was found to be 2.8 x 10^{-6} M. Kannan and John reported a new method of single step attachment of 2,5-dimercapto-1,3,4-thiadiazole (DMT), 5-amino-2-mercapto-1,3,4-thiadiazole (AMT) stabilized AuNPs on Au electrode surface and used it for electrochemical sensing of AA [68]. The modified electrode enhances the oxidation current of AA by twice and in addition more than 200 mV negative shifts in the oxidation potential in contrast to bare Au electrode. Kalimuthu and John demonstrated the size dependent electrocatalytic oxidation of AA using various sizes (2.6, 12.6, 20, 40 and 60 nm) of citrate stabilized AuNPs incorporated into 3-MPTS sol-gel network on Au electrode [51]. Since the surface area of 2.6 nm AuNPs modified electrode was higher than other AuNPs, it shows less overpotential and increased current response for AA oxidation. The AuNPs modified electrodes resolve the oxidation peak of AA and UA and interestingly the peak separation was identical (180 mV) irrespective of the size of AuNPs though the oxidation potentials of them were shifted to more positive potentials.

Recently, a new kind of AuNPs modified electrode was reported by self-assembling AuNPs to the surface of L-cysteine modified glassy carbon electrode [156]. The modified electrode showed an excellent electrocatalytic activity towards uric acid (UA) and AA with nearly 0.31 V separation between the oxidation potentials of them. The anodic currents of UA and AA at the AuNPs modified electrode were 6 and 2.5 fold to that of the bare GCE, respectively. Using DPV technique, a highly selective and simultaneous determination of UA and AA has been explored at the modified electrode. DPV peak currents of UA and AA increased linearly with their concentration at the range of 6.0×10^{-7} to 8.5×10^{-4} mol L^{-1} and 8.0×10^{-6} to 5.5×10^{-3} mol L^{-1}, respectively. The proposed method was applied for the detection of UA and AA in human urine with satisfactory result.

5.3. Electrochemical Sensors for Uric Acid

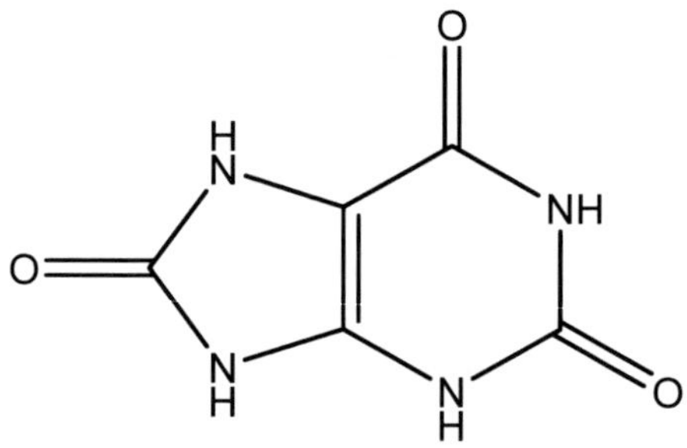

Uric acid

Uric acid (UA) is the primary end product of catabolism of purine nucleosides adenosine and guanosine and has often been regarded as a key biomarker in evaluation of physiological wellbeing [157,158]. In healthy human, UA is filtered and removed from the blood by the kidneys and excreted through urine and hence kidney diseases are known to affect uric acid levels. The normal UA levels range from 4.1 to 8.8 and 250–750 mg dl^{-1} in serum and urinary excretion, respectively [159]. Abnormal level of UA in blood stream leads to several diseases and disorders such as gout, uremia, leukemia, pneumonia, hyperuricemia and the Lesch–Nyhan syndrome [160,161]. Gout results from the deposition of monosodium urate crystals in a variety of soft tissues throughout the body especially in joints resulting in a very painful inflammatory condition. Furthermore, recent findings have suggested that mild hyperuricemia may have a pathogenic role in the development of hypertension, vascular disease, and renal disease [162-165]. Therefore, in order to diagnose patients suffering from a series of disorders associated with altered purine metabolism, the screening of UA in human physiological fluids is an indispensable target of measurement.

During the initial stage of development of UA sensor, researchers used uricase enzyme (UOx) based electrodes for the determination of UA where UOx serves as a molecular recognition element. In the enzyme based electrodes UOx will oxidize UA to allantoin in the presence of O_2 and gives away CO_2 and H_2O_2 as side products. The equation for the enzymatic oxidation of UA is:

$$\text{Uric acid} + O_2 + H_2O \xrightarrow{\text{Uricase}} \text{Allantoin} + H_2O_2 + CO_2 \qquad (7)$$

Here UA concentration is indirectly determined by measuring the increased level of CO_2 or decreases level of O_2. Another alternative method for the determination of UA is amperometric determination H_2O_2 and these indirect gas sensing devices have severe drawbacks as we seen in the case of glucose sensing [166-168]. To overcome these drawbacks, nowadays researchers are using chemically modified electrodes, especially AuNPs fabricated electrodes for determining UA concentration.

Yogeswaran et al., designed a new bimetallic nanoparticles (Au and Pt) modified electrodes for simultaneous determination of AA, EP and UA [169]. First, a composite film comprising of functionalized multiwall carbon nanotubes and nafion was formed on the GC electrode. Then Au and Pt NPs were electrochemically deposited on to the composite film modified GC electrode. The voltammetric peaks of AA, EP and UA are well resolved with the peak separations of 222 mV and 131 mV respectively. Lu et al., demonstrated the determination of UA on GC electrode electrodeposited with AuNPs and DNA [170]. Clean GC electrode was immersed into a AuNPs colloidal solution and a potential of +1.5 V is applied for 60 min for the deposition of AuNPs. Then the electrode was dipped into a DNA solution (0.1 mg/ml) and a potential of +1.5 V is applied for 30 min to electrodeposit DNA. Finally, DNA/AuNPs modified electrode excellently separates the voltammetric signals of UA, NEP and AA. Li et al., electrodeposited AuNPs on the GC electrode modified with the ultrathin overoxidized polypyrrole film [171]. The modified determines the UA in the presence of EP and AA with a lowest detection limit of 1.2×10^{-8} M.

5.4. Electrochemical Sensors for Neurotransmitters

Neurological research has identified over 50 kinds of neurotransmitters. Scientists have found that several neurotransmitters are directly related to mental health problems. The important neurotransmitters are dopamine, serotonin epinephrine and norepinephrine.

5.4.1. Dopamine

Dopamine (DO) was discovered by Arvid Carlsson and Jils-Ake Hillarp at the Laboratory for Chemical Pharmacology of the National Heart Institute of Sweden, in 1952.

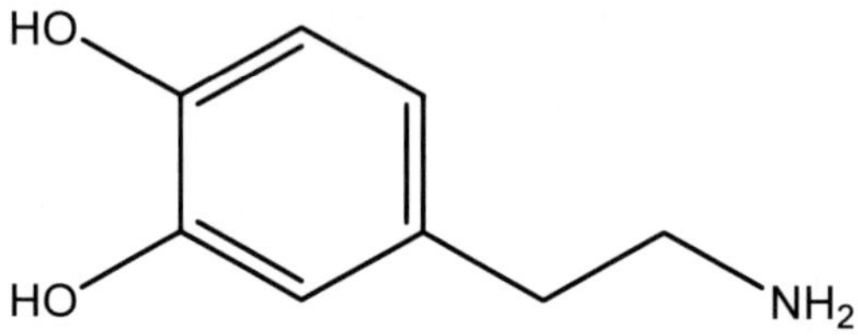

Dopamine

It was named Dopamine because it was a monoamine, and its synthetic precursor was 3,4-dihydroxyphenylalanine (L-DOPA). He was awarded Nobel Prize in 2000 along with Eric Kandel and Paul Greengard in Medicine for showing that dopamine is not just a precursor of noradrenaline and adrenaline, but also neurotransmitter as well. DO is a type of neurotransmitter naturally produced in by the human body. It is also a neurohormone released by the hypothalamus. It is a chemical messenger that is similar to adrenaline and affects the brain processes that control movement, emotional response, and the capacity to feel pleasure and pain. It is vital for performing balanced and controlled movements [172,173]. In the extra-cellular fluid of the central nervous system, the basal DO concentration is very low (0.01-1μM). Abnormal levels of DO have been linked with Parkinson's disease, Tourette's syndrome, Schizophrenia, attention deficit hyperactive disorder and generation of pituitary tumours [174-176].

5.4.2. Serotonin

Serotonin (5-hydroxytryptamine, or 5-HT) is a monoamine neurotransmitter synthesized in serotonergic neurons in the central nervous system (CNS) and enterochromaffin cells in the gastrointestinal tract of animals including humans. In the central nervous system, serotonin plays an important role as a neurotransmitter in the modulation of anger, aggression, temperature regulation, muscle contraction, sleep, sexuality, appetite, endocrine regulation and metabolism, as well as stimulating vomiting [177-179].

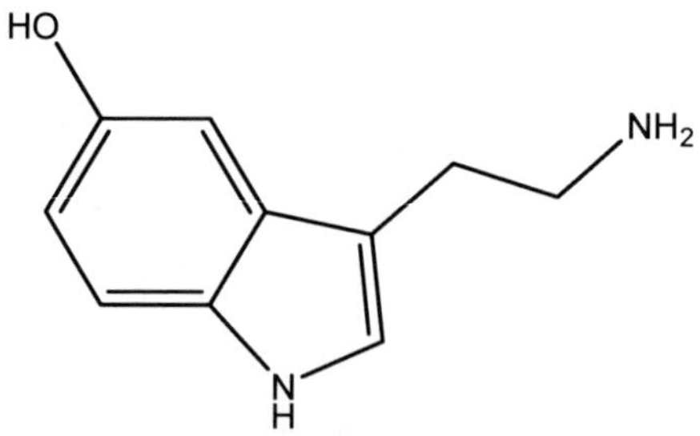

Serotonin

5.4.3. Epinephrine

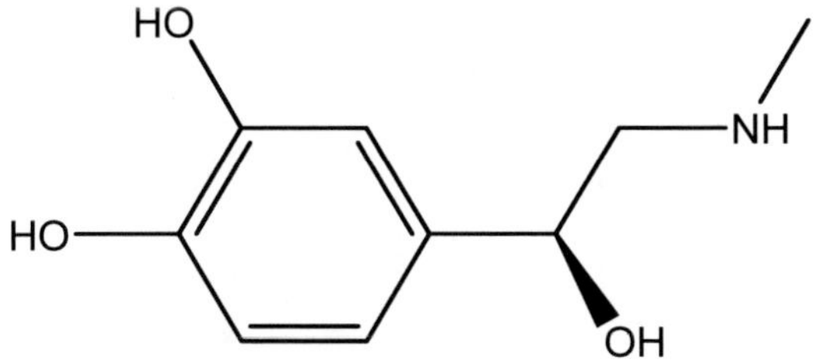

Epinephrine

Epinephrine (EP), a neurotransmitter, widely called as adrenaline is a hormone secreted by the medulla of the adrenal glands. It is as an important chemical mediator for conveying nerve impulse in the mammalian central nervous systems. It is also known as 'fight' or 'flight' hormone and when secreted into the bloodstream, it rapidly prepares the body for action in emergency situations[180, 181]. The hormone boosts the supply of oxygen and glucose to the brain and muscles, while suppressing other non-emergency bodily processes (digestion in particular) [2]. It increases heart rate and stroke volume, dilates the pupils, and constricts arterioles in the skin and gastrointestinal tract while dilating arterioles in skeletal muscles. It elevates the blood sugar level by increasing catabolism of glycogen to glucose in the liver, and at the same time begins the breakdown of lipids in fat cells. Like some other stress hormones, epinephrine has a suppressive effect on the immune system. Further, EP is used as a drug to treat cardiac arrest and bronchodilator for asthma patients [180].

5.4.4. Norepinephrine

Norepinephrine (NE) or noradrenaline is a catecholamine which plays a dual role as a hormone and a neurotransmitter. Along with epinephrine, NE is also underlies the fight-or-flight response, directly increasing heart rate, triggering the release of glucose from energy stores, and increasing blood flow to skeletal muscle. However, when NE acts as a drug it will increase blood pressure. It is released from the adrenal medulla into the blood as a hormone, and is also a neurotransmitter in the central nervous system and sympathetic nervous system where it is released from noradrenergic neurons [180,181].

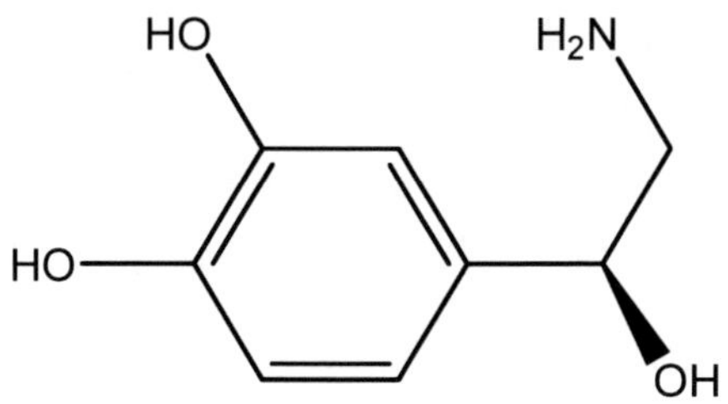

Norepinephrine

So far we have seen the significance of the very important neurotransmitters. In the second part we are going to see how the concentration of these neurotransmitters are electrochemically determined by AuNPs modified electrode.

Kumar et al., demonstrated the electrochemical determination of DO using AuNPs incorporated poly (3,4-ethylenedioxythiophene) (PEDOT) modified GC electrode [182]. Using Brust two-phase method PEDOT stabilized AuNPs was synthesized. Then by applying the potential, AuNPs/PEDOT is electrochemically deposited on to the electrode surface where the conducting PEDOT provides the matrix for the incorporation of AuNPs. The above modified electrode shows a selective sensing of DO in the presence of AA with a lowest detection limit of 2 nM. Gopalan et al., prepared a polymer film of 4-aminothiophenol (ATP) on GC electrode and AuNPs are electrochemically deposited into the polymer matrix of ATP by electrochemical reduction of $HAuCl_4$ solution [183]. This electrode simultaneously determines the concentration of AA and DO. Further, it is used to determine the concentration of DO in the commercially available dopamine hydrochloride injection. Zuo et al., reported a seed mediated growth of AuNPs on ITO surface and then modified with cyclodextrin by immersing AuNPs modified electrode in 1 mM DMF solution containing cyclodextrin [184]. The modified electrode selectively senses DO in the presence of AA with a lowest detection limit of 3.1 x 10^{-6} M. AuNPs was covalently attached to the free thiol group of cysteamine which was attached to the GC electrode surface by continuous electrochemical potential cycling [185]. Selective sensing of DO in the presence of high concentration of AA was achieved at this electrode. In the DPV experiment the peak current of DO was linear in the concentration range of 1.0 x 10^{-8} mol L^{-1} to 2.5 x 10^{-5} mol L^{-1} with a detection limit of 4.0 x 10^{-9} mol L^{-1}. Further the electrode was practically used for determining the concentration of DO in the injection. A new electrochemical biosensor for DO and 5-HT was developed by Li et al., using AuNPs modified GC electrode [186]. Initially, overoxidized polypyrrole film was prepared on GC surface by electropolymerization of pyrrole followed by electrochemical deposition of AuNPs. The modified electrode shows well resolved voltammetric peaks for DO and 5-HT with a detection limit of 1.0 x 10^{-9} M and 1.5 x 10^{-8} M for 5-HT and DO, respectively. The designed sensor has been successfully applied for the determination of 5-HT and DA in human blood serum and obtained satisfactory results. Goyal et al., reported the simultaneous determination of DO and 5-HT in the presence of high concentration of AA using ITO electrode modified with seed mediated growth of AuNPs [187]. The lowest detection limit of 0.5 nM and 3.0 nM was achieved for DO and 5-HT, respectively. The adequacy of this method was evaluated by applying it to the determination of the content of dopamine in dopamine hydrochloride injections. The proposed procedure was also successfully applied to simultaneously determine DO and serotonin in human serum and urine.

Wang et al., proposed a method for covalently immobilizing AuNPs on the mixed SAM of dithiothreitol (DTT) and dodecanethiol (DDT) on Au electrode [188]. The modified electrode shows good voltammetric response towards EP. The lowest detection limit achieved was 6.0 x 10^{-8} M. AuNPs covalently attached to cysteamine modified GC electrode for sensing EP was reported by Yang et al [189]. The modified electrode shows an excellent electrocatalytic activity for the oxidation of EP in the presence of AA. The catalytic current of EP linearly increases for the concentration range of 1.0 x 10^{-7} to 5.0 x 10^{-4} mol L^{-1} with a detection limit of 4.0 x 10^{-8} mol L^{-1}. Li et al., demonstrated the determination of EP along with UA using AuNPs incorporated into the overoxidized polypyrrole film with a detection limit of 3.0 x 10^{-8} M [171]. The preparation and characterization of an electrodeposited DNA membrane doped with AuNPs for the design of biosensors was demonstrated by Lu et al [190]. This work described the preparation and characterization of an electrodeposited DNA membrane doped with AuNPs for the design of biosensors. The AuNPs were electrochemically deposited on the surface of DNA layer formed on the GC electrode surface. This electrode was successfully used for the selective determination of norepinephrine (NE) in the presence of AA. The reversibility of the electrode oxidation reaction of NE is significantly improved in result of 200 mV negative shift of the voltammetric peak potential on the AuNPs electrode, and a large increase in the peak current in contrast to bare electrode. A detection limit of 5 nM NE is obtained by using DPV in static solutions. The co-existence of a large excess of AA does not interfere with the detection. This electrode shows excellent sensitivity, good selectivity and antifouling properties.

REFERENCES

[1] Cox, M. M.; Nelson, D. L.; *Lehninger Principles of Biochemistry*; 4th ed.; W.H. Freeman & Company: New York, 2004; pp 1-14.
[2] Metzler, D. E.; *Biochemistry-The chemical reactions of living cells*; 2nd ed.; Elsevier Academic Press: San Diego, CA, 2003; pp 1-39.
[3] Fotopoulou, M. A.; Loannou, P. C. *Anal. Chim. Acta* 2002, *462*, 179-185.
[4] Garrido, E. M.; Lima, J. L.; Cristina, D. M. *J. Pharmaceut. Biomed.* 1997, *15*, 845-849.
[5] Du, J. X.; Shen, L. H.; Lu, J. R. *Anal. Chim. Acta* 2003, *489*, 183-189.
[6] Zhang, L.Y.; Qv, S. F.; Wang, Z. L.; Cheng, J. K. *J. Chromatogr. B* 2003,*792*, 381-385.
[7] Wei, S. L.; Song, G. Q.; Li, J. M. *J. Chromatogr. A* 2005, *1098*, 166-171.
[8] Canizares, P.; de Castro, L. *Anal. Chim. Acta*. 1995, *317*, 335-341.
[9] Sorouraddin, M. H.; Manzoori, J. L.; Kargarzadeh, E. *J. Pharmceut. Biomed.* 1998, *18*, 877-881.
[10] Michalowski, J.; Halaburda, P. *Talanta* 2001, *55*, 1165-1171.
[11] Bakker, E.; Qin, Y. *Anal. Chem*. 2006, *78*, 3965-3984.
[12] Pingarron, J. M.; Sedeno, P.Y.; Cortes, A. G. *Electrochim. Acta* 2008, *53*, 5848-5866.
[13] Clark, L.; Lyons, C. *Ann. NY Acad. Sci*. 1962, *102*, 29-45.
[14] Cammann, K. *Fresenius Z Anal. Chem*. 1977, *287*, 1-9.
[15] Albery, W. J.; Craston, D. H. In *Biosensors, Fundamentals and Applications*; Turner, A. P. F.; Karube, I.; Wilson, G. S.; Ed.; Oxford University Press: Oxford, 1987; PP 180
[16] Theavenot, D. R.; Toth, K.; Durst, R. A.; Wilson, G. S. *Pure Appl. Chem*. 1999, *71*, 2333-2348.
[17] Mohanty S. P.; Kougianos, E. *Biosensors: A Tutorial Review*, University of North Texas, Denton, TX 76203
[18] Bergveld, P.; Thevenot, D. R. In *Advances in Biosensors, Supplement 1*; Turner, A. P. F. Ed.; JAI Press: London, UK, 1993; pp 31.
[19] Wang, J. *Analyst* 2005,*130*, 421-426.
[20] Daniel, M. C.; Astruc, D. *Chem. Rev*. 2004, *104*, 293-346.
[21] Shipway, A. N.; Katz, E.; Willner, I. *Chemphyschem*. 2000, *1*, 18-52.
[22] Luo, X.; Morrin, A.; Killard, A. J.; Smyth, M. R. *Electroanalysis* 2006, *18*, 319-326.
[23] Faraday, M. *Philos. Trans*. 1857, *147*, 145-181.
[24] Turkevich, J.; Stevenson, P. C.; Hillier, J. *Discuss. Faraday Soc*. 1951, *11*, 55-75.
[25] Frens, G. *Nature*, 1972, *241*, 20-22.

[26] Frens, G. *Nature Phys. Sci.* 1973, *241*, 19-22.
[27] Giersig, M.; Mulvaney, P. *Langmuir* 1993, *9*, 3408-3413.
[28] Brust, M.; Walker, M.; Bethell, D.; Schiffrin, D. J.; Whyman, R. *J. Chem. Soc., Chem. Commun.* 1994, 801-802.
[29] Brust, M.; Fink, J.; Bethell, D.; Schiffrin, D. J.; Kiely, C. J. *J. Chem. Soc., Chem. Commun.* 1995, 1655-1656.
[30] Brown, K. R.; Natan, M. J. *Langmuir* 1998, *14*, 726-728.
[31] Brown, K. R.; Walter, D. G.; Natan, M. J. *Chem. Mater.* 2000, *12*, 306-313.
[32] Mossmer, S.; Spatz, J. P.; Moller, M.; Aberle, T.; Schmidt, J.; Burchard, W. *Macromolecules* 2000, *33*, 4791-4798.
[33] Sau, T. K.; Pal, A.; Jana, N. R.; Wang, Z. L.; Pal, T. *J. Nanopart. Res.* 2001, *3*, 257-261.
[34] Mallick, K.; Wang, Z. L.; Pal, T. J. *J. Photochem. Photobiol.* 2001, *140*, 75-80.
[35] Reed, J. A.; Cook, A.; Halaas, D. J.; Parazolli, P.; Robinson, A.; Matula, T. J.; Griezer, F. *Ultrason. Sonochem.* 2003, *10*, 285-289.
[36] Okitsu, K.; Yue, A.; Tanabe, S.; Matsumoto, H.; Yobiko, Y. *Langmuir* 2001, *17*, 7717-7720.
[37] Chen, W. Cai, W. P.; Liang, C. H.; Zhang, L. D. *Mater. Res. Bull.* 2001, *36*, 335-342.
[38] Mizukoshi, Y.; Okitsu, K.; Maeda, Y.; Yamamoto, T. A.; Oshima, R.; Nagata, Y. *J. Phys. Chem. B* 1997, *101*, 7033-7037.
[39] Henglein, A.; Meisel, D. *Langmuir* 1998, *14*, 7392-7396.
[40] Bronstein, L.; Chernyshov, D.; Valetsky, P.; Tkachenko, N.; Lemmetyinen, H.; Hartmann, J.; Forster, S. *Langmuir* 1999, *15*, 83-91.
[41] Mafume, F.; Kohno, J. Y.; Takeda, Y.; Kondow, T. *J. Phys. Chem. B* 2002, *106*, 7575-7577.
[42] Zhang, J.; Kambayashi, M.; Oyama, M. *Electroanalysis* 2005, *17*, 408-416.
[43] Nabok, A.; *Organic and inorganic nanostructures*; Artech House: London, 2005; pp 13-59.
[44] Li, J.; Wu, Z.; Wang, H.; Shen, G.; Yu, R. *Sens. Actuat. B-Chem.* 2005, *110*, 327-334.
[45] Liu, Z.; Liu, J.; Shen, G.; Yu, R. *Electroanalysis* 2006, *18*, 1572-1577.
[46] Sivanesan, A.; John, S. A. *Electrochim. Acta* 2007, *52*, 8118-8124.
[47] Abdelrahman, A. I.; Mohammad, A. M.; Okajima, T.; Ohsaka, T. *J. Phys. Chem. B* 2006, *110*, 2798-2803.
[48] Wang, M.; Wang, L.; Wang, G.; Ji, X.; Bai, Y.; Li, T.; Gong, S.; Li, J. *Biosens. Bioelectron.* 2004, *19*, 575-582.
[49] Jia, J.; Wang, B.; Wu, A.; Cheng, G.; Li, Z.; Dong, S. *Anal. Chem.* 2002, *74*, 2217-2223.
[50] Jena, B. K.; Raj, C. R. *Chem. A Euro. J.* 2006, *12*, 2702-2708.
[51] Kalimuthu, P.; John, S. A. *J. Electroanal. Chem.* 2008, *617*, 164-170.
[52] Ozsoz, M.; Erdem, A.; Kerman, K.; Ozkan, D.; Tugrul, B.; Topcuoglu, N.; Ekren, H.; Taylan, M. *Anal. Chem.* 2003, *75*, 2181-2187.
[53] Feng, J. J.; Zhao, G.; Xu, J. J.; Chen, H.Y. *Anal. Biochem.* 2005, *342*, 280-286.
[54] Mena, M. L.; Sedeno, P. Y.; Pingarron, J. M. *Anal. Biochem.* 2005, *336*, 20-27.
[55] Xu, Y. Y.; Bian, C.; Chen, S.; Xia, S. *Anal. Chim. Acta* 2006, *561*, 48-54.
[56] Manso, J.; Mena, M. L.; Sedeno, P. Y.; Pingarron, J. M. *Anal. Biochem.* 2008, *375*, 345-353.

[57] Raj, C. R.; Abdelrahman, A. I.; Ohsaka, T. *Electrochem. Commun*. 2005, *7*, 888-893.
[58] Zhang, S.; Zheng, F.; Wu, Z.; Shen, G.; Yu, R. *Biosens. Bioelectron*. 2008, *24*, 129-135.
[59] Stolarczyk, K.; Bilewicz, R. *Electrochim. Acta* 2006, *51*, 2358-2365.
[60] Olson, L. G.; Lo, Y. S.; Beebe, T. P.; Harris, J. M. *Anal. Chem*. 2001, *73*, 4268-4276.
[61] Ko, W. B.; Yun, J. M.; Jo, S.W.; Shon, Y. S. *Ultrasonics* 2006, *44*, e363-e366.
[62] Cheng, W.; Dong, S.; Wang, E. *Chem. Mater*. 2003, *15*, 2495-2501.
[63] Wang, Y.; Qian, W.; Tan, Y.; Ding, S.; Zhang, H. *Talanta* 2007, *72*, 1134-1140.
[64] Zhao, J.; Bradbury, C. R.; Huclova, S.; Potapova, I.; Carrara, M.; Fermin, D. J. *J. Phys. Chem. B* 2005, *109*, 22985-22994.
[65] Kakkassery, J. J.; Abid, J. P.; Carrara, M.; Fermin, D. J. *Faraday Discuss*. 2004, *125*, 157-169.
[66] Bradbury, C. R.; Zhao, J.; Fermin, D. J. *J. Phys. Chem. C* 2008, *112*, 10153-10160.
[67] Zhao, J.; Bradbury, C. R.; Fermin, D. J. *J. Phys. Chem. C* 2008, *112*, 6832-6841.
[68] Kannan, P.; John, S. A. *Nanotechnology* 2008, *19*, 085602-085611.
[69] Andreescu, S.; Luck, L. A.; *Anal. Biochem*. 2008, *375*, 282-290.
[70] Du, Y.; Luo, X. L.; Xu, J. J.; Chen, H. Y. *Bioelectrochemistry* 2007, *70*, 342-347.
[71] Sugunan, A.; Thanachayanont, C.; Duttaa, J.; Hilborn, J. G. *Sci. Technol. Adv. Mat*. 2005, *6*, 335-340.
[72] Fukuoka, A.; Araki, H.; Kimura, J. I.; Sakamoto, Y.; Higuchi, T.; Sugimoto, N.; Inagaki, S.; Ichikawa, M. *J. Mater. Chem*. 2004, *14*, 752-756.
[73] Bore, M. T.; Pham, H. N.; Switzer, E. E.; Ward, T. L.; Fukuoka, A.; Datye, A. K. *J. Phys. Chem. B* 2005, *109*, 2873-2880.
[74] Yu, J. J.; Lu, S.; Li, J. W.; Zhao, F. Q.; Zeng, B. Z. *J. Solid State Electrochem*. 2007, *11*, 1211-1219.
[75] Fendler, J. H.; Meldum, F. *Adv. Mater*. 1995, *7*, 607-632 and references therein.
[76] Heath, J. R.; Knobler, C. M.; Leff, D. V. *J. Phys. Chem. B* 1997, *101*, 189-197.
[77] Chi, L. F.; Rakers, S.; Hartig, M.; Fuchs, H.; Schmid, G. *Thin Solid Films* 1998, *327–329*, 520-523.
[78] Bourgoin, J. F.; Kergueris, C.; Lefevre, E.; Palacin, S. *Thin Solid Films* 1998, *327–329*, 15-519.
[79] Li, W.; Xu, R.; Wang, L.; Cui, H.; Xi, S. *Mol. Cryst. Liq. Cryst*. 1999, *337*, 185-188.
[80] Burghard, M.; Philipp, G.; Roth, S.; Klitzing, K. V.; Pugin, R.; Schmid, G. *Adv. Mater*. 1998, *10*, 842-845.
[81] Sastry, M.; Patil, V.; Mayya, K. S.; Paranjape, D. V.; Singh, P.; Sainkar, S. R. *Thin Solid Films* 1998, *324*, 239-244.
[82] Ganguly, P.; Paranjape, D. V.; Patil, K. R.; Chaudhari, S. K.; Kshirsagar, S. T. *Ind. J. Chem. A* 1992, *31*, F42-F45.
[83] Sastry, M.; Kumar, A.; Mukherjee, P. *Colloids Surf. A* 2001, *181*, 255-259.
[84] Zhai, L.; McCullough, R. D. *J. Mater. Chem*. 2004, *14*, 141-143.
[85] Liu, F. K.; Changb, Y. C.; Koa, F. H.; Chub, T. C.; Daia, B. T. *Microelectron. Eng*. 2003, *67–68*, 702-709.
[86] Danckwerts, M.; Novotny, L. *Phys. Rev. Lett*. 2007, *98*, 026101-026104.
[87] Maduraiveeran, G.; Ramaraj, R. *Electrochem. Commun*. 2007, *9*, 2051-2055.
[88] John, S. A. *J. Electroanal. Chem*. 2005, *579*, 249-256.

[89] Ramanavicius, A.; Ramanaviciene, A.; Malinauskas, A. *Electrochim. Acta*. 2006, *51*, 6025-6037.
[90] Privett, B. J.; Jae, H. S.; Schoenfisch, M. H. *Anal. Chem*. 2008, *80*, 4499-4517.
[91] Noguer, T.; Marty, J. L. *Anal. Lett*. 1997, *30*, 1069-1080.
[92] Vidal, J. C.; Ruiz, E. G.; Castillo, J. R. *Microchim. Acta*, 2003, *143*, 93-111.
[93] Ahuja, T.; Mir, I. A.; Kumar, R. D. *Biomaterials* 2007, *28*, 791-805.
[94] Yuqing, M.; Jianrong, C.; Xiaohua, W. *Trends in Biotechnology*, 2004, *22*, 227-231.
[95] Perez, J. P. H.; Cabarcos, E. L.; Ruiz, B. L. *Biomol. Eng*. 2006, *23*, 233-245.
[96] Ofir, Y.; Samanta, B.; Rotello, V. M. *Chem. Soc. Rev*. 2008, *37*, 1814-1825.
[97] Wallace, G. G.; Smyth, M.; Zhao, H. Trends in *Anal. Chem*. 1999, *18*, 245-251.
[98] Bremle, G.; Persson, B. Gorton, L. *Electroanalysis* 1991, *3*, 77-86.
[99] Antiochia, R.; Lavagnini, I. *Anal. Lett*. 2006, *39*, 1643-1655.
[100] Willner, I.; Riklin, A. *Anal. Chem*. 1994, *66*, 1535-1539.
[101] Bardea, A.; Katz, E.; Buckmann, A. F.; Willner, I. *J. Am. Chem. Soc*. 1997, *119*, 9114-9119.
[102] Zhang, S.; Wang, N.; Yu, H.; Niu, Y.; Sun, C. *Bioelectrochemistry* 2005, *67*, 15-22.
[103] Zaborsky, O. R.; Ogletree, J. *Biochem. Biophys. Res. Commun*. 1974, *61*, 210-216.
[104] Yoon, H. C.; Hong, M. Y.; Kim, H. S. *Anal. Chem*. 2000, *72*, 4420-4427.
[105] Yoon, H. C.; Kim, H. S. *Anal. Chem*. 2000, *72*, 922-926.
[106] Nakamura, S.; Hayashi, S.; Koga, K. *Biochim. Biophys. Acta* 1976, *445*, 294-308.
[107] Zhang, S.; Wang, N.; Yu, H.; Niu, Y.; Sun, C. *Sens. Actuat. B-Chem*. 2005, *109*, 367-374.
[108] Losada, J.; Armada, M. P. G. *Electroanalysis* 2001, *13*, 1016-1021.
[109] Zhang, S.; Yang, W.; Niu, Y.; Sun, C. *Anal. Chim. Acta* 2004, *523*, 209-217.
[110] Yang, W.; Wang, J.; Zhao, S.; Sun, Y.; Sun, C. *Electrochem. Commun*. 2006, *8*, 665-672.
[111] Bautista, F. M.; Campelo, J. M.; Garcia, A.; Jurado, A.; Luna, D.; Marinas, J. M.; Romero, A. A. *J. Mol. Catal. B-Enzym*. 2001, *11*, 567-577.
[112] Zhang, F.; Cho, S. S.; Yang, S. H.; Seo, S. S.; Cha, G. S.; Nam, H. *Electroanalysis* 2006, *18*, 217-222.
[113] Zhao, S.; Zhang, K.; Bai, Y.; Yang, W.; Sun, C. *Bioelectrochemistry* 2006, *69*, 158-163.
[114] Wu, B. Y.; Hou, S. H.; Yin, F.; Li, J.; Zhao, Z. X.; Huang, J. D.; Chen, Q. *Biosens. Bioelectron*. 2007, *22*, 838-844.
[115] Hoshi, T.; Sagae, N.; Daikuhara, K.; Takahara, K. *J. Anzai, Mat. Sci. Eng. C* 2007, *27*, 890-894.
[116] Luo, X. L.; Xu, J. J.; Du, Y.; Chen, H.Y. *Anal. Biochem*. 2004, *334*, 284-289.
[117] Sheng, Q. L.; Shen, Y.; Zhang, H. F.; Zheng, J. B. *Chinese J. Chem*. 2008, *26*, 1244-1250.
[118] Guang, C. X.; Ying, Q.; Juan, Z. S.; Yong, Z. X. *Acta Chim. Sinica* 2007, *65*, 337-343.
[119] Fernandes, R.; Wu, L. Q.; Chen, T.; Yi, H.; Rublov, G. W.; Ghodssi, R.; Bentley, W. E.; Payne, G. F. *Langmuir* 2003, *19*, 4058-4062.
[120] Li, J.; Yu, J.; Zhao, F.; Zeng, B. *Anal. Chim. Acta* 2007, *587*, 33-40.
[121] Miscoria, S. A.; Barrera, G. D.; Rivas, G. A. *Electroanalysis* 2005, *17*, 1578-1582.

[122] Reach, G.; Wilson, G. S. *Anal. Chem.* 1992, *64*, 381A-386A.
[123] Wang, J. *Chem. Rev.* 2008, *108*, 814-825.
[124] Clark, L. *U.S. Patent* 1970, 33, *539*, 455.
[125] Guilbault, G.; Lubrano, G. *Anal. Chim. Acta* 1973, *64*, 439-455.
[126] Cass, A. E. G; Davis, G.; Francis, G.; Hill, H. A.; Aston, W.; Higgins, I. J.; Plotkin, E.; Scott, L.; Turner, A. P. *Anal. Chem.* 1984, *56*, 667-671.
[127] Hill, H. A. O.; *Eur. Pat. Appl.* EPO 1984, 125,139 A2, *14*, 45-46.
[128] Frew, J.; Hill, H. A. *Anal. Chem.* 1987, *59*, 933A-944A.
[129] Marcus, R. A.; Sutin, N. *Biochim. Biophys. Acta* 1985, *811*, 265-322.
[130] Degani, Y.; Heller, A.; *J. Phys. Chem.* 1987, *91*, 1285-1289.
[131] Ohara, T.; Rajogopalan, R.; Heller, A. *Anal. Chem.* 1994, *66*, 2451-2457.
[132] Miscoria, S. A.; Barrera, G. D.; Rivas, G. A. *Sens. Actuators B-Chem.* 2006, *115*, 205-211.
[133] Retama, J. R.; Ruiz, B. L.; Cabarcos, E. L. *Biomaterials* 2003, *24*, 2965-2973.
[134] Li, T.; Yao, Z. H.; Ding, L. *Sens. Acutat. B-Chem.* 2004, *101*, 155-160.
[135] Retama, J. R.; Cabarcos, E. L.; Ruiz, B. L. *Talanta* 2005, *68*, 99-107.
[136] Patel, H.; Li, X.; Karan, H. I. *Biosens. Bioelectron.* 2003, *18*, 1073-1076.
[137] Lawrence, N. S.; Deo, R.; Wang, J. *Anal. Chem.* 2004, *76*, 3735-3739.
[138] Hodak, J.; Etchenique, R.; Calvo, E. J. *Langmuir* 1997, *13*, 2708-2716.
[139] Calvo, E. J.; Etchenique, R.; Pietrasanta, L.; Wolosiuk, A. *Anal. Chem.* 2001, *73*, 1161-1168.
[140] Guo, S.; Wang, E. *Anal. Chim. Acta* 2007, *598*, 181-192.
[141] Liu, S. Q.; Leech, D.; Ju, H. X. *Anal. Lett.* 2003, *36*, 1-19.
[142] Xiao, Y.; Patolsky, F.; Katz, E.; Hainfeld, J. F.; Willner, I. *Science* 2003, *299*, 1877-1881.
[143] Chen, X.; Li, J.; Li, X.; Jiang, L. *Biochem. Biophys. Res. Commun.* 1998, *245*, 352-355.
[144] Vertegel, A. A.; Siegel, R. W.; Dordick, J. S. *Langmuir* 2004, *20*, 6800-6807.
[145] Zhao, J.; O'Daly, J. P.; Henkens, R. W.; Stonehurner, J.; Crumbliss, A. L. *Biosens. Bioelectron.* 1996, *11*, 493-502.
[146] Willner, I.; Willner, B. *Pure Appl. Chem.* 2002, *74*, 1773-1783.
[147] Kang, X.; Mai, Z.; Zou, X. ; Cai, P. J. Mo, *Anal. Biochem.* 2007, *369*, 71-79.
[148] Wu, B. Y.; Hou, S. H.; Yin, F.; Zhao, Z .X.; Wang, Y. Y.; Wang, X. S.; Chen, Q. *Biosens. Bioelectron.* 2007, *22*, 2854-2860.
[149] Sun, Y.; Bai, Y.; Yang, W.; Sun, C. *Electrochim. Acta* 2007, *52*, 7352-7361.
[150] Xue, M. H.; Xu, Q.; Zhou, M.; Zhu, J. J. *Electrochem. Commun.* 2006, *8*, 1468-1474.
[151] Luo, X. L.; Xu, J. J.; Zhang, Q.; Yang, G. J.; Chen, H. Y. *Biosens. Bioelectron.* 2005, *21*, 190-196.
[152] Du, D.; Ding, J.; Cai, J.; Zhang, A. *Sens. Actuat. B-Chem.* 2007, *127*, 317-322.
[153] Du, Y.; Luo, X. L.; Xu, J. J.; Chen, H. Y. *Bioelectrochemistry* 2007, *70*, 342-347.
[154] Tee, E. S.; Ismail, N. M.; Nasir, A. M.; Kahtijah, I. *Nutrient composition of Malayisan foods*; 4th Ed.; Malaysian Food Composition Database Programme: Kuala Lumpur, 1997; pp 310.
[155] Zhang, L.; Jiang, X.; *J. Electroanal. Chem.* 2005, *583*, 292-299.
[156] Hu, G.; Ma, Y.; Guo, Y.; Shao, S. *Electrochim. Acta* 2008, *53*, 6610-6615.
[157] Smith, T. E. In *Textbook of Biochemistry with Clinical Correlations*; Devlin, T. M.; Ed.; Wiley-Liss: New York, 1992; pp 929.

[158] Dryhurst, G. *Electrochemistry of Biological Molecules*; Academic Press: New York, 1977; pp 71-185.
[159] Kissinger, P. T.; Pachla, L. A.; Reynolds, L. D.; Wright, S. *J. Assoc. Off. Anal. Chem.* 1987, *70*, 1-14.
[160] Yamanaka, H.; Togashi, R.; Hakoda, M.; Terai, C.; Kashiwazaki, S.; Dan, T.; Kamatani, N. *Adv. Exp. Med. Biol.* 1998, *431*, 8-13.
[161] Iseki, K.; Oshiro, S.; Tozawa, M.; Iseki, C.; Ikemiya, Y.; Takishita, S.; Signi, W. *Hypertens Res*. 2001, *24*, 691-697.
[162] Zen, J. M.; Jou, J. J.; Hangovan, G. *Analyst* 1998, *123*, 1345-1350.
[163] Selby, J. V.; Friedman, G. D.; Quesenberry, C. P. *Am J Epidemiol*. 1990, *131*, 1017-1027.
[164] Jossa, F.; Farinaro, E.; Panico, S.; Krogh, V.; Celentano, E.; Galasso, R.; Mancini, M.; Trevisan, M. *J Hum Hypertens*. 1994, *8*, 677-681.
[165] Puig, J. P.; Ruilope, L. M. *J Hypertens*. 1999, *17*, 869-872.
[166] Miland, E.; Ordieres, A. J. M.; Blanco, P. T.; Smyth, M. R.; Fagain, C. O. *Talanta* 1996, *43*, 785-796.
[167] Kuwabata, S.; Nakaminami, T.; Ito, S. I.; Yoneyama, H. *Sens. Actuat. B-Chem*. 1998, *52*, 72-77.
[168] Luo, Y. C.; Do, J. S.; Liu, C. C. *Biosens. Bioelectron*. 2006, *22*, 482-488.
[169] Yogeswaran, U.; Thiagarajan, S.; Chen, S. M. *Anal. Biochem*. 2007, *365*, 122-131.
[170] Lu, L.; Lin, X. *Anal. Sci*. 2004, *20*, 527-530.
[171] Li, J.; Lin, X. Q.; *Anal. Chim. Acta*, 2007, *596*, 222-230.
[172] Jose, P. A.; Eisner, G. M.; Felder, R. A. *Pharm. Therap*. 1998, *80*, 149-182.
[173] Michel, C. D.; Montastruc, J. L.; Tran, M. A. *Hypertens. Res*. 1995, *18*, S119-S124.
[174] Inone, A.; Nakata, Y. *Jpn. J. Pharm*. 2001, *86*, 376-380.
[175] Li, D.; Sham, P. C.; Owen, M. J.; He, L. *Hum. Mol. Gen*. 2006, *15*, 2276-2284.
[176] Kienast, T.; Heinz, A. *CNS Neurol. Disord.: Drug Targets* 2006, *5*, 109-131.
[177] Van, N. J. M.; Janssens, W. J.; Vanhoutte, P. M. *Pharm. Res. Commun*. 1985, *17*, 585-608.
[178] Wise, T. N.; Arnold, L. M.; Maletic, V. *CNS Spectrums* 2005, *10*, 1-13.
[179] Woodley, D.W. *Dis. Nervous Syst*. 1960, *21*, 87-96.
[180] Berg, J. M.; Tymoczko, J. L.; Stryer, L. *Biochemistry*; 5th Ed.; W. H. Freeman: New York, 2002; pp 603-605.
[181] Mathews, C. K.; Holde, K. E. V.; Ahern, K. G. *Biochemy*; 3rd Ed.; Benjamin Cummings: San Francisco, 1999; pp 374.
[182] Kumar, S. S.; Mathiyarasu, J.; Phani, K. L. *J. Electroanal. Chem*. 2005, *578*, 95-103.
[183] Gopalan, A. I.; Lee, K. P.; Manesha, K. M.; Santhosh, P.; Kim, J. H.; Kanga, J. S. *Talanta* 2007, *71*, 1774-1781.
[184] Zuo, F.; Luo, C.; Zheng, Z.; Ding, X.; Peng Y. S. *Chem. Lett*. 2008, *37*, 434-435.
[185] Hu, G. Z.; Zhang, D. P.; Wu, W. L.; Yang, Z. S. *Colloids Surface B* 2008, *62*, 199-205.
[186] Li, J.; Lin, X. *Sens. Actuat. B-Chem*. 2007, *124*, 486-493.
[187] Goyal, R. N.; Gupta, V. K.; Oyama, M.; Bachheti, N. *Talanta* 2007, *72*, 976-983.
[188] Wang, L.; Bai, J.; Huang, P.; Wang, H.; Zhang, L.; Zhao, Y. *Electrochem. Commun*. 2006, *8*, 1035-1040.
[189] Yang, Z.; Hu, G.; Chen, X.; Zhao, J.; Zhao, G. *Colloids Surface. B* 2007, *54*, 230-235.
[190] Lu, L. P.; Wang, S. Q.; Lin, X. Q. *Anal. Chim. Acta* 2004, *519*, 161-166..

In: Nanostructured Materials for Electrochemical Biosensors ISBN: 978-1-60741-706-4
Editors: U. Yogeswaran; S. Kumar; S. Chen ©2009 Nova Science Publishers, Inc.

Chapter 5

WET CHEMICAL DEPOSITION OF METAL NANOPARTICLES AND METAL OXIDE NANOSTRUCTURED FILMS ON ELECTRODE SURFACES FOR BIOELECTROANALYSIS

***Jingdong Zhang*[*1] *and Munetaka Oyama*[†2]**
[1] Huazhong University of Science and Technology, Wuhan, China.
[2] Kyoto University, Kyoto, Japan.

ABSTRACT

Seed-mediated growth of metal nanoparticles on electrode surfaces has been introduced. Using this wet chemical method, gold nanoparticles were successfully deposited on various electrode substrates such as indium tin oxide (ITO) and glassy carbon. The as-prepared gold nanoparticle-modified electrodes showed catalytic activity toward the oxidation of small biomolecules such as dopamine, ascorbic acid, uric acid, epinephrine and norepinephrine, which could improve the sensitivity or selectivity of bioelectroanalysis. The deposited gold nanoparticles were also biocompatible for immobilization of biomacromolecules, namely hemoglobin and myoglobin, on which the direct electron transfer of redox proteins was realized and reagentless H_2O_2 biosensors were provided.

On the other hand, liquid phase deposition (LPD) has been demonstrated as a flexible wet chemical method for preparing metal oxide nanostructured films on electrode surfaces. By the LPD process, electroactive titanium dioxide (TiO_2) films were prepared on graphite, glassy carbon and ITO. The electrochemical properties of such LPD TiO_2 films were dependent upon the film thickness controlled by the deposition time. The LPD technique was easily combined with other techniques, e.g., seed-mediated growth, which could provide metal/metal oxide composite nanomaterials. Moreover, hybrid nanostructured films were facilely obtained by doping dyes, surfactants and other

---

* College of Chemistry and Chemical Engineering, Huazhong University of Science and Technology, Wuhan 430074, China. Tel: +86-27-87792154, Fax: +86-27-87543632, E-mail: zhangjd@mail.hust.edu.cn.
† Department of Material Chemistry, Graduate School of Engineering, Kyoto University, Nishikyo-ku, Kyoto, 615-8520, Japan.Tel. +81-75-383-3074, Fax: +81-75-383-3074, E-mail: m.oyama@kx8.ecs.kyoto-u.ac.jp

materials into the LPD films. These dopants improved the electron transfer kinetics at LPD films by reducing the film resistance and thus making the hybrid films useful for bioelectroanalysis.

1. INTRODUCTION

Metal and semiconductor nanoparticles exhibit attractive properties in electrode modification by increasing the surface area, enhancing the electrode conductivity, facilitating the electron transfer and improving the analytical sensitivity and selectivity [1], thus attracting great research interest for electrochemical analysts. The preparation of nanoparticle-modified electrodes includes the synthesis of nanoparticles and attachment of the nanomaterials to electrodes. There are numerous approaches to fabricating nanomaterials on electrode surfaces, depending on the exact material and substrate. The modified electrodes usually exhibit different electrochemical and electrocatalytic characteristics even if there is a slight change in the modification procedure. Therefore, it is necessary to discover different nano electrode materials as well as novel attachment approaches. Among these, gold nanoparticles are the most popular metal nanomaterials to be attached on electrodes because they provide promising applications to catalysis and biology [2]. Because gold tends to covalently bond with some organic molecules, the traditional gold nanoparticle-modified electrodes are usually fabricated by assembling gold nanoparticles on electrode surfaces using organic linker molecules such as thiols [3-9] and polymers [10,11]. However, these organic layers may reduce the surface conductivity and affect the catalytic reactivity of the nanoparticles [12]. Thus, binder-free attachment of gold nanoparticles onto an electrode surface is desirable. The traditional binder-free approach, namely electrodeposition [13], is expected to avoid this problem. However, it is difficult to control the particle size uniformly in electrodeposition, which usually leads to many large particles appearing with the nanoparticles, because of the fast deposition rate and short deposition time.

Titanium dioxide (TiO_2) is well-known as one of the most important semiconductor materials providing extensive applications ranging from photocatalytic water splitting to electrochromic devices [14,15]. In electrochemistry, TiO_2 is an excellent electrode material which plays an important role [16,17]. TiO_2 electrodes, especially nanostructured TiO_2 electrodes, have been applied to a wide range of devices, including solar cells, photoelectrocatalysis and electrochemical sensors. TiO_2 electrodes can generally be obtained by four representative methods: (1) electrodeposition of TiO_2 on a titanium substrate, (2) thermal pyrolysis of titanium to form a TiO_2 film, (3) dipping the electrode in a TiO_2 sol-gel, and (4) coating the electrode with a commercial TiO_2 suspension [18-21]. However, these preparation methods have some limitations. For example, the first two methods can only be used with a titanium substrate, while the last two methods require high temperature to reinforce the stability of the film on substrates. Therefore, it is necessary to develop a new convenient method for preparing a TiO_2 nanostructured electrode.

In this chapter, we would like to introduce two wet chemical methods, namely a seed-mediated growth approach and a liquid phase deposition process, which have been successfully utilized to modify electrode surfaces with gold nanoparticles or TiO_2 nanostructured films. Because both methods are "soft", the particle size or film thickness is easily controlled by deposition time, which is particularly useful for providing tunable electrochemical performances for bioelectroanalysis.

2. SEED-MEDIATED GROWTH OF GOLD NANOPARTICLES ON ELECTRODE SURFACES

2.1. Fabrication of Gold Nanoparticle-Modified Electrodes with Seed-Mediated Growth Approach

Actually, the seed-mediated growth approach was first proposed and developed for the synthesis of metal nanorods or nanowires in solution [22-26]. The procedure begins with the synthesis of metallic nanospheres (nanoseeds) by chemical reduction of a metal salt with a strong reducing agent such as sodium borohydride. These seeds are then added to a growth solution containing metal salt, a weak reducing agent (e.g., ascorbic acid), and a rodlike micellar template (cetyltrimethylammonium bromide, CTAB). The seeds serve as nucleation sites for nanorod and nanowire growth (Figure 1A).

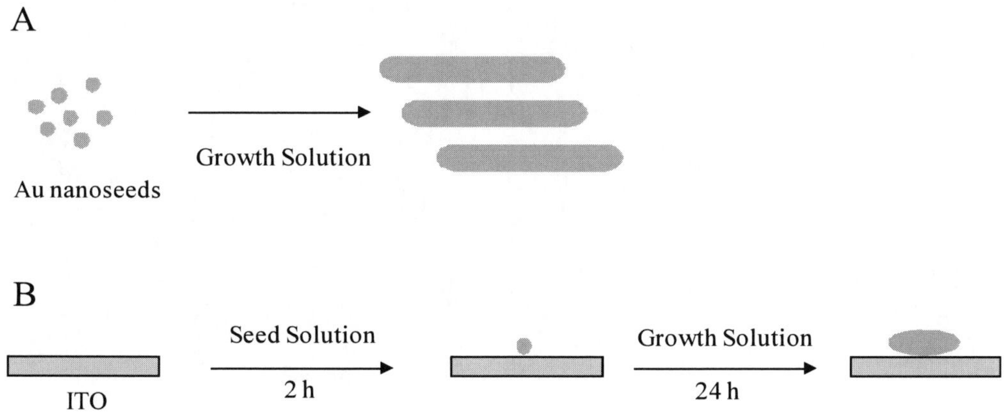

Figure 1. Schemes of the seed-mediated growth method (A) for preparing Au nanorods, and (B) for modifying an ITO surface with gold nanoparticles.

Interestingly, while such a seed-mediated growth approach was applied to the electrode modification by immersing an electrode substrate (e.g., indium tin oxide (ITO)) into the gold nanoseed solution followed by treating in the growth solution (Figure 1B), gold nanoparticles and nanorods could be firmly attached and grown on the electrode surface [27, 28]. Figure 2 displays the typical surface morphology of the seed-mediated growth of gold nanoparticles and nanorods on an ITO surface observed by scanning electron microscopy (SEM). As can be seen, some rod-shaped gold nanoparticles having a width of 25-30 nm and a length of 100-800 nm appear as well as nanospheres having a diameter of 50-60 nm. Of course, the seed-mediated growth procedure is important for such a modification. If immersing the ITO only into the seed solution, no nanoparticles or nanorods as shown in Figure 2 could be observed on the electrode surface before contact with the growth solution. On the other hand, if immersing the ITO only into the growth solution without treating in the seed solution, only aggregated large gold crystals could be observed very sparsely.

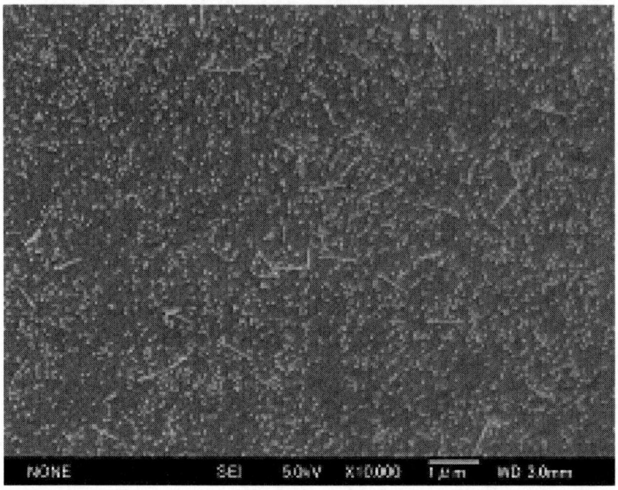

Figure 2. SEM image of ITO surface modified with gold nanoparticles and nanorods.

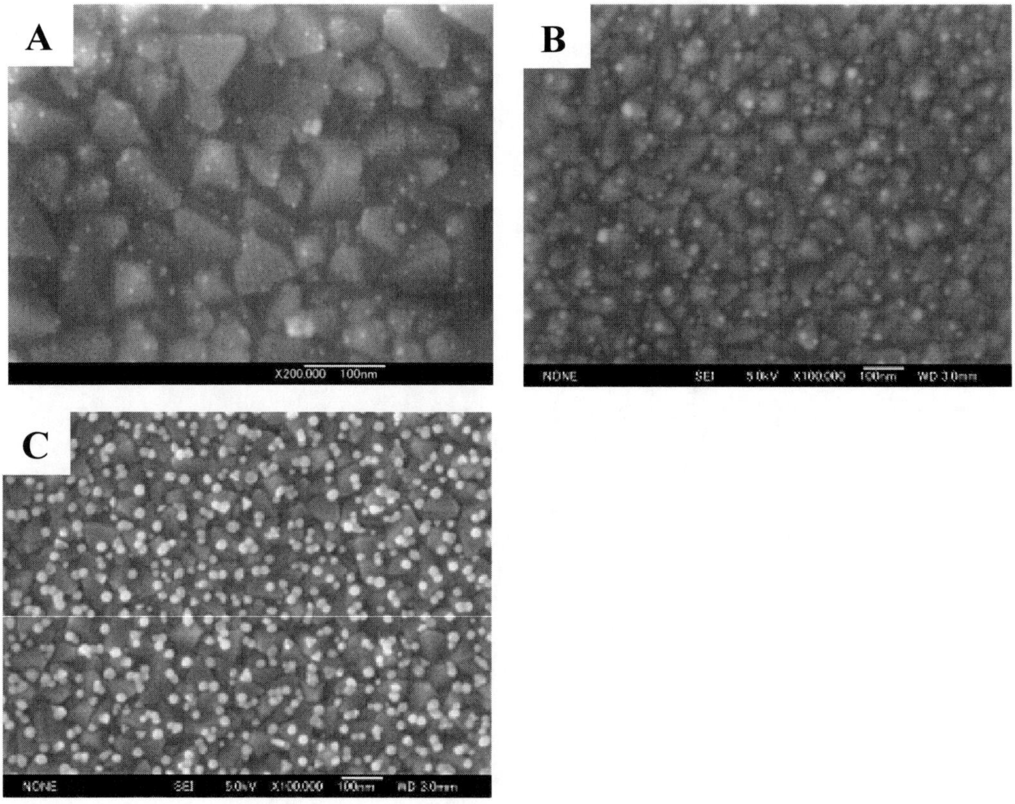

Figure 3. SEM images of gold nanoparticle arrays fabricated on nanostructured ITO substrates in (A) 0-min, (B) 15-min and (C) 24-h growth time. Reproduced from [29], copyright 2005, with permission from Elsevier.

Moreover, a uniform nanoparticle-modified electrode could be prepared by a modified seed-mediated growth approach [29], which also consisted of two modification steps. In the first modification step, an Au complex was adsorbed on the ITO substrate surface when the ITO was immersed in the $AuCl_4^-$ solution. When $NaBH_4$ was added into the precursor complex solution, Au(III) in solution or adsorbed on the substrate surface was reduced to Au. The defects in the nanostructured ITO surface provided active sites for the strong adsorption of the $AuCl_4^-$, which was then reduced to gold nanoparticles by $NaBH_4$, resulting in nanoparticles dispersed on the ITO. Fig. 3A shows a typical SEM image of an ITO surface after the first modification procedure. As can be seen, the presence of many gold nanoparticles having a diameter of 4 ± 1 nm dispersed on the nanostructured ITO surface is confirmed. After treating the substrate in the growth solution for 15 min following the first modification step, the size of the gold nanoparticles on the ITO surface is increased to 14 ± 2 nm (Fig. 3B). The particle size can be further increased with growth time. Fig. 3C shows an SEM image of the gold nanoparticle arrays after 24-h growth, in which the size of the gold nanoparticles is estimated to be 22 ± 2 nm. Meanwhile, the growth phenomenon was also observable during the growth procedure. With increasing growth time up to 24 h, the substrate became more and more pinkish while the growth solution remained transparent, indicating the reduction of CTAB-capped gold ions by ascorbic acid and the growth of nanoparticles on the Au nanoseed-attached substrate. In contrast, if either of the modification procedures was omitted, the growth phenomenon was not observed, and no gold nanoparticles dispersed on the ITO surface were displayed in the SEM image.

The growth of gold nanoparticles on ITO substrates by this process was monitored by cyclic voltammetry. The cyclic voltammograms of gold nanoparticle arrays prepared under different deposition times exhibit the characteristic oxidation and subsequent reduction peaks of Au (Fig. 4A). The peak currents of the nanoparticle arrays are seen to increase with growth time. The active area of the deposited gold nanoparticles is estimated by assuming that Au has an area of 450 $\mu C/cm^2$ for the reduction peak near +0.9 V [30,31]. Fig. 4B illustrates the calibration curve of the gold area versus growth time. As recognized from this result, up to 30 min, the active area of deposited gold nanoparticles is almost linearly increased with growth time; whereas after 1 h, the growth of the gold nanoparticles becomes slow. However, after 24-h growth, large amounts of CTAB were adsorbed on the nanoparticles to form a thick surfactant layer. Thus the growth reaction between the nanoparticles on the electrode surface and the growth solution was inhibited, and no further increase in the particle size could be observed. If the surfactant layer adsorbed on the grown nanoparticle surface was removed by water cleaning, the particle size of the 24-h nanoparticle arrays could grow further by repeatedly treating the electrode in the growth solution. Fig. 5 shows the SEM images of the gold nanoparticle arrays after two or three repeated treatments in the growth solution. The growth time for each treatment was 24 h, and the electrode was thoroughly washed with water between each repeated treatment. As can be seen, the particle size was obviously increased with the increasing time of the repeated growth treatment. However, with increasing time of the repeated treatment, the monodispersity of the nanoparticles on the electrode surface was decreased; namely, the particle size differences became larger, indicating that the nanoparticles did not grow uniformly. This might be influenced by the particle position on the defect sites of the nanostructured electrode surface. Although some gold nanoparticles began to coalesce into a connected film after three repeated treatments (Figure 5B), the stability of the nanoparticle arrays decreased. In some parts of the nanoparticle arrays (24 h×3 growth), some particles were found to peel off the electrode surface.

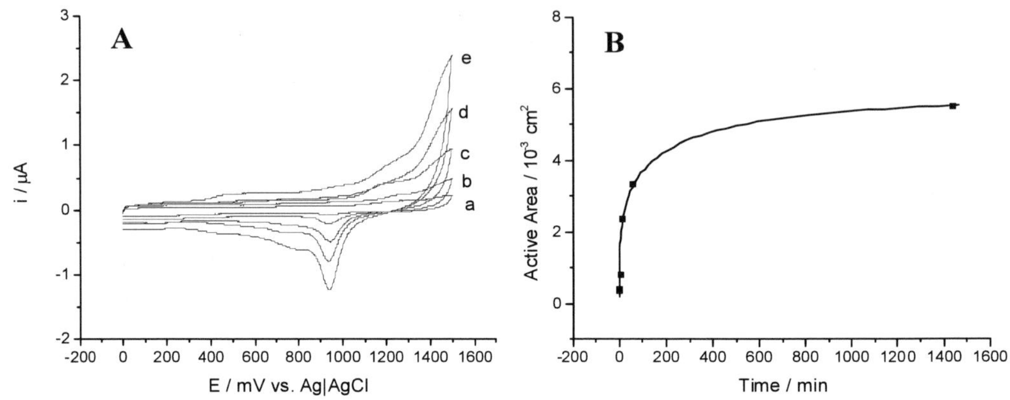

Figure 4. (A) Cyclic voltammograms in 0.5 M H_2SO_4 at 0.1 V/s for gold nanoparticle arrays prepared in (a) 0-min, (b) 5-min, (c) 15-min, (d) 1-h and (e) 24-h growth time. (B) Increase in the active area of the Au nanoparticles deposited on nanostructured ITO substrates with growth time. Reproduced from [29], copyright 2005, with permission from Elsevier.

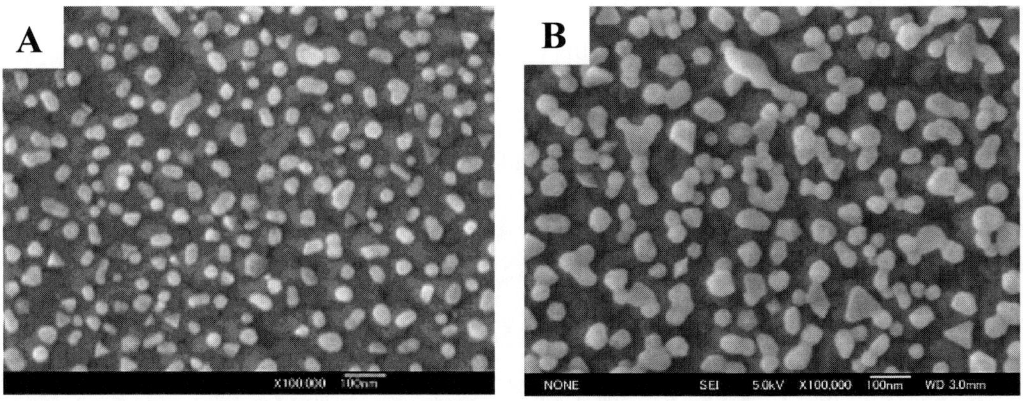

Figure 5. SEM images of gold nanoparticle arrays fabricated on ITO substrates in (A) 24-h ×2 and (B) 24-h ×3 growth time. Reproduced from [29], copyright 2005, with permission from Elsevier.

In addition, modifying the electrode with the seed-mediated growth of gold nanoparticles is not limited by the electrode substrate. For example, if a glassy carbon is used instead of ITO, gold nanoparticles could also be attached and grown on the glassy carbon electrode surface using the seed-mediated growth method [32]. Figure 6 illustrates the attachment of gold nanoparticles directly on the glassy carbon electrode surface with the seed-mediated growth method. Of course, the morphology of the modified electrode is sensitive to the substrate which may impact the adsorption of gold nanoseeds and determine the growth of gold nanoparticles.

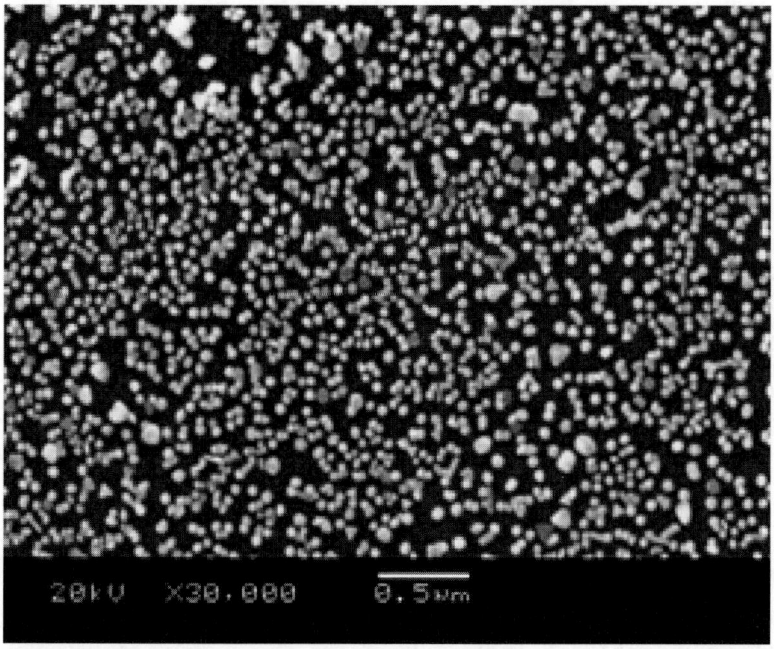

Figure 6. SEM image of glassy carbon electrode surface modified with gold nanoparticles prepared with the seed-mediated growth approach. Reproduced from [32], copyright 2007, with permission from the Japan Society for Analytical Chemistry.

2.2. Electrocatalytic Activity of Gold Nanoparticles Toward Small Biomolecules

Uric acid (UA) and ascorbic acid (AA) are important electroactive biomolecules appearing in biochemical and biomedical processes. On a bare ITO electrode, both UA and AA show very sluggish $2H^+$ and 2e electron-transfer kinetics. Figure 7A shows the cyclic voltammograms of 1 mM UA in 0.1 M PBS (pH 7.4) at a scan rate of 0.1 V/s on bare and gold nanoparticle-modified ITO electrodes. The oxidation peak of UA on bare ITO appears at 1.04 V. At an Au/ITO electrode, the oxidation peak of UA shifts negatively to 0.80 V accompanied by an enhancement of 1.37 μA in the peak current compared to that of bare ITO. These results illustrate the favorable electrocatalytic activity of both gold nanoparticle-modified electrodes toward the oxidation of UA by reducing the oxidation overpotential and increasing the peak current.

AA has a similar catalytic behavior on an Au/ITO electrode (Figure 7B). Compared with bare ITO, the oxidation peak potential of AA shifts from 1.05 V to a more negative position at 0.89 V on Au/ITO, while the peak current is increased by 1.32 μA.

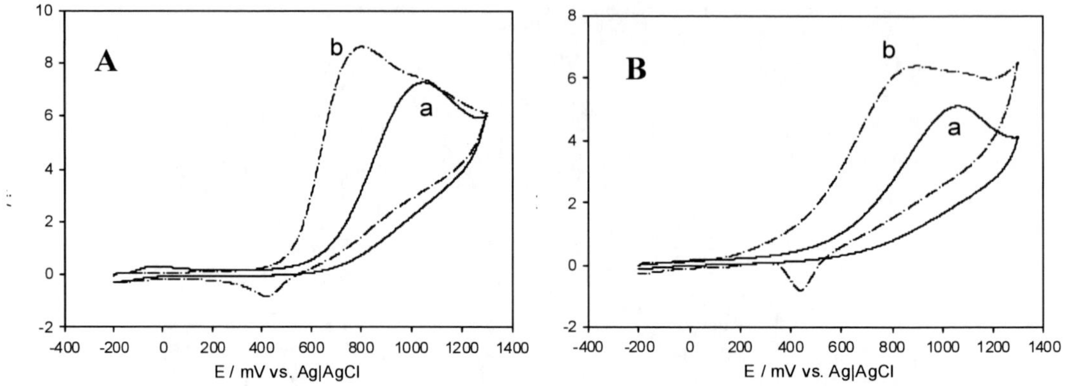

Figure 7. Cyclic voltammograms of (A) 1 mM UA and (B) 1 mM AA in 0.1 M PBS (pH 7.4) at (a) ITO and (b) Au/ITO electrodes. Scan rate: 0.1 V/s. Reproduced from [34], copyright 2005, with permission from Wiley-VCH.

Similarly, the cyclic voltammograms of catecholamine neurotransmitters dopamine (DA), norepinephrine (NE) and epinephrine (EP) on bare and gold nanoparticle-modified ITO electrodes were measured and are illustrated in Figure 8. As can be seen, the voltammetric responses of DA, NE and EP are significantly improved on a gold nanoparticle-modified ITO electrode compared with bare ITO.

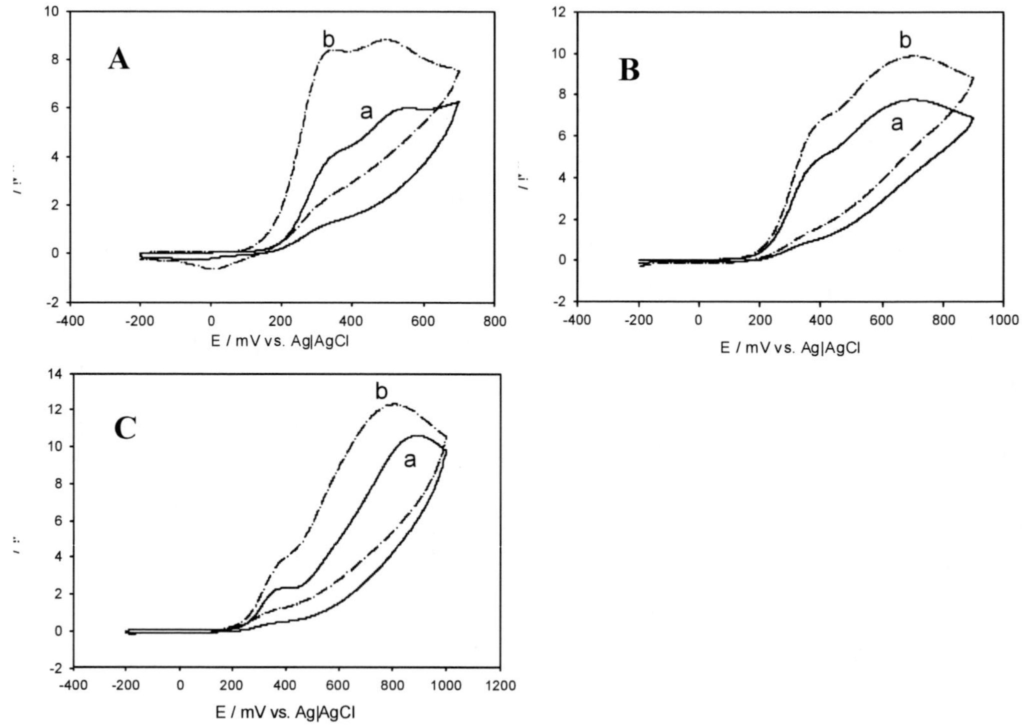

Figure 8. Cyclic voltammograms of (A) 1 mM DA, (B) 1 mM NE and (C) 1 mM EP in 0.1 M PBS (pH 7.4) at (a) ITO and (b) Au/ITO electrodes. Scan rate: 0.1 V/s. Reproduced from [34], copyright 2005, with permission from Wiley-VCH.

The electrochemical determination of neurotransmitters has suffered from AA present in the mammalian central nervous system because of the close oxidation potentials and the reaction between AA and the oxidation products of the neurotransmitters. Therefore, improvement in the detection selectivity and sensitivity for neurotransmitters in the presence of AA has attracted much attention [33]. Considering that the potential difference between EP and AA on ITO is smaller than those of the other two catecholamine neurotransmitters, a mixture of EP and AA was selected as a model to demonstrate the electroanalytical application of the gold nanoparticle-modified ITO electrode with a more sensitive and selective method, namely square wave voltammetry [34]. Figure 9 illustrates the selective determination of EP in the presence of 1 mM AA in 0.1 M PBS (pH 7.4) on the bare ITO and Au/ITO electrodes. On the bare ITO, a linear relationship exists between the peak current and the concentration of EP in the range of $5.0 \times 10^{-5} - 2 \times 10^{-3}$ M. The linear regression equation is expressed as $i_p/\mu A = 0.0378 + 0.9513C/mM$ (correlation coefficient r = 0.9961). On the Au/ITO, a linear relationship exists between the peak current and the concentration of EP in the range of $5.0 \times 10^{-6} - 2 \times 10^{-3}$ M. The linear regression equation is $i_p/\mu A = 0.1897 + 1.3199C/mM$ (r = 0.9977). The detection limit (S/N = 3) of EP on the bare ITO is 1.1×10^{-5} M, which is improved to 1.8×10^{-6} M on the Au/ITO.

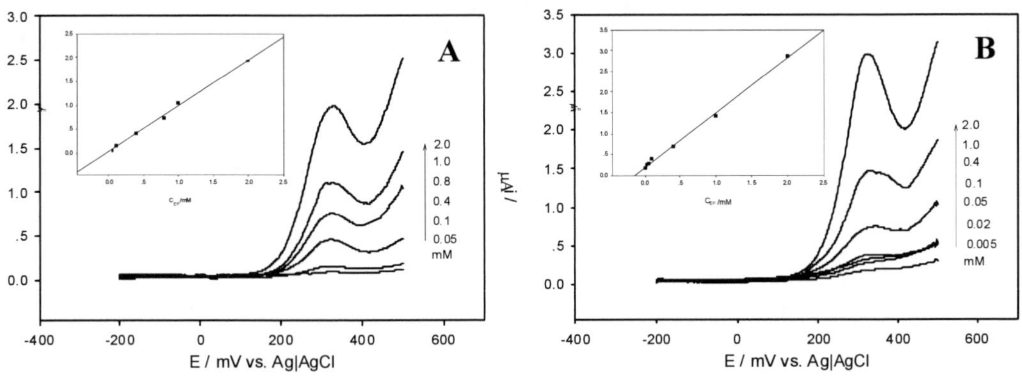

Figure 9. Square wave voltammograms of mixtures containing different amounts of EP and 1 mM AA in 0.1 M PBS (pH 7.4) at (A) bare ITO and (B) Au/ITO electrodes. Pulse height: 25 mV. Frequency: 15 Hz. Scan increment: 2 mV. Inset: Linear relationship between the peak current and the concentration of EP. Reproduced from [34], copyright 2005, with permission from Wiley-VCH.

Furthermore, considering the self-assembled monolayer (SAM)-modified planar gold electrodes showing high selectivity and sensitivity, fast response or anti-fouling properties for voltammetric determination of small biomolecules, the gold nanoparticle-modified ITO electrode prepared using the seed-mediated growth method was employed for the assembly of a monolayer of 3-mercaptopropionic acid (MPA) to clarify its electrocatalytic activity toward small molecules [35]. Figure 10 shows the scheme of two- and three-dimensional MPA monolayers, and Figure 11 illustrates the electrochemical behavior of small biomolecules such as NADH, AA, UA and DA on bare and modified electrodes. The cyclic voltammetric results indicated that the three-dimensional MPA monolayer promoted the electron transfer between NADH and the electrode (Figure 11A), which was similar to the effect of a two-dimensional MPA monolayer assembled on a planar gold electrode. However, regarding the electrooxidation of AA, although the two-dimensional MPA monolayer exhibited a blocking effect, the three-dimensional MPA monolayer showed an obvious promotion (Figure 11B). The catalytic activity of the three-dimensional MPA monolayer toward UA (Figure 11C) and DA (Figure 11D) was also observed, which was attributed to its three-dimensional structure that might effectively prevent poisoning of the electrode surface by the oxidation products. The electrocatalytic activity of a three-dimensional monolayer assembled on as-prepared gold nanoparticles is not only useful in bioelectroanalysis but also advantageous in understanding the fundamental properties of a three-dimensional monolayer on a nano scale.

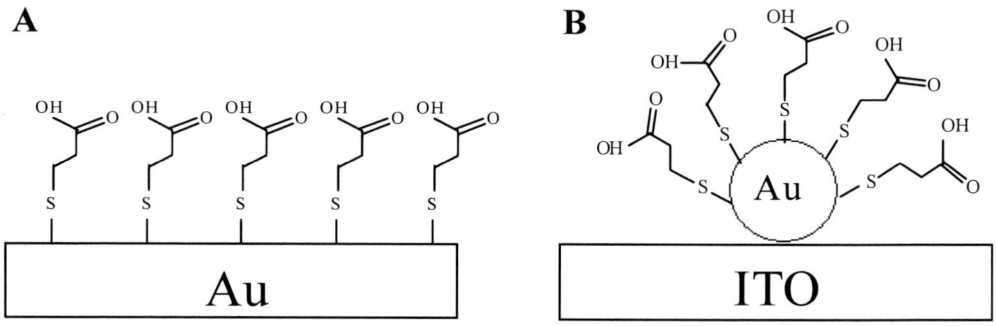

Figure 10. Scheme of (A) two-dimensional MPA monolayer assembled on planar gold surface and (B) three-dimensional MPA monolayer assembled on gold nanoparticle-modified ITO. Reproduced from [35], copyright 2007, with permission from Elsevier.

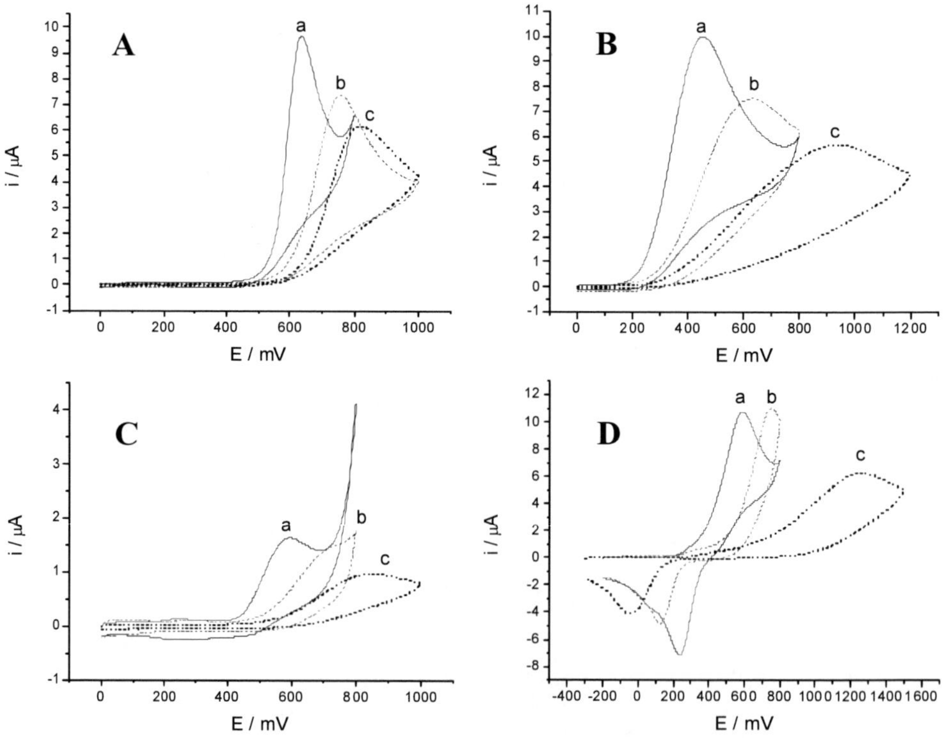

Figure 11. Cyclic voltammograms for 1 mM (A) NADH, (B) AA, (C) UA and (D) DA on MPA monolayer-modified gold nanoparticle arrays (a), gold nanoparticle arrays (b) and bare ITO electrode (c). Scan rate: 0.1 V/s. Reproduced from [35], copyright 2007, with permission from Elsevier.

2.3. Biosensors Based on Proteins Immobilized on Gold Nanoparticles

Myoglobin (Mb) and hemoglobin (Hb) are typical redox heme proteins playing important roles in protein electrochemistry. However, due to the extended three-dimensional structure and the resulting inaccessibility of the electroactive center or its adsorption onto and subsequent passivation of the electrode surface, Mb or Hb usually exhibits sluggish electron transfer at conventional electrodes. Great efforts have been made to promote and improve the direct electron transfer between protein and electrode. Among these, nanoparticle-modified electrodes are found to have good biocompatibility that allows them to effectively facilitate or promote the electron transfer between proteins and electrodes. The direct electrochemistry of heme proteins has been successfully studied on metal nanoparticles [36-40], carbon nanotubes [41] and colloidal gold [42] modified electrodes.

Among various nanomaterials, gold nanoparticles are the most intensively studied and utilized metal nanoparticles in electrochemistry due to their stable physical and chemical properties, useful catalytic activities and small dimensional size [43]. When Mb was immobilized on a gold nanoparticle-modified ITO electrode by casting Mb solution on the working surface of an Au/ITO electrode, stable and well-behaved voltammetric responses for Mb could be obtained [44]. Figure 12 illustrates the cyclic voltammograms of Mb immobilized on Au/ITO and bare ITO electrodes. It can be seen that Mb shows a pair of well-behaved redox peaks on the Au/ITO electrode. From the integration of the cathodic peak of Mb/Au/ITO, the surface coverage (Γ) of active Mb in the film is estimated to be 5.05×10^{-10} mol/cm^2 according to $\Gamma = Q/nFA$, where Q is the charge, n the electron transfer number, F the Faraday constant and A denotes the geometric area of the working electrode. On the other hand, although the characteristic waves for the Mb Fe(III)/Fe(II) redox couple also appear in the cyclic voltammogram of an Mb/ITO electrode in acetate buffer solution (curve b in Figure 12), both the reduction and oxidation peak currents on the Mb/ITO are obviously lower as compared with the Mb/Au/ITO. The surface coverage of active Mb in Mb/ITO is estimated to be 3.47×10^{-10} mol/cm^2, which is improved by about 46% in the presence of gold nanoparticles. Apparently, the coverage increase of electroactive Mb on an Au/ITO surface can be attributed to the fact that the deposited gold nanoparticles on ITO provide more active area for Mb immobilization. Moreover, the gold nanoparticles on the electrode surface may permit protein molecules to orient in conformations more favorable for direct electron transfer with the active sites closer to the conducting electrode [45], also resulting in more electroactive Mb in the film immobilized on Au/ITO. Therefore, a promoted electrochemical response is observed on Mb/Au/ITO. Furthermore, the Mb/Au/ITO electrode showed effective catalytic activity toward the reduction of H_2O_2. In pH 7.0 buffer, this electrode exhibited a quick and linear amperometric response to the addition of H_2O_2 over the concentration range of 2.5×10^{-6} to 5×10^{-4} M, which provided a new Mb-based biosensor for the detection of H_2O_2 (Figure 13).

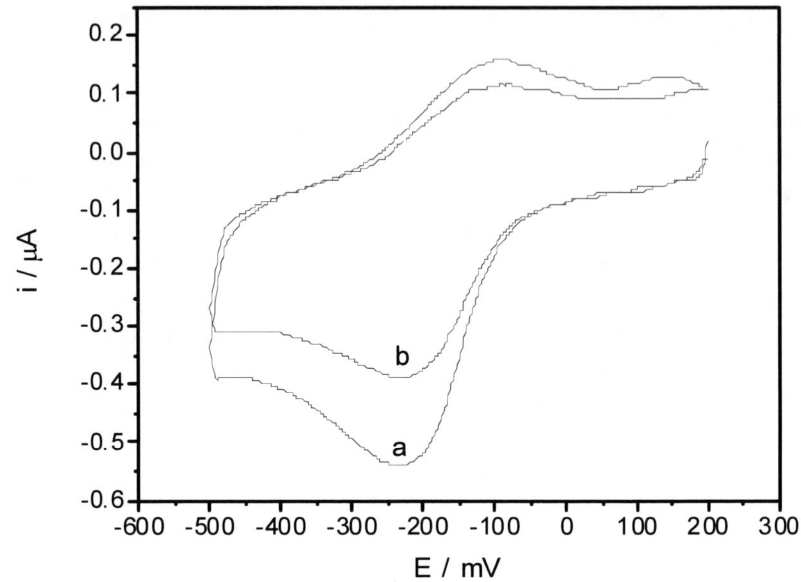

Figure 12. Cyclic voltammograms of (a) Mb/Au/ITO and (b) Mb/ITO electrodes in pH 4.0 acetate buffer at 0.1 V/s. Reproduced from [44], copyright 2005, with permission from Elsevier.

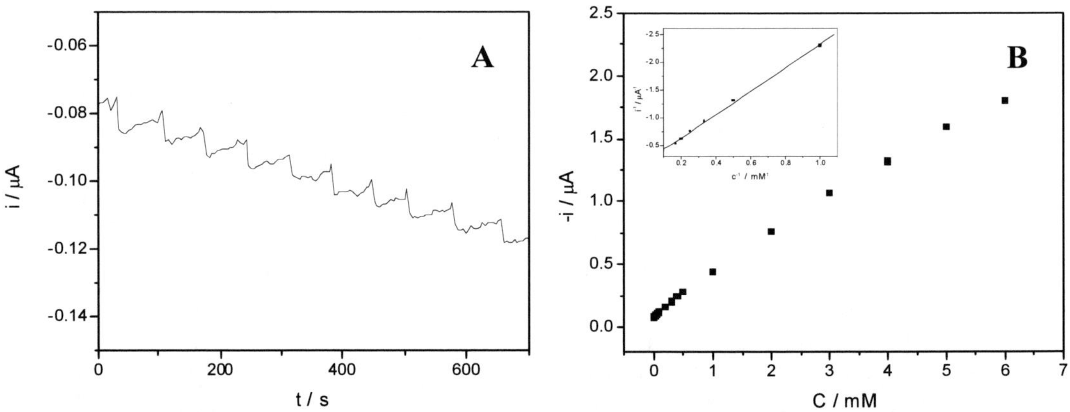

Figure 13. (A) Chronoamperometric response of Mb/Au/ITO electrode at -0.4 V in pH 7.0 phosphate buffer while successively injecting 10 μM H_2O_2. (B) Plot of catalytic current vs. H_2O_2 concentration. Inset: Linear calibration curve of 1/i vs. $1/C_{H_2O_2}$. Reproduced from [44], copyright 2005, with permission from Elsevier.

On an Au/ITO electrode, Hb exhibited similar electrochemical behavior to Mb if Hb was immobilized on the electrode surface by casting the Hb solution thereon. However, when Hb was immobilized on Au/ITO by adsorption of Hb on a modified electrode, no direct voltammetric response for Hb could be seen. This was because the adsorption of Hb on the modified electrode did not provide a sufficient amount of protein. However, the adsorptive immobilization of Hb on a gold nanoparticle-modified ITO electrode could be observed by electrochemical impedance measurements using an $[Fe(CN)_6]^{3-}/[Fe(CN)_6]^{4-}$ redox probe (Figure 14) [46]. By the simulation program, the charge transfer resistance (R_t) value of bare ITO is estimated to be 77.43 kΩ, which is decreased to 15.97 kΩ after the gold nanoparticles modification, indicating effectively improved heterogeneous electron transfer kinetics between the redox couple and the electrode interface, attributed to the deposition of the gold nanoparticles. However, the R_t value of the Au/ITO electrode is increased to 79.05 kΩ after Hb is immobilized, confirming the formation of an Hb layer adsorbed on the electrode surface, which exhibits a barrier effect on the electron transfer kinetics. If we estimate the apparent surface coverage (θ) according to $\theta = 1- R_t/R_t'$, where R_t and R_t' represent the charger transfer resistance of the electrode before and after immobilization, respectively, the coverage of Hb on the Au/ITO surface is about 80%. In a comparison, the coverage of Hb on a bare ITO surface is estimated to be 71% according to the change in the R_t value of ITO, which is decreased to 267.30 kΩ after Hb is immobilized thereon. Therefore, the gold nanoparticle-deposited surface is more advantageous for the adsorptive immobilization of Hb. On the other hand, although the direct electrochemical behavior of Hb could not be observed on this adsorptive immobilized Hb/Au/ITO electrode, the effective catalytic activity of Hb toward the reduction of H_2O_2 was achieved on this electrode (Figure 15), attributed to the improved electron transfer of Hb by the gold nanoparticles. Thus, the electrode exhibited a quick and linear response to the addition of H_2O_2 over a wide concentration range from 1×10^{-5} to 7×10^{-3} M (Figure 16). The peroxidase-like activity but low cost of Hb as well as the low detection limit, good reproducibility and stability of this electrode provide a novel and promising Hb-based biosensor for the detection of H_2O_2.

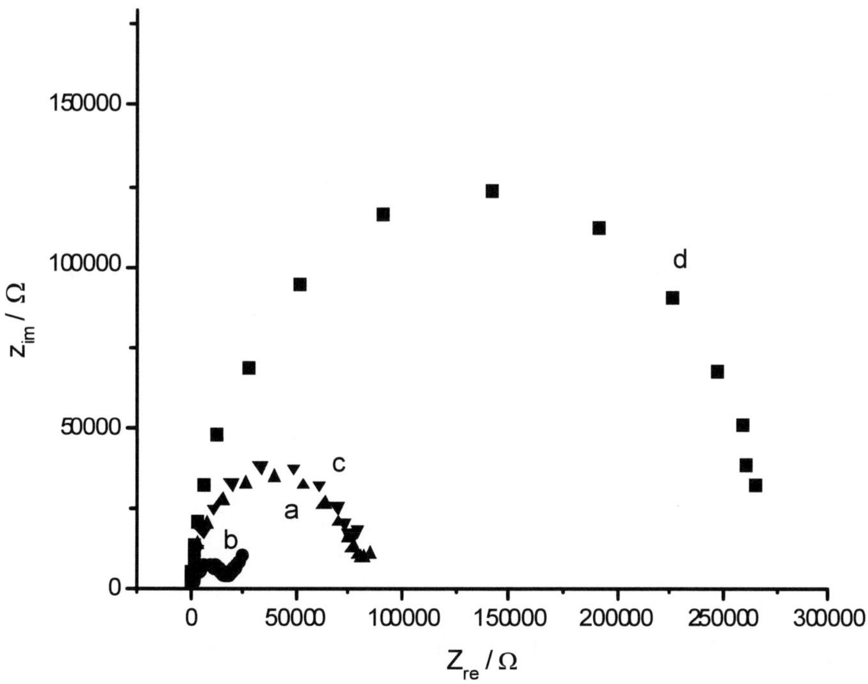

Figure 14. Electrochemical impedance spectra of (a) bare ITO, (b) Au/ITO, (c) Hb/Au/ITO and (d) Hb/ITO electrodes in 0.1 M PBS (pH 7.0) containing 0.5 mM $K_3[Fe(CN)_6]/K_4[Fe(CN)_6]$. Applied potential: 0.225 V. Frequency range: 100 kHz – 100 mHz. Reproduced from [46], copyright 2004, with permission from Elsevier.

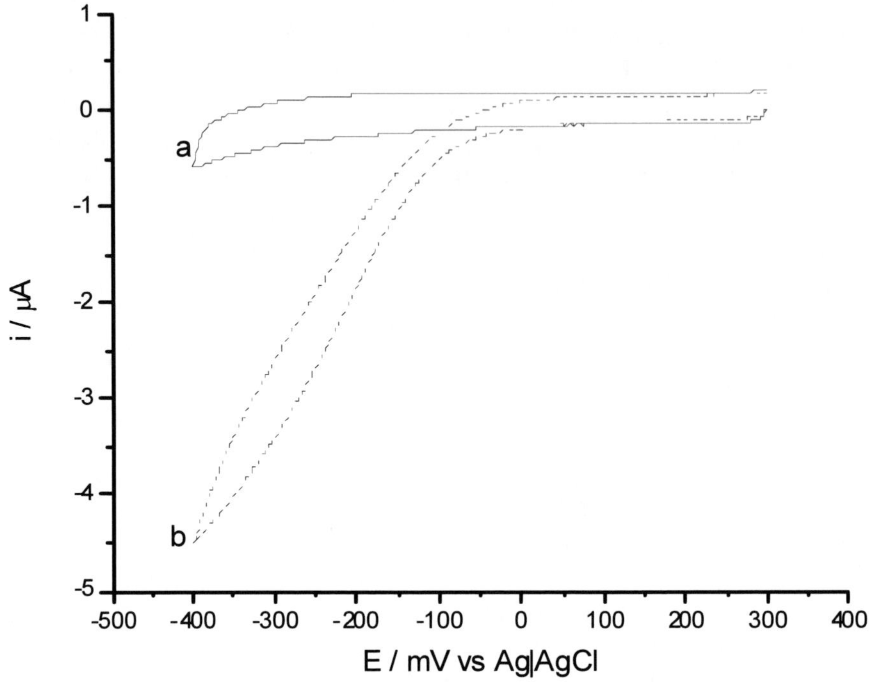

Figure 15. Cyclic voltammograms recorded using an Hb/Au/ITO electrode (a) before and (b) after adding 2 mM H_2O_2 into PBS (pH 7.0). Scan rate: 0.1 V/s. Reproduced from [46], copyright 2004, with permission from Elsevier.

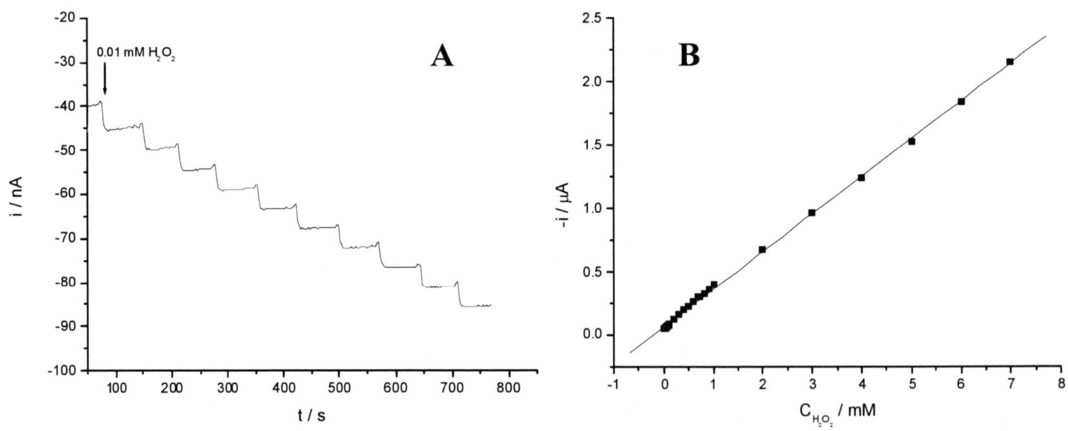

Figure 16. (A) Chronoamperometric response of Hb/Au/ITO electrode at -0.3 V in pH 7.0 phosphate buffer while successively injecting 10 μM H_2O_2. (B) Linear calibration of catalytic current obtained with the Hb/Au/ITO electrode vs. H_2O_2 concentration. Reproduced from [46], copyright 2004, with permission from Elsevier.

3. LIQUID PHASE DEPOSITION OF TiO_2 ON ELECTRODE SURFACES

3.1. Preparation of TiO_2 Film Electrodes with Liquid Phase Deposition Process

Liquid phase deposition (LPD) process is the formation of oxide thin films from an aqueous solution of a metal–fluoro complex which is slowly hydrolyzed by adding fluoride scavengers such as boric acid or aluminum metal [47], namely

$$H_{(n-m)}MF_n + m/2H_2O \rightleftharpoons MO_{m/2} + nHF \quad (1)$$

$$H_3BO_3 + 4HF \rightleftharpoons HBF_4 + 3H_2O \quad (2)$$

$$Al + 6HF \rightleftharpoons H_3AlF_6 + 1.5H_2 \quad (3)$$

Compared with traditional methods for the preparation of the oxide film, the LPD technique is advantageous because no vacuum, no high temperature, no expensive apparatus and no special substrate are required. Using this LPD process, various metal oxide films such as TiO_2, SiO_2, V_2O_5, SnO_2, FeOOH and $SrTiO_3$ have been successfully prepared from aqueous solutions at room temperature [48-55]. Because the LPD technique has no requirement for the substrate, oxide film electrodes could be obtained if conductive substrates were employed. Based on this method, TiO_2 film electrodes were provided by treating conductive substrates such as graphite [56], glassy carbon [57] and ITO in an aqueous solution of $(NH_4)_2TiF_6$ and H_3BO_3. Figure 17 shows the morphological structures of LPD TiO_2 films on graphite prepared within different deposition times. As can be seen, the film morphology is strongly influenced by deposition time. With increasing deposition time from 5 h to 40 h, the particle size was increased from tens of nanometers to hundreds of nanometers, due to the accumulation of deposited particles. Meanwhile, the film thickness increased with deposition time. When the deposition time was less than 5 h, the LPD film was very thin, and the substrate surface was not thoroughly covered by TiO_2. When the deposition time was increased to 10 h, the film became thicker and the entire surface was almost covered by highly dense TiO_2 particles. When the deposition time reached 20 h, some cracks appeared in the film. These cracks were generated by the internal stress of the film due to contracting of the film by dissociation of water in the drying procedure. With increasing deposition time from 20 h to 40 h, the film thickness was further increased, which increased the internal stress of the film, resulting in deeper and wider cracks. Moreover, the as-prepared LPD TiO_2 films are electroactive and exhibit the characteristic voltammetric response of TiO_2 increasing with the increase in film thickness controlled by deposition time (Figure 18).

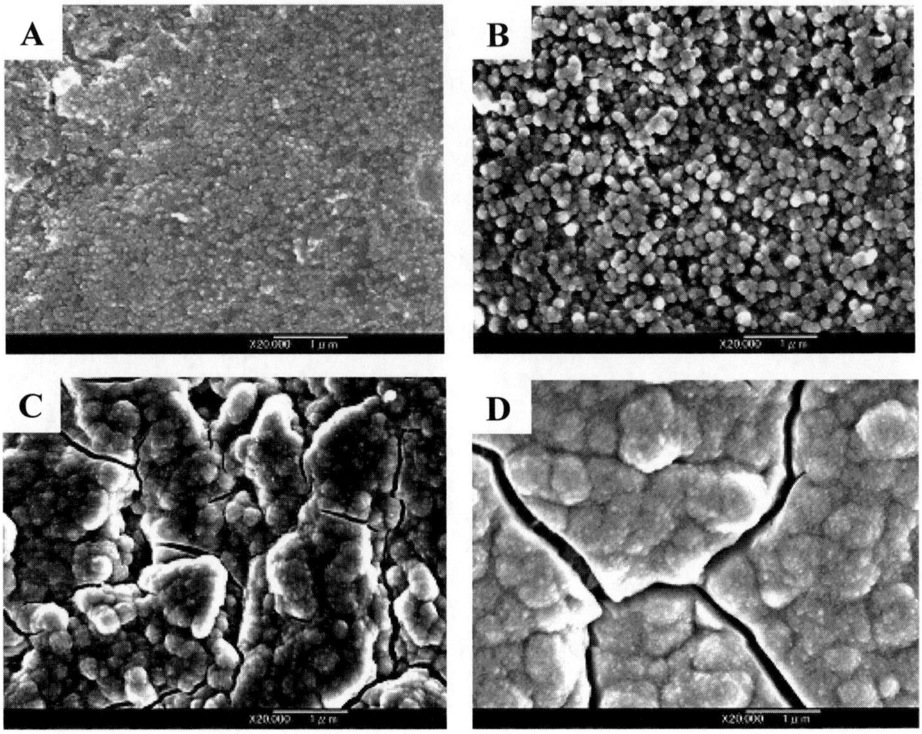

Figure 17. SEM images of LPD TiO_2 films on graphite prepared from 0.1 M $(NH_4)_2TiF_6$ and 0.2 M H_3BO_3 for different deposition times: (A) 5 h; (B) 10 h; (C) 20 h; (D) 40 h. Reproduced from [56], copyright 2004, with permission from Elsevier.

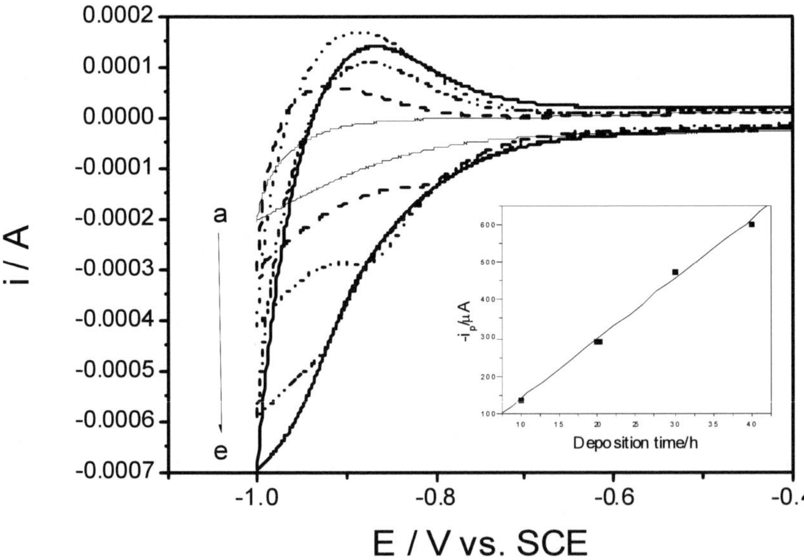

Figure 18. Cyclic voltammograms of TiO_2 electrodes prepared from 0.1 M $(NH_4)_2TiF_6$ and 0.2 M H_3BO_3 for (a) 5 h, (b) 10 h, (c) 20 h, (d) 30 h and (e) 40 h. The electrolyte was 0.2 M phosphate at pH 6.0. Inset: Linear increase in cathodic peak current with deposition time. Reproduced from [56], copyright 2004, with permission from Elsevier.

3.2. Doping LPD TiO_2 Films with other Materials

The LPD TiO_2 film electrodes possess useful catalytic activity toward some organic molecules such as maleic acid, nitrobenzene, etc. However, due to the semiconductive property of TiO_2, the LPD film inhibits the electron transfer on the electrode surface, which might limit the applicability of TiO_2 film acting as an electrode material. Thus, preparing composite nanostructured films by doping other materials into the LPD films may improve the features of the LPD film electrodes.

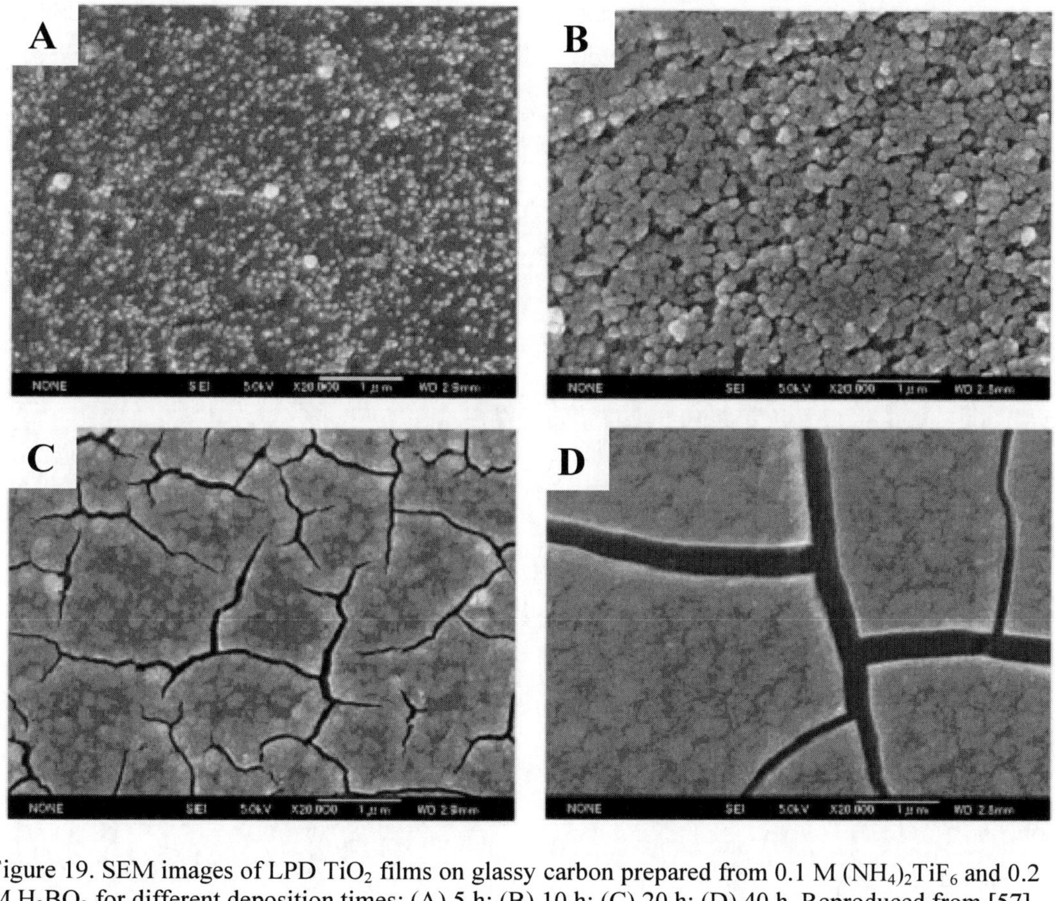

Figure 19. SEM images of LPD TiO_2 films on glassy carbon prepared from 0.1 M $(NH_4)_2TiF_6$ and 0.2 M H_3BO_3 for different deposition times: (A) 5 h; (B) 10 h; (C) 20 h; (D) 40 h. Reproduced from [57], copyright 2008, with permission from Springer.

The first example is the preparation of TiO_2-Au interface by seed-mediated growth of gold nanoparticles on LPD TiO_2 films [58]. Figures 19 and 20 compare the SEM images of LPD TiO_2 films deposited on glassy carbon surface before and after attaching gold nanoparticles with the seed-mediated growth approach. As can be seen, nanostructured TiO_2-Au interfaces are successfully prepared on the electrode surface based on the incorporation of the seed-mediated growth approach and the LPD process. Both the thickness of the TiO_2 film and the size of the gold nanoparticles can be easily controlled by adjusting the chemical reaction time. Moreover, the attached gold nanoparticles showed an obvious influence on the electron transfer on the LPD film electrode. Figure 21A shows the cyclic voltammograms of bare and modified GC electrodes in phosphate buffer solution (pH 7.0) containing 0.5 mM $K_3[Fe(CN)_6]/K_4[Fe(CN)_6]$. As can be seen, the redox peaks of $[Fe(CN)_6]^{3-}/[Fe(CN)_6]^{4-}$ observed on bare GC disappeared on the TiO_2 film, indicating that the TiO_2 film is inactive for the electron transfer between the redox probe and the electrode. When gold nanoparticles were attached on the LPD film, the redox peaks were observed again. Moreover, the stronger peak currents observed at this TiO_2-Au electrode relative to the bare GC electrode implied that the TiO_2-Au interface provided a highly active surface area for reaction and that additional $[Fe(CN)_6]^{3-}/[Fe(CN)_6]^{4-}$ was trapped in the mesoporous film. In agreement with this result, the electrochemical impedance spectra measured in $[Fe(CN)_6]^{3-}/[Fe(CN)_6]^{4-}$ solution indicated that the charge transfer resistance (R_t) for a bare GC was drastically increased after coating a LPD TiO_2 film but significantly decreased when gold nanoparticles were deposited on the TiO_2 film, indicating that the extremely sluggish heterogeneous electron transfer kinetics of $[Fe(CN)_6]^{3-}/[Fe(CN)_6]^{4-}$ at the TiO_2 film was dramatically improved after gold nanoparticles were attached and grown on the surface.

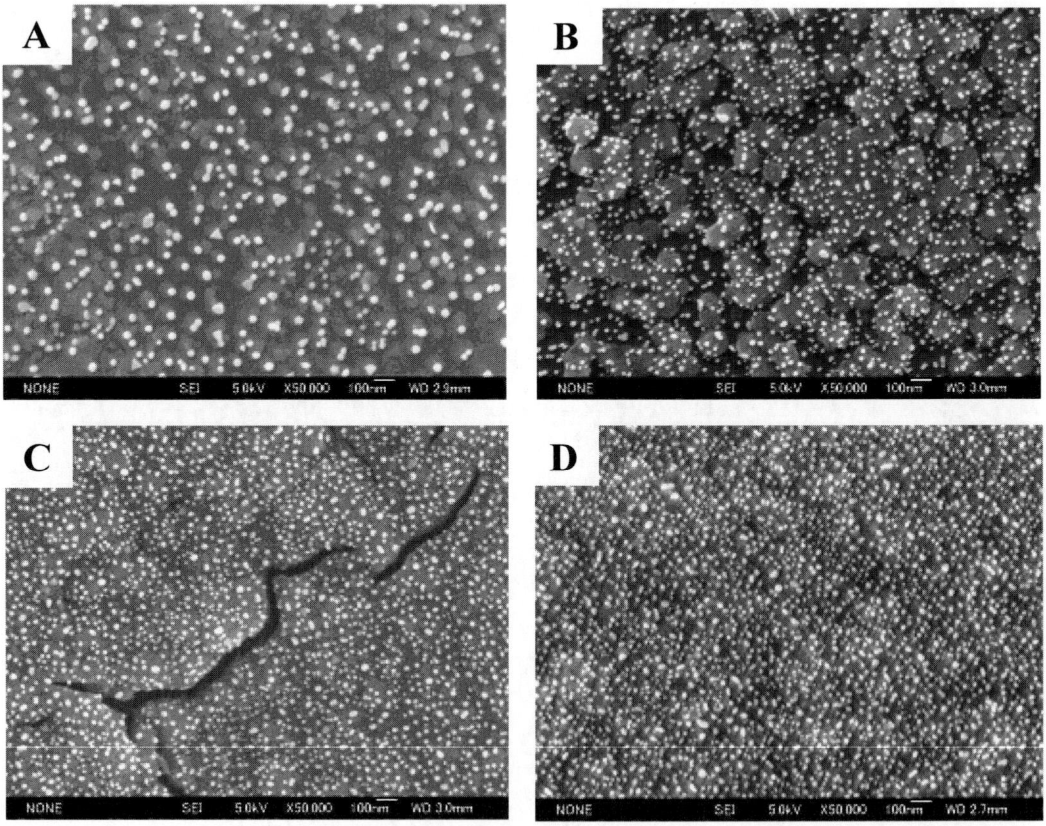

Figure 20. SEM images of seed-mediated growth of gold nanoparticles on LPD TiO_2 films. The LPD films deposited on glassy carbon from 0.1 M $(NH_4)_2TiF_6$ and 0.2 M H_3BO_3 for different deposition times: (A) 5 h; (B) 10 h; (C) 20 h; (D) 40 h. (C) Reproduced from [58], copyright 2005, with permission from the Electrochemical Society.

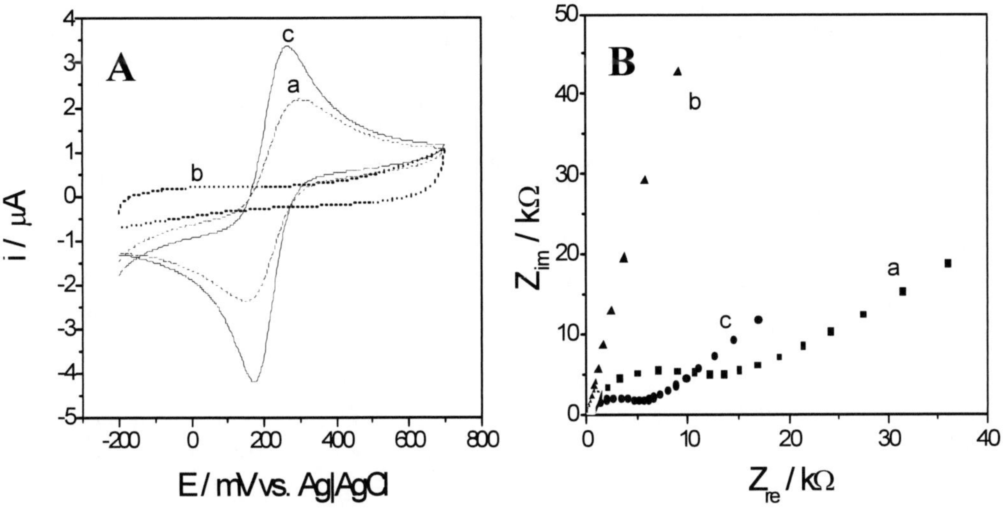

Figure 21. (A) Cyclic voltammograms at 0.05 V/s and (B) electrochemical impedance spectra at 0.23 V in 0.1 M phosphate buffer solution (pH 7.0) containing 0.5 mM $K_3[Fe(CN)_6]/K_4[Fe(CN)_6]$ for (a) bare glassy carbon, (b) TiO_2 film and (c) Au/TiO_2 film. Reproduced from [58], copyright 2005, with permission from the Electrochemical Society.

On the other hand, doping of organic materials into LPD TiO_2 films to form organic/inorganic hybrid thin films has also attracted much attention, which may explore a new one-step route to the preparation of hybrid films and has expanded the application domains of LPD films. For example, alkyl sulfate and alkylbenzene sulfonate surfactants/TiO_2 hybrid films have been prepared to observe the influences of surfactant on the formation and properties of an LPD film [59]. By employing LPD TiO_2 as a base thin-film matrix and poly-L-lysine (PL) as an organic compound/binder that can interact with acidic proteins to form protein-PL complexes, a hybrid film with protein recognition ability has been prepared [60]. Gutiérrez-Tauste et al. have described the preparation of methylene blue (MB)/TiO_2 hybrid thin films by the LPD technique applied to the fabrication of light-activated colorimetric oxygen indicators [61]. TiO_2 hybrid film-modified electrodes can be obtained when conductive substrates are utilized. Figure 22 shows the voltammetric response of an MB/TiO_2 hybrid thin LPD film deposited on glassy carbon. As could be observed for the MB/TiO_2 hybrid film, prior to the redox peaks of TiO_2, a pair of redox peaks assigned to the cathodic and anodic processes of MB was observed at a middle point potential (E_m) of -0.25 V (vs SCE) [62]. MB in such an LPD hybrid film showed a stable electrochemical response, although a small amount of the doped MB did not obviously affect the morphology of the LPD film. The electroactivity of MB could improve the features of the LPD film electrode. As illustrated in Figure 23, although the electron transfer of $K_3[Fe(CN)_6]$ on a glassy carbon surface was completely inhibited by the TiO_2 film, the catalytic response of $K_3[Fe(CN)_6]$ caused by MB was observed on the MB/TiO_2 hybrid films. With the increasing concentration of $K_3[Fe(CN)_6]$, the cathodic peak current was increased, while the anodic peak current was decreased, illustrating the catalytic reduction of $K_3[Fe(CN)_6]$ by MB in the LPD film.

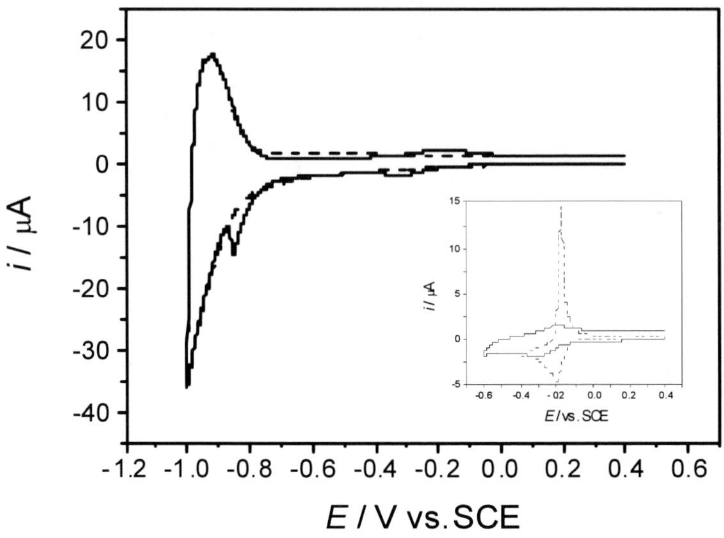

Figure 22. Cyclic voltammograms of LPD MB/TiO_2 (solid line) and TiO_2 (dashed line) films. Inset: Comparison between cyclic voltammograms of MB/TiO_2 hybrid film (solid line) and 0.5 mM MB solution (dashed line) recorded on GC electrodes. Supporting electrolyte: 0.1 M PBS (pH 7.0). Scan rate: 50 mV/s. LPD deposition time: 20 h. Reproduced from [62], copyright 2008, with permission from Elsevier.

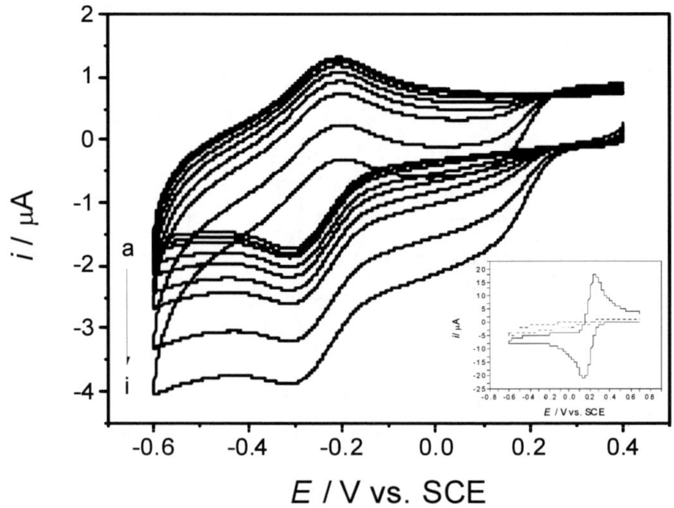

Figure 23. Cyclic voltammograms of LPD MB/TiO_2 film in 0.1 M PBS (pH 7.0) containing (a) 0; (b) 1; (c) 2; (d) 4; (e) 6; (f) 8; (g) 10; (h) 15; (i) 20 mM $K_3Fe(CN)_6$. Inset: Cyclic voltammograms of bare GC (solid line) and LPD TiO_2 film (dashed line) in 0.1 M PBS (pH 7.0) containing 5 mM $K_3Fe(CN)_6$. Reproduced from [62], copyright 2008, with permission from Elsevier.

3.3. Bioelectroanalysis Based on LPD Films

As mentioned above, although the LPD TiO_2 film electrodes possess useful catalytic activity toward some organic molecules, the semiconductive property of TiO_2 resulted in the inhibition of LPD film to the electron transfer on the electrode surface. Thus, directly utilizing a TiO_2-LPD film electrode for bioelectroanalysis is limited. However, the hybrid TiO_2-LPD film may be useful for such an application because the electron transfer performance of the film is significantly improved by doping with other materials. One example is the construction of the H_2O_2 sensor based on an MB/TiO_2 hybrid film-modified electrode. It is known that H_2O_2 is an important analyte appearing as the side product of some enzymatic reactions. Thus, construction of an H_2O_2 sensor has always been one of the main topics among various biosensors. H_2O_2 biosensors based on dyes such as Prussian blue (PB) [63-66] and MB [67-70] with or without incorporation of hydrogen peroxidase (HPR) have been developed because these dyes can mediate the electron transfer between HPR and electrode or directly catalyze the reduction of H_2O_2 acting as an "artificial peroxidase". Figure 24 shows the electrochemical response of H_2O_2 in different concentrations on the MB/TiO_2 film electrode. The results confirmed the catalytic activity of this hybrid film for the reduction of H_2O_2 and indicated that the cathodic peak current was linearly proportional to the concentration of H_2O_2 in the range of 3-20 mM, demonstrating the promising application of the MB/TiO_2 hybrid film in the preparation of biosensors.

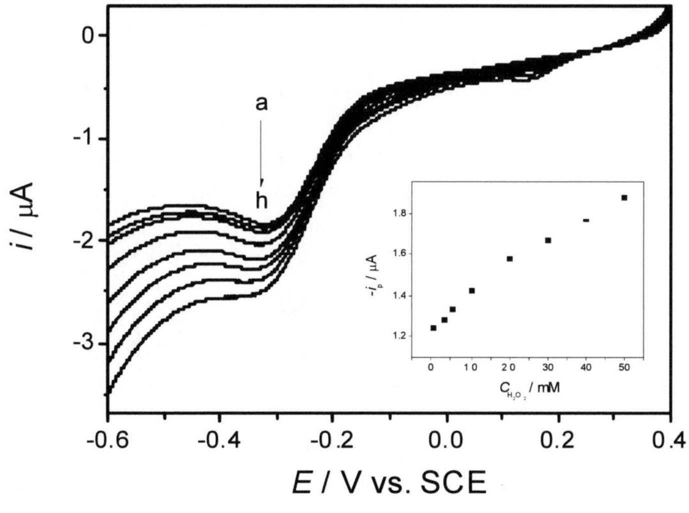

Figure 24. Linear sweep voltammograms of LPD MB/TiO_2 film in 0.1 M PBS (pH 7.0) containing (a) 0; (b) 3; (c) 5; (d) 10; (e) 20; (f) 30; (g) 40; (h) 50 mM H_2O_2. Inset: Plot of peak current versus H_2O_2 concentration. Scan rate: 0.05 V/s. Reproduced from [62], copyright 2008, with permission from Elsevier.

Another example is using sodium dodecylsulfonate (SDS)-doped TiO_2 film for fabricating an Hb-based H_2O_2 biosensor [71]. For the Hb/SDS/TiO_2 film, a drastic increase in the reduction current was observed in the presence of H_2O_2. In contrast, there was no distinct peak when using the Hb/TiO_2 electrodes in the presence of H_2O_2, but leading only to a cathodic current increase. This result demonstrates that the SDS-doped TiO_2 film improved the electron transfer of biomolecules, which provides an excellent biocompatible platform for biomaterial immobilization and construction of electrochemical biosensors.

4. CONCLUSION

This chapter introduced two wet chemical methods for preparing nanoparticle-modified electrodes. At first, the seed-mediated growth of metal nanoparticles on electrode surfaces was described. Using this wet chemical method, gold nanoparticles were successfully deposited on various electrode substrates such as ITO and glassy carbon. The as-prepared gold nanoparticle-modified electrodes showed catalytic activity toward the oxidation of small biomolecules such as dopamine, ascorbic acid, uric acid, epinephrine and norepinephrine, which could improve the sensitivity or selectivity of bioelectroanalysis. The deposited gold nanoparticles were also biocompatible for immobilization of biomacromolecules, namely hemoglobin and myoglobin, on which the direct electron transfer of redox proteins was realized and reagentless H_2O_2 biosensors were provided.

On the other hand, liquid phase deposition (LPD) was demonstrated as a flexible wet chemical method for preparing metal oxide nanostructured films on electrode surfaces. By the LPD process, electroactive titanium dioxide (TiO_2) films were prepared on graphite, glassy carbon and ITO. The electrochemical properties of such LPD TiO_2 films were dependent upon the film thickness controlled by the deposition time. The LPD technique was easily combined with other techniques, e.g., seed-mediated growth, which could provide metal/metal oxide composite nanomaterials. Moreover, hybrid nanostructured films were facilely obtained by doping dyes, surfactants and other materials into the LPD films. These dopants improved the electron transfer kinetics at LPD films by reducing the film resistance and thus making the hybrid films useful for bioelectroanalysis.

5. REFERENCES

[1] Katz, E.; Willner, I.; ; Wang, J. *Electroanalysis* 2004, *16,* 19-44.
[2] Shipway, A.N.; Katz, E.; Willner, I. *ChemPhysChem* 2000, *1,* 18-52.
[3] Doron, A.; Katz, E.; Willner, I. *Langmuir* 1995, *11,* 1313-1317.
[4] Grabar, K. C.; Brown, K. R.; Keating, C. D.; Stranick, S. J.; Tang, S. L.; Natan, M. J. *Anal. Chem.* 1997, *69,* 471-477.
[5] Musick, M. D.; Pena, D. J.; Botsko, S. L.; McEvoy, T. M.; Richardson, J. N.; Natan, M. J. *Langmuir* 1999, *15,* 844-850.
[6] Lahav, M.; Gabai, R.; Shipway, A. N.; Willner, I. *Chem. Commun.* 1999, 1937-1938.
[7] Harnisch, J. A.; Pris, A. D.; Porter, M. D. *J. Am. Chem. Soc.* 2001, *123,* 5829-5830.
[8] Cheng, W.; Dong, S.; Wang, E. *Anal. Chem.* 2002, *74,* 3599-3604.
[9] Lowe, L. B.; Brewer, S. H.; Kramer, S.; Fuierer, R. R.; Qian, G.; Agbasi-Porter, C. O.; Moses, S.; Franzen, S.; Feldheim, D. L. *J. Am. Chem. Soc.* 2003, *125,* 14258-14259.
[10] Rubin, S.; Bar, G.; Taylor, T. N.; Cutts, R. W.; Zawodzinski, Jr. T. A. *J. Vac. Sci. Technol. A* 1996, *14,* 1870-1877.

[11] Hrapovic, S.; Liu, Y.; Enright, G.; Bensebaa, F.; Luong, J. H. T. *Langmuir* 2003, *19,* 3958-3965.
[12] Yu, A.; Liang, Z.; Cho, J.; Caruso, F. *Nano Lett.* 2003, *3,* 1203-1207.
[13] El-Deab, M.S.; Ohsaka, T. *Electrochem. Commun.* 2002, *4,* 288-292.
[14] Bavykin, V.; Friedrich, J. M.; Walsh, F. C. *Adv. Mater.* 2006, *18,* 2807-2824.
[15] Chen, X.; Mao, S. S. *Chem. Rev.* 2007, *107,* 2891-2959.
[16] Grätzel, M. *Nature* 2001, *414*, 338-344.
[17] Tian, M.; Wu, G.; Adams, B.; Wen, J.; Chen, A. *J. Phys. Chem. C* 2008, *112,* 825-831.
[18] Oliva, F. Y.; Avalle, L. B.; Santos, E.; Camara, O. R. *J. Photochem. Photobio. A* 2002, *146,* 175-188.
[19] Khan, S. U. M.; Al-Shahry, M.; Ingler Jr., W. B. *Science* 2002, *297,* 2243-2245.
[20] Zoppi, R. A.; Trasferetti, B. C.; Davanzo, C. U. *J. Electroanal. Chem.* 2003, *544,* 47-57.
[21] Taghizadeh, A.; Lawrence, M.F.; Miller, L.; Anderson, M.A.; Serpone, N. *J. Photochem. Photobio. A* 2000, *130,* 145-156.
[22] Jana, N. R.; Gearheart, L.; Murphy, C. J. *J. Phys. Chem. B* 2001, *105,* 4065-4067.
[23] Johnson, C. J.; Dujardin, E.; Davis, S. A.; Murphy, C. J.; Mann, S. *J. Mater. Chem.* 2002, *12,* 1765-1770.
[24] Murphy, C. J.; Jana, N. R. *Adv. Mater.* 2002, *14,* 80-82.
[25] Nikoobakht, B.; El-Sayed, M. A. *Chem. Mater.* 2003, *15,* 1957-1962.
[26] Gao, J.; Bender, C. M.; Murphy, C. J. *Langmuir* 2003, *19,* 9065-9070.
[27] Zhang, J.; Kambayashi, M.; Oyama, M. *Electrochem. Commun.* 2004, *6,* 683-688.
[28] Kambayashi, M., Zhang, J.; Oyama, M. *Cryst. Growth Des.* 2005, *5,* 81-84.
[29] Zhang, J.; Oyama, M. *Anal. Chim. Acta* 2005, *540,* 299-306.
[30] Finklea, H. O. In *Electroanalytical Chemistry;* Bard, A. J.; Rubinstein I.; Ed.; Marcel Dekker: New York, 1996; Vol. 19, p. 110.
[31] Evans, U.; Colavita, P. E.; Doescher, M. S.; Schiza, M.; Myrick, M. L. *Nano Lett.* 2002, *2,* 641-645.
[32] Cui, Y.; Yang, C.; Zeng, W.; Oyama, M.; Pu, W.; Zhang, J. *Anal. Sci.* 2007, *23,* 1421-1425.
[33] Raj, C. R.; Okajima, T.; Ohsaka, T. *J. Electroanal. Chem.* 2003, *543,* 127-133.
[34] Zhang, J.; Kambayashi, M.; Oyama, M. *Electroanalysis* 2005, *17,* 408-416.
[35] Zhang, J.; Oyama, M. *Electrochem. Commun.* 2007, *9,* 459-464.
[36] Lvov, Y.; Munge, B.; Giraldo, O.; Ichinose, I.; Suib, S. L.; Rusling, J. F. *Langmuir* 2000, *16,* 8850-8857.
[37] Li, Q.; Luo, G.; Feng, J. *Electroanalysis* 2001, *13,* 359-363.
[38] Cao, D.; He, P.; Hu, N. *Analyst* 2003, *128,* 1268-1274.
[39] He, P.; Hu, N.; Rusling, J. F. *Langmuir* 2004, *20,* 722-729.
[40] He, P.; Hu, N. *Electroanalysis* 2004, *16,* 1122-1131.
[41] Zhao, G. C.; Zhang, L.; Wei, X. W.; Yang, Z. S. *Electrochem. Commun.* 2003, *5,* 825-829.
[42] Liu, S.; Ju, H. *Electroanalysis* 2003, *15,* 1488-1493.
[43] Daniel, M. C.; Astruc, D. *Chem. Rev.* 2004, *104,* 293-346.
[44] Zhang, J.; Oyama, M. *J. Electroanal. Chem.* 2005, *577,* 273-279.
[45] Liu, S.; Leech, D.; Ju, H. *Anal. Lett.* 2003, *36,* 1-19.
[46] Zhang, J.; Oyama, M. *Electrochim. Acta* 2004, *50,* 85-90.

[47] Niesen, T. P.; De Guire, M. R. *Solid State Ionics* 2002, *151,* 61-68.
[48] Deki, S.; Aoi, Y.; Hiroi, O.; Kajinami, A. *Chem. Lett.* 1996, 433-434.
[49] Deki, S.; Aoi, Y.; Miyake, Y.; Gotoh, A.; Kajinami, A. *Mater. Res. Bull.* 1996, *31,* 1399-1406.
[50] Tsukuma, K.; Akiyama, T.; Imai, H. *J. Non-Crys. Solids* 1997, *210,* 48-54.
[51] Deki, S.; Yoshida, N.; Hiroe, Y.; Akamatsu, K.; Mizuhata, M.; Kajinami, A. *Solid State Ionics* 2002, *151,* 1-9.
[52] Gao, Y.; Masuma, Y.; Yonezawa, T.; Koumoto, K. *Mater. Sci. Eng. B* 2003, *99,* 290-293.
[53] Huang, C. J.; Chen, J. R.; Huang, S. P. *Mater. Chem. Phys.* 2001, *70,* 78-83.
[54] Shimizu, K.; Imai, H.; Hirashima, H.; Tsukuma, K. *Thin Solid Films* 1999, *351,* 220-224.
[55] Ozawa, N.; Kumazawa, Y.; Yao, T. *Thin Solid Films* 2002, *418,* 102-111.
[56] Zhang, J.; Yang, C.; Chang, G.; Zhu, H.; Oyama, M. *Mater. Chem. Phys.* 2004, *88,* 398-403.
[57] Zhang, J.; Oyama, M. *J. Appl. Electrochem.* 2008, *38,* 1421-1426.
[58] Zhang, J.; Oyama, M. *Electrochem. Solid State Lett.* 2005, *8,* E49-E52.
[59] Li, L.; Mizuhata, M.; Deki, S. *Appl. Surf. Sci.* 2005, *239,* 292-301.
[60] Tatemichi, M.; Sakamoto, M.; Mizuhata, M.; Deki, S.; Takeuchi, T. *J. Am. Chem. Soc.* 2007, *129,* 10906-10910.
[61] Gutiérrez-Tauste, D.; Domènech, X.; Domingo, C.; Ayllón, J. A. *J. Photochem. Photobio. A* 2007, *187,* 45-52.
[62] Zhang, J.; Zheng, Y.; Jiang, G.; Yang, C.; Oyama, M. *Electrochem.Commun.* 2008, *10,* 1038-1040.
[63] Li, Z.; Chen, J.; Li, W.; Chen, K.; Nie, L.; Yao, S. *J. Electroanal. Chem.* 2007, *603*, 59-66.
[64] Wang, Q.; Zhang, L.; Qiu, L.; Sun, J.; Shen, J. *Langmuir* 2007, *23,* 6084-6090.
[65] Wang, G.; Zhou, J.; Li, J. *Biosens. Bioelectron.* 2007, *22,* 2921-2925.
[66] Zhao, W.; Xu, J. J.; Shi, C. G.; Chen, H. Y. *Langmuir* 2005, *21,* 9630-9634.
[67] Yao, H.; Li, N.; Xu, S.; Xu, J. Z.; Zhu, J. J.; Chen, H. Y. *Biosens. Bioelectron.* 2005, *21,* 372-377.
[68] Yang, X.; Chen, X.; Zhang, X.; Yang, W.; Evans, D. G. *Sens. Actuators B* 2008, *129,* 784-789.
[69] Gu, T.; Hasebe, Y. *Anal. Chim. Acta* 2004, *525,*191-198.
[70] Santos, A. S.; Durán, N.; Kubota, L. T. *Electroanalysis* 2005, *17,* 1103-1111.
[71] Jiang, G.; Tang, H.; Zhu, L.; Zhang, J.; Lu, B. *Sens. Actuators B* 2009, *138*, 607-612.

In: Nanostructured Materials for Electrochemical Biosensors ISBN: 978-1-60741-706-4
Editors: U. Yogeswaran; S. Kumar; S. Chen ©2009 Nova Science Publishers, Inc.

Chapter 6

BIOSENSOR FABRICATION BASED ON METAL OXIDES NANOMATERIALS

***Abdollah Salimi*[*1,2]*, Rahman Hallaj*[1]*, Abdollah Noorbakhash*[1] *and Saied Soltanian*[2]**

[1]Department of Chemistry, University of Kurdistan, Sanandaj-Iran
[2]Research Center for Nanotechnology, University of Kurdistan, Sanandaj-Iran

ABSTRACT

The immobilization of biomolcules especially, enzymes on electrode surfaces is one of the main factor that affects the performance of biosensors. To improve the characteristics of an enzyme sensor, such as sensitivity, response time, dynamic range, enzymes should be deposited on the electrode substrate as an ultrathin film. Different materials and several methodologies have been used for immobilization of thin enzyme films on the electrode surfaces. Due to advantageous of nanomaterials such as, high surface area, favorable electronic properties and electrocatalytic effect they have been considerable attention for construction of electrochemical enzyme biosensors. Among the inorganic materials, metal oxide nanoparticles are suitable matrixes and novel candidates for immobilization of enzymes and proteins due to their high electrical conductivity, wide electrochemical working window, high biocompatibility, excellent substrate adhesion and stable chemical, electrochemical and physical properties.This review discusses main techniques and methods which use for preparation different nanoscale metal oxides and their applications for construction of electrochemical biosensors. Various applications of the metal-oxide nanoparticles based biosensors for detection different analytes are described.

* Corresponding adsress: Tel: +98-871-6624001, Fax: +98-871-6624008, E-mail:absalimi@uok.ac.ir or absalimi@yahoo.com (A. Salimi)

1. INTRODUCTION

Numerous efforts have been focused on the development of biosensors in recent years because of their applications in biological and chemical analysis, clinical detection, environmental monitoring and food processing industries.Biosensors combine a biological recognition element that responds to the substrate being measured with a transducer whose function is to convert an observed change into a measurable signal. The biological element can be either a biocatalyst (enzymes, microorganisms, tissue material or a bioligand (antibody, nucleic acid, lipid layers). Typically the biorecognition element can be attached directly to the transducer or retained within a carrier material, which is subsequently deposited at the transducer surface [1,2]. The rapid progress in nanoscience and nanotechnology introduced a fast growth in the field of electrochemical biosensors during the past years [1-3]. The electrochemical studies of enzymes and proteins in solution were often frustrated by adsorption and denaturation of biomolcules on electrode surfaces and highly irreversible electron reactions that may have been related to electrode fouling. Considerable attention has been devoted to immobilization of biomolcules especially enzymes on electrode surfaces for development of electrochemical biosensors and biotechnological processes. The choice of immobilization process is important because the active sites of the biorecognition element should not be compromised. Furthermore, the immobilization process also affects the lifetime of the biosensor in terms of storage and operational stability. Direct electrochemistry of redox proteins or enzymes is of immense interest both for the fundamental study of electron transfer of proteins or enzymes and for the development of highly selective bioelectrocatalyst and biosensors [4,5]. It is difficult for enzymes and proteins to directly exchange electron with electrodes surface, because they usually have large and complex structure [6]. In addition, the redox centers deeply immerse in the bodies and three dimensional structures hinder interaction with the electrode, the adsorptive denaturation of proteins onto electrodes and the unfavorable orientations at the electrode [7]. Therefore, the immobilization of proteins/enzymes on the electrode surfaces is a usual approach to achieve enhanced interfacial electron transfer. However, the surfaces of the unmodified electrodes are incompatible materials that, in general, proteins undergo denaturation upon immobilization on bare or unmodified electrodes and consequently lose their bioactivities. Furthermore in most cases enzyme is hardly exhibits heterogeneous electron transfer process, which means that electron transfer, is very slow. Therefore, no detectable current appears at conventional electrodes, even when rather large overvoltages are applied. These inhibitions can be overcome by modifying electrodes with mediators and promoters [8,9] or incorporating enzymes and proteins into various films on modified electrode surfaces for observing direct electron transfer. Direct electron transfer was not often a general future of the biosensors, and mediators that shuttle electrons between enzymes and electrodes were employed. A mediator plays the role of electron transfer agent, facilitating electron transfer from the enzyme reaction to the electrode surface by diffusion. There are several methods for biosensor fabrication using electron transfer mediator. Commonly used mediators are organic dyes [10,11] ferrocence derivatives [12] metal complexes [13,14] and similar compounds. Mediators are efficient at promoting a good response from an enzyme reaction under low overpotential. However sometimes they affect the response due to reaction interference or redox catalytic side reactions. Also, many kinds of mediators are known to be toxic to enzyme, leading to enzyme deactivation. Therefore, biosensors based on direct electron transfer have been proposed to overcome the problems of mediator systems. The control of electrode surface structure was the key step to reversible protein voltammery. In particular minimization of adsorptive surface denaturation of proteins and enzymes and cleanliness of the electrode surface was found to be essential to facilitating direct electron exchange between redox biomolcules and electrodes. The incorporation, direct electrochemistry and electrocatalytic activity of enzymes in different polymer and biopolymer films [15-17] lipid film [18], membranes [19], water soluble surfactants [20,21], organic material film [22], liquid crystal film [23], silica sol-gel film [24], cationic polyelectrolytes [25] layer by layer covalent attachment [26,27], dendrimer [28] and self assembled monolayers [29,30] have been investigated. For more reported systems only little reversible electrochemical behavior of the immobilized enzymes was observed and their catalytic activity was low. In addition, direct adsorption of biomolcules onto naked surfaces of bulk materials results in their denaturation and loss of bioactivity. Hence, it is pertinent to explore and develop a new and suitable matrix for entrapment of biological molecules on electrode surfaces.

During enzymes or proteins immobilizing on solid substrates, it is important to keep high electroactivity of the protein or enzyme immobilized on the electrode surface. The unfavorable orientation or direct adsorption of biomolcules onto a metal electrode surface may dramatically decrease their catalytic activity of electrode. However, due to rapid protein denaturation during contact with metals, and propensity of metal surfaces to adsorb organic contaminates, the electron exchange rate decay rapidly, unless special electrode surface modification procedures are under taken in order to increase process sustainability and rate. The performance of biosensor mainly depends on the properties of the bioactive layer associated with the transducer. In order to retain its high electroactivity, different supporting materials have been used for the immobilization of enzymes and proteins. Application of nanoparticles have been reported in different biosensing devices using various transduction methods such as colorimertic [31], surface plasmon resonance [32], electrochemical [33,34] fluorescent [35] magnetic [36] and surface enhanced Raman scattering [37]. Owing to low cost, simple design, high selectivity and sensitivity of electrochemical biosensors, the fabrication of nanomaterials based biosensors has been an attractive and popular subject. Direct electron communication between enzyme-active sites and electrodes may also be facilitated by nanoscale morphology of the electrode. The adsorption of such biomolcules onto the surface of nanoparticles can retain their bioactivity due to the biocompatibility of nanoparticles. Since most of the nanoparticles are normaly charged, they can electrostatically adsorb biomolcules with different charges [38]. The combination of biological molecules and novel nanomaterials components is of great importance in the processes of developing new nanoscale devices for future biological, medical and electronic applications [39, 40]. The combination of nanometer materials and biomolcules is of interest in these fields, because nanoparticles can play an important role in immobilization of biomolcules due to their large specific surface area, excellent biocompatibility and good conductivity [41]. A large number of nanomaterials such as carbon nanotubes [42-48], carbon nanofibers [49] clay nanoparticles [50,51], nanometer-sized gold particles [52-56] and platinum nanoparticles [57,58] also have been shown to be suitable for the incorporation of enzymes and proteins. Among these, inorganic nanostructured materials are more promising because of their regular structure, high active surface area of protein bonding and good chemical and thermal stability. Finding of suitable supporting matrix for the immobilization of enzymes is key step in development of enzyme base electrodes. A suitable supporting matrix should be stable for immobilization or integration of biological molecules in the host matrix and efficiently retaining the functionality of the biomolcules. The synthesis of highly ordered metal oxide matrix for enzyme immobilization has become attractive due to its fascinating properties such as high ratio surface area, uniform open pore structure, as well as chemical and thermal stability. Various metal oxide particles and nanoparticles such as manganeous oxide [59], zirconium oxide [60], titanium oxide [61,62], tungsten oxide [63], iridium oxide [64], iron oxide [65], zinc oxide [66], cobalt oxide [67], copper oxide [68] and nickel oxide [69] have been used successfully for immobilization and direct electrochemistry of enzymes and proteins. Electrochemical co-deposition of enzyme and supporting matrix is a convenient single step method which is fast and well controlled [70]. Due to structure stability and small size of metal oxide nanoparticles, they provided a favorable microenvironment for redox proteins and enzymes in order to transfer electrons with underlying electrodes. The aim of this chapter is to review the various metal oxide nanoparticles have been used for immobilization of different enzymes and proteins and their application for direct electron transfer kinetics of immobilized biomolcules entrapped them. The application of prepared nano- biocomposite materials for construction of third generation biosensor and bioelectronics devices without using electron transfer mediators investigate.

2. Electrochemical Applications of Metal Oxides and Metal Oxide Nanoparticles

Metal oxide, oxyhydroxide and their relevant metal alloys are extensively used in many different areas such as corrosion protective coating, electrochemical capacitors in the electronic industry, magnetic nanostructures, photochemical energy conversion, lithium ion batteries and display technology [71-75]. Moreover, metal oxide films are the most interesting class of materials in electrocatalysis. They widely used as anode for electrooxidation of various organic molecule, ozone and oxygen evolution [76]. Furthermore, metal oxide films has been used as pH sensing materials [77,78]. Since, metal oxides are indirect band-gap semiconductor with electrical and optical properties that are exploited for many different applications such as oxygen storage, electrochemical capacitor and super capacitors [79-82], transparent conducting electrodes [83,84], electrochromic materials [85,86] and semiconductor photoelectrodes [87]. In addition , due to low production cost , high stability, good electrical properties, low resistively, and remarkable redox properties, metal oxide particles and nanoparticles are suitable for the application in gas sensors [88-90], litium ion bateries and Li- ion storage materias [91,92]. Electrocatalytic activity of metal oxide or mediators immobilized onto metal oxide film is a new challenge in sensor fabrication and electrode modification technologies [93-98]. Detection of hydrogen peroxide which is a byproduct in an enzymatic reaction is important in the field of biosensor fabrication [99]. The electrodes modified with metal oxide film have been successfully used for either electrocatalytic oxidation or reduction of hydrogen peroxide [100-103].

Enzyme immobilization is considered as an important factor in biosensor technologies. Great attempts are in progress for finding novel materials for fabrication electrochemical biosensors . Due to electrical, optical, biocompatible properties, structure stability and small size of inorganic nanoparticles [104,105] they provide a favorable microenvironment for immobilization of redox proteins and enzymes. The direct electron transfer of immobilized enzymes with underlying electrodes can be applied for biosensor fabrication and electrochemical catalysis of various substances.Furthermore, due to large surface area of inorganic nanomaterials they can immobilize more enzyme molecules and provide direct electron transfer between the active cites of enzyme and electrode. Among the inorganic materials, metal oxide particles or nanoparticles are suitable matrixes and novel candidates for immobilization of enzymes and proteins due to their high electrical conductivity, wide electrochemical working window, excellent substrate adhesion and stable chemical, electrochemical and physical properties. Furthermore, magnetic metal oxide particles(micro and nano sizes) functionalized with redox units were employed for reversibly activate electrocatalytic and bioelectrocatalytic processes by magneto-induced attraction and retraction of the active units to and from the electrode surface respectively [106]. It has been reported that bioelectrocatalytic processes and amplification of biosensing responses of biosensors are enhanced when magnetic metal oxide particles functionalized with DNA , and pyrroloquinolin quinine(PQQ) [107,108]. Small dimensions of inorganic nanomaterials lead to increasing the current density on the electrode surface, allowing the investigation of fast charge transfer kinetics. In addition, small pores in metal oxide could act as substrate-transport channels to decrease the mass transfer resistance for efficient biocatalytic processes. Biocatalytic activities of biosensors depend on the metal oxide nanomaterials morphologies and particle sizes. The existence of nanosize effects offers a new possibility to control reactivity by controlling the particle size and morphology. Metal oxide nanomaterials with various size can be formed into different morphologies such as nanoparticles [109] nanofibers [110] nanotubes [111], nano porous [112], nanowires [113,114] and nanosheets [115] using different synthesis processes.

3. Synthesis of Metal Oxide Particles and Nanoparticles

Oxide nanoparticles are essential for fabrication of different materials such as, semiconductors, superconductors, sensors, biosensors and many other devices in a future nanotechnology. Therefore a general synthetic access is needed for their large-scale preparation. From the scientific point of view, transforming the manifold of technically relevant oxidic materials into 1D nanostructure offers fundamental opportunity for investigation the effect of size and dimensionality on their collective optical, magnetic and electronic propertie [116]. During the final decade of the last century, vest knowledge about the synthesis of metal oxide nanoparticles was collected, with new insights and discoveries emerging almost on a daily basis. Moreover, physical and chemical properties of substances can be considerably altered when they are exhibited on a nanoscopic scale, and this phenomenon opens up a completely new perspective for material design.

Metal oxide nanostructures have been fabricated using different methods and preparation conditions. The most promising technique is sol-gel processing in combination with dip-coating technique.This method enables us to prepare spinel oxide thin film electrodes at ambient temperature with high level of doping and large surface area [117,118]. The physical and chemical vapor deposition is another technique for metal oxide preparation [119,120].

Thermal salt decomposition [121,122], spray pyrolysis [123] plasma sputtering [124] powder immobilization [125] and γ-irradiation [126] methods have also been used for metal oxide preparation. Oxidation of metal salts with oxidizing agents has also been used for metal oxide formation [127,128]. Most of these techniques except sol-gel method require relatively high temperature during the preparation procedure. Low temperature methods are attractive, because they are convenient, compatible with a wide range of substrate materials. They also favor the production of high effective surface area. Several metal oxide materials were synthesized through sol-gel process, which used to immobilize proteins and realize their direct electron transfer [129,130]. In sol-gel process the reaction is performed with strong acid or organic solvents, which are unfavorable condition to biomolcules immobilization and biosensors fabrications [131]. In addition, there are more disadvantages for using this technique such as creaking of the prepared surfaces and difficulty in film formation due to inefficient functional groups on the surface. These disadvantages limit the application of this technique [132]. To overcome these limitations, electrodeposition is chosen as an alternative method to prepare metal oxide nanomaterials. This method is the most prospective technique to generate desirable films by controlling experimental conditions. Electrochemical procedures are widely used in order to obtain new oxide materials with specific chemical, physical and magnetic properties. Using electrodeposition technique for preparation of oxide filmsn offers several advantageous in comparison to other deposition techniques. Very thin layer of metal oxide nanomaterials with high surface area, specific composition , controlled morphology and a good adhesion between the deposited film and the substrate can be easily prepared by electrochemical techniques are main advantages of electrodeposition[133].The physical properties of electrodeposited metal oxide films can be easily modulated by means of the various experimental parameters affecting the electrodeposition process such as, electrolyte composition, applied potential, pH, temperature, current density, time of deposition time and electrode substrate. The cathodic and anodic electrodeposition [97,134,135] and cyclic voltammetry [136-138] have been successfully used for preparation and immobilization of metal oxide particles or nanoparticles on the electrode surfaces. The anodic oxidation of metals has been used for formation a uniform film of metal oxide nanomaterials [139]. Figure 1, shows the SEM images of different metal oxide nanomaterials which uniformly distributed and deposited on the electrode surfaces. As shown a uniform film of metal oxide particles with average size 150 nm for NiOx nanoparticles, 60 nm for cobalt oxide nanoparticles, 100 nm for nanotubular TiO_2 and 50 nm for zinc oxide have been electrodeposited on the surface different electrode materials. Furthermore, electrodeposition techniques have been used for preparation mixed metal oxide materials. Anodic electrodeosition has been employed for preparation Co+Ni [140] and Mn +Co [141] mixed oxide materials. The electrocatalytic synergism of mixed metal oxide has attracted considerable attention in view of their potential applications in electrocatalysis.

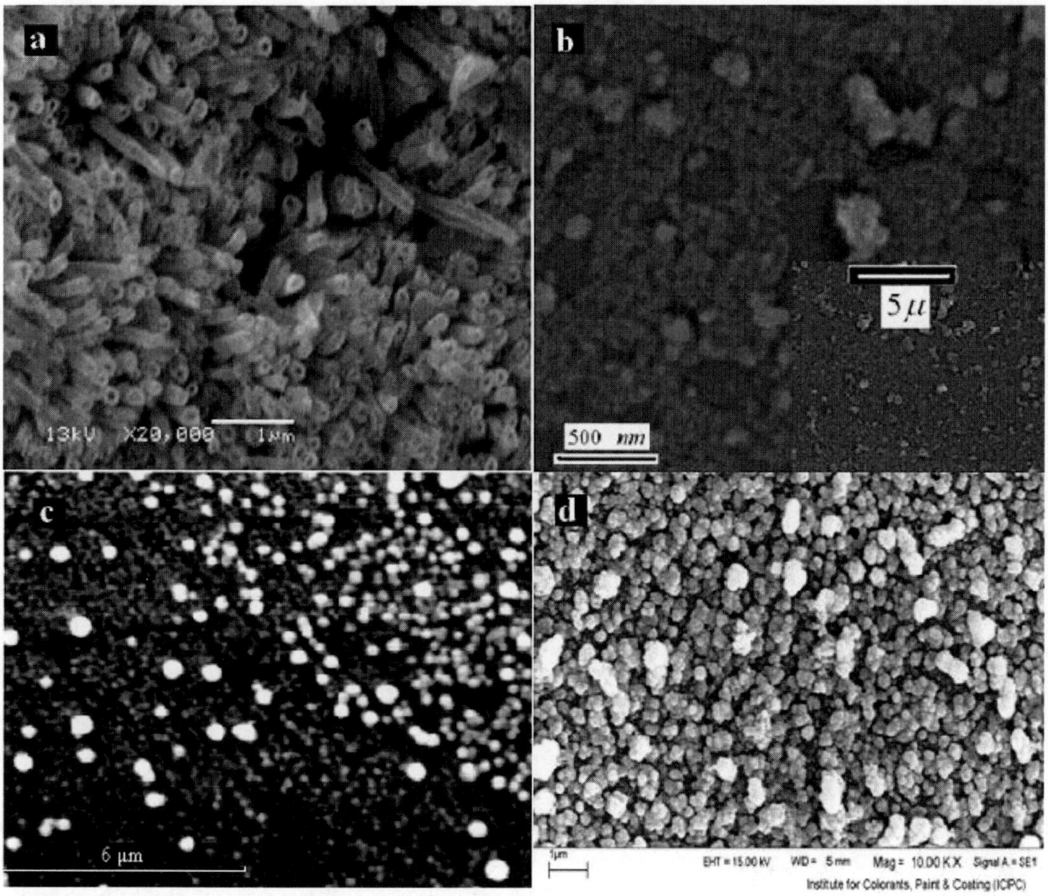

Figure 1. SEM images of different electrodeposited metal oxide nanoparticles; TiO2 nanotube arrays grown on Ti substrate(a); cobalt oxide nanoparticles onto glassy carbon electrode (b); nickel oxide nanoparticles(c) and zinc oxide nanoparticles;;Reproduced from references [138],[102],[137] and [135] with permission from Elsevier.

4. Electrochemical Biosensors Based on Metal Oxide Nanoparticles

The fundamental aspects of an electrochemical biosensor involve the enzyme immobilization onto an electrode surface and the formation of efficient electrical communication between enzyme and the electrode while retaining the enzymatic stability and bioactivity [142]. To achieve this goal, one of the promising ways is to employ nanostructure material for preparation of biosensors. The emerging sensor technology based on nanoparticles and nanocomposites with biological molecules is much beneficial for direct and real applications. The ability to tailor the size and structure and properties of nanomaterials offers excellent prospects for designing novel sensing systems and enhancing the performance of bioanalytical devices [143]. Among these nano-scale materials metal oxide are attracting considerable interest in bioanalytical area as they can combine properties of high surface area, non toxicity, biocompatibility, ease of fabrication, optical transparency, chemical and photochemical stability as well as excellent electrocatalytic activity [144]. Furthermore, metal oxide is important materials due to their versatile properties such as, high temperature superconductivity, ferromagnetism, piezoelectricity and simiconductivity [145]. The films formed by metal oxide nano materials typical reveals porous structure, which can greatly enhance the active surface area available for protein binding and facilate direct electron transfer process between metalloenzymes and the electrodes. Electron transfer between redox proteins and electrodes have been extensively studied, because of their important roles not only in biotechnology and physiological processes but also in the development of biofuel cells and bioelectronic devices. Furthermore, direct electron transfer of enzymes and proteins have been attracting more attention due to their importance in understanding of intrinsic thermodynamic and kinetics behaviors of biomolecules, more importantly, in the practical development of third generation biosensors for different substrates without using redox mediators. Probe immobilization is the key-step in biosensor construction. The conventional methods for biomolcules immobilization are physical adsorption, covalent attachment, cross-linking and entrapment in gels or membranes.

The enzyme can be successfully entrapped within the biocompatible metal oxide materials by using simple procedure, without the need of complicated and time consuming covalently attachment process. During the past decade, different types of enzymes or proteins films have been developed to achieve direct electron transfer with metal oxide covered electrodes. In addition, small pores in metal oxide could act as substrate-transport channels to decrease the mass transfer resistance for efficient biocatalytic processes. Electrical contacting of redox enzymes with electrodes is a key process in construction of third generation biosensors. The active centers of enzymes are surrounded by considerably thick insulating protein shells and enzymes resulted in lack of direct electron communications with electrodes. Nanoscale materials are suitable for enhancing the electron transfer between the active center of enzymes and electrodes acting as electron transfer mediators or electrical nanowires [146]. The immobilized enzymes are used as analytical reagents to measure substrate molecules by catalyzing the turnover of these species to detectable products. Furthermore, direct electron transfer utilize metal oxide thin films that immobilize the enzymes and proteins , inhibit the denaturation of the protein and assorption of the passivating impurities on the electrode and may control other factors such as orientation and bioactivity.

In this chapter, we review the recent progress in the development of different metal oxide nanoparticles with various shapes and size for fabrication of biosensors. The development of metal oxide nanomaterials surface film for direct electron exchange between electrodes and redox enzymes and proteins will be summarizing. The electrochemical properties, stability and biocatalytic activity of the proposed biosensors will be discussed. The biocompatibility of the metal oxide nanomaterials for enzymes and biomolecules will be evaluated. We will briefly describe some techniques for the investigation of proteins and enzymes when adsorbed to the electrode surfaces. Cyclic voltammetry, impedance spectroscopy, UV-visible spectroscopy and surface imaging techniques were used for surface characterization and bioactivity measuring.

4.1. Zinc Oxide Nanomaterial for Biosensors Fabrication

As a typical n-type metal oxide semiconductor, ZnO possesses many unique optical and electrical properties for applications in many important area such as chemical sensors, heterogenous catalysis and solar cells [147]. ZnO nanoparticles have been exploited as a potential material for biosensing because of their unusual properties including high surface are, high catalytic efficiency, nontoxicity, chemical and photochemical stability, optical transparency, electrochemical activity, high electron communication, biocompatibility and strong adsorption stability [148,149]. Zinxc oxide with higher isoelectric point (p*I*= 9.5) , can be used for adsorption of proteins with lower isoelectric point where the protein immobilization is driven by electrostatic interaction [150] . Different nano-scale materials of ZnO have been used for direct electron transfer of enzymes and fabrication third generation biosensor. Various ZnO nanostructures such as nanorods [151], nanowires [152] nanobelts [153] nanoring [154] nanosheet [155] and radial nanoarray [156] have been prepared. But there are fewer reports on ZnO porous nanostructures and their applications in biosensing [157]. The cholesterol oxidase (ChOx) immobilized in zinc oxide nanoparticles -chitosan (CHIT) composite film onto inidium-tin oxide (ITO) glass plate has been used for fabrication of sensitive cholesterol biosensor [148].vThe mechanism of nano ZnO-CHIT electrode fabrication and immobilization of cholesterol oxidase into nanocomposite is shown in Fig.2.

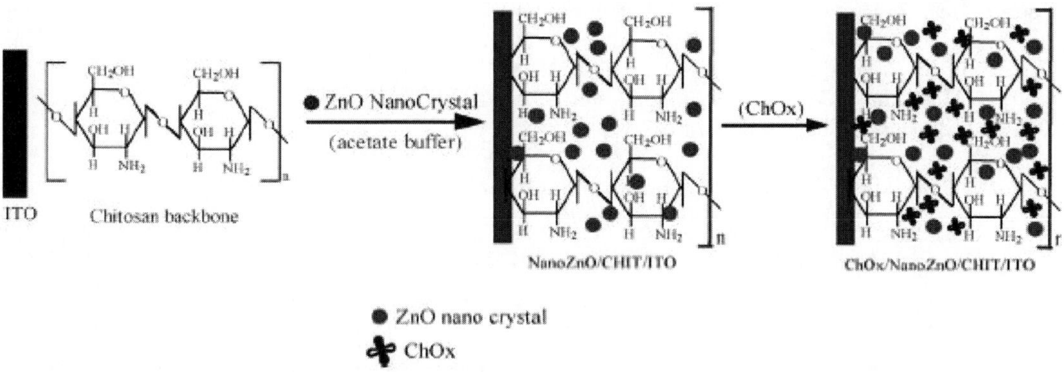

Figure 2. The mechanism for preparation of Nano ZnO-CHIT electrode and immobilization of ChOx onto NanoZnO-CHIT Nanocomposite , Reprinted from Analytica Chimica Acta, 616, R. Khan, A. Kaushik, P. R. Solanki, A.A. Ansari, M.K. Pandy, B.D. Malhotra, Zinc oxide nanoparticles –chitosan composite film for cholesterol biosensor, 209,Copyright(2008) with permission fom Elsevier.

It appears that the nanocomposite film provides a biocompatible environment to the ChOx enzyme and ZnO nanoparticles act as an electron mediator resulting in a accelerated electron transfer between enzyme and electrode. Figure 3A shows the surface morphology of CHIT/ITO, nanoZnO-CHIT/ITO and ChOx/ nanoZnO-CHIT/ITOelectrodes using SEM images.After ChOx immobilization the porous morphology of nano-ZnO-CHIT changes into regular form due to electrostatic interaction between nano-ZnO-CHIT and cholesterol oxidase.Figure 3B shows the biochemical reaction of the biosensor for cholesterol detection.

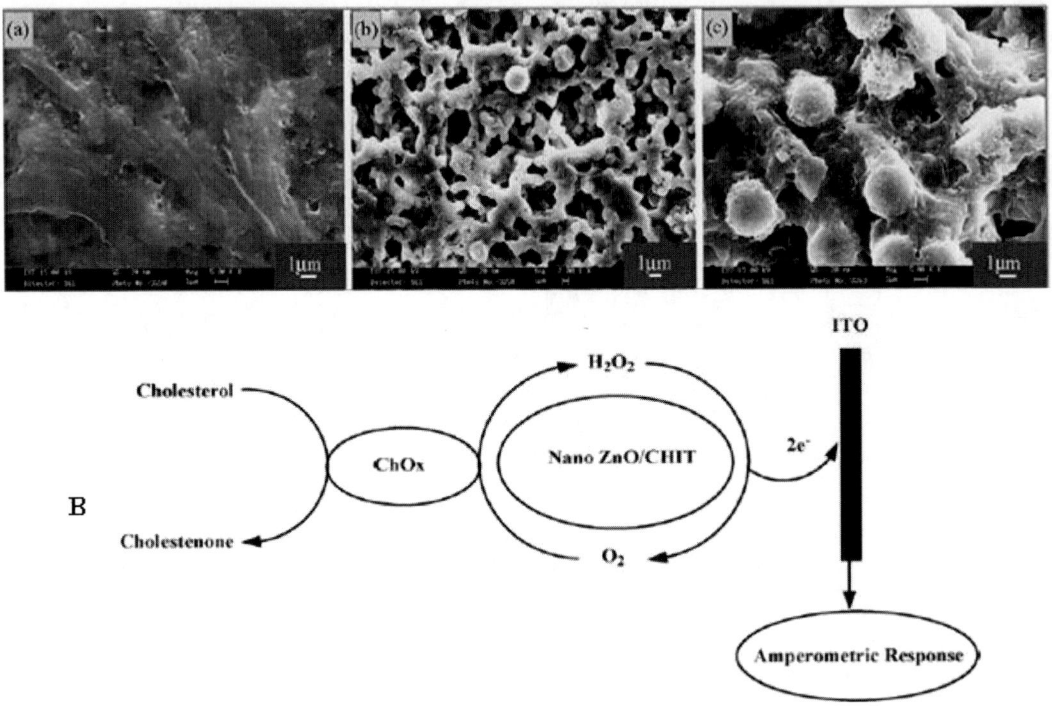

Figure3. (A) SEM images of; CHIT/ITO electrode (a) NanoZnO-CHIT/ITO electrode (b) and ChOx/NanoZnO-CHIT/ITO bioelectrode (c). (B) Biochemical reaction of the biosensor to cholesterol. Reprinted from Analytica Chimica Acta, 616, R. Khan, A. Kaushik, P. R. Solanki, A.A. Ansari, M.K. Pandy, B.D. Malhotra, Zinc oxide nanoparticles –chitosan composite film for cholesterol biosensor, 209,211,Copyright (2008) with permission fom Elsevier.

The $[Fe(CN)_6]^{3-/4-}$ has been used as electrocatalyst for oxidation of hydrogen peroxide arises to the enzymatic reaction between ChOx and cholesterol. The oxidation peak of $[Fe(CN)_6]^{3-/4-}$ redox couple increase with increasing cholesterol concentration results in increasing the concentration of hydrogen peroxide during enzymatic reaction. Glassy carbon electrode modified with nanoshheet-based ZnO microspheres has been used for immobilization and direct electron transfer of hemoglobin [149].The fabricated biosensor displayed good performance for detection of hydrogen peroxide and nitrite with a wide linear range. The SEM image of porous nanoshet-based ZnO microsphere is shown in Fig.4A.

As shown the thickness of these nanosheets is about 20 nm. There are numerous nanoscaled cavities on the surface of ZnO microspheres. The size of the cavity is about several hundred nanometers, which is accessible for the enzymes to sequester in the cavities or bind on the surface. Furthermore the cavities may provide a protective microenvironment for the enzymes to retain their enzymatic stability and activity by limiting the conformational change and unfolding of the entrapped enzyme. The FTIR spectra of hemoglobine (Hb) and Hb-ZnO- nafion composite film is shown in Fig.4B. The similarities of two spectra suggested that Hb retained the essential features of its native secondary structure in ZnO nafion composite film, and revealed the excellent biocompability of ZnO nafion composite film. Cyclic voltammetry response of the biosensor at different scan rates was shown in Fig.5.

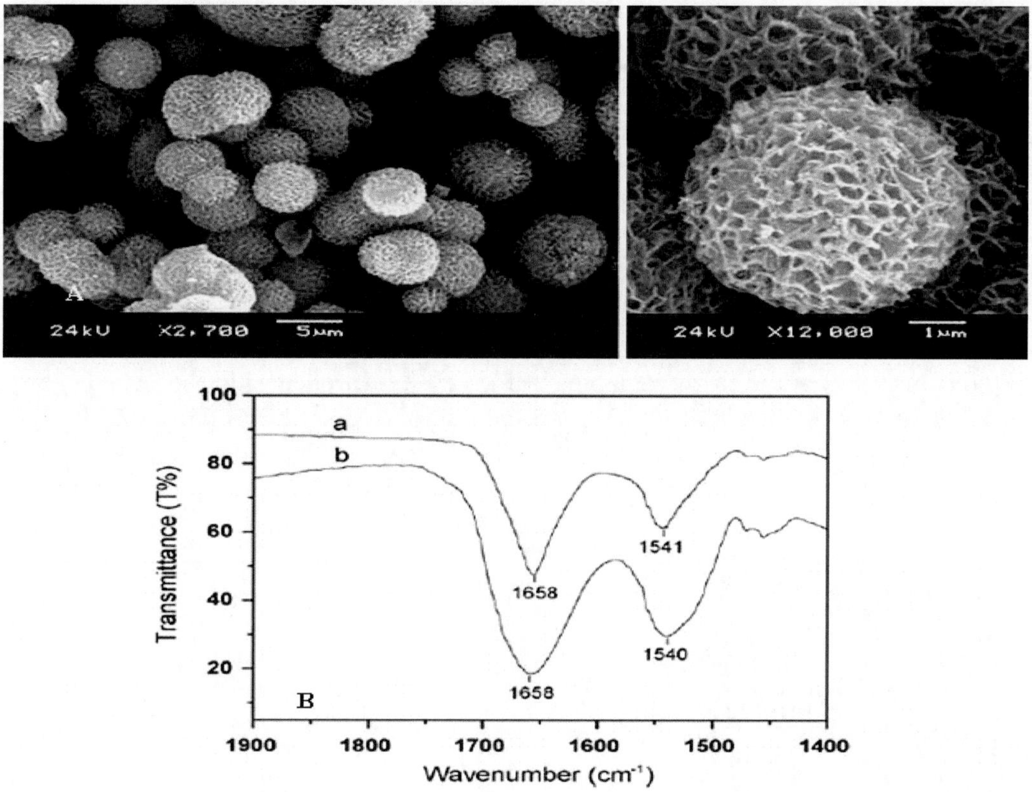

Figure4. (A) SEM imagesof prepared porous nanosheet-based ZnOmicrosphere with different magnification. (B) FTIR spetra of hemoglobine (Hb) and Hb-ZnO- nafion composite film. (Reprinted from Biosensors and Bioelectronics 24, X. Lu, H. Zhang, Y. Ni, Q. Zhang, J. Chen, Porous nanosheet-based ZnO microspheres for the construction of direct electrochemical biosensors, 95, Copyright (2008) with permission fom Elsevier.

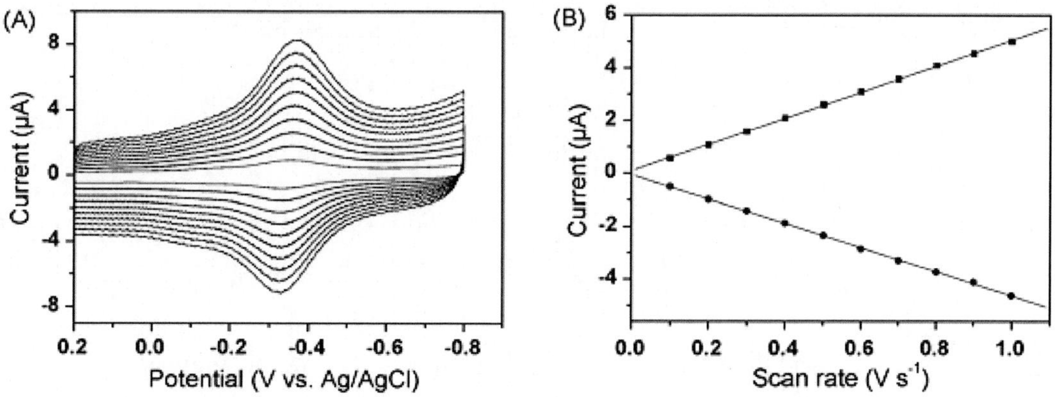

Figure 5. (A) CyclicvoltammogramsofHb–ZnO–Nafion/GC in pH 7.0 PBS with scan rates from 0. 1to 1.0 Vs^{-1} (B) Plot of cathodic and anodic peak currents vs.scan rates. (Reprinted from Biosensors and Bioelectronics 24, X. Lu, H. Zhang, Y. Ni, Q. Zhang, J. Chen, Porous nanosheet-based ZnO microspheres for the construction of direct electrochemical biosensors,96, Copyright (2008) with permission fom Elsevier.

A well defined voltammogram for direct electron transfer of Hb was observed.The high value of electron transfer rate constant (k_s) , 3.2 s^{-1} suggesting faster elec tron transfer process at this metal-oxide nanomaterial. Is The surface concentration of electroactive Hb(Γ) is about 1×10^{-10} mol cm^{-2} which is 5 times higher than of the theoretical monlayer coverage,which indicates that multilayer of hemoglobin in the three-dimensional composite film participated in the electron transfer process. The apparent Michaelis-Menten constant K_M was estimated to be 143 μM, indicating that Hb entrapped in the nanocomposite film possesses high peroxidase like activity. Porous nanomaterials provide a larger surface are available for protein bending and decrease the diffusion distance for the substrate to access the immobilized enzyme.Graphite electrode modified with electrodeposited ZnO nanoparticles use for immobilization of myoglobin(Mb) [158].Electrodeposition of ZnO film was performed potentiostatically at -0.6 V for 5 min in a mixed solution of 20 mM $Zn(NO_3)_2$ nd 0.1% SDS without stirring at 60°C. The AFM image of electrodeposited ZnO shows a uniform film of zinc oxide adsorbed on the electrode surface (Fig. 6A).

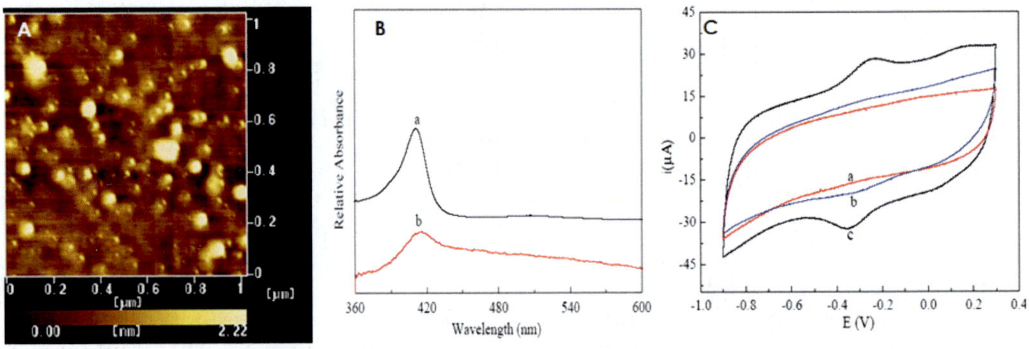

Figure 6. (A)AFM image of electrodeposited ZnO nanoparticles(B) UV-Vis spectra of Mb in pH 7 PBS (a) and on an ITO glass slide deposited with ZnO nanoparticles(b).CVs of ZnO (a), Mb (b), and Mb-ZnO (c)modified GE in PBS (pH 7.0); scan rate, 100 mV s^{-1} (Reprinted from Analytical Biochemistry , 350, G. Zhao, J. J. Xu, H. Y. Chen, Interfacing Myoglobine to graphite electrode with an electrodeposited nanoporous ZnO film,147, Copyrights (2006) with permission fom Elsevier.

In order to su attach the protein molecules to the electrode surface, the graphite electrode modified with ZnO film incubated in a 3 mg/mL myoglobin solution (pH 7) for about 10 h. Recorded cyclic voltammogram of biosensor shows direct electron transfer of myoglobin on the ZnO nanoparticles (Fig.6 B). The Soret band is sensitive to variation of the microenvironment around the heme site and can give helpful information on whether proteins have been denatured [159]. Figure 6C, shows the UV-Vis spectra of Mb in pH 7 PBS and on an ITO glass slide deposited with ZnO nanoparticles.For Mb adsorbed on electrodeposited ZnO film the soret band is located at 413 nm, with shifts only 2 nm in comparison to natural Mb in solution(411 nm). This result suggests that ZnO film is a good matrix to supply a friendly microenvironment to immobilize Mb and retain its bioactivity. Direct voltammetry of microperoxidase immobilized onto ZnO nanoparticles is investigated [160]. Due to semiconductor characteristic of ZnO nanoparticles, the catalytic ability of the immobilized microperoxidase toward hydrogen peroxide reduction greatly promoted, by irradiating the microperoxidase/ZnO nanoparticles co-modified electrode with UV light for 4 h. The photovoltaic effect of ZnO nanoparticles improved the catalytic activity of microperoxidase.

With immobilizing tyrosinase onto ZnO nanoparticles, a mediator free phenol biosensor was fabricated [161]. The fabricated biosensor has shows good response for p-cresol, phenol and catechol detection using amperometric technique. The apparent Michaelis -Menten constant K_M for immobilized tyrosinase was calculated. The K_M values were 21, 23 and 40 μM for p-cresol, phenol and catechol respectively, which are lower than values reported for free enzyme in solution (700 μM, using phenol as substrate). This result indicates excellent biocompability of ZnO nanoparticle to tyrosinase enzyme. Due to importance of glucose detection for diagnosing diabetics, different glucose biosensors based on metal oxide nanoparticles have been fabricated. Thin films of ZnO nanoroads and nanocombs have been used for fabrication of glucose biosensor [162,163]. TheXRD patterns, SEM, TEM, and high resolution TEM images of produced nanocomb are shown in Fig.7. The ZnO nanocombs were prepared by a vapor phase transport method.

The stems of nanocombs are ribbons with thickness of about 50 nm, the length of the main stems reaches several tens of micrometers. The branching nanorods grow on one side of nanoribbon with a diameter of about 200nm. The distance between two adjacent nanorods is about 500 nm.

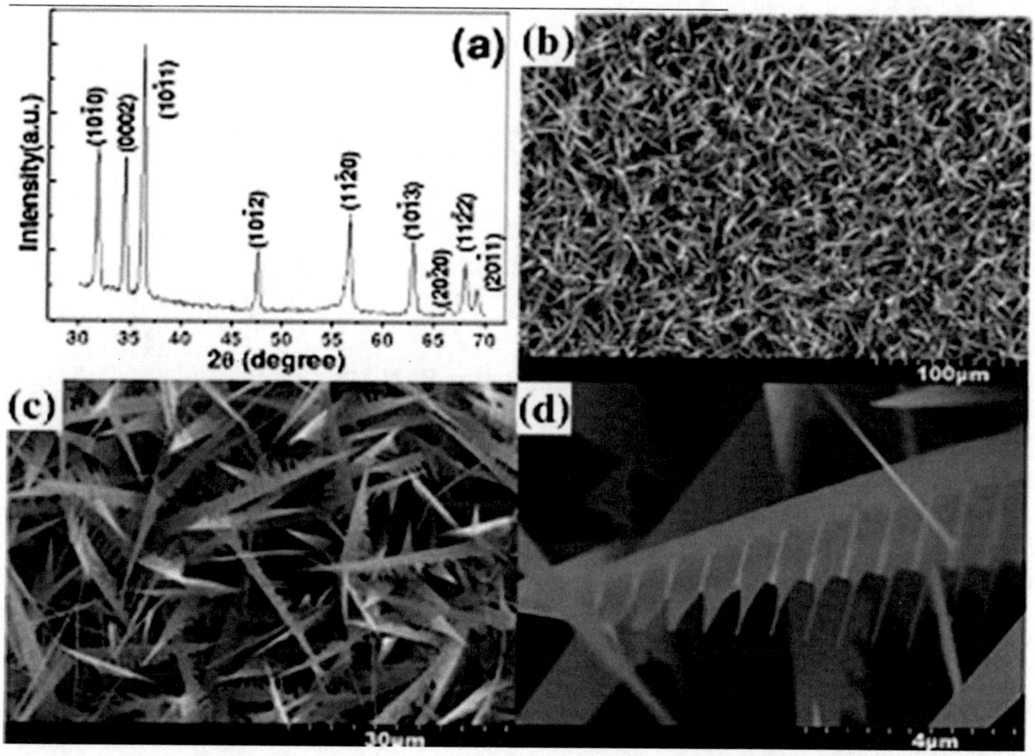

Figure 7. (a) XRD pattern of ZnOnano combs and SEM images of ZnO Nanocombs with (b) low, (c) medium, and (d) high magnifications, respectively (Reused with permission from J.X. Wang, X.W. Sun, A. Wei, Y. Lei, X.P. Cai, C.M. Li, Z.L. Dong, Appl. Phys. Lett. 2006, 88, 233106. Copyrights 2006 American Institute of Physics"

To fabricate the glucose biosensor, the GOx solution was dropped onto the surface of ZnO nanocombs /gold electrode. ZnO nanocombs are positively charged and display electrostatic interaction with negartively charged GOx. Fig.8 shows the CV curves of

Nafion/GOx/ZnO /gold electrode in PBS with 0.0 and 0.3 mM glucose, compared to buffer solution without glucose, indicating the response of the biosensor to glucose. As we can see a weak shoulder peak appeares at about 0.6 V on the CV curve for Nafion/GOx/ZnO/gold electrode in PBS with 3 mM glucose. The K_M value 2.19 mM indicating the high affinity of ZnO glucose biosensor. This peak can be attributed to hydrogen peroxide generated during glucose oxidation by glucose oxidase.

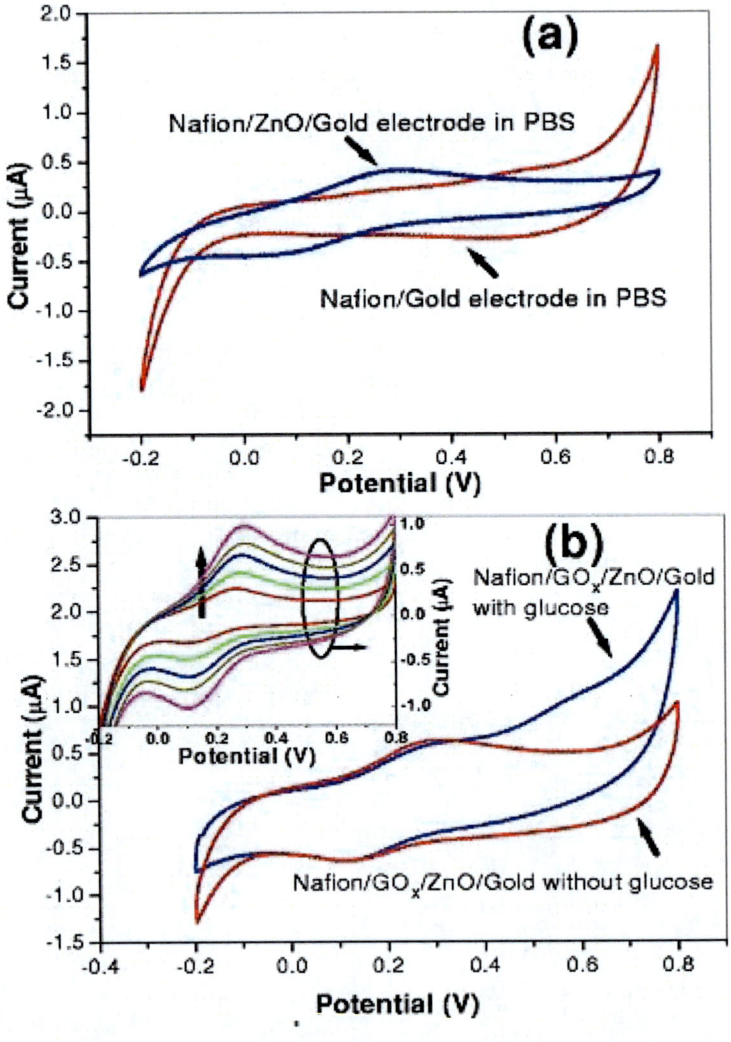

Figure 8. (a) Cyclic voltammograms of Nafion/gold electrode andNafion/ZnO/gold electrode blue in0.01M, pH 7.4 PBS buffer at scan rate of 50 mV/s.(b)Cyclic voltammograms of nafion / GOx/ZnO/gold electrode in the same buffer solution in the absence and presence of 3 mM glucose.Inset is the CVcurves recorded at various scan rates of 20,40,60,80,and100 mV/s in same buffer solution,(Reused with permission from; J.X. Wang, X.W. Sun, A. Wei, Y. Lei, X.P. Cai, C.M. Li, Z.L. Dong, Appl. Phys. Lett. 2006, 88, 233106. Copyrights 2006 American Institute of Physics"

A highly sensitive glucose biosensor based on immobilization of glucose oxidase (GOx) onto tetragonal pyramid-shaped (TPSP) ZnO nanostructure is prepare [164]. TPSP- ZnO nanostructure exhibits favorable biocompability for facilitating the electron transfer between

GOx and electrode.The high value for electron transfer rate constant k_s, 7.5 ± 0.4 s^{-1}, indicate the high ability of TPSP- ZnO nanostructure for direct electron transfer of immobilized enzyme. The immobilized GOx preserves its natural structure and bioactivity and display better responses to glucose than those from other morphological ZnO nanoparticles. To verify the effect of GOx on TTRSP-ZnO, N_2 adsorption isotherms before and after GOx loading are evaluated .The surface area of ZnO decreases upon the immobilization treatment. The surface area of the TPSP-ZnO calculated from N_2 adsorption isotherm is about 41 m^2g^{-1}.This value decreases to 24 m^2g^{-1} by loading GOx (about 60%) of that befor enzyme loading, indicating that GOx intercalates into the pores of ZnO [165]. The AFM images of the TPSP-ZnO befor and after GOx loadind shown in Fig.9 A and B.

After GOx immobilization, the surface pores of TPSP-ZnO can not be observed and the diameter of the ZnO slightly increased, indicating the immobilization of GOx onto nanostructure. Based on the AFM and N_2 isotherm investigation, GOx not only adsorbed on the surface of TPSP-ZnO, but also intercalated into the pores of ZnO. The recorded cyclic voltammograms of GOx enzyme immobilized onto ZnO nanostructure is shown in Fig.9C. The reversible redox behavior indicates, direct electron transfer of GOx.Fabricated biosensor has also been used for detection of glucose. GOx catalyzes the oxidation of glucose to produce gluconolactone and hydrogen peroxide, and oxygen is used as the electron acceptor [166]

$$\text{GOx (FAD)} + 2e^- \leftrightarrows +2H^+ \quad \text{GOx (FADH}_2\text{)} \qquad (1)$$

$$\text{GOx (FADH}_2\text{)} + O_2 \rightarrow \text{GOx (FAD)} + H_2O_2 \qquad (2)$$

Upon glucose addition, the electrocatalytic reaction is restrained to the enzyme catalyzed reaction between the oxidized form of glucose oxidase and glucose.

$$\text{Glucose} + \text{GOx (FAD)} \rightarrow \text{gluconolactone} + \text{GOx (FADH}_2\text{)} \qquad (3)$$

During glucose addition to oxygen saturated solution the reduction current response of the biosensor decreased, which resulted from the electrocatalytic reaction restrained to the enzyme catalyzed reaction between the oxidized form of GOD and glucose. With increasing glucose concentration the catalytic reduction current of oxygen decreased.

Another application of Zinc oxide nanostructure is immobilization of uricace onto ZnO nanorod and fabrication a sensitive biosensor for uric acid detection [167]. The biosensor successfully used for micromolar detection of uric acid in the presence serious interferences, glucose, ascorbic acid, and l-cysteine. The apparent K_M value for the uric acid biosensor is 0.238 mM, showing high affinity of the biosensor. Direct electron transfer of SOD at a physical vapor deposited zinc oxide nanoparticles surface was investigated [168]. In comparison to SOD immobilized onto ZnO nanodisks [169], the electron transfer rate constant is small and a quasi- reversible electrochemical behavior observed. A novel superoxide anion ($O_2^{-\bullet}$) biosensor based on direct electron transfer of copper-zinc-superoxide dismutase(Cu,Zn-SOD) at zinc oxide nanodisk surface was fabricated [169]. A ZnO nanodisks films was electrodeposited on the ITO glase plate from 0.1 mM $Zn(NO_3)_2$ solution containing 0.1 mM KCl at applied potential of -0.9 verses Ag/AgCl for 20 min, and then sintered at 773 K for 05-1.5 h. By immersing the ZnO film modified electrode into PBS (pH 7.2) containing of Cu, Zn-SOD (0.2 mM) for 0.5 -3 h at 3°C in a refrigerator biosensor fabricates. The SEM image of electrodeposited ZnO nanodisks is shown in Fig.10A.

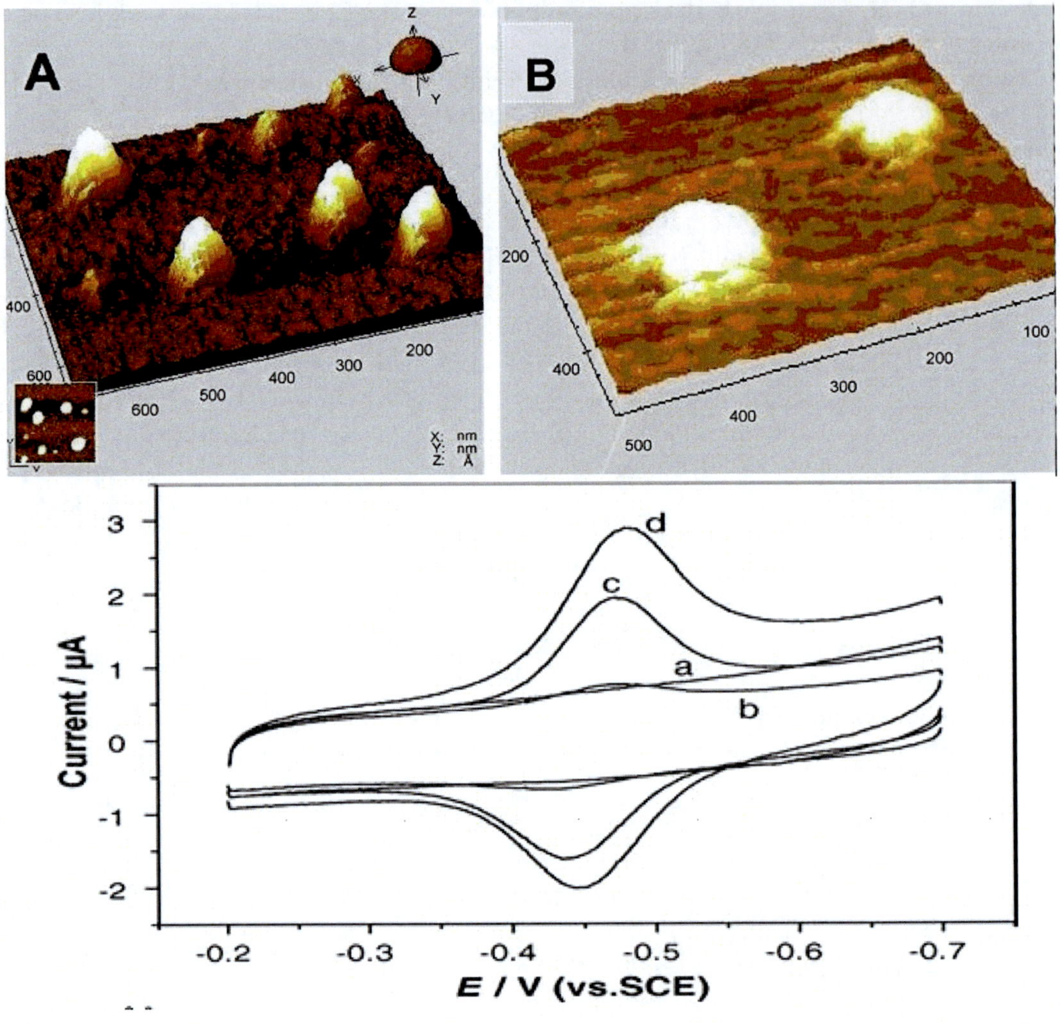

Figure 9. AFM images of TPSP-ZnO before (A)and after(B)GOD loading.(C) Cyclic voltammograms of TPSP-ZnO/Nafion (a), GOD/Nafion (b)GOD/spherical ZnO/ Nafion (c) and GOD/TPSP-ZnO/Nafion (d) modified in 0.1M pH 7.0 PB at $0.1 Vs^{-1}$(Reprinted from Biosensors and Bioelectronics ,24, Z. Dai, G. Shao, J. Hong, J. Bao, J. Shen, Immobilization and direct electrochemistry of glucose oxidase on a tetragonal pyramid-shaped porous ZnO nanostructure for a glucose biosensor, 1288,1289, Copyrights (2009) with permission fom Elsevier.

As can be seen the ZnO nanodisks are typically 50-80 nm in thickness and several micrometers in dimensions. Many nanodisks are rather regular hexagons , and the contrast on a hole sheet is homogenous. For investigating the direct electron transfer of SOD onto ZnO nanodisks the cyclic voltammograms of ZnO nanodisks and ZnO nanodisks-SOD in phosphate buffer solution free of SOD recorded .As shown a well defined redox couple for immobilized enzyme observed (Fig.10B). Furthermore, the CVs remained essentially unchanged on consecutive potential scanning up to 1000 cycles at a sweep rate of 20 mVs^{-1}, indicating that immobilized SOD onto ZnO nanodisks was stable. According to the Laviron procedure [170], the electron transfer rate constant (k_s) of immobilized enzyme is estimated to be 17± 2 s^{-1}, reveals that the direct electron transfer of SOD is strikingly enhanced at the nanostructured ZnO surface.The behavior of adsorbed SOD was confirmed by electrochemical impedance spectroscopy (EIS) technique.

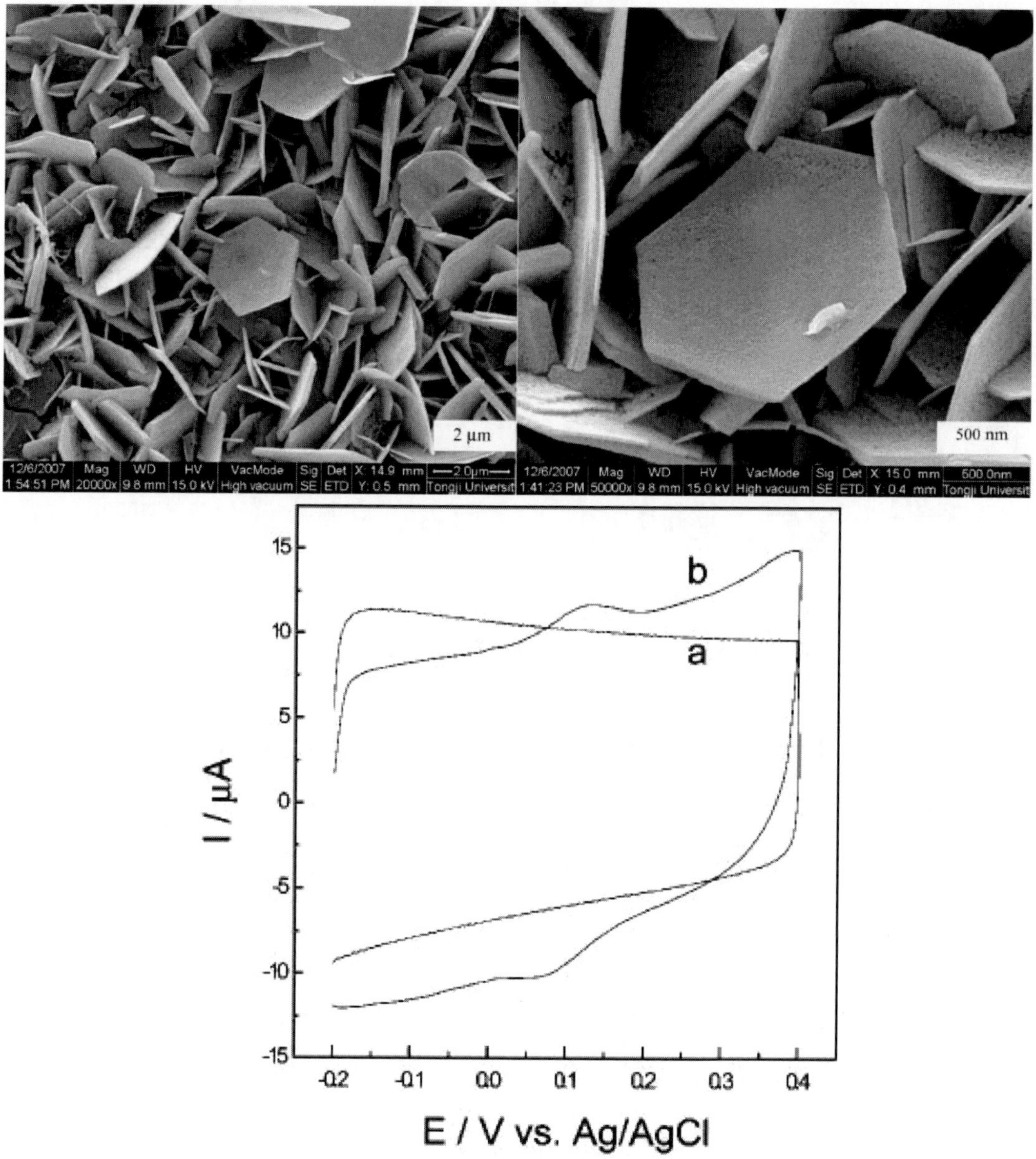

Figure 10.(A) SEM images of electrodeposited ZnOx nanodisk onto ITO electrode, (B) CVs obtained at (a) bare ZnO nanodisks film and (b) ZnO/SOD film in 25 mM PBS (pH 7.2); Potential scan rate, 500 mV s-1(Adapted with permission from; Z. Deng, Q. Rui, X. Yin, H. Liu, Y. Tian, Anal. Chem. 2008, 80, 5839-5846.Copyright 2008 American Chemical Society)

Figure 11 shows the Nyquist plots obtained at bare ZnO nanodisk film and ZnO/SOD electrode in 0.1 M KCl solution containing 0.1 M $[Fe(CN)_6]^{3-/4-}$.

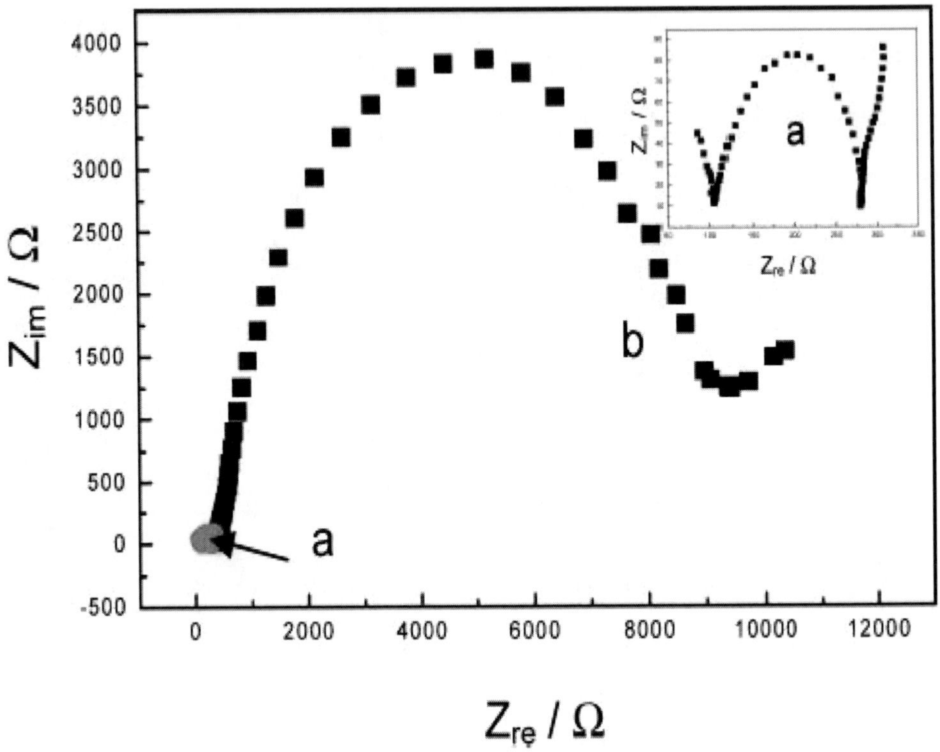

Figure 11. Nyquist plots obtained at (a) bare ZnO nanodisks film (enlarged in the inset) and (b) ZnO/SOD electrode in 0.1 M KCl solution containing 1 mM $[Fe(CN)6]^{3-/4-}$. EIS conditions: potential, 0.25 V; alternative voltage, 5 mV; frequency range, 0.1-105 Hz. (Adapted with permission from; Z. Deng, Q. Rui, X. Yin, H. Liu, Y. Tian, Anal. Chem. 2008, 80, 5839-5846.Copyright 2008 American Chemical Society)

The charge transfer resistance (Rct) of the redox couple is 174 Ωat ZnO nanodisk film, while it increases to 9.7 KΩ after SOD immobilized onto ZnO nanodisks.These results indicate that adsrorbed SOD might inhibit the electrochemical communications between the electron transfer indicator and nanostructured ZnO electrode. The SOD immobilized onto ZnO nanodisks catalyzes the dismutation of $O_2^{-\cdot}$ to O_2 and H_2O_2 via a cyclic oxidation - reduction electron transfer. Therefore, the third generation biosensor for superoxide developed. Figure 12 A shows the cyclic voltammograms of ZnO/SOD electrode in the absence and presence of $O_2^{-\cdot}$.

Both currents in the oxidation and reduction regionsincreased in the presence of superoxide.The observed increase in the anodic and cathodic currents responses of the ZnO/SOD electrode in the presence of $O_2^{-\cdot}$ can be ascribed to the oxidation and reduction of $O_2^{-\cdot}$, respectively, which are effectively mediated by the SOD confined on the electrode. The following reaction mechanism could explain the enhanced oxidation current.

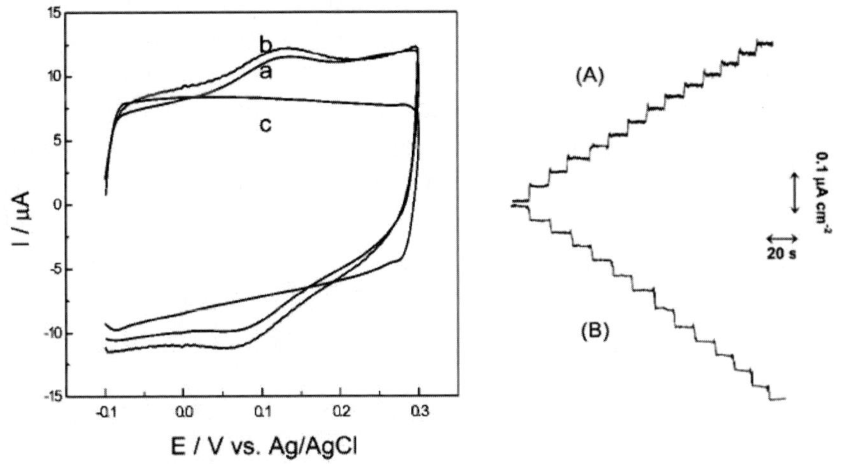

Figure 12. (left) Cvs obtained at ZnO/SOD (a,b) and bare ZnO nanodiscks(c) electrodes in the absence (a) and presence (b,c) of 30 mM $O_2^{-\cdot}$ in pH 7.2, scan rate 500mVs^{-1}.(Right)Typical amperometric responses of the ZnO/SOD to successive additions of 4 μL of KO_2 (10 μM) at applied potentials of (A) +300 and (B)0.0 mV (Adapted with permission from; Z. Deng, Q. Rui, X. Yin, H. Liu, Y. Tian, Anal. Chem. 2008, 80, 5839-5846. Copyright 2008 American Chemical Society)

$$\text{SOD (Cu (I))} - e^- \rightarrow \text{SOD (Cu (II))} \quad (4)$$

$$\text{SOD (Cu(II))} + O_2^{-\cdot} \rightarrow \text{SOD (Cu (I))} + O_2 \quad (5)$$

Similary the reduction current is enhanced in the cathodic scan according to the following reactions:

$$\text{SOD(Cu(II))} + e^- \rightarrow \text{SOD(Cu(I))} \quad (6)$$

$$\text{SOD(Cu(I))} + O_2^{-\cdot} \xrightarrow{H^+} \text{SOD (Cu (II))} + H_2O_2 \quad \textbf{(7)}$$

Amperometric responses of ZnO/SOD to successive addition of $O_2^{-\cdot}$ at applied potential of +0.3 and 0.0 V are displayed in Fig.12 A&B. As shown a well defined steady state response current are obtainedat both potential step and the currents increased stepwise with successive addition of superoxide. Due to high loading ability of ZnO nanomaterials for enzymes immobilization it can be used for entrapment of enzymes and preparation various medical biosensors. A sensitive cholesterol biosensor based on immobilization of cholesterol oxidase (ChOx)onto zinc oxide nanoporous thin film was also fabricated [171].The ChOx/ZnO/Au bioelectrode is sensitive to the detection of cholesterol in 25-400 mg/dl range. A relative low value of enzyme kinetic parameter, K_M 2.1 mM indicates enhanced enzyme affinity of ChOx to cholesterol. Zinc oxide-chitosan nanobiocomposite film onto ITO coated glass has also been used to immobilize urease(Urs) and glutamate dehydrogenase (GLDH) enzyme [172].The presence ZnO nanoparticles in chitosanincreasing surface are and electron transfer kinetics. The proposed biosensor has been successfully used for urea detection. The sensitivity, liner concentration range, and detection limit of the biosensor were, 9.4 μA/mg dl^{-1} ,3 mg dl^{-1},5-100 mg dl^{-1} and 10 s, respectively. The K_M, 0.82 mM, indicates high affinity of the biosensor to urea. The cyclic voltammograms of Urs-GLDH/ZnO-Chitosan/ITO bioelectrode in solution contaning $Fe(CN)_6^{-3}$ in the presence different urea concentration is shown hown in Fig.13a. As shown with increasing urea concentration the anodic peak current increased. The selectivity of the biosensor has been estimated by comparing magnetide of current response by adding different concentrations of interferences (50 mM ascorbic acid, 5 mM of lactic acid, 100 mM of uric acid, 5 mM glucose and 5mM cholesterol). The results indicated that the biosensor response is not significantly affected in the presence these interferences. Figure 13b shows the electrochemical reaction of the biosensor in the presence urea, zinc oxide nanoparticles and and electron transfer mediator.

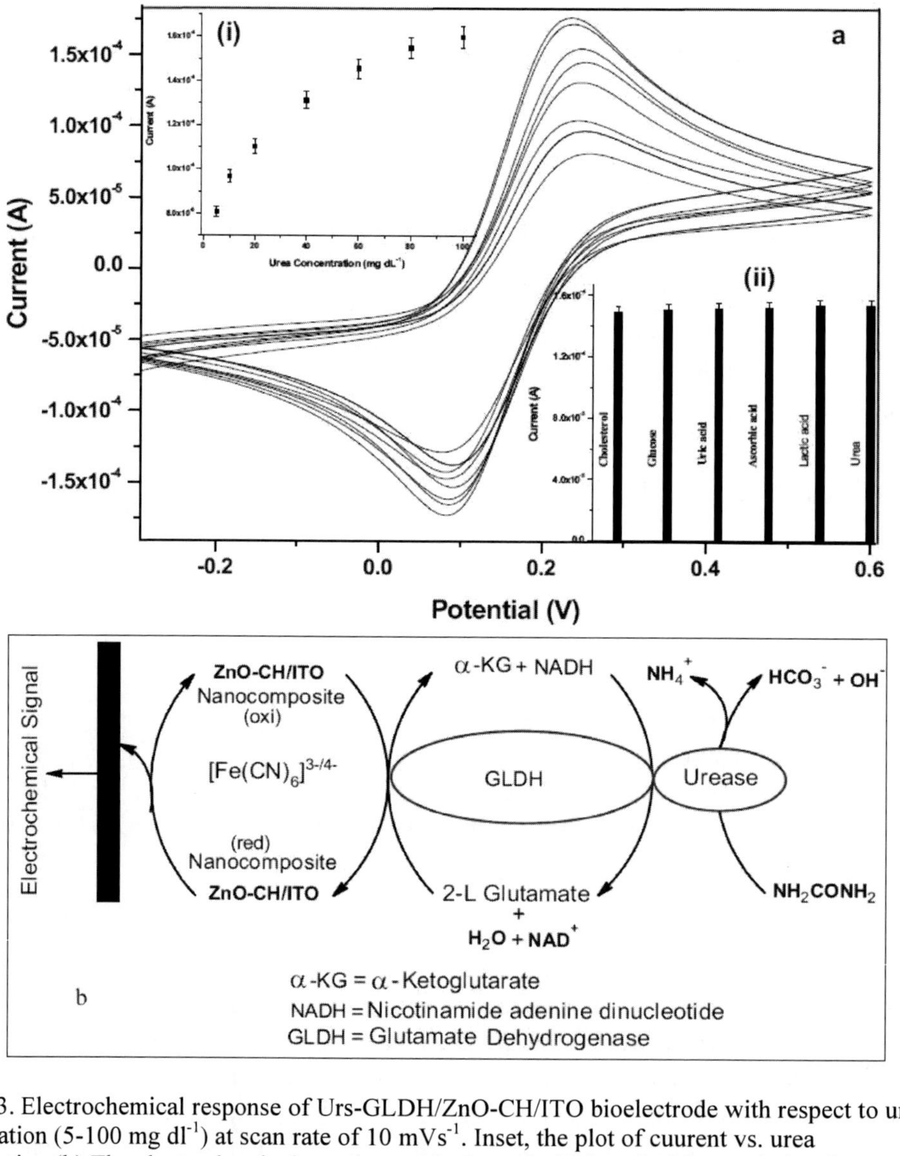

Figure 13. Electrochemical response of Urs-GLDH/ZnO-CH/ITO bioelectrode with respect to urea concentration (5-100 mg dl^{-1}) at scan rate of 10 mVs^{-1}. Inset, the plot of cuurent vs. urea concentration.(b) The electrochemical reaction at bioelectrode.(Reused with permission from P.R. Solanki, A.Kaushik, A.A. Ansari, G. Gumana, B.D. Malhotra, Applied Physics Letters, 93, 2008, 163903. Copyrights 2008 American Institute of Physics"

Recently we used glassy carbon electrode modified with electrodeposited ZnO nanoparticles for electrooxidation of guanine [135]. The guanine oxidation product(8- oxo-guanine) adsorbed strongly and irreversibly on zinc oxide bnanoparticles. The modified electrode shows a pair of well defined, nearly reversible and surface controlled redox couple at wide pH range (2-12) based on the following electrochemical process.

$$\text{8-oxo-guanine} \leftrightharpoons \text{2- amino 1-H purine 6,8- dione} + 2H^+ + 2e^- \qquad (8)$$

The surface coverage (Γ) and heterogeneous electron transfer rate constant (k_s) of adsorbed redox couple were about 9.5×10^{-9} mol cm^{-2} and 3.18 (±0.20) s^{-1}, respectively, indicating the high loading ability of ZnOx nanoparticles toward guanine oxidation product and great facilitation of the electron transfer between redox couple and ZnOx nanoparticles. The modified electrode exhibited excellent electrocatalytic activity toward L-cysteine oxidation. The k_{cat} for L-cysteine oxidation was found to be $4.20(\pm0.20)\times10^3$ M^{-1}s^{-1}. The catalytic oxidation current allows the amperometric detection of L-cysteine at potential of 0.5 V with detection limit of 50 nM, linear response up to 20 μ M and sensitivity of 215.4 nA.μ A^{-1}cm$^{-2.}$ This results indicate ZnO nanoparticles modified electrodes are suitable microenvironment for observation and stabilization of unusual and unstable redox couples.

4.2. Titanium Oxide Nanomaterial for Biosensors Fabrication

Titanium oxide, $TiO_{2,}$ a wide band gap semiconductor have application in different area such as water and air purification, solar cells, batteries, photovoltaic, photocatalysis systems and catalyst support [173,174]. Recently, there are a considerable interests for TiO_2 films since they have high surface area, optical transparency, excellent biocompability, and relatively good effective conductivity. Furthermore, TiO_2 nanoparticles also widely used in biomedical and bioengineering fields due to their strong oxidizing properties, chemical inertness and nontoxicity. With immobilization of biomolecules onto titanium oxide nanomaterials, not only the photocatalytic capacities of TiO_2 retain, but also the bioactivity of biomolecules enhanced. Morevere, TiO_2 nanoparticles possess specific ability to advance photochemical applications and can efficiently separate photogenerated charges that could facilitate some redox chemical reactions with attached biomolecules [175] .Thin mesoporous films of TiO_2 deposited at electrode surfaces allow molecular redox system and redox proteins to be immobilized and connected to the electrode [176,177]. Titanium dioxide can be formed into different morphologies such as nanoparticles, nanofibers, nanotubes and nanosheets [178,179]. Various TiO_2 nano-scale materials were used to immobilize proteins or enzymes on electrode surfaces for either mechanistic study of the proteins or fabricating of electrochemical biosensors. Direct electron transfer of heme proteins (cytochrom C, myoglobin and hemoglobin) assembeled onto nanocrystaline TiO_2 has been studied [7]. TiO_2 film could not only offer a friendly platform to assemble protein molecule but also enhance the electron transfer process between protein molecules and the electrode. Indium tin oxide (ITO) modified with a nanocomposite containing multilayers of TiO_2 nanoparticles and phytic acid, has been used as support material for immobilization of hemoglobin and cytochrom *c* [180]. Cyclic voltammograms of Hb immobilized onto a 10 layer of TiO_2-phytate film in pH

5.5 at different scan rates is shown in Fig.14. A redox couple with formal potential of 0.01 *vs* SCE observed for immobilized hemoglobin. This value is more positive than reported value in the literature (0.25V), due to phytate- hemoglobin interaction. With increasing the layer TiO_2-phytate layers (40 layers), the nanocomposite act as insulating film and redox activity of adsorbed hemoglobin deminesed.

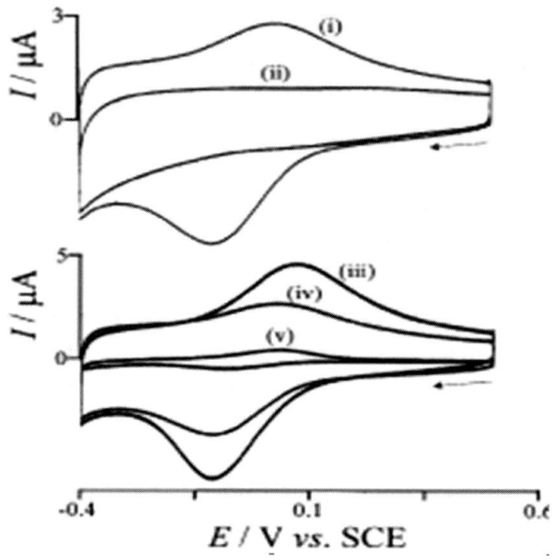

Figure 14. (A) Cyclic voltammograms 0.1M phytate film with phosphate buffer at pH 5.5 for:(i) 10-layer TiO_2 surface adsorbed hemoglobin; (ii) 40-layer TiO_2.(B)Cyclic voltammograms are also compared for a 10-layer TiO_2 phytate film with surface adsorbed hemoglobin at scan rates of :(iii) 0.1; (iv) 0.05; (v) 0.01Vs^{-1}(Reprinted from Electrochemistry Communications, 6, C.A. Paddon, F. Marken, Hemoglobin adsorption into TiO2 phytate multi-layer films:paeticle size and conductivity effects ,1251, Copyrights (2004), with permission from Elsevier.

Pores produced from aggregates of 6-10 nm diameter of TiO_2 nanoparticles seemed to be sufficient for the bulk immobilization. Protiens such as cytochrome *c* readly adsorb into a mesoporous TiO_2-phytate composite host [181]. Methemoglobin is immobilized into thin porous TiO_2 films at ITO electrode surface [182]. TiO_2 film with 40 nm particle size are also produced.The pore size in this film is sufficient for methemoglobin (ca. 6 nm diameter) to diffuse into the porous structure and to remain immobilized in electrochemically active form. The electrochemical reduction of methemoglobin immobilized onto TiO_2 nanoparticles was observed in two steps (Fig. 15).

A quasi-reversible voltammetric signal at formal potential of -0.16V vs.SCE is consistent with the Fe(III)/Fe(II) one electron reduction of the hemin unit in methemoglobin [28].

$$Fe(III)(Hb) + e^- (ITO) \leftrightharpoons Fe(II)Hb \qquad (9)$$

A second reduction is observed at a potential ca. -0.5V *vs.* SCE.This reduction peak current is relatively small for 1 layer TiO_2 film but almost enhanced one order of magnetide for the 10 layer TiO_2 film electrode. This reduction identified for Fe(III)/Fe(II) redox couple with electron conduction through the bulk TiO_2 film. This reduction requires the transport of electrons through the porous oxide and therefore occurs at more negative potential which is sufficient concentrations of electrons are available in the TiO_2 film.

$$Fe(III)(Hb) + e^{-}(TiO_2)) \rightarrow Fe(II)Hb \quad (10)$$

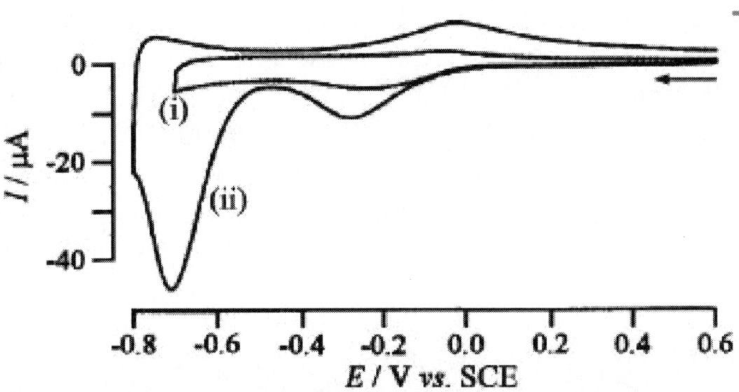

Figure 15. Cyclic voltammograms obtained for the reduction of adsorbed methemoglobin on (i) a bare ITO electrode and (ii) an ITO electrode covered with 1 layer of 40 nm diameter TiO_2 nanoparticles immersed in aqueous 0.1 M KCl (Reprinted from Bioelectrochemistry, 20, E.V. Milson, H.A. Dash, T.A. Jenkis, M.Opallo, F. Marken, The effects of conductivity and electrochemical doping on the reduction of methemoglobin immobilized in nanoparticles TiO_2 films,223, Copyrights(2007) with

The other nanocomposite was used for immobilization of large redox proties (methemoglobin) is cellulose-nanofibril-TiO_2 nanoarticles [183]. The TiO_2 nanophase is creating conducting pathways for electrons in a relatively open cellulose structure. Zhang et al. investigated the direct electrochemistry and bioelectrocatalytic activity of HRP immobilized in TiO_2 nanoparticles film on pyrolytic graphite electrode [184]. The electron exchange between the enzyme and pyrolytic graphite electrode was greatly enhanced in the TiO_2 nanoparticle film microenvironment. The heterogeneous electron transfer rate constant (k_s) was 72± 9 s^{-1}. This large k_s value of HRP- TiO_2 nanopartickes confirms the enhancement of electron transfer rate by TiO_2 nanoparticles film. Furthermore, the formal potential of HRP in titanium oxide film was more negative than that in other films such as polyacrylamide, tributhylmethyl phosphonium chloride, and didodecyldimethylammonium bromide and carbon nanotubes due to different interactions of film components with protein. The low value of K_M, 0.2 mM for hydrogen peroxide as substrate, indicating excellent biocompability of nanocomposite for entrapment of tyrosinase enzyme onto titania sol-gel nanocomposite film [185]. This titania matrix could supplies a good environment for enzyme loading, which results in a high sensitivity of 15.78 $\mu A \mu M^{-1}$ cm^{-2} for monitoring phenol with detection limit of 10 nM. TiO_2 nanotubes fabricated by low cost anodic oxidation of the Ti substrate possess large surface areas and good uniformity and conformability over large areas, desirable for electrochemical biosensor design. With immobilization of horseradish peroxidase onto Au-modified titanium dioxide nanotube arrays a sensitive biosensor for H_2O_2 detection was fabricated [138]. The immobilized HRP exhibits high biological activity and good stability. The amperometric response of the developed biosensor to H_2O_2 concentration has long-range linearity.The interaction of anticancer drugs with DNA and RNA bases in the presence nano-titanium dioxide enhanced [186]. The resutts indicated that the presence of TiO_2 nanoparticles can obviously increase the binding affinity of dacarbazine to DNA and specific DNA bases and significantly enhanced detection sensitivity. Figure 16 shows SEM images of TiO_2 nanotubes prepared by oxidation of Ti foil in a 1:8 acetic acid -water solution containing 1.0 vol% hydrofluoric acid at 20 V for 45min, forming TiO_2 nanotube arrays on the Ti substrate. As shown the average pore diameter is 80 nm and thickness is 29 nm [187]. With co-adsorption of HRP and thionine(Th) onto TiO_2 nanotubes highly sensitive biosensor for H_2O_2 detection was fabricated. The amperometric response and calibration curve of the biosensor for hydrogen peroxide detection is hown in Fig.16 A and B. The direct voltammetry and electrocatalytic activity of cytochrom *c* and hemoglobin adsorbed onto titania nanoparticles/ITO electrode have been investigated [188]. The spectroelectrochemical application of the prepared film was investigated. Due to ability of HbFe(II) on TiO_2 to bind oxygen and there after react with nitric oxide to form HbFe(III) it can be used as an aerobic optical sensor for nitric oxide, NO.

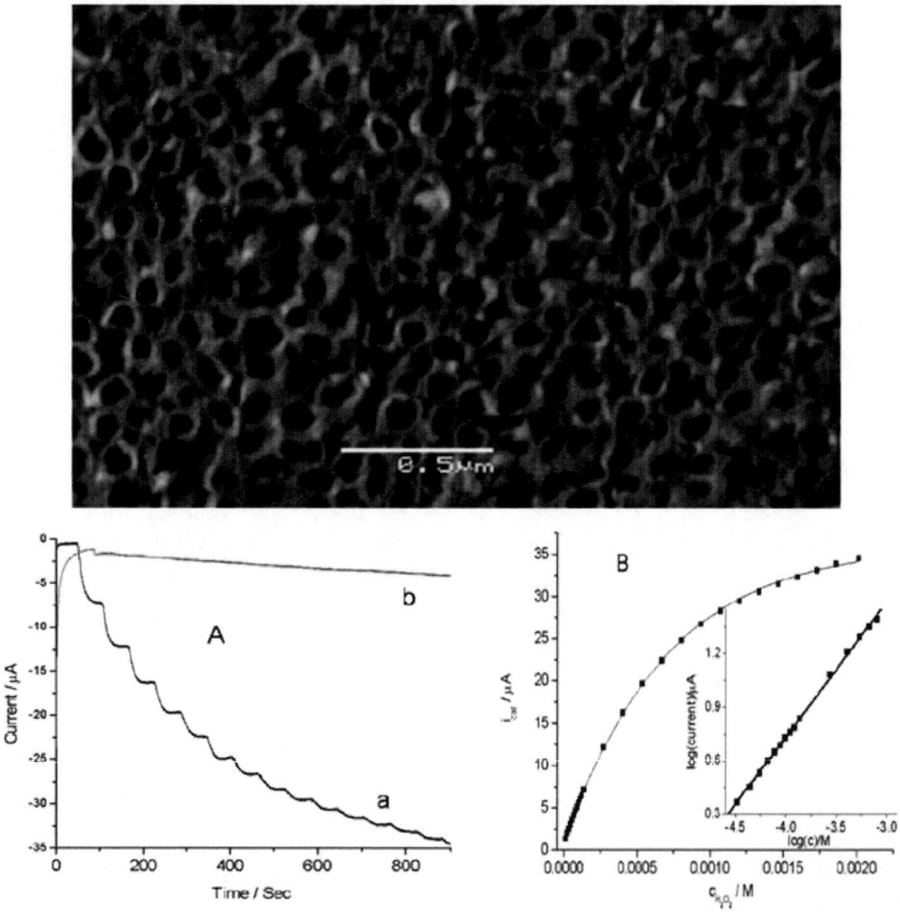

Figure 16, SEM image of TiO_2 nanotubes prepared by anodic oxidation of Ti substrate in an acetic acid solution containing 1.0 vol % HF at 20 V for 45 min.(A) Amperometric response of (a) Th/HRP/ TiO_2 and (b) Th/ TiO_2 at-450 mV upon successive additions of 0.134 mM H_2O_2 into 0.1M PB at pH 6.8. (B) Plot of the reduction current versus the H_2O_2 (Adapted with permission from; S. Liu, A. Chen, Langmiur 2005, 21, 8409-8413.Copyright 2000 American Chemical Society).

4.3. Iron Oxide Nanomaterial for Biosensors Fabrication

As one of the most important materials, magnetite (Fe_3O_4) nanoparticles and their thin films have attracted a lot of attentions, due to their interesting magnetic properties and potential applications in the field of biology, pharmacy, diagnostics , drug delivery, hyperthermia treatments, MRI contrast enhancement agents,purification of biomolecules, cell separation, biosensors and enzymatic assays [189-197]. The successful applications of magnetic nanoparticles in the immobilization of biomolcular have also been reported [198,199].Duo to good biocompatibility, strong superparamagnetic, low toxicity and easy preparation process, magnetic nanoparticles has been used to immobilize enzyme in different matrices such as hydrophobic sol-gel materials and biopolymer chitosan [200,201]. Due to high surface area and bioaffinity of nanomaterials as adsorbents, protein adsorption onto nanosize magnetic matrices have been investigate [202,203]. Furthermore, immobilization of lipase, ribonuclease, lysozyme, penicillin G acylase a, glucose oxidase and *Saccharomyces cerevisiae* mandelated dehydrogenase on magnetic nanoparticles was studied [204- 208]. The immobilization of protein or enzymes on magnetic nanoparticles has attracted much attention, which may afford an important platform for fabricating electrochemical biosensors and bioreactors. Direct voltammery of hemoglobineonat the glassy carbon electrode modified with electrodeposited chitosan/ Fe_3O_4 nanoparticles was investigated [209]. Multilayer film was formed firstly by electrodeposited chitosan / Fe_3O_4 nanoparticles thin film and then layer by layer assembly using phytic acid. Layer by layer deposition was used for multilayer formation of Fe_3O_4/ chitosan.(Fig.17A).

For the immobilization of hemoglobin (Hb), the (Fe_3O_4)/chitosan-phytic acid)$_n$ modified electrodes (phytic acid was the outer layer) were dipped into Hb solution (3 mg ml^{-1} , pH 7) for about 10 h in order to attach protein.The cyclic voltammograms of (Fe_3O_4)/chitosan-phytic acid)$_n$ and Hb-(Fe_3O_4)/chitosan-phytic acid)$_n$ modified electrodes recorded in pH 7 as shown in the Figure 17B. As can be seen no redox response observerd for (Fe_3O_4)/chitosan-phytic acid)$_4$, however, Hb-(Fe_3O_4)/chitosan-phytic acid)$_n$ isplayed a pair of well defined redox peaks at about Epc= -0.408V, Epa=-0.288 V, which is in accordance with the characteristic of Fe(III)/Fe(II) redox couple of heme protein.

When multilayer film containes no Fe_3O_4 nanoparticles, the redox peak of Hb is also observed , but the current value is much smaller than that for the film containing Fe_3O_4.This results indicating that magnetic nanoparticles in the film could increase the adsorbtion ability for protein and /or favor the orientation of Hb. The biosensor shows excellent activity With immobilizing of myoglobin onto poly-dimethyldiallylammonium chloride)(PDDA)/ Fe_3O_4@ SiO_2 nanoparticles a high sensitie biosensor for hydrogen peroxide was fabricated [210]. Figure 18 showed the TEM image of the obtained Fe_3O_4 nanoparticles with the size ranging from 10 to 20 nm.

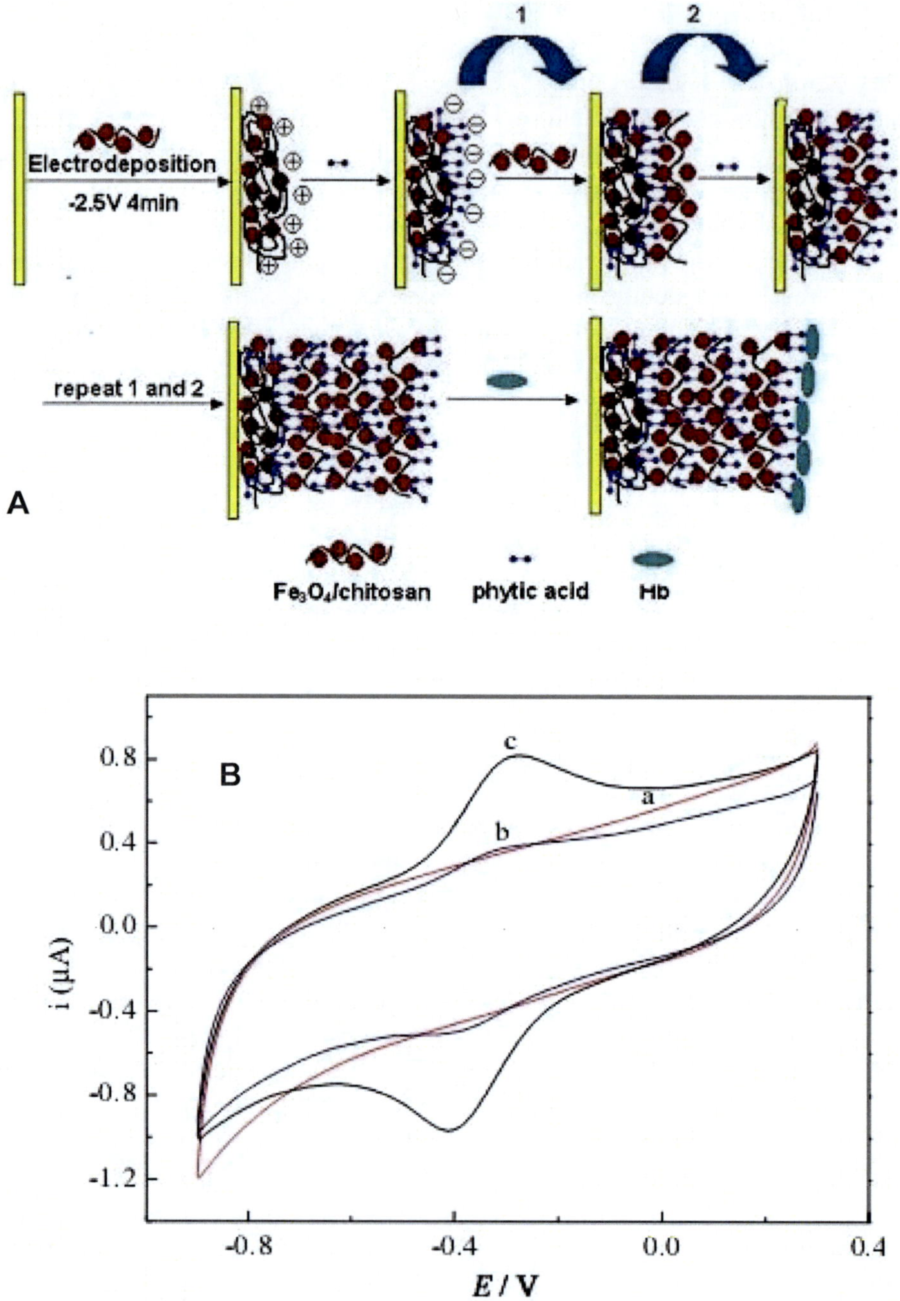

Figure 17 (A) Layer by layer assembly process of Hb/(Fe_3O_4 /chitosan–phytic acid) film. (B) CVs of (Fe_3O_4 /chitosan–phytic acid)4 (a); Hb/(chitosan–phytic acid) $_4$ and Hb/(Fe_3O_4 /chitosan–phytic acid) $_4$ modified GCE at pH 7.0 PBS, scan rate 100 mVs^{-1} (Reprinted from Electrochemistry Communications ,8, G. Zhao, J.J. Xu, H. Y. Chen, Fabrication, characterization of Fe3O4 multilayer film and its application in promoting direct electron transfer of hemoglobin,149,152, Copyrights (2005) with permission from Elsevier.

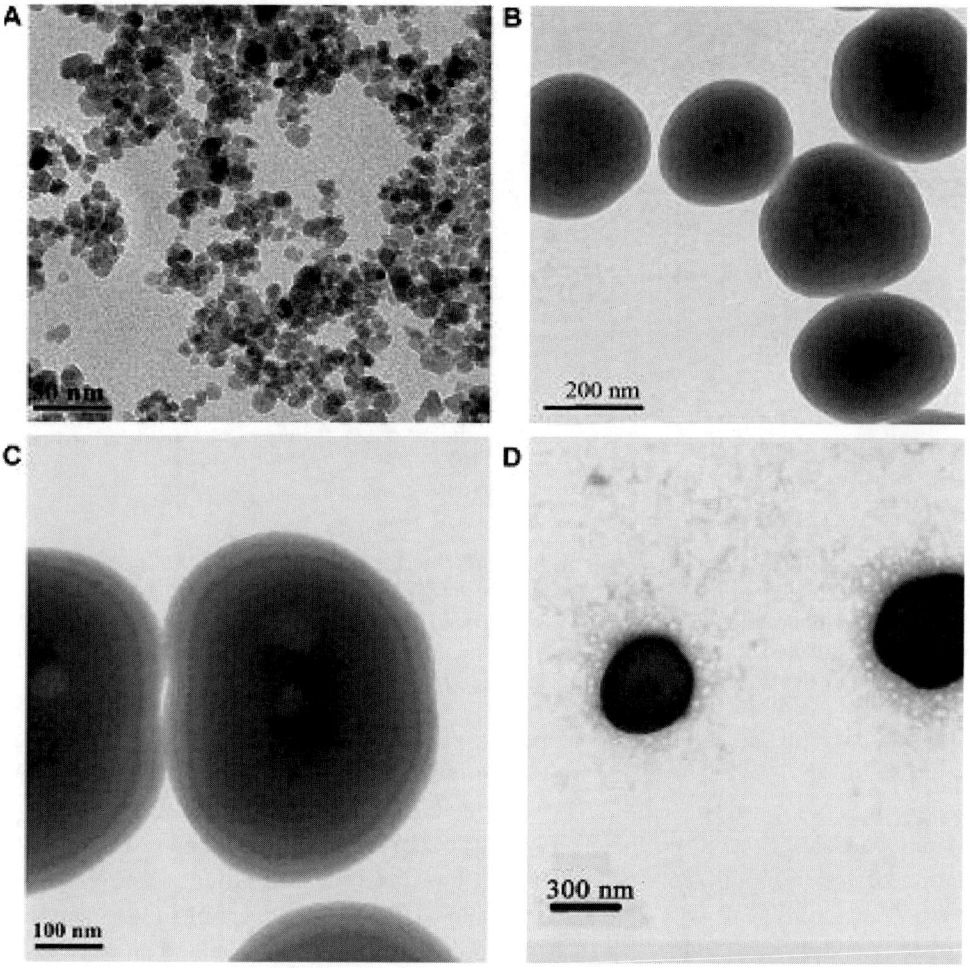

Figure 18.TEM of the Fe_3O_4 (A), Fe_3O_4 @SiO2 (B),PDDA–modified Fe_3O_4 @ SiO_2 nanoparticles(C),and Mb/ Fe_3O_4 @SiO_2 nanocomposite(D) (Reprinted from Electrochemistry Communications ,10, Q. Xu, X.J. Bian, L.L. Li, X.Y. Hu, M.Sun, D. Chen, Y. Wang, Myoglobin immobilizaed on Fe_3O_4 @ SiO_2 magnetic nanoparticles:direct elwcreon transfer, enhanced thermostability and electroactivity,997, Copyrights (2008) with permission from Elsevier.

Silica was precipitated from sodium silicate solution with the addition of hydrochloric acid and then deposited on Fe_3O_4 nanoparticles to form a SiO_2 coating layer. It could be observed that the obtained Fe_3O_4@SiO_2 nanoparticles were well dispersed with the average size of about 400-500 nm .The silica coating could prevent the aggregation and the partial exposure of naked Fe_3O_4 which would damage the activity of biological substances. Due to isoelectric point of myoglobin, P_I =7.2, it has negatively charged in pH 7.5 solution and it has affinity to positively charged (PDDA). The immobilized myoglobin surrounding the Fe_3O_4@SiO_2 magnetic nanoparticles was clearly visible in the TEM image (Fig.18 D). It is quite different from the smooth and uniform surfaces of the particles coated in the absence of enzyme (Fig.18 C). An other technique for evaluation of immobilized myoglobin is electrochemical impedance spectroscopy (EIS). Nyquist plot of EIS for Mb/ Fe_3O_4@SiO_2/GCE and Fe_3O_4@SiO_2/GCE shown in the Fig.19.

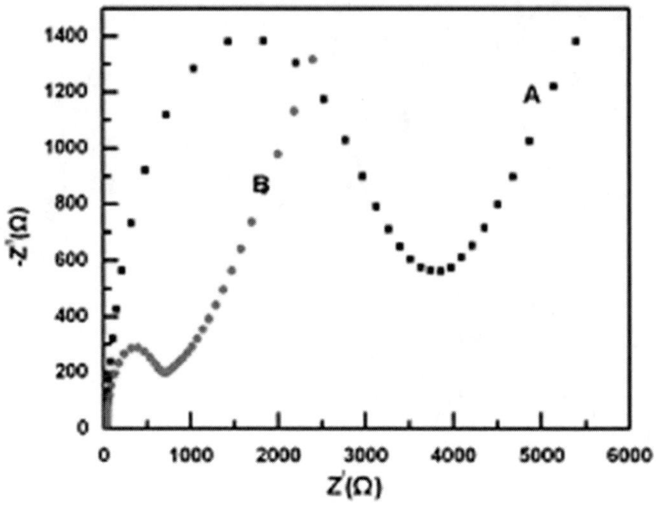

Figure19. Electrochemical impedance spectrograms of Mb/ Fe_3O_4 @SiO_2 /GCE(A) and Fe_3O_4@SiO_2 /GCE(B) in the presence of 5mM Fe(CN)63- /Fe(CN)64- and 0.10 molL KNO_3 . ((Reprinted from Electrochemistry Communications ,10, Q. Xu, X.J. Bian, L.L. Li, X.Y. Hu, M.Sun, D. Chen, Y. Wang, Myoglobin immobilizaed on Fe_3O_4@SiO_2 magnetic nanoparticles:direct elwcreon transfer, enhanced thermostability and electroactivity,998, Copyrights (2008) with permission from Elsevier.

The increase in diameter of the semicircle for Mb/ Fe_3O_4@SiO2/GCE electrode, indicating that Mb has been successfully immobilized onto nanoparticles. The biosensor shows excellent redox response to H_2O_2 with detection limit of 0.55 mM and K_M 0.045mM. Fe_3O_4 nanoparticles coated with acrylic acid copolymer was synthesized and used for fabrication of Hb immobilized electrochemical biosensor [211]. Direct electron transfer of Hb at this nanocomposite was studied by Gong and Lin. A reversible redox reaction for Fe(III)/Fe(II) couple was found. The surface concentration (Γ) of adsorbed hemoglobin is 2.567×10^{-10} molcm^{-2}, which is calculated according to the equation Q=nFA Γ, where n is the number of electron transferred ,F is faraday constant and A is the surface area of the electrode and Q is the passed charge. The biosensor has been successfully used for detection of trichloroacetic acid based on the following mechanism [212].

$$\text{HbFe (III)} + e^- \leftrightharpoons \text{HbFe(II)} \quad (11)$$

$$\text{HbFe(II)} + \text{RCl} \rightarrow \text{HbFe(III)} + R^{\cdot} + Cl^- \quad (12)$$

$$\text{HbFe(II)} + R^{\cdot} + H^+ \rightarrow \text{HbFe(III)} + \text{RH} \quad (13)$$

The voltammetric response of the biosensor in the presence of different trichloroacetic acid (TCA) concentration is shown in the Fig.20. With increasing the trichloroacetic acid concentration the cathodic peak current is increased.A novel glucose biosensor was fabricated by entrapping GOD in chitosan composite dopped with ferrocene monocarboxylic acid modified magnetic core-shell and Fe_3O_4@SiO_2 nanoparticles [213]. Figure 21 shows the response of biosensor to successive addition of glucose. The biosensor kept its original sensitivity after 4 weeks.

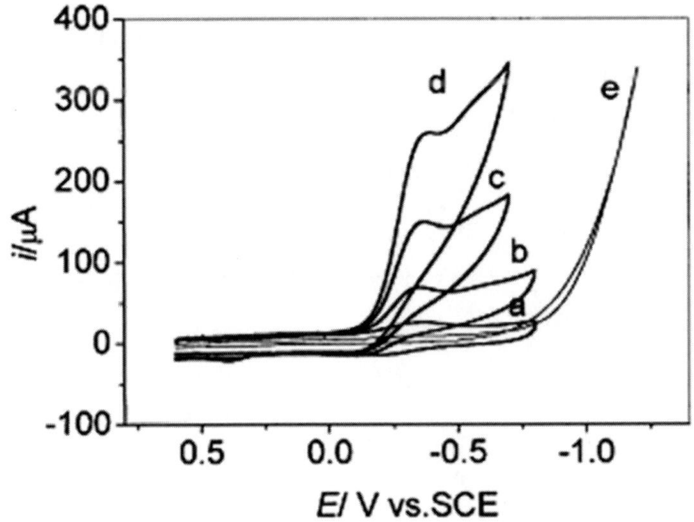

Figure 20. Cyclic voltammograms of Hb/ Fe_3O_4 /PIGE in the absence of TCA (a) and in the presence of 7.44 (b); 19.6 (c) and 36.1 mmol l-1 TCA (d) and cyclic voltammogram of $Fe_3O_4$4 /PIGE in the presence of 47.6 mmoll-1 TCA (e) in PBS Solution pH 5.9 and Scan rate 500mVs-1 (Reprinted from Microchemical Journal, 75, J. Gong, X. Lin, Facilated electron transfer of hemoglobin embedded in nanosized Fe3O4 matrix based on paraffin impregnated graphite electrode and electrochemical catalysis for trichloroacetic acid, 56, Copyrights(2003) with permission from Elsevier.

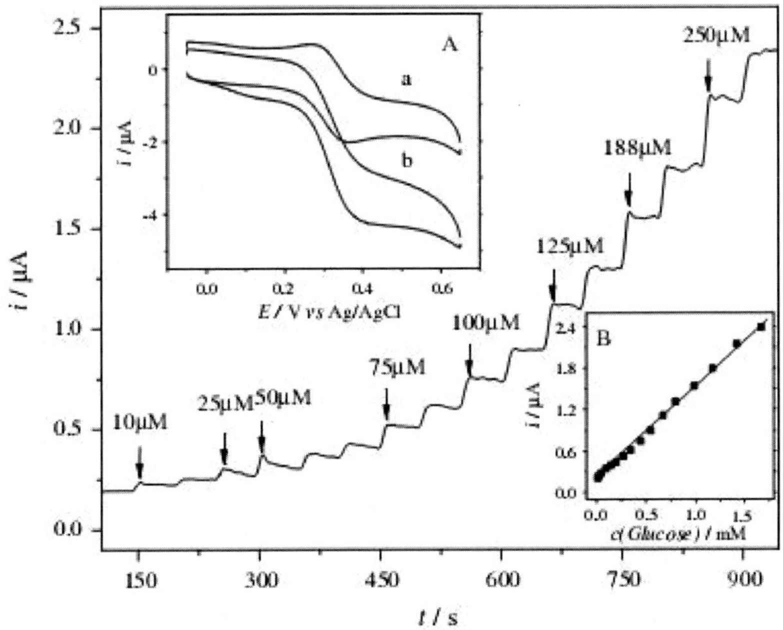

Figure 21. Typical amperometric response of the biosensor to successive addition of glucose into stirring PBS at potential +350 mV. Inset:(A) Cyclic Voltammograms of GOD entrapped in FMC-AFSNPs/CS composite film in absence (a) and presence (b) of 2.5mM glucose in PBS at 100mV/s.(B) Recorded calibration curve. (Reprinted from Electrochemistry Communications, 9, J. Qiu, H. Peng, R. Liang,Ferrocene-modified Fe_3O_4@SiO_2 magnetic nanoparticles as building blocks for construction of reagentless enzyme –based biosensors,2737, Copyrights(2007) with permission from Elsevier.

Covalently attachment GOD enzyme to amino modified magnetic nanoparticles was used to prepare bioactive magnetic nanoparticles with glucose sensing capabilities [200].Figure 22 shows the preparation of amino-modified magnetic nanoparticles and covalent attachment of glucose oxidase to them.

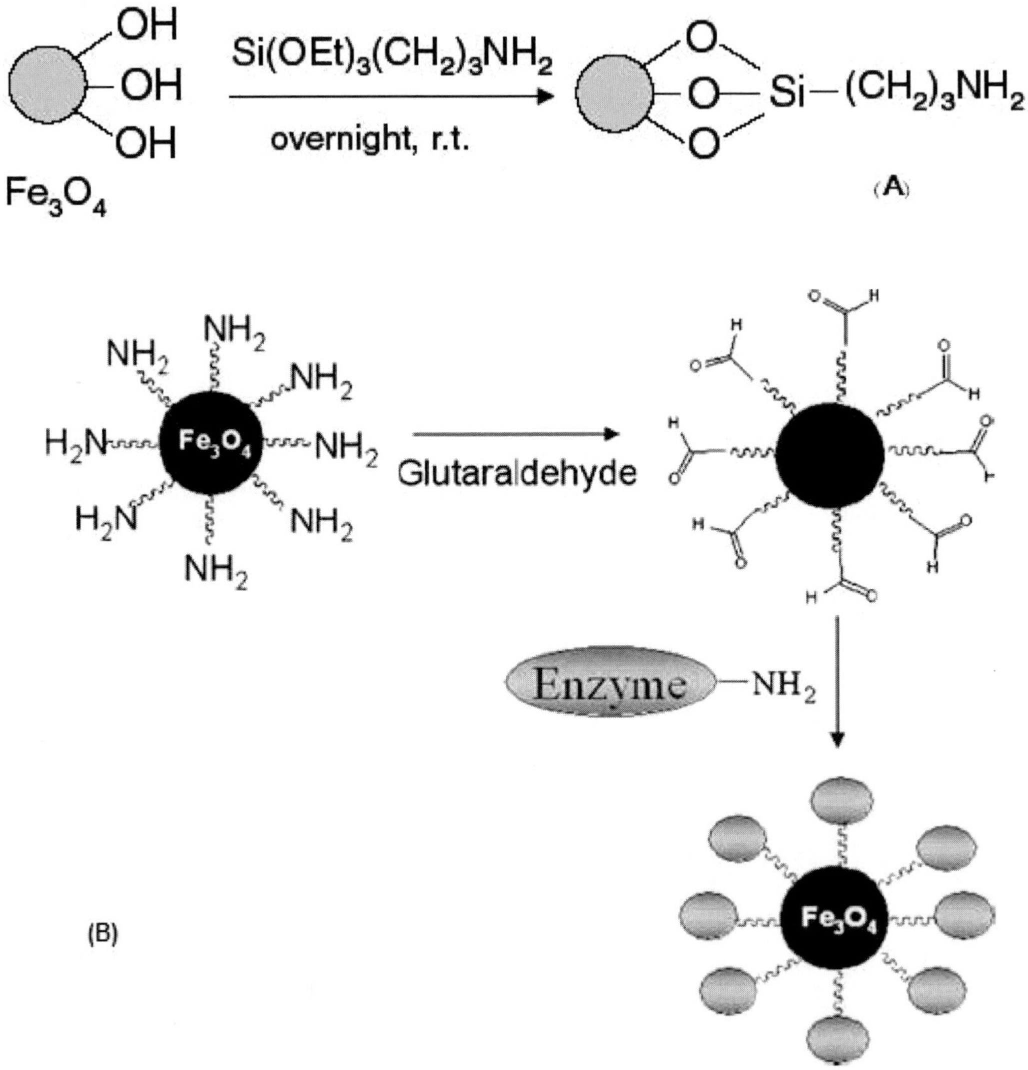

Figure 22. (A) Preparation of amino-modified magnetic nanoparticles, (B) Covalent conjugation of glucose oxidase to amino functionalized magnetic nanoparticles(Analytical Bioanalytical Chemistry, 380, 606-613, Glucose oxidase-magnetite nanoparticle biocongugate for glucose sensing, : L.M. Rossi, A.D. Quach, Z.Rosenzweig ,Schemes 1 and 2: With kind permission of Springer Science)

The enzymatic activity of GOD coated Fe_3O_4 was investigated by monitoring of oxygen consumption during the enzymatic oxidation of glucose. With immobilization of tyrosinase onto Fe_3O_4-chitosan nanocomposite a sensitive biosensor for detection phenolic compounds was developed [214]. The large surface area of Fe_3O_4 nanoparticles and the porous morphology of chitosan led to high loadinglevel of enzyme, the entrapped enzyme could retain its bioactivity. Catechol has been used as a phenolic compound model to investigate the electrochemical sensing characteristics of the proposed biosensor. Figure 23 shows the recorded cyclic voltammograms of buffer solution containing 0.1 mM of catechol at bare glassy carbon electrode (GCE), chitosan- Fe_3O_4 nanoparticles, tyrosine-chitosan- GCE and tyrosinase-chitosan- Fe_3O_4 nanoparticles.

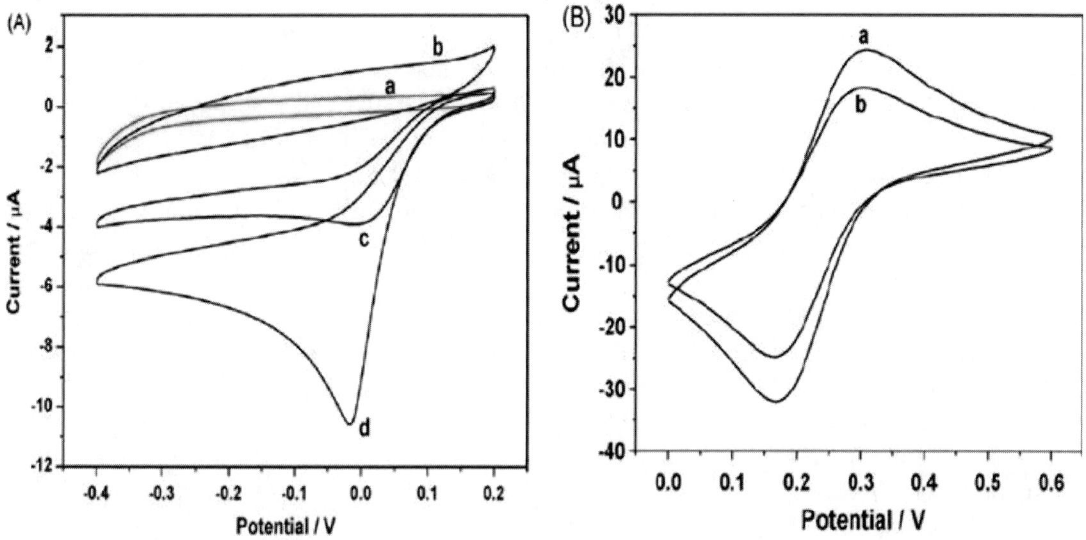

Figure 23. (A) Cyclic voltammograms of 0.1mM catechol at (a) GCE; (b) chitosan-Fe_3O_4-GCE; (c) chitosan-tyrosinase-GCE and (d) chitosan- Fe_3O_4 - tyrosinase-GCE, scan rate: $50mVs^{-1}$; supporting electrolyte: PBS (pH 6.5). (B) Cyclic voltammograms of chitosan- Fe_3O_4-GCE (curve a) and chitosan-GCE (curve b) in 0.5 mM $[Fe(CN)_6]^{3-/4-}$ + 0.5 M KNO_3 solution, scan rate: 100 mVs^{-1}(Reprinted from Biosensors and Bioelectronics , 23, S. Wang, Y. Tan, D. Zhao, G. Liu, ,Amperometric tyrosinase biosensor based on Fe_3O_4 nanoparticles-chitosan nanocomposite,1784, Copyrights(2008) with permission from Elsevier.

It indicates that a well defined reduction peak at the potential of -0.02 V was observed at, tyrosine-chitosan- GCE and tyrosinase-chitosan- Fe_3O_4 nanoparticles modified glassy carbon electyrodes. As shown in the Fig.23 the redox response of biosensor in the presence of magnetic nanoparticles increased. The Fe_3O_4 nanoparticles play an important role in immobilizing tyrosinase and enhancing the enzyme catalytic sites accessible to catechol molecules.The observed reduction peak was attributed to the direct reduction of quinone librated from the enzyme -catalyzed reaction on the electrode surface based on the following enzymatic reaction [215].

$$\text{Catechol} + \text{Tyrosinase} (O_2) \rightarrow \text{o-Quinone} + H_2O \quad (14)$$

$$\text{o- Quinone} + 2H^+ + 2e^- \rightarrow \text{catechol} \quad (15)$$

The proposed biosensor has been used for nanomolar detection of various phenolic compounds (phenol, p-cresol and phenol). Above results indicates that Fe_3O_4 nanoparticles played an important role in immobilizing tyrosinase and enhancing the enzyme catalytic sites accessible to substrate molecules. By introducing Fe_3O_4 nanoparticles onto Multi-walled carbon nanotubes (MWCNTs) a new kind of nanocomposite for fabrication of biosensors was prepared. Horseradish peroxidase (HRP) was employed as a model enzyme to demonstrate the final performance of the nanostructured biosensor [216]. The Fe_3O_4-MWCNTs-HRP multilayer films were grown on the electrode by successive dipping the electrode into the solution of Fe_3O_4-MWCNTs and HRP. The biosensor showed satisfactory stability, good biocompability and excellent catalytic activity toward hydrogen peroxide reduction at reduced overpotential. The K_M value of the biosensor was 0.31 mM, indicating that the HRP immobilized in multilayers films retains its bioactivity and has a high affinity to H_2O_2.

The application of magnetic nanoparticles for various material loading, dual biosensing and electrocatalytic and bioelectrocatalytic processes have been reported [217-221]. The duel analysis of two substrates was done by the application of two enzyme(glucose oxidase GOx, and lactate dehydrogenase, LDH) a relay ferrocene monolayer functionalized Au electrode, relay NAD^+-cofactor functionalized Fe_3O_4 nanoparticles and using external magnetic field. The recorded cyclic voltammograms of the system that lacks two substrates, while the external magnet position was above or below the electrochemical cell. When the external magnet is above the working electrode only redox process of the ferocene (Fc) monolayer observed. With changing magnetic position to below working electrode, the cofactor faunctionalized magnetic particles attracts the electrode, and redox response of PQQ was also observed. The observed cyclic voltammograms of Fc-monolayer functionalized Au-electrode in the presence NAD^+-PQQ-functionalized magnetic particles in the potential range of -0.1 to +0.6 V is shown. When the magnet is positioned above the cell, the electrocatalytic current correspondingto the Fc-mediated bioelectrocatalyzed oxidation of glucose by GOD is observed. Upon shifting the magnet to below the electrochemical cell the anodic current is observed at the potentials values that PQQ is oxidized. In the presence of LDH, lactate reduces the NAD^+- cofactor associated with the magnetic particles. Magnetic nanoparticles were used for activation of soluble redox enzyme with electron transfer mediator bound to electrode surfaces. In such systems the bioelectrocatalytic process includes diffusional steps as well as electrochemical reaction of surface confined mediator. The bioelectrocatalytic system contains GOD and glucose as diffusional components and ferrocene monolayer confined to the electrode surface as electron mediating interface has been used by Katz et. al [219](Fig.24).

Hydrophobic magnetic nanoparticles allow the selective On and Off switching of the diffusional part of the process. When the magnetic nanoparticles are retracted from the electrode surface, upon applied potential for ferrocene oxidation, the mediated bioelectrocatalytic oxidation of glucose by GOx should proceed, and electrocatalytic anodic currents are generated. Upon the magnetic attraction of the nanoparticles to the electrode the hydrophobic thin film isolates the ferrocene-functionalized surface from the soluble enzyme substrate, resulting in the inhibition of the bioelectrocatalytic process (Fig.24).Therefore, use of functional magnetic nanoparticles and external magnetic field provides a novel concept in development of bioelecrocatalytic processes. The attraction of functionalized magnetic nanoparticles to electrode surfaces can be used for concentrate seprate of analytes [106].

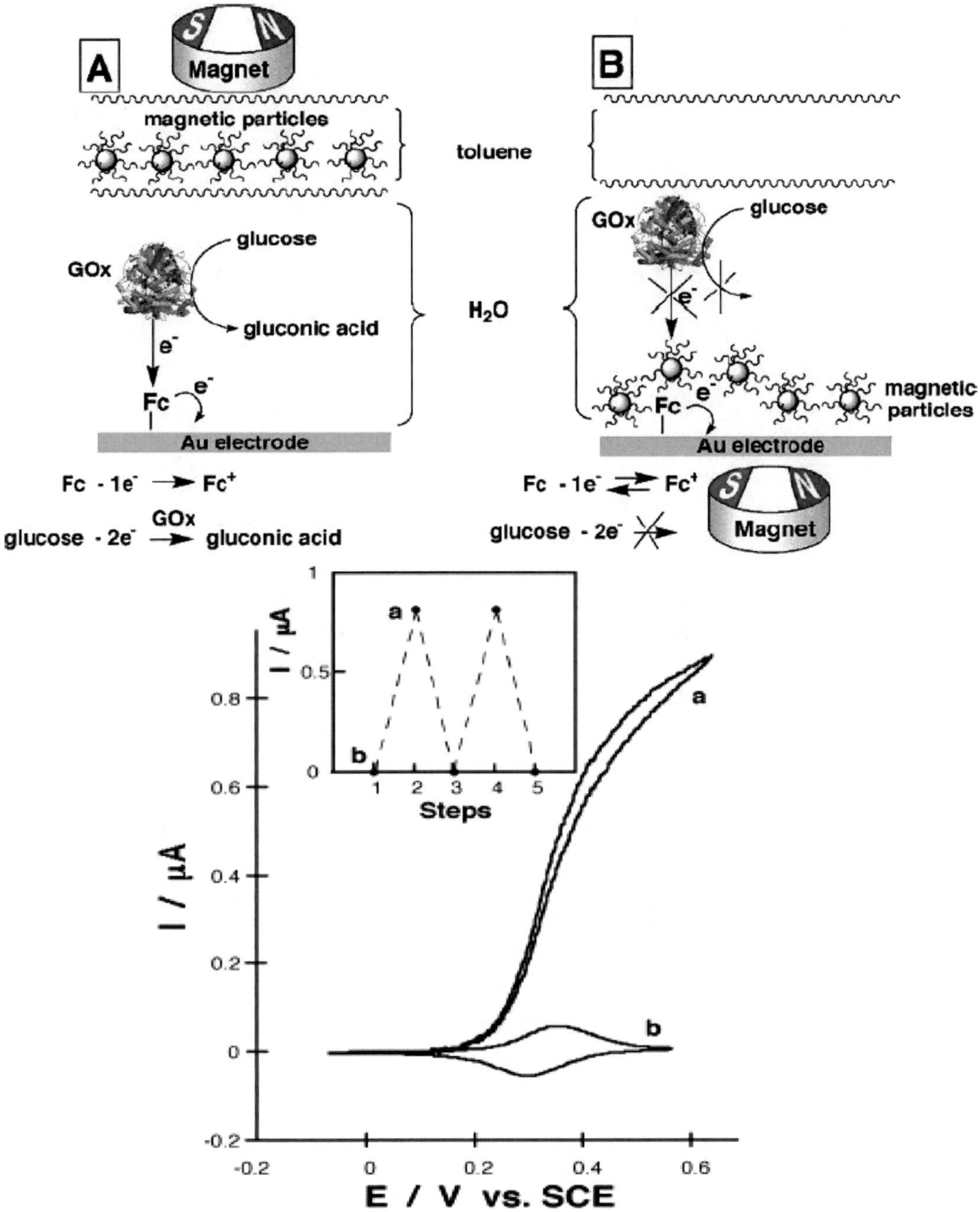

Figure 24. Magneto-controlled reversible “ON”-”OFF” switching of the bioelectrocatalytic oxidation of glucose by GOx using the hydrophobic magnetic nanoparticles. CVs of the system consisting of the surface confined ferrocene, glucose oxidase, 1 mg mL^{-1}, and glucose, 80 mM,dissolved in the aqueous phase (a) when the magnetic nanoparticles are retracted from the electrode surface and (b) when the magnetic nanoparticles are attracted to the electrode surface. Potential scan rate 5 mV s^{-1}. Inset: The reversible switch of the current generated by the system at *E*) 0.5 V. “Adapted with permission from; E. Katz, R. Baron, I. Wilner, J. Am. Chem. Soc. 2005, 127, 4060-4070.Copyright 2005 American Chemical Society”

4.4. Manganese Oxide Nanomaterial for Biosensors Fabrication

Manganese dioxide (MnO_2) has been proved to be a catalytic substance to promote disproportionation of hydrogen peroxide to oxygen and water [222,223]. The electrocatalytic properties of $MnO_2$for oxygen reduction in alkaline solution is also investigated [224]. Glassy carbon and carbon paste modified with microparticles of MnO_2 have been used for micromolar detection of H_2O_2 [223,225]. The application of manganese dioxide modified carbon substrate and screen printed electrodes for biosensors fabrication was reported [226,227]. In comparison to MnO_2 powder, the manganese oxide nanoparticles were found to have more and special reaction activity [228]. The MnO_2 nanoparticles based modified electrodes have been used successfully as sensitive sensor for hydrogen peroxide detection [229,230]. The MnO_2 nanoparticles dispersed in dihexadecyl hydrogen phosphate (DHP) composite has been used for fabrication of high sensitive sensor for hydrogen peroxide detection [229], that produced in the enzymatic reaction (in the presence glucose oxidase). Furthermore, the ability of hydrogen peroxide sensor for fabrication of choline oxidase biosensor was evaluated [230]. Various biosensor were fabricated with immobilization of enxymes or proteins onto MnO_2 nonmaterial. A sensitive biosensor for H_2O_2 detection was fabricated base on intercalation of methelyne blue (MB) into manganese oxide layer coimmobilized with horseradish peroxidase (HRP). The MB- MnO_2 material can be used as electron transfer mediator and it can efficiently shuttle electrons from the electrode to HRP [231]. The third generation biosensors for hydrogen peroxide fabricated based on direct voltammery of HRP immobilized onto manganese dioxide nanosheets and nanoparticles [232,233]. The detection limit and K_M of the prepared biosensors were 2.1×10^{-7}, 7.8×10^{-8} M, and 0.127 mM and 0.044 mM. These results implying that the HRP/ MnO_2 nanoparticles modified electrodes exhibit higher affinity for hydrogen peroxide. Alternative adsorption of oppositely charged polyions was developed as a novel technique for ultrathin film assembly [234]. A multilayer film of MnO_2 nanoparticles with polycation, poly (dimethyl diallyl-ammonium)(PDDA) or myoglobin and sodium poly (styrensulfonate) (PSS) was used for electrocatalytic reduction of oxygen [235]. Based on this process films of Mb and MnO_2 up to 30 nm thick on rough pyrolytic graphite electrode could be constructed. As shown in the Figure 25 a, the reversible redox couple for proteins heme Fe(III)/Fe(II) with 10 electroactive layers of protein was observed. The electrocatalytic activity of the modified electrode for oxygen reduction was investigated (Fig. 25 b).

As shown for PG/PSS/PDDA/ MnO_2 $(Mb/ MnO_2)_{10}$ electrode in the presence of oxygen an increase in Fe(III) reduction peak and disappearance of the Fe(II) oxidation peak was observed, which indicating the catalytic reduction of oxygen. The direct uncatalyzed reduction of oxygen was observed at more negative potential at the surface of PG/PSS/PDDA/MnO_2 electrode. Electrodeposition was used for modification of graphite electrode with nanocomposite containing poly (diallyl dimethyl ammonium) (PDDA) and manganese oxide nanoparticles [236]. Direct voltammetry of glucose oxidase onto electrodeposited nanocomposite was investigated [237]. The biosensor has been used for glucose detection based on decreasing of chathodic peak currents of oxygen. Furthermore, a nonenzymatic glucose sensor based on electrodeposition of MnO_2 onto carbon nanotubes was fabricated [238]. MnO_2 nanoparticles were found to have special reaction activity and they react with produced hydrogen peroxide in enzymatic reaction. The O_2 and Mn^{2+} are reaction products and two H^+ was consumed [239]. The pH change induced by the hydrogen ions consumed can be monitored by the ion selective filled effect transistor (ISFET). This method can be used for development of oxidase based FET biosensors, especially for biosensors with little or no pH change during the enzymatic reaction such as lactate oxidase [240]. Layer by layer deposition technique has been proposed to prepare lactate biosensor on the gate of an ISFET. MnO_2 nanoparticles were introduced as an oxidant to react with hydrogen peroxide, which results in a sensitive pH change in the sensitive membrane of the enzyme-field effect transistors (ENFET) with the lactate addition. With the deposition of manganeous oxide nanoparticles and lactate oxidase (LOD) on the ion selective field effect transistor the sensitivity of lactate biosensor is increased. The Structure of ISFET and biosensor response is shown in Figure 26. A typical response of the $(PDDA/MnO_2 /PDDA/LOD)_3$ modified enzyme-field effect transistors (ENFET) is shown in Fig.26 (curve a). As can be seen with the addition of lactate, the concentration of H^+ near the sensitive gate surface decreased and open circuit potentialshifts to more negative values. For $(PDDA /LOD)_n$ modified ENFET with the addition of lacate a small response observed. As shown with MnO_2 nanoparticles the sensitivity of the ENFET is 50 times higher than that biosensor without metal oxide nanoparticles(16.84 mV mM^{-1} vs. 0.34 mV mM^{-1}). The dynamic range of the lactate biosensor is extended up to 6.0 mM with detection limit 8.0 μM.

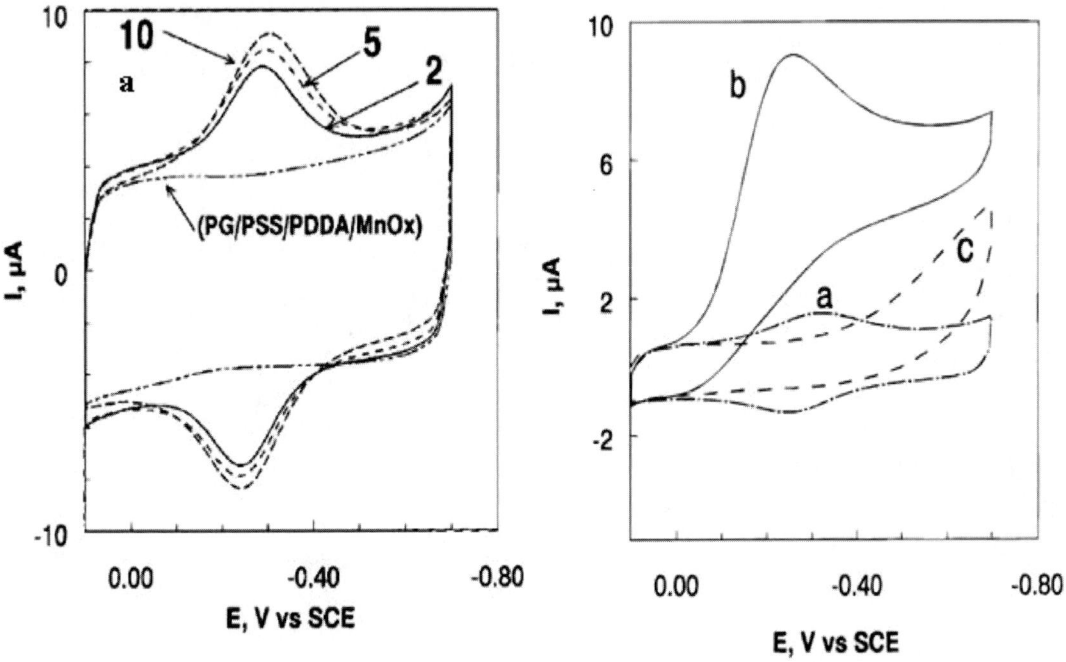

Figure 25. (a) CVs of PG/PSS/PDDA/ MnO_2 (Mb/MnO_2) *n* films with *n*) 2, 5, and 10 at scan rate 0.3 V s^{-1} in pH 5.5 buffer. (b). CVs of PG/PSS/PDDA/ MnO_2 (Mb/M MnO_2) 10 films (a) without oxygen, (b) with oxygen present, and (c) direct reduction of oxygen on the PG/PSS/PDDA/ MnO_2 electrode in pH 5.5 buffer at 0.05 V s^{-1}(Adapted with permission from ; Y. Lvov, B. Munge, O. Giraldo, I. Ichinose, S.L. Suib, J.F. Rusling, Langmiur 2000, 16, 8850-8857.Copyright 2000 American Chemical Society).

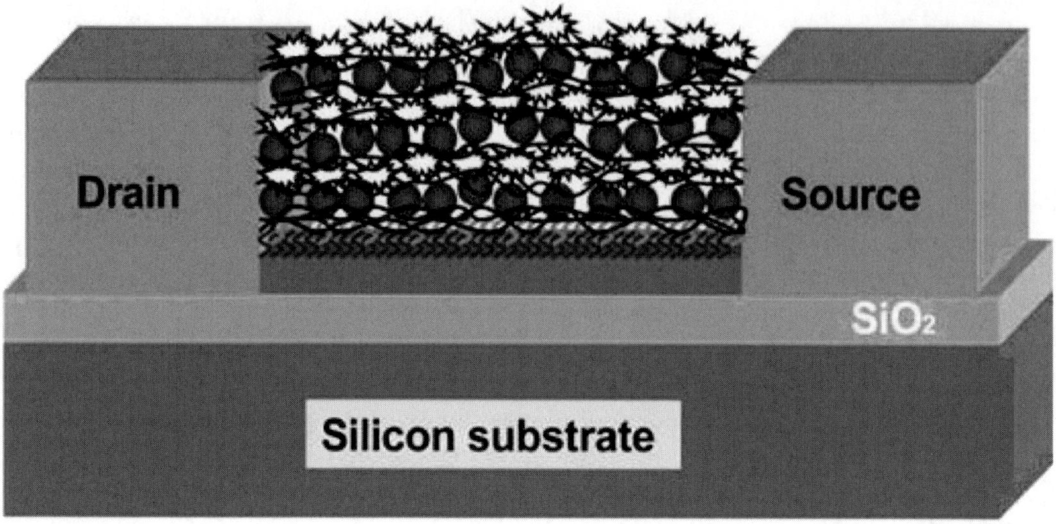

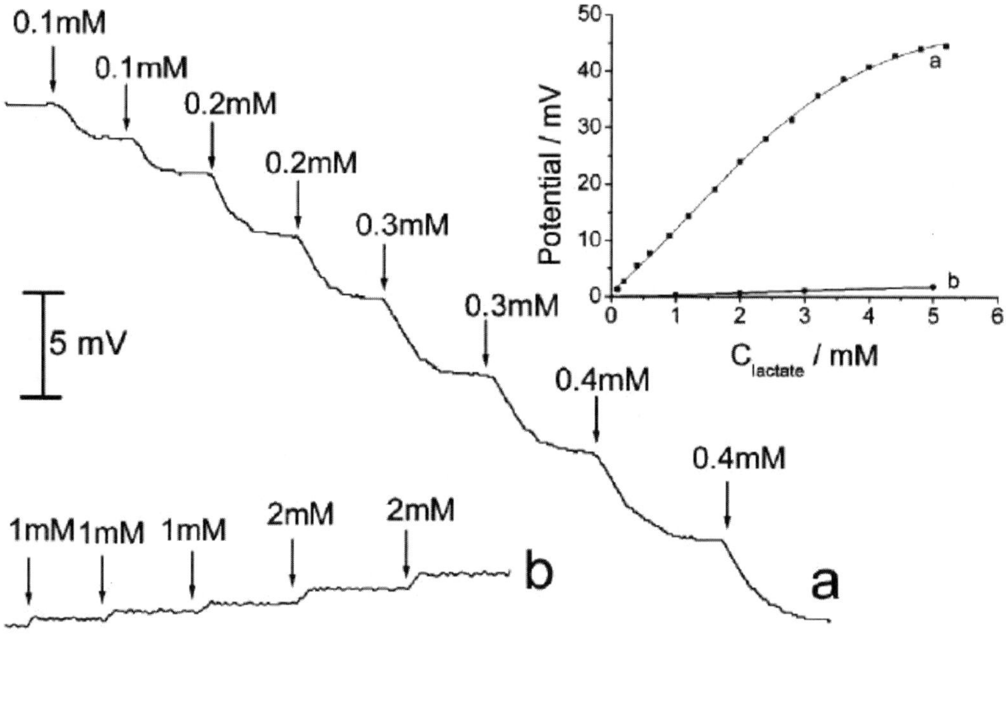

Figure 26. Structure of an ISFET. The MnO_2 nanoparticles and LOD are layer-by-layer self-assembled on top of the sensitive membrane.Successive response of the three-multilayer film based ENFETwith (a) and without (b) MnO_2 nanoparticles to lactate in 10 mM PBS(pH 7.4). Inset: calibration curve of theENFET with (a) and without (b) MnO_2 nanoparticles to lactate (J.J. Xu, W. Zhao, X. L. Luo, H.Y. Chen, Chem. Commun. 2005, 792-794; Reproduced with permission of The Royal Society of Chemistry).

4.5. *Nickel* Oxides for Biosensors Fabrication

Nickel and nickel coated electrode have various applications in the field of electrochromic, electroanalytical chemistry, electrocatalysis and electroanalysis [241-245]. Most analytical applications of nickel electrodes are based on the Ni $(OH)_2/NiO(OH)$ redox couple. Nickel based chemically modified electrode have been used for detection of aliphatic alcohols [246], acetylcholine [247] and carbohydrates [248]. Recently we reported the application of nickel oxide modified carbon composite electrode for picomolar detection of insulin [249] enzymeless detection of glucose [250] and aminoacids [251]. Based on unique properties of nickel oxide nanoparticles, they can be used for immobilization of biomolecules. The easy preparation, electroinactivity in physiological pH solutions and high porosity are advantages of nickel oxide nanomatyerials for bimolecules entrapment. The electrochemical techniques have been used for nickel oxide formation [249-251]. Figure 27 shows the consequence cyclic voltammograms of carbon composite electrode modified with nickel powder. In alkaline solution, nickel dissolution and oxide formation was obtained [252]. The cyclic voltammogram of Ni-powder modified carbon electrode shows a redox couple with anodic and cathodic peak potentials of 0.45 and 0.35 V, respectively. These values correspond to $Ni(OH)_2/NiO(OH)$ redox couple [253]. This system can be used as electrocatalyst for various substances. The direct voltammetry and electrocatalytic properties of different biomolcules (glucose oxidase, catalase and hemoglobin) immobiliz onto electrodeposited nickel oxide nanoparticles were also investigated in our group [248-250]. The direct voltammetry and electrocatalytic properties of different biomolcules (glucose oxidase, catalase and hemoglobin) immobilization onto electrodeposited nickel oxide nanoparticles was investigated in our group[254-256]. The electrodeposition of metallic nickel was carried out using constant potential (-0.8 V vs. reference electrode for 5 min) in pH 4 acetate buffer solution containing 1mM nickel nitrate. Then, the modified electrode was immersed in buffer solution containing 5 mg ml^{-1} of glucose oxidase and potential was hold at -0.8 V for 15 min. Fig. 28 shows the cyclic voltammograms of glucose oxidase-NiO modified GC electrode in pH 7 at different scan rates. The formal potential of glucose oxidase redox center ($FAD/FADH_2$) immobilized on NiO nanoparticles is close to the standard electrode potential of $FAD/FADH_2$ redox couple at pH 7 [257], indicating that GOx molecules preserved their native structures after immobilized on nickel oxide nanoparticles. The heterogeneous electron transfer rate constant (k_s) of glucose oxidase immobilized onto the nickel oxide nanoparticles (k_s) was 25.2 ± 0.5 s^{-1}.This value is higher than reported values for immobilized GOD in other nanomaterials. Long term stability is the most important property for this biosensor. A pair of well defined and stable redox peaks obtained for adsorbed GOx in pH range 2-10. The stability of GOx-nickel oxide film electrodes was investigated by recording consequence potential cycling. The peak height and peak potential of the immobilized enzyme remained nearly unchanged and amount of 90% of GOx remaining on the electrode surface after 250 cycles. Furthermore, the biosensor shows 95% of its initial current response to glucose after intermitted use over 10 days. Thus, high stability of the biosensor is related to the interaction between GOx and nickel oxide, the high chemical stability of nickel oxide nanoparticles, and strong adsorption of GOx on nickel oxide films.

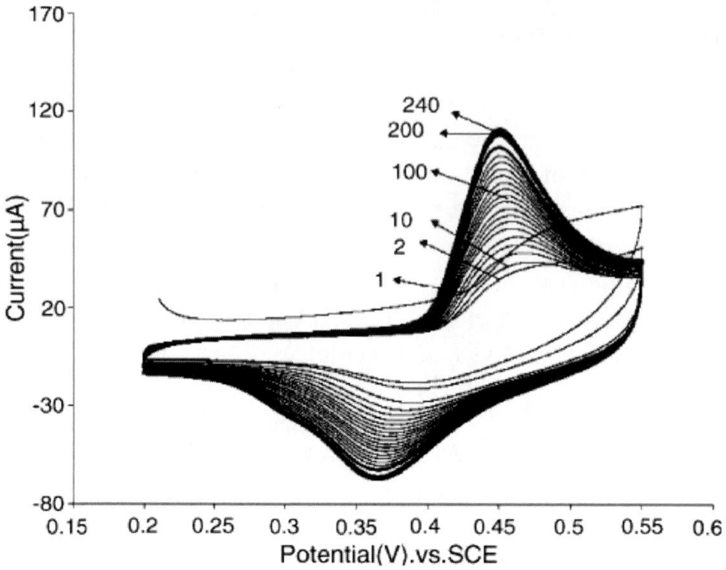

Figure 27.Cyclic voltammograms of Ni-powder modified CCE in 0.1 M NaOH Solution at scan rate $100mVs^{-1}$. The cycle numbers are written on the voltammograms. Reprinted from Electrochimica Acta, 51 A.Salimi, M. Roushani, R. Hallaj, Micromolar determination of sulfur oxoanions and sulfide ata renewable sol–gel carbon ceramic electrode modified with nickel powder, 1954, Copyrights(2006) with permission from Elsevier.

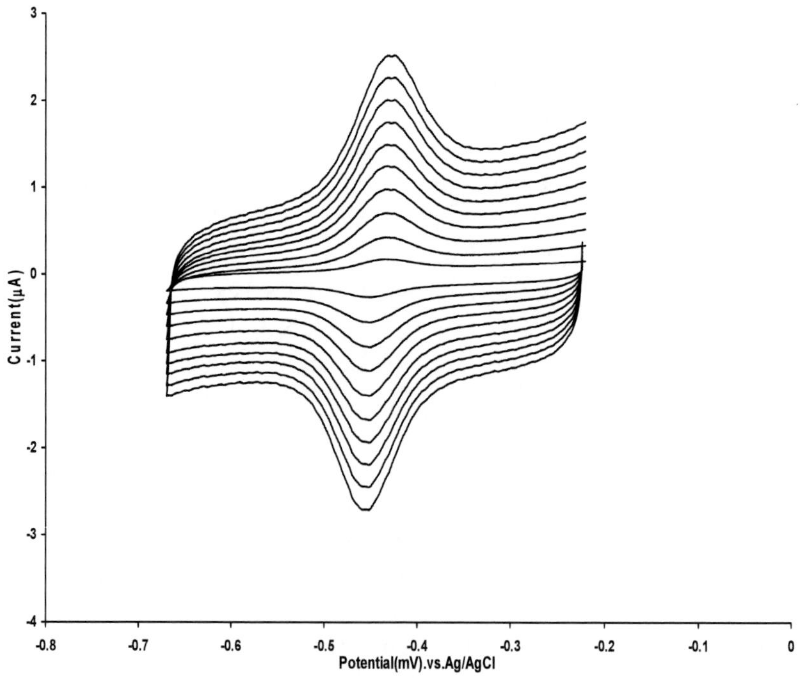

Figure 28. CVs of GOx /NiOx modified GC electrode at various scan rate in pH 7 PBS, from inner to outer, 10, 20, 30, 40, 50, 60, 70, 80, 90 and $100mVs^{-1}$. Reprinted from Biosensors and Bioelectronics, 22, A.Salimi, E. Sharifi, A. NoorBakhash, S. Soltanian, Immobilization of glucose oxidase on electrodeposited nickel oxide nanoparticles: Direct electron transfer and electrocatalytic activity,3148,Copyeight (2007) ,with permission from Elsevier.

Therefore, the GOx-nickel oxide modified glassy carbon electrode, can be used as a biosensor due to its long term stability and excellent electron transfer rate constant. The bioactivity of the biosensor was evaluate by recording cyclic voltammograms in buffer solution containing 0.5 mM of ferrocenemethanol and different concentration of glucose (Fig.29). The coverage of active enzyme Γ_{ET}, was estimated to be 9.45×10^{-13} mol cm^{-2}

The biosensor ability for oxidation of glucose was investigated by recording cyclic voltammograms of GOX/NiO nanoparticles modified in the presence of different glucose concentration (Fig.30). Inset of Fig.30 shows the plot of catalytic oxidation currents vs. glucose concentration at potential of 0.9V.

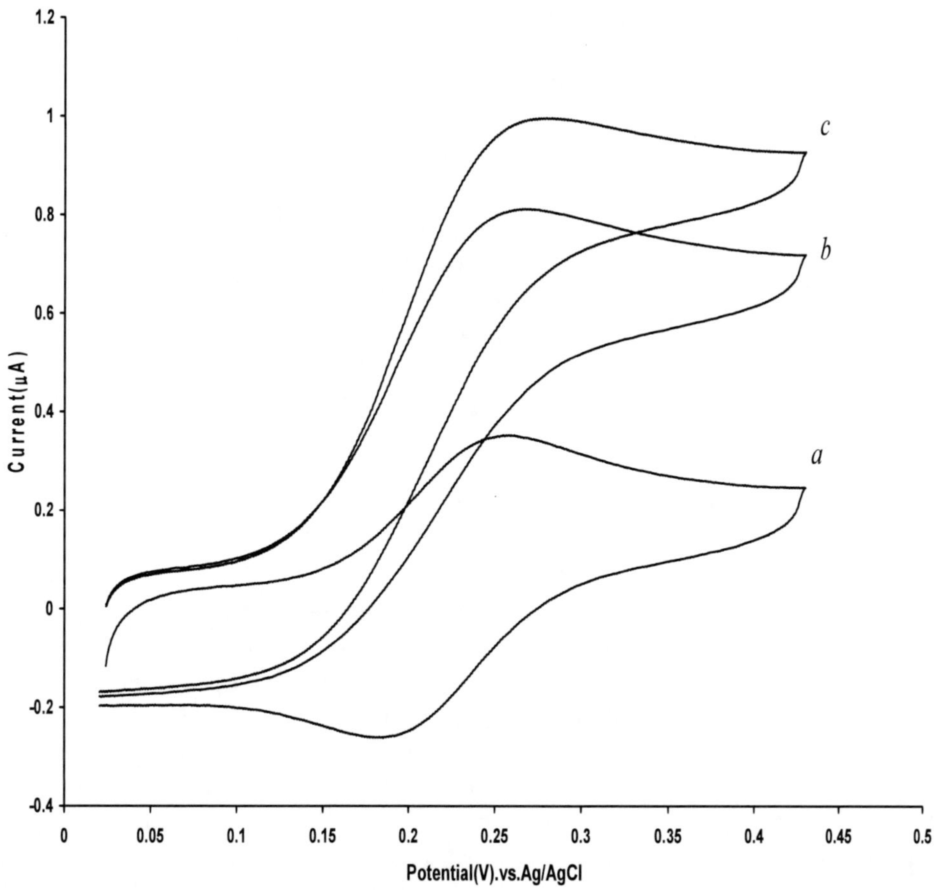

Figure 29. CVsof GOx/NiO modifiedGCelectrode in PBS, pH 7 containing 0.5mM ferrocenemethanol (a) in the absence, (b) and (c) in the presence 10 and 20 mM of glucose, scan rate $10 mVs^{-1}$ Reprinted from Biosensors and Bioelectronics, 22, A.Salimi, E. Sharifi, A. NoorBakhash, S. Soltanian, Immobilization of glucose oxidase on electrodeposited nickel oxide nanoparticles: Direct electron transfer and electrocatalytic activity,3150,Copyeight (2007) ,with permission from Elsevier.

The bioelectrocatalytic currents levels off when glucose concentration is 25 mM to a maximum value of I_{cat}^{sat}=1100 nA. The maximum turnover rate of the GOx to be TR_{max} =10

s^{-1} (electrons generated by one glucose oxidase per second) was calculated based on the following equation [258].

$$TR_{max} = I_{cat}^{sat} / (F.n.\, \Gamma_{ET}) \quad (16)$$

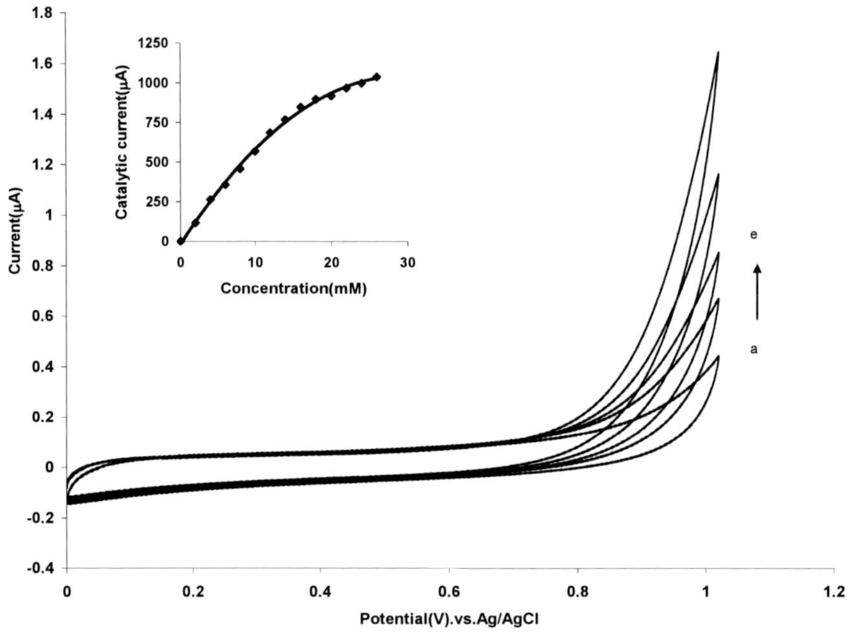

Figure 30, CVs of GOx/NiOx modified GC electrode in PBS, pH 7at scan rate $20 mVs^{-1}$, without (a), (b) 2, (c) 4, (d) 8 and (e) 18mM of glucose. Inset, plot of the catalytic current vs. glucose concentration at $E = 0.9$V. Reprinted from Biosensors and Bioelectronics, 22, A.Salimi, E. Sharifi, A. NoorBakhash, S. Soltanian, Immobilization of glucose oxidase on electrodeposited nickel oxide nanoparticles: Direct electron transfer and electrocatalytic activity,3151,Copyeight (2007) ,with permission from Elsevier.

Due to high biocompability of NiOx nanoparticles, we investigate the direct electron transfer processes of immobilized hemoglobin and catalase onto glassy carbon electrodes modified with nickel oxide nanosize materials [255,256].

Cyclic voltammetry was used for immobilization of biomolecules and nickel oxide nanoparticles onto glassy carbon and ITO electrodes. Figure 31, shows UV-visible spectra of catalase in pH 7.0 phosphate buffer solutions and catalase immobilized onto electrodeposited nickel oxide film at ITO glass electrode. The absorption bond of catalase nickel oxide film (Curve b) is 402 nm similar to that of catalase in pH buffer solution (Curve a), indicating no observable denaturation of catalase on the NiO film. The GC/NiOx nanoparticles /hemoglobin and GC/NiOx nanoparticles/catalase displayed heme Fe(III)/Fe(II) redox couple.The electron transfer rate constant was 5.2 ± 0.5 and $3.7 \pm 0.5\ s^{-1}$ for hemoglobin and catalase immobilized film. The biosensors showed excellent catalytic activity toward hydrogen peroxide, oxygen and nitrite.

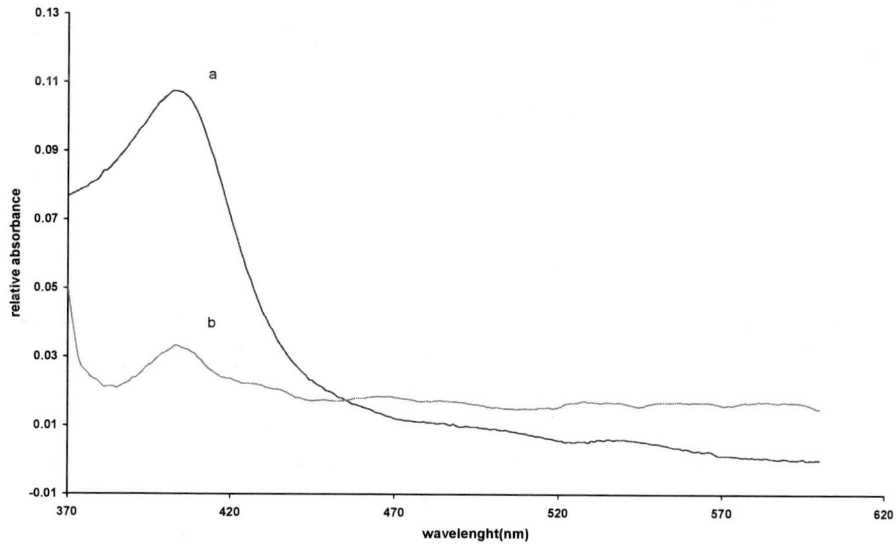

Figure 31-UV- visible spectra of catalase in PBS (pH 7)phosphate buffer solution(curve a) and Cat-NiO film on ITO electrode(curve b). Reprinted from Biophysical Chemistry, 125, A.Salimi, E. Sharifi, A. NoorBakhash, S. Soltanian, Direct electrochemistry and electrocatalytic activity of catalase immobilized onto electrodeposited nano-scale islands of nickel-oxide ,542, Copyright(2007), with permission from Elsevier.

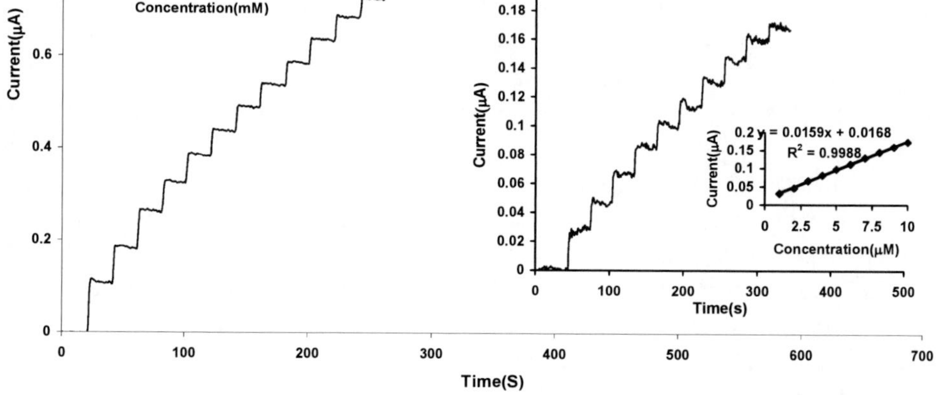

Figure 32. Amperometric response of rotating Cat/NiO modified GC electrode to H_2O_2, conditions -0.3 V constant potential, pH 7.0 and rotation speed is 2000 rpm, (A) successive addition of 100μM and (B) 1μM : insets plot of chronoamperometric current vs, H_2O_2 concentration and linear calibration curve for determination of K_M. Reprinted from Biophysical Chemistry, 125, A.Salimi, E. Sharifi, A. NoorBakhash, S. Soltanian, Direct electrochemistry and electrocatalytic activity of catalase immobilized onto electrodeposited nano-scale islands of nickel-oxide ,546, Copyright(2007), with permission from Elsevier.

Figure 32 shows the amperometric response of the biosensor in the presence of different hydrogen peroxide concentration. As shown a well defined response was observed after hydrogen peroxide addition. The values of K_M, 0.96 mM for hemoglobin and 1.37 mM for catalase indicates the immobilized biomolecules into nickel oxide nanoparticles retained their native activity.

Direct voltammetry of other immobilized biomolecules onto nickel oxide nano-scale materials was reported. The immobilized tyrosinase enzyme shows direct electron transfer with electron transfer rate contant; $1.15\pm 0.04\ s^{-1}$ [259]. Furthermore, stable redox response for direct electron transfer of immobilized cytochrome *c* onto nanometer size nickel oxide particles was observed [260,261]. Direct voltammetry, stability and electrocatalytic activity of myoglobin immobilized onto nickel oxide film was investigated [262]. The fabricated biosensor has been successfully used for micromolar detection of hydrogen peroxide. Since NiOx nanoparticles is a biocompatible material with high isoelectric point (IEP 10.7), it can be used as suitable adsorber for adsorption of biomolecules with low IEP.The Glucose oxidase immobilized onto NiO hollow nanospheres has been used as sensitive amperometric biosensor for glucose detection[263]. These results indicate that nickel oxide nanomaterials are good candidate for immobilization biomolecules and fabrication third generation of biosensors.

4.6. Cobalt Oxides for Biosensors Fabrication

Cobalt-oxide(CoOx) based materials have been widely used for construction of electrochromic thin films [264], energy storage system [265], magnetoresistive devices [266] and heterogeneous catalysis [45]. Furthermore, Co_3O_4 and other cobalt based oxides materials are also showed excellent electrocatalytic activity toward various compounds, ozone and oxygen evolution [267]. The electrocatalytic property of the cobalt-oxide film is very much depends on the deposition method. Various methods such as, spray pyrolysis, plasma sputtering, thermal salt decomposition, powder immobilization, γ-irradiation , and sol-gel technique have been used so far for cobalt oxide synthesis[121,126,268-271]. Electrochemical techniques are suitable methods to preparation of thin film with specific composition, morphology and good adhesion between the deposited film and the substrate. Electrodeposition techniques have been used for preparation of cobalt oxide or oxyhydroxide layers on the surface of gold and GC electrode [133, 272,273]. The cobalt-oxide modified electrode showed catalytic activity toward oxidation different organic molecules such as, glucose, cysteine, hydroquinone, methanol and propylamine as model compounds [95, 96,133,274]. Recently we used electrodeposited cobalt oxide nanoparticles for nanomolar detection of hydrogen peroxide and arsenic [102, 275]. The cyclic voltammogram and SEM image of cobalt-oxide nanoparticles electrodeposited onto glassy carbon electrode was shown in Fig. 33. The excellent electrocatalytic activity of nanoparticles cobalt oxide redox couple indicating the high ability of materials for electroanalysis purposes (Fig. 34).As shown cobalt oxide nanoparticles display high electrocatalytic activity toward hydrogen peroxide and arsenic (III) in physiological pH solution at reduced overpotential.

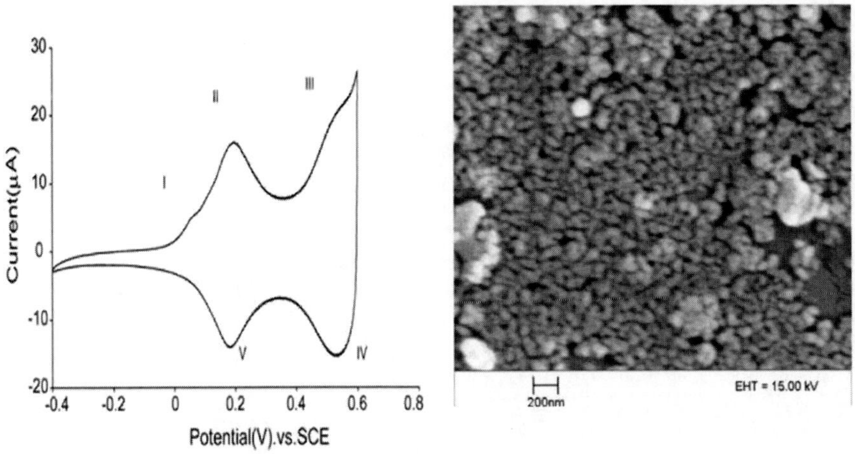

Figure 33. (A) CV response of GC electrode modified with CoOx Nanoparticles in pH 12 solutions at v = 20 mVs^{-1}. (B) SEM image of the electrodeposited CoOx on GC electrode. Reprinted from Analytica Chimica Acta, 594, A. Salimi, R. Hallaj, H. Mamkhezri, S. Soltanian, Nanomolar detection of hydrogen peroxide on glassy carbon electrode modified with electrodeposited cobalt oxide nanoparticles,26,Copyrights(2007) and J. Electroanalytical Chemistry, 619-620, A.Salimi, R.Hallaj, H. MamKhezri, S.M.T. Hosaini, "Electrochemical properties and electrocatalytic activity of FAD immobilized onto cobalt oxide nanoparticles : Application to nitrite detection,33, Copyrights (2008) with permission from Elsevier.

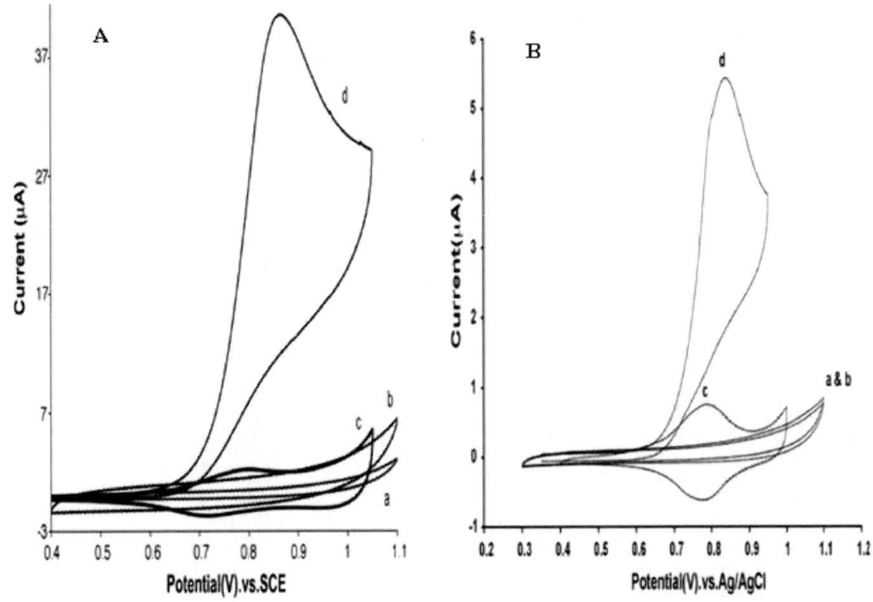

Figure 34. (A)Cyclic voltammograms of CoOx nanoparticles modified GC electrode in pH=7 solution at scan rate of $20mVs^{-1}$ In the absence (c) and presence of 40 µM H_2O_2 (d). (a) and (b) are same as (c) and (d) for bare GC electrode. Reprinted from Analytica Chimica Acta, 594, A. Salimi, R. Hallaj, H. Mamkhezri, S. Soltanian, Nanomolar detection of hydrogen peroxide on glassy carbon electrode modified with electrodeposited cobalt oxide nanoparticles, 28, Copyrights (2007)with permission from Elsevier. (B) As (A) for 70 µM arsenic (III). Reprinted from Sensors and Actuators B, 129, A. Salimi, H. MamKhezri, R. Hallaj,S. Soltanian, "Electrochemical detection of an ultratrace amount of arsenic (III) at glassy carbon electrode modified with cobalt oxide nanoparticles, 248, Copyrights(2008) with permission from Elsevier.

As shown, a reversible redox couple for immobilized protein was observed. Furthermore, the absorption bond of hemoglobin cobalt- oxide film (Curve b) is 407 nm similar to that of hemoglobin in pH buffer solution (Curve a), indicates no observable denaturation of hemoglobin happened on cobalt oxide film. The immobilized hemoglobin shows excellent stability at wide pH range with high electron transfer rate constant, $1.4 \pm 0.1\ s^{-1}$.

However, the application of cobalt- oxide nanomaterials for immobilization of biomolecelus and biosensor fabrication is rare. Recently we used electrodeposited cobalt-oxide nanoparticles for immobilization of hemoglobin [67]. The UV-visible spectrophotometric analysis and voltammetric studied indicates the immobilization of Hb onto cobalt-oxide nanoparticles (Figure 35).

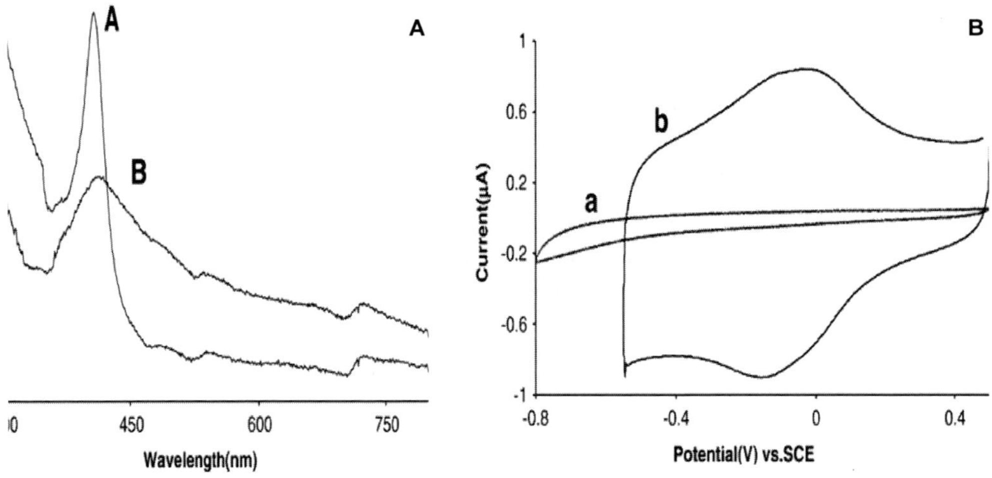

Figure 35. UV–visible spectra of catalase in PBS (pH 7) phosphate buffer solution (curveA) and Hb-CoOx film on ITO electrode (curveB).(B) CVs of glassy carbon electrode modified with cobalt oxide nanoparticles (a) and Glassy carbon electrode modified with cobalt oxide nanoparticles and Hb (b) , electrolyte is PBS (pH7), scan rate is 100 mVs^{-1}(Reprinted from Biophysical Chemistry, 62, A.Salimi, R. Hallaj, S. Soltanian, Immobilization of hemoglobin on electrodeposited cobalt-oxide nanoparticles: Direct voltammetry and electrocatalytic activity,124,125, Copyrights(2007) with permission from Elsevier.

Similar to other proteins and enzymes containing the heme group, the immobilized hemoglobin onto cobalt-oxide nanoparticles have ability to electrocatalytic reduction of H_2O_2 and O_2 based on the following equations:

$$HbFe(III) + H^+ + e^- \rightarrow HbHFe(II) \quad (17)$$

$$2HbHFe(II) + H_2O_2 \rightarrow HbFe(III) + 2H_2O \quad (18)$$

The recorded cyclic voltammograms of biosensor in the presence of different concentration of oxygen and hydrogen peroxide is shown in Fig.36.

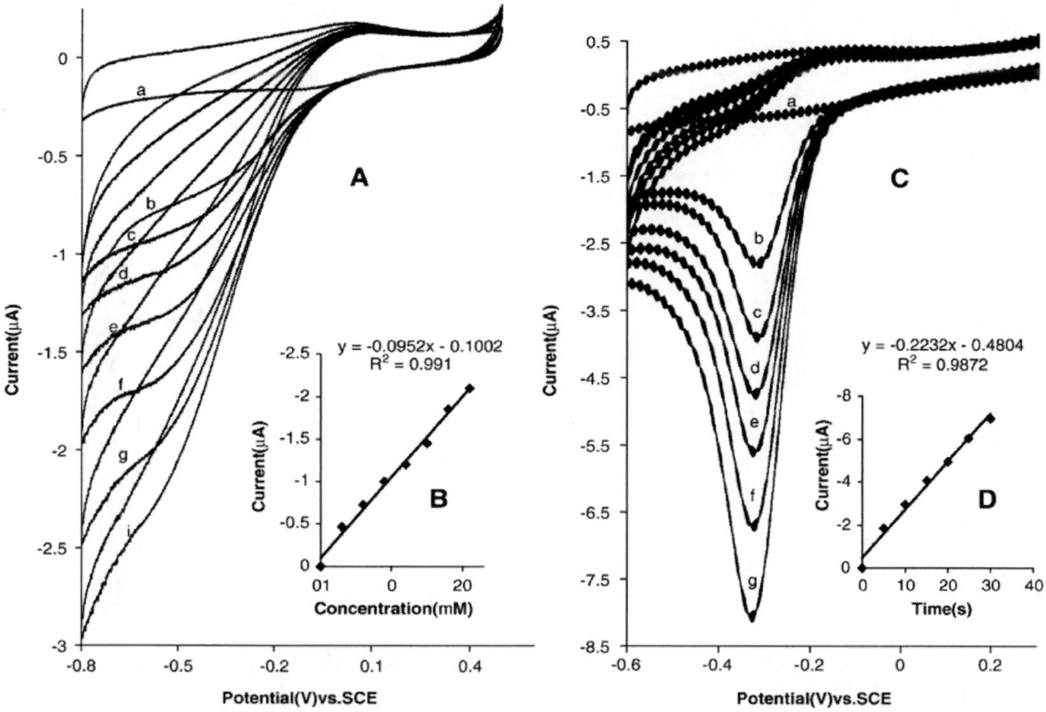

Figure 36.(A) Cyclic voltammetry response of Hb/CoOx modified GC electrode in the presence different concentration of H_2O_2 inPBS (pH7) at scanrate $20mVs^{-1}$, (a) 0.0 (b) 3 (c) 6 (d) 9 (e) 12 (f) 15 (g) 18 and (i) 21mM. (B) The plot of catalytic current vs. H_2O_2 concentrations. (C) Recorded CVs of Hb/CoOx modified GC electrode for different bubbling time of oxygen (a) 0.0 (b) 6 (c) 12 (d) 18 (e) 24 (f) 30 and (g) 36s. (D) Plot of peak current vs. bubbling times of oxygen. Reprinted from Biophysical Chemistry, 62, A.Salimi, R. Hallaj, S. Soltanian, Immobilization of hemoglobin on electrodeposited cobalt-oxide nanoparticles: Direct voltammetry and electrocatalytic activity, 127, Copyrights (2007) with permission from Elsevier.

Due to high biocompability and large surface are of cobalt oxide nanoparticles it can be used for immobilization of other biomolecules. Flavin adenine FAD is a flavoprotein coenzyme that plays an important biological role in many oxidoreductase processes and biochemical reactions. The immobilized FAD onto different electrode surfaces provides a basis for fabrication of sensors, biosensors, enzymatic reactors and biomedical devices. The electrocatalytic oxidation of NADH on the surface of graphite electrode modified with immobilization of FAD was investigated [276]. Recently we used cyclic voltammetry as simple technique for cobalt-oxide nanoparticles formation and immobilization flavin adenine dinucleotide (FAD) [277]. Repeated cyclic voltammograms of GC/ CoOx nanoparticles modified electrode in buffer solution containing FAD is shown in Fig.37A.

The reduction and oxidation of FAD are -0.48 V and -0.44V, respectively. With increasing the cycles number, the redox peak currents of FAD is found to be increased obviously. This behavior might be due to formation, growth and adsorption of FAD film on the cobalt oxide film. The FAD/CoOx (nano particles) /GC electrode shows a quasireversible redox couple FAD/$FADH_2$ with electron transfer rate constant of was 0.8 ± 0.1 $s^{-1.}$ Recorded CVs of FAD/ CoOx nanoparticles/ GC modified electrode in buffer solution containing different nitrite concentration is shown in inset of Fig.37A. As can be seen with increasing nitrite concentration the chatodic peak current increases and anodic peak currents decresed and at higher nitrite concentration disappeared. These results indicate excellent electrocatalytic activity toward nitrite reduction in physiological pH solution.

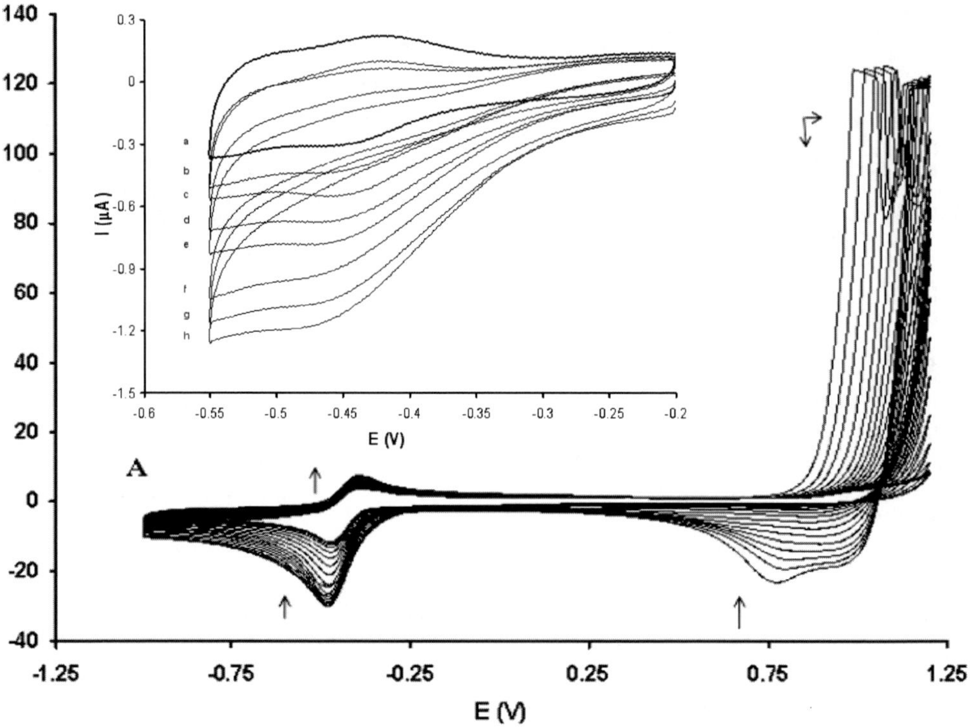

Figure 37. Consecutive CVs of GC electrode modified with electrodeposited CoOx nanoparticles in PBS (pH7) containing 5 mg ml FAD, scan rate $0.1Vs^{-1}$. Inset, shows the recorded cyclic voltammograms of FAD/CoOx nanoparticles/GCelectrode in the presence different nitrite concentration. (Reprinted from J. Electroanalytical Chemistry, 619-620, A.Salimi, R.Hallaj, H. MamKhezri, S.M.T. Hosaini, "Electrochemical properties and electrocatalytic activity of FAD immobilized onto cobalt oxide nanoparticles : Application to nitrite detection,33,36, Copyrights (2008) with permission from Elsevier.

4.7. Other Metal- Oxides Nanomaterials for Biosensors Fabrication

Direct and facile electron exchange between redox proteins and electrodes is important for development of biosensors and bioreactors. Due to biocompability, large surface area and high isoelectric point of metal oxide nanomaterials, they have been used as friendly environments for direct voltammetry and bioelectrocatalytic activity of biomolecules. Recently rare metal oxide nanoparticles successfully used for immobilization of biomolecules and biosensor fabrication. Metal oxides with tetravalent metal are good candidates for biomolcules immobilization. Hydrogen peroxide biosensors were fabricated based on immobilization of hemoglobine, myoglobin and zirconium oxide (ZrO_2) nanoparticles on glassy carbon and pyrolytic graphite (PG) electrodes [60]. The UV-Visible spectra and voltammetric studies suggested that proteins immobilized onto ZrO_2 nanoparticles retained their bioactivity and native structures (Fig. 38). The biosensors were successfully used for hydrogen peroxide detection. The low values of Michaelis-Menten constant ,K_M, 0.31 mM for ZrO_2/Hb/PG, 1.77 mM for ZrO_2- chitosan /Hb/GC and 1.53 mM for ZrO_2 - chitosan /Mb/GC suggested that the immobilized biomolecules into zirconium oxide nanoparticles retained their native activity. Furthermore, direct voltammetry and thermal stability of hemoglobin immobilized on a nanometer-size zirconium dioxide modified pyrolytic graphite electrode was studied [278]. For preparation biosensor, first ZnO_2 nanoparticles dispersed in DMSO. Then aqueous mixture of Hb solution and zirconium dioxide suspension was spread onto the surface of pyrolytic graphite electrode. Hb/ ZrO_2/DMSO/PG electrode shows excellent electrocatalytic activity toward hydrogen peroxide reduction. On the ZrO_2 nanoparticles Hb retains its bioactivity and displays a high affinity to H_2O_2. The electron transfer rate constant (k_s) was estimated based on theLaviron theory [170], is 7.9± 0.93 s-1, suggesting a reasonably fast electron transfer between the immobilized hemoglobin and the electrode due to the presence zirconium oxide nanoparticles. Low value of K_M 0.31 mM indicate high affinity of the biosensor to hydrogen peroxide. With immobilization of oligonucleotide onto MWCNTs/ ZrO_2 nanoparticles/chitosan -modified electrode, a high sensitive biosensor for detection of target DNA was fabricated [279]. Nanoporous niobium oxide exhibits good electronic and photacatalytic activity, and it can be applicable in biotechnology and electronic devices [280,281]. Due to highly ordered and narrow pore size of Nb_2O_5 nanomaterials, they are good candidate for biomolecules immobilization.

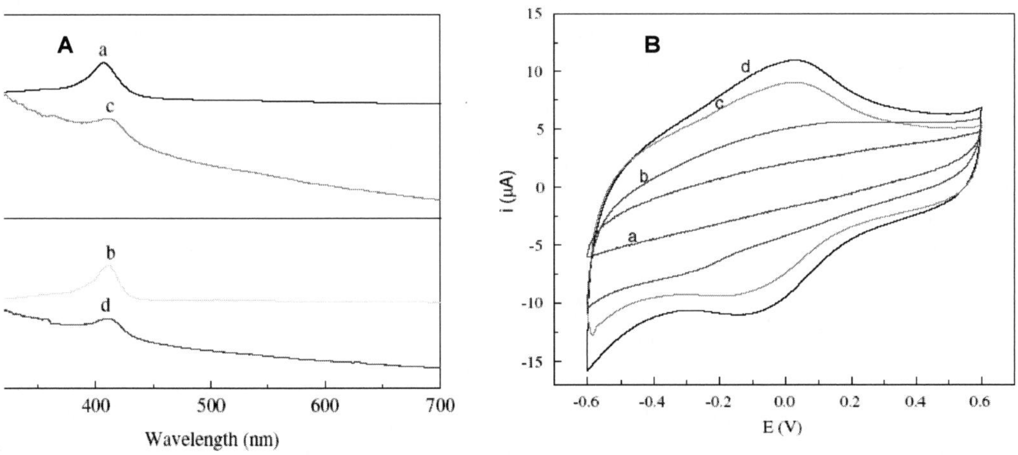

Figure 38 (A) UV–Vis spectra for: Hb (a), Mb (b) in PBS (pH 6.0), Hb/ ZrO_2/chitosan (c) and Mb/ZrO_2/chitosan (d) assembled layers on ITO glass (B) Cyclic voltammograms of bare (a), Hb/chitosan (b), Hb/ ZrO_2/ chitosan (c), Mb/ ZrO_2/chitosan (d) modified GCE in 25 mmol l^{-1} PBS (pH 6.0), scan rate: 100 mV s^{-1}.(Reproduced from Electrochemistry Communications, 7, G. Zhao, J.J. Feng, J.J. Xu, H.Y. Chen, " Direct electrochemistry and electrocatalysis of heme proteins immobilized on self assembled ZrO_2 film,726,727, Copyright (2005) with permission from Elsevier.

The direct voltammetry and bioelectrocatalytic activity of cytochrom *c*, HRP immobilized onto niobium oxide (Nb_2O_5) mesoporous matrix at inidium-tin oxide (ITO) electrode was investigated [282,283].The electron transfer rate constant of cytochrom *c* is 0.28 s^{-1} , reflective of the intrinsic electron transfer rate. In addition mesoporous niobium oxide offers a good environment for enzyme loading as well as substrate diffusion, tresulting in high sensitivity and long-term stability. Prepared biosensors have been successfully used for hydrogen peroxide detection.The Cyt *c* and HRP immobilized onto Nb_2O_5 nanoparticles retains their bioactivity and displays a high affinity to H_2O_2, producing a novel hydrogen peroxide biosensor for a quick measurement of H_2O_2 down to 0.1 μM. Carbon paste electrode modified with alchol dehydrogenase (ADH), nicotinamide adenine dinucleotide (NAD+) cofactor and meldola,s blue (MB) adsorbed on silica gel coated with niobium oxide has been used as sensitive amperometric biosensor for ethanol detection [284]. Figure 39, shows the mechanism of biosensor response.

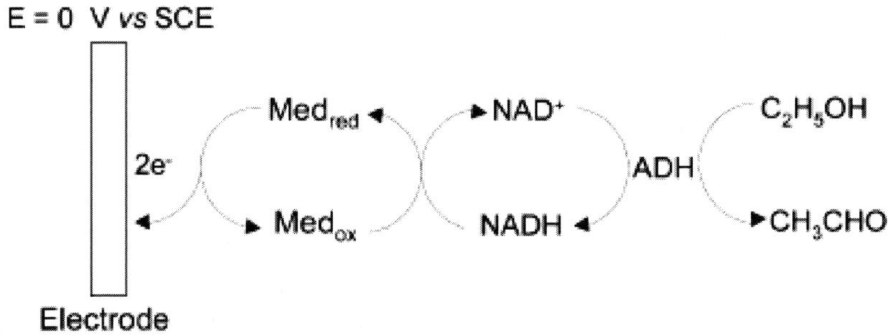

Figure 39. The mechanism of ADH/NAD/MB-based biosensor response for ethanol (Reprinteed from J. Electroanalytical Chemistry , 547, A.S. Santos, R.S. Freire, L.T. Kubota, Highly stable amperometric biosensor for ethanol based on Meldola's blue adsorbed on silica gel modified with niobium oxide ,137, Copyright(2003) with permission from Elsevier.

As shown the enxyme catalyzes the oxidation of ethanol to acetaldehyde in the presence NAD^+, and produced NADH can be detected amperometrically based on the following mechanism.

$$CH_3CH_2OH + NAD^+ \xrightarrow{ADH} CH_3CHO + NADH + H^+ \quad (19)$$

$$NADH \xrightarrow{\text{Electrode}} NAD^+ + H^+ + e^- \quad (20)$$

The other metal oxide for biosensor fabrication is cerium oxide nanoparticles. Nanocomposite containing nano-porous cerium oxide (CeO_2) and chitosan has been used for immobilization of single stranded DNA(ssDNA).The prepared DNA biosensor was used for determination the amount of colorectal cancer target DNA sequence, using methylene blue as redox indicator[285].The established biosensor has high detection sensitivity a relatively wide linear range and the ability to discriminate completely complementary target sequence. Electrodeposited mesoporous tungsten oxide (WO_3) was also used for adsorption of hemoglobin and fabrication a third generation biosensors for hydrogen peroxide detection [286].The WO_3/Hb modified graphite electrode shows excellent electrocatalytic activity toward hydrogen peroxide, nitrite and trichloroacetic acid. The K_M values of the biosensor for hydrogen peroxide and nitrite, 0.11 mM and 1.84 mM indicates high affinity of Hb adsorbed onto WO_3 nanoparticles to H_2O_2 and nitrite. Antimony oxide Sb_2O_3 is an important metal oxide semiconductor that has been uased as industrial catalyst. A new derivative of Sb_2O_3 is antimony oxide bromide (AOB) $Sb_8O_{10}(OH)_2Br_2$ contain two additional hydroxyl groups, has better biocompatibility for immobilization of proteins. Lu and coworkers reported the preparation of nanocomposite containing antimony oxide bromide nanorods and chitosan for biosensor fabrication. With immobilization of HRP onto nanocomposite a mediatorless third generation HRP biosensor was fabricated [287]. The STM and SEM images of antimony oxide nanoroads is shown in Fig. 40 A. A pair of well defined redox couple for immobilized enzyme at HRP/Chitosan/AOB/GC was observed (Fig.40 B).As shown for HRP/Chitosan/ /GC much smaller redox peaks observed. This result indicates AOB nanoroads play an important role in facilitating the direct electron transfer of HRP. The biosensor showed excellent electrocatalytic activity toward H_2O_2 reduction. The K_M value is 7.5 μM indicating the HRP immobilized onto nanocomposite possessed high affinity to H_2O_2. Tin oxide nanocrystalline film SnO_2, has a bond gap (330 nm) and an isoelectric point (IEp 5) is more conducting than zinc and titanium oxide. Therefore, it can be used for protein immobilization and biosensor construction. Direct voltammetry of cytochrom *c* cand hemoglobin immobilized onto SnO_2 nanoparticles was investigated [288].Voltammetric response of Cyt-c and Hb immobilized onto tin oxide nanoparticles is shown in Fig.41A.

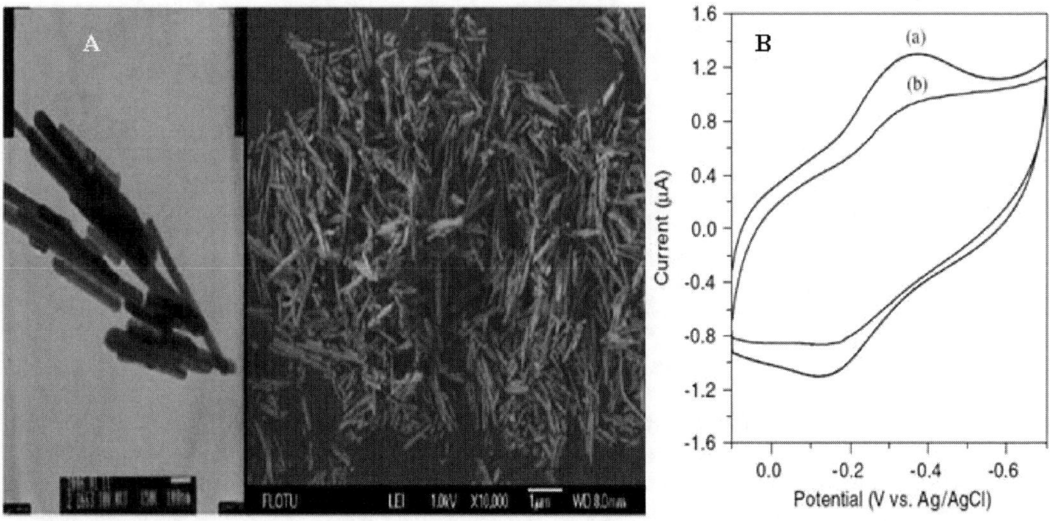

Figure 40. (A)TEM (left) and SEM (right) images of AOB nanorods.(B)Cyclic voltammograms of HRP (equal amount HRP) at different modified electrodes in pH 7.0 PBS with scan rate $0.02Vs^{-1}$: (a) HRP–Chi–AOB/GC and (b) HRP–Chi/GC.(Reprinted from Biomaterials 27, X. Lu, Z. Wen,Hydroxyl-containing antimony oxide bromide nanorods combined with chitosan for biosensors, 5742, 5744, Copyright(2006) with permission from Elsevier.

Electron transfer rate constants of 1.0 ± 0.03 s^{-1} and 0.53 ± 0.03 s^{-1} were determined for Cyt-c/ SnO_2 and Hb/SnO_2 electrodes.The electrochemically active Hb can be used as sensing element for NO detection(Fig.41 B). As shown with increasing NO concentration the formal potential of the adsorbed Hb sfhifted to positive potential values. Carbon nanotube modified with SnO_2 nanoparticles has been used for immobilization of urecase [289]. The modified electrode can be used as a reagentless, sensitive and selective biosensor for uric acid detection.Tin oxide nanoparticles was also used for glucose biosensor fabrication based on direct electron transfer of immobilized glucose oxidase [290].

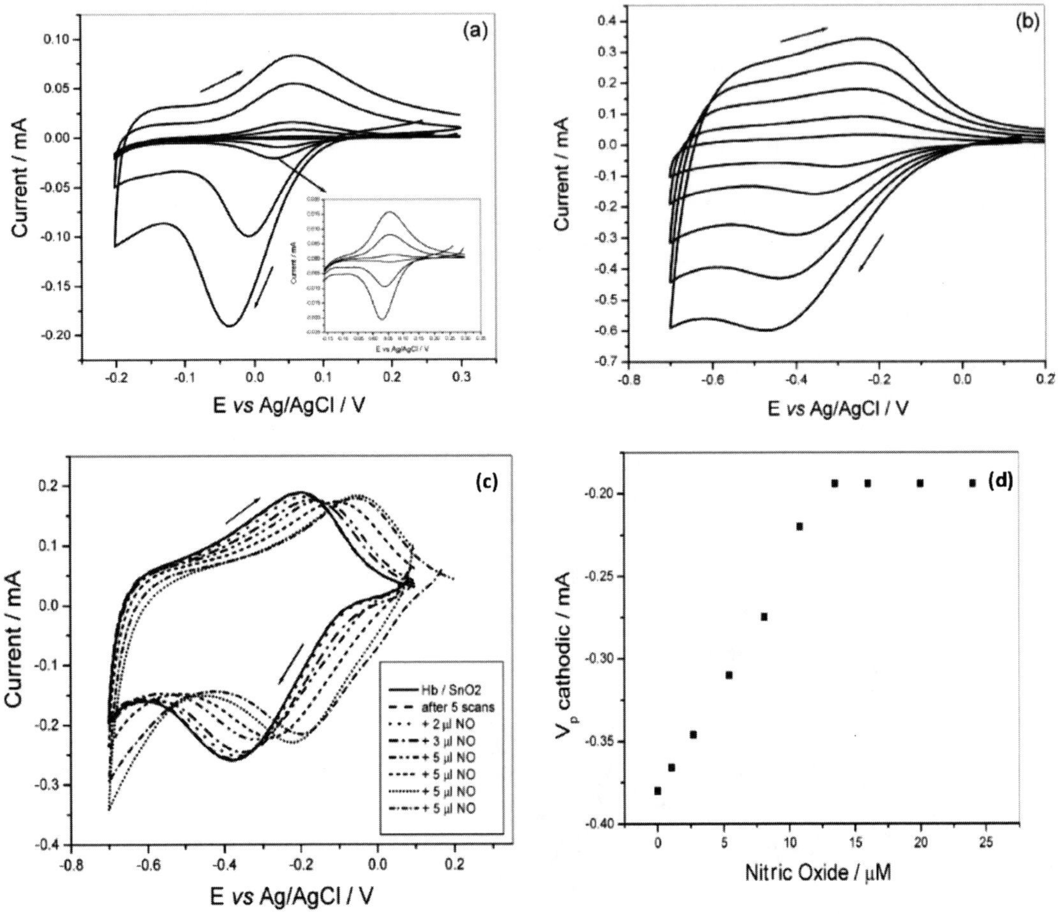

Figure 41. CVs of (a) Cyt-*c* immobilized on a mesoporous SnO_2 electrode in a pH 7 PBS, at 1, 5, 10, 50, and 100 mV s^{-1} (from lowest to highest peak currents) and (b) Hb immobilized on mesoporous SnO_2 electrode in a pH 7 PBS at 10, 25, 50, 75, and 100mVs^{-1} (from lowest to highest peak currents). (c) CVs obtained for a Hb/SnO_2 electrode in a pH 7, PBS before and after the addition of increasing amounts (1-13 μM) of NO-saturated buffer solution at a scan rate of 0.05 V s^{-1} (d)Plot of the cathodic peak potential Ep versus the NO concentration obtained from CV data (Adapted with permission from, E. Topoglidis, Y.Astuti, F. Duriaux, M. Gratzel, J.R. Durrant, Langmiur 2003, 19, 6894-6900.Copyright 2003 American Chemical Society.)

5. CONCLUSIONS

This chapter has addressed recent advances in the application biomolcules immobilized onto metal oxide nanoparticles for fabrication of biosensors. Electrochemical contacting of redox enzymes or proteins with electrode surfaces is a key step in construction of third generation reagent-free biosensors. We have described a variety of metal oxide nanoparticles

/ biomaterial for electrical contacting. The films formed by metal oxide nano materials have typical porous structure, which can greatly enhance the active surface area available for protein binding and facilate electron transfer process between metalloenzymes and the electrodes. Due to electrical properties, optical transparency, biocompatiblility, non toxicity, ease of fabrication, chemical, physical and photochemical stability, high isoelectric point, high porosity and small size of metal oxide nanoparticles they provided a favorable microenvironment for redox proteins and enzymes to direct electron transfer with underlying electrodes and their application for fabrication of third generation biosensors. Furthermore, due to biocompability of nanomaterials the immobilized biomolcules can retain their bioactivity and using of nanoparticles increased the surface area of the particles, thus increasing the number and acticity of enzyme molucles in the nanoparticle formulation. In addition most of the metal oxide nanoparticles carry charges; they can electrostatically adsorb biomolcules with opposite charges. The combination of biological molecules and novel nanomaterials components is of great importance in the processes of developing new nanoscale devices for future biological, medical and electronic applications. The remarkably facilated electron transfer of immobilized enzymes onto metal oxide nanomaterials with their intrinsic catalytic activity esentially allowed us to develop high sensitive third generation biosensors. By applying nanotechnology for advanced enzyme immobilization technique the electron transfer from enzyme to the transducers is increasing. Such strategies lowering opertating potential, increasing enzyme stability, extending activity, decreasing the rate of enzyme denaturation and eliminating interferences. In addition biosensors based on direct voltammetry of enzymes onto nanomaterials can offer higher sensitivity. Further research into the optimization of novel metal oxide nanomaterials or mixed metal oxide nanomaterials for enzyme based biosensor fabrication also promising. Biosensors fabricated based on metal oxide nanomaterials promise for widespread clinical use as well as diagnostics monitoring for at home applications.

ACKNOWLEDGMENTS

This research was supported by Iranian Nanotechnology Initiative and Research Office of University of Kurdistan.

REFERENCES

[1] Majid, E.; Harapovic, S.; Liu, Y.L.; Male, K.B.; Luong, J.H.T. *Anal. Chem.* 2006, *78*, 762-769.

[2] Lad, U.; Khokhar, S. ; Kale, G. *Anal. Chem.* 2008, *80*, 7910-7917.

[3] Harapovic, S.; Majid, E.; Liu, Y.L.; Male, K.B.; Luong, J.H.T. *Anal. Chem.* 2006, *78*, 55504-5512.

[4] Rusling, J.F. *Acc. Chem. Res.* 1998, *31*, 363-369.

[5] Heller, A. *Acc. Chem. Res.* 1999, *23*, 128-134.

[6] Rodrigues, L.G.; Wedd, A.G.; Bond, A.M. *J. Electroanal. Chem.* 1991, *312*, 131-140.

[7] Li, Q.; Luo, G.; Feng, J. *Electroanalysis.* 2001, *13*, 359-363.

[8] Schuhmann, W.; Ohara, T.J.;Schimdt, H.L.; Heller, A. *J. Am. Chem. Soc.* 1991, *113*, 1394-1397.

[9] Yabuki, S. ; Mizutani, F. ; Hirata, Y. *Sens. Actuators B.* 2000, *65* , 49-51.

[10] Kim S.H., Song, S.H.; Yao, Y.J. *Biotechnol. Bioprocess Eng.* 2005, *10*, 47-51.

[11] Ghica, M.E.; Brett, C.M.A.; *Anal. Chim. Acta.* 2005, *532*, 145-151.

[12] Shan, D.; Yao, W.; Xue, H. *Biosens. Bioelectron.* 2007, *23*, 432-437.

[13] Kotzian, P.; brazdilova, P.; RezkovaK. Kalcher, S.; Vytras, K.; *Electroanalysis.* 2006, *18*, 1499-1504.

[14] Warren, S.; McCormac, T.; Dempsey, E. *Bioelectrochemistry.* 2005, *67*, 23-35.

[15] Li, M.; Deng, C.; Zie, Q.; Yang, Y.; Yao, S. *Electrochim. Acta.* 2006, *51*, 5478-5486.

[16] Pan, D.; Chen, J.; Yao, S.; Nie, L.; Xia, J.; Tao, W. *Sens. Actuators.* 2005, *104*, 68-74.

[17] Hung, H.; Hu, N.; Zhou, Y. G. *Anal. Biochem.* 2002, *308*, 141-151.

[18] Zhang, Z.; Chouchane, S.; Magiliozzo, R.S.; Rusling, J.F. *Anal. Chem.* 2002, *74*, 163-170.

[19] Fan, C.; Wang, H.; Sun, S.; Zhu, D.; Wagner, G.; Li, G. *Anal. Chem.* 2001, *73*, 2850-2854.

[20] Liu, X. ; Xu, Y. ; Ma, X. ; Li, G. *Sens. Actuators B.* 2005, *106*, 284-288.

[21] He, X.; Zhu, L. *Electrochem. Commun.* 2006, *8*, 615-620.

[22] Arrigant, D.W.M. ; Bartlett, P.N. *Biosens. Bioelectron.* 1998, *13*, 293-304.

[23] Chen, X.; Xie, H.; Kong, J.; Deng, J.; *Biosens. Bioelectron.* 2001, *16*, 115-120.

[24] Wang, Q.; Lu, G.; Yang, B. *Biosens. Bioelectron.* 2004, *19*, 1269-1275.

[25] Ferreyra, N.; Coche- Guerente, L.; Labbe, P. *Electrochim. Acta.* 2004, *49*, 477-484.

[26] Yang, W.; Wang, J.; Zhao, S.; Sun, Y.; Sun, C. *Electrochem. Commun.* 2006, *8*, 665-672

[27] Sun, Y. Yan, F.; Yang, W.; Sun, C. *Biomaterials.* 2006, *27*, 4042-4049.

[28] Shen, L. Hu, N. *Biochem. Biophys. Acta.* 2004, 1*608*, 22-33.

[29] Losic, D.; Gooding, G.G.; Shapter, J.G.; Hibbert, D.B.; Short, K. *Electroanalysis.* 2001, *13* , 1385-1393.

[30] Wen, Z.H.; Ye, B.X.; Zhou, X.Y. *Electroanalysis.* 1997, *9*, 641-644.

[31] Elghanian, R.; Storhoff, J.J.; Mucic, R.C.; Letsinger, R.L.; Mirkin, C.A. *Science.* 1997, *227*, 1078-1081.

[32] He, L.; Musick, M.D.; Nicewarner, S.R.; Salinas, F.G. Benkovic, S.J. Natan, M.G. Keating, C.D. *J.Am. Chem. Soc.* 2000, *122*, 9071-9077.

[33] Willner, I.; Willner, B.; Katz, E. *Bioelectrochemistry.* 2007, *70*, 2-11.

[34] Scodeller, P.; Flexer, V.; Szamocki, R.; Calvo, E.J.; Tognalli, N.; Troiani, H.; Fainstein, A. *J. Am. Chem. Soc.* 2008, *130*,12690-12697.

[35] Maxwell, D.J.; Taylor, J.R.; Nie, S.M. *J.Am. Chem. Soc.* 2002, *124*, 9609-9612.

[36] Perez, J.M.; Simeone, F.J.; Tsourkas, A.; Josephson, L.; Weissleder, R. *Nano. Lett.* 2004, *4*, 119-122.

[37] Doering, W.E.; Piotti, M.E.; Natan, M. *J. Advans. Mater.* 2007, *19*, 3100-3108.

[38] Luo, X.; Morrin, A. Killard, A.J.; Smyth, M. R. *Electroanalysis.* 2006, *18*, 319-326.

[39] Willner, I. *Science.* 2002, *98*, 2407-2408.

[40] Shipway, A.N.; Katz, E.; Willner, I. *Chem. Phys. Chem.* 2000, *1*, 18-52.

[41] Zhang, S.; Wang, N.; Niu, Y.; Sun, C. *Sens. Actuators B.* 2005, *109*, 367-373.

[42] Zhao, G. C.; Zhang, L.; Wei, X.W.; Yang, Z.S. *Electrochem. Commun.* 2003, *5*, 825-829.

[43] Zhao, Y. D.; Zhang, W.D.; Chen, H.; Luo, Q. M.; Li, S.F.Y. *Sens. Actuators B*. 2002, *87*, 168-172.

[44] Wang, J. Li, M.; Shi, Z.; Li, N.;. Gu, Z. *Anal. Chem*. 2002,*741*,993-1997.

[45] Salimi, A.; Noorbakhash, A.; Ghadermarzi, M. *Anal. Biochem*. 2005, *344*, 16-24.

[46] Salimi, A.; Noorbakhash, A.; Ghadermarzi, M. *Sens. Actuators B*. 2007, *344*, 16-24.

[47] Weigel, M. Ch.; Tritscher, E.; Lisdat, F. *Electrochem. Commun*. 2007, *9*, 689-693.

[48] Cheng, W.; Jin, G.; Zhang, Y. *Sens. Actuators B*. 2006, *114*, 40-46.

[49] Vamvakaki, V.; Tsagaraki, K.; Chaniotakis, N. *Anal. Chem*. 2006, *78*, 5538-5542.

[50] Liu, Y.; Liu, H.; Hu, N. *Biophys. Chem*. 2005, *117*, 27-37.

[51] Shumyantseva, V.V.; Ivanov, Y.D.; Bistolas, N.; Scheller, F.W.; Archakov, A.I.; Wollenberger, U. *Anal.Chem*. 2004, *76*, 6046-6052.

[52] Liu, Y.; Liu, H.; Hu, *Biophys. Chem*. 2005, *17*, 27-37.

[53] Zhang, S.; Wang, N.; Niu, Y.; Sun, C. *Sens. Actuators B*. 2005, *109*, 367-374.

[54] Gu, H.Y.; Yu, A.M.; Chen, H.Y. *J. Electroanal. Chem*. 2001, *516*, 119-126.

[55] Xiao, Y.; Potolsky, F.; Katz, E.; Hainfeld, J.F.; Willner, I. *Science*. 2003, *229*, 1877-1881.

[56] Katz, E.; Willner, I. *Angewandte Chemi*. 2004, *43*, 6042-6108.

[57] Yang, M.; Yang, Y.; Liu, Y.; Shen, G.; Yu, R. *Biosens. Bioelectron*. 2006, *21*, 1125-1131.

[58] Bahshi, L. Frasconi, M. Tel-Vered, R.; Yehezkcli, O. Willner, I. *Anal. Chem*. 2008, *80*, 8253-8259.

[59] Lvov, Y .; Munge, B. Giraldo, O.; Ichinose, I.; Suib, S.; Rusling, J.F. *Langmuir*. 2000, *16*, 8850-8857.

[60] Zhao, G.; Feng, J.J.; Xu, J.J.; Chen, H.Y. *Electrochem. Commun*. 2005, *7*, 724-729.

[61] Li, Q.; Luo, G.; Feng, J.; Zhou, Q.; Zhang, L.; Zhu, Y. *Electroanalysis*. 2001, *13*, 413-416.

[62] Topoglidis, E.; Campbell, C.J.; Cass, A. E.G.; Durrant, J.R. *Electroanalysis*. 2006, *18*, 882-887.

[63] Feng, J.J.; Xu, J.J.; Chen, H.Y. *Electrochem. Commun*. 2005, *8*, 77-82.

[64] Rodriguez, M.C.; Rivas, G.A. Electroanalysis. 1999, *11*, 558-564.

[65] Zhao, G.; Xu, J. J.; Chen, H.Y. *Electrochem. Commun*. 2006, *8*, 148-154.

[66] Zhang, C.L.; Liu, M.C.; Li, P.; Xian, Y.Z.; Cheng, Y.X.; Zhang, F.F.; Wang, X.L.; Jin, L.T. Chin. *J. Chem*. 2005,*23*, 144-148.

[67] Salimi, A.; Hallaj, R. ; Soltanian, S. *Biophys. Chem*. 2007, *62*, 122-131.

[68] Remirez, C.P. ; Caruana, D.J. *Electrochem. Commun*.2006, *8*, 450-454.

[69] Chen, X.; Fu, C.; Wang, Y.; Yang, W.; Evans, D.G. *Biosens. Bioelectron*.2008, *24*, 356-361.

[70] Cosnier, S. *Appl. Biochem. Biotech*. 2000, *89*, 127-134.

[71] Zaman, H.; Yamada, A. Fukuda, H.; Ueda, Y. *J. Electrochem. Soc*. 1998, *145*, 565-568.

[72] Jyoko, Y.; Kashiwabara, S.; Hayashi, Y. *J. Electrochem. Soc*. 1997, *144*, L5-L8.

[73] Cassella, I. G.; Gatta, M. *J. Electroanal. Chem*. 2002, *534*, 31-38.

[74] Wang, G. X.; Chen, Y.; Konstantinov, K.; Yao, J.; Ahn, J.H.; Liu, H.K.;. Dou, S.X. *J. Alloys Compounds*. 2002, *340*, L5-L10.

[75] Liu, Y.; Wang, M.; Zhao, F.; Xu, Z.; Dong, S. *Biosens. Bioelectron*. 2005, *21*, 984-988.

[76] Trasatti, S.; in : *J. Lipkowski*, N.Ross (Eds.) Transition metal oxides: Versatile Materials for electrocatalysis ,*VCH publishers Inc*, New York, 1994.

[77] Silva, G.M. da.; Lemos; S.G.; Pocrifka, L.A.; Marreto, P.D.; Rosario, A.V.; Pereira, E.C. *Anal. Chim. Acta*. 2008, *616*, 36-41.
[78] Gill, E.; Arshak, K.; Arshak, A.; Korostynska, O. *Microsyst. Technol*. 2008, *14*, 499-507.
[79] Chou, S.L.; Wang, J. Z.; Chew, S.Y.; Liu, H.K.; Dou, S. X. *Electrochem. Commun*. 2008, *10*, 1724-1727.
[80] Toupin, M. ; Brousse, T. ; Belanger, D. *Chem. Mater*, 2004, *16*, 3184-3190.
[81] Jow, T.R.; Zheng, J.P. *J. Electrochem. Soc*. 1998, *145*, 49-52.
[82] Shinde, V.R.; Mahadik; S.B.; Gujar, T.P.; Lokhande, C.D. *Appl. Surf. Sci*. 2006, *252*, 7487-7492.
[83] Budianu, E.; Purica, M.; Iacomi, F.; Baban, C.; Prepelita, P.; Manea, E. *Thin Solid Films*, 2008, *516*, 1629-1633.
[84] L. Dennany, E.J. O'Reilly, T.E. Keyes, R.J. Forster, *Electrochem. Commun*. 2006, *8*, 1588-1594.
[85] H. Kamal, E.K. Elmaghraby, S.A. Ali,K. Abdel Hady, *Thin Solid Films*. 2005, *483*, 330-339.
[86] Garcia-Miquel, J.L.; Zhang, Q. Allen, S.J.; Rougier, A.; Blyr, A.; Davies, H.O.; Jones, A.C.; Leedham, T.J.; Williams, P.A.; Impey, S.A. Thin Solid Film. 2003, *424*, 165-170.
[87] Sayama, K.; Oi, T.; Abe, R.; Yanagida, M.; Sugihara, H.; Iwasaki, Y. Solar. *Energy Mater. Solar Cells*, 2006, *90*, 2429-2437.
[88] 82 . Wu, R. J.; Wu, J. G.; Tsai, T.K.; Yeh, C.T. *Sens. Actuators B*, 2006, *120*,104-109.
[89] Tabata, S.; Higaki, K. Ohnishi, H.; Suzuki, T.; Kunihara, K.; Kobayashi, M. *Sens. Actuators B*. 2005, *109*, 190-193.
[90] Yamauura, H.; Moriya, K.; Miuro, N.; Yamazoe, N. *Sens. Actuators B*. 2000, *65*, 39-41.
[91] Wang, G.X.; Chen, Y.; Konstantino, K.; Yao, J.; Ahn, J.; Liu, H.K.; Dou, S.X. J. *Alloys Comp*. 2002, *340*, L5-L10.
[92] Kim, H.; Kim, M.G.; Shin, T.J.; Shin, H.J.; Cho, J. *Electrochem. Commun*. 2008, *10*, 1669-1672.
[93] Yavuz, Y.; Koparal, A.S. *J. Hazardous Mater. B*. 2006,*136*, 296-302.
[94] Feng, Y.J.; Li, X.Y. *Water Reserarch*. 2003, *37*, 2399-2407.
[95] Fan, L.F.; Wu, X.Q.; Guo, M.D.; Gao, Y.T. *Electrochim. Acta*..2001, *52* , 3654-3659.
[96] Jafarian, M.; Mahjani, M.G.; Heli, H.; Gobal, F.; Khajehsharifi,H.; Hamedi, M.H. *Electrochim. Acta*. 2003, *48*, 3423-3429.
[97] Casella, I. G. *J. Electroanal. Chem*. 2002, *520*, 119-125.
[98] Manea, F. ; Radovan, C.; Schoonman, J. *J. Appl. Electrochem*. 2006, *36*, 1075-1081.
[99] Wang, J. *Electroanalyasis*. 2001, *13*, 983-988.
[100] Lo, P.H.; Kumar, S.A.; Chen, S.M. *Colloids Surfac.B*. 2008, *66*, 266-273.
[101] Yang, X.; Chen; X.; Zhang, X.; Yang, W.; Evans, D.G. *Sens. Actuators B*. 2008, *129*, 784-789.
[102] Salimi, A.; Hallaj, R.; Mamkhezri, H.; Soltanian, S. *Anal. Chim. Acta*. 2007, *594*, 24-31.
[103] Miao, X.M.; Uan, R.; Chai, Y.Q.; Shi, Y.T.; Yuan, Y.Y. *J. Electroanal. Chem*. 2008, *612*, 157-163.
[104] Shipway, A. N.; Katz, E.; Willner, I. *Chem. Phys. Chem*. 2000, *1*, 18-52.
[105] Wu, B.Y.; Hou, S.H.; Yin, F.; Li, J.; Zhao, Z.X.; Huang, J.D.; Chen;Q.; *Biosens. Bioelectron*. 2007, *22*, 838-844.

[106] Willner, I.; Katz, E. *Angew. Chem., Int. Ed.* 2003, *42*, 4576-4588.
[107] Weizmann, Y.; Patolsky, F.; Katz, E.; Willner, I. *J. Am. Chem. Soc.* 2003, *125*, 3452-3454.
[108] Katz, E.; Lioubashevski, O.; Willner, I. *J.Am. Chem. Soc.* 2005, *127*, 3979-3988.
[109] Feng, K.J.; Yang, Y. H.; Wang, Z. J.; Jiang, J.H.; Shen, J.L.; Yu, R. Q. *Talanta.* 2006, *70*, 561-565.
[110] Liu, A. *Biosens. Bioelectron.* 2008, *24*, 167-177.
[111] Satishkumar, B.C.; Govindaraj, A.; Nath, M.; Rao, C.N.R. *J. Mater. Chem.* 2000, *10*, 2115-2119.
[112] Liu, C. ; Yang, X. ; Yang, B. ; Yan, Y. ; Yan, Y. ; Qian, Y. *Matter. Lett.* 2005, *59*, 1409-1412.
[113] Wang, H.; Xu, C.; Cheng, F.; Jiang, S. *Electrochem. Commun.* 2007, *9*, 1212-1216.
[114] Izu, N.; Shin, W.; Murayama, N.; Kanzaki, S. *Sens. Actuators B.* 2002, *87*, 95-98.
[115] Lee, J. Y.; Liang, K.; Hyeok An, K.; Le, Y. H. *Synthetic Metals.* 2005, *150*, 153-157.
[116] Patzke, G.R.; Krumeich, F.; Nesper, R.; *Angew. Chem.Int.Ed.* 2002, *41*, 2446-2461.
[117] Svegl, F.; Orel, B.; Grabec-Svegl, I.; Kaucic, V. *Electrochim. Acta.* 2000, *45*, 4359-4371.
[118] Drasovean, R.; Monteiro, R.; Fortunato, E.; Musat, V. *J. Non-Crystalline Solids.* 2006, *352*,1479-1485.
[119] Maruyama, T. ; Arai, S. *J. Electrochem. Soc.*1996, *143*, 1383-1386.
[120] Cheng, C.S.; Serizawa, M.; Sakata, H.; Hirayama, T. *Mater. Chem. Phys.* 1998, *53*, 225-230.
[120] DaSilva, L.M.; Boodts, J.F.C.; Faria, L.A. D. *Electrochim Acta.* 2001, *46*, 1369-1375.
[121] Hamdani, M.; Koening, J.F.; Chartier, P. *J. Appl. Electrochem.* 1988, *18*, 561-567.
[122] Wen, S.; Lee, J.W. ; Yeo, I. H. ; Park, J. ; Mho, S. *Electrochim. Acta* .2004, *50*, 849-855.
[123] Schumacher, L.C.; Holzhueter, I.B. Hill, I.R. ; Dignam, M.G. *Electrochim. Acta.* 1990, *35*, 975-984.
[124] Jiang, S.P.; Tseung, A.C.C. *J. Electrochem. Soc.* 1990, *137*, 764-769.
[125] Ni, Y. ; Ge, X. ; Zhang, Z. ; Liu, H. ; Zhu, Z. ; Ye, Q. *Mater. Res.Bull.* 2001, *36*, 2283-2288.
[126] Liu, Z.H.; Ooi, K.; Kanoh, H.; Tang, W.P.; Tomida, T. *Longmuir.* 2000, *16*, 4154-4164.
[127] Lee, H.Y.; Goodenough, J.B. *J. Solid State Chem.* 1999, *144*, 220-223.
[128] Choi, H.N. ; Kim, M.A.; Lee, W.Y. *Anal. Chim. Acta.* 2005, *537*, 179-187.
[129] Dai, Z.H.; Liu, S.Q.; Ju, H.X.; Chen, H.Y. *Biosens. Bioelectron.* 2004, *19*, 861-867.
[130] Yiu, H.H.P.; Wright, P.A.; Botting, N.P. *J.Mol.Cat.B:Enzyme.* 2001, *15*, 81-92.
[131] Feng, J.J.; Xu, J. J.; Chen, H. Y. *Electrochem. Commun.* 2006, *8*, 77-82
[132] Casella, I.G.; Gatta, M.; *J. Electroanal. Chem.* 2002, *543*, 31-38.
[133] Escudero, M.J.; Rodrigo, T.; Mendoza, L.; Cassir, M.; Daza, L. *J. Power Sources,* 2005, *140*, 81-87.
[134] Hallaj, R. ; Salimi, A. ; Akhtari, K. ; Soltanian, S. ; Mamkhezri, H. *Sens. Actuators B.* 2009, 135, 632–641
[135] Casella, I.G.; Guascito, M. R. *J. Electroanal. Chem.*1999, *476*, 54-63.
[136] Giovanelli, D.; Lawrence, N.S. Wilkins, S.J.; Jiang, L.; Jones, T.G.J.; Compton, R.G. *Talanta.* 2003, *61*, 211-220.

[137] Kafi, A.K.M.; Wu, G.; Chen, A. *Biosens. Bioelectron.* 2008, *24*, 566-571.
[138] Cui, X.; Li, Z.; Yang, Y.; Zhang, W.; Wang, Q. *Electroanalysis*. 2008, *20*, 970-975.
[139] Wu, G.; Li, N.; Zhou, D.R.; Mitsuo, K.; Xu, B. Q. *J. Solid State Chem.* 2004, *177*, 3682-3692.
[140] Chuang, P.Y.; Hu, C.C. *Mater. Chem. Phys*. 2005, *92*, 138-145.
[141] Zang, J.F.; Li, C.M.; Cui, X.Q.; Wang, J.X.; Sun, X.W.; Dong, H.; Sun, C.Q. *Electroanalysis*. 2007, *19*, 1008-1014.
[142] Wang, J. *Analyst*. 2005, *130*, 421-426.
[143] Lu, X.; Wen, Z.; Li, J. *Biomaterials*. 2006, *27*, 5740-5747.
[144] J.A. Rodriguez, Fernandez-Garcia,in,M. Synthesis, properties and applications of oxide nanomaterials, Wiley-Interscience , 2007.
[145] Yang, J.; Zhang, R.; Xu, Y.; He, P.; Fang, Y. *Electrochem. Commun.* 2008, *10*, 1889-1892.
[146] Vayssieres, L. Advanced Mater.2003, 15, 464-466.
[147] Khan, R.; Kaushik, A.; Solanki, P. R.; Ansari, A.A.; Pandy, M.K.; Malhotra, B.D. *Anal. Chim. Acta*. 2008, *616*, 207-213
[148] Lu, X. ; Zhang, H. ; Ni, Y. ; Zhang, Q. J. Chen, *Biosens. Bioelectron*. 2008, *24*, 93-98.
[149] Kumar, S.A.; Chen, S.M. *Anal. Lett*. 2008, *41*, 141-158.
[150] Cheng, B.; Sumalski, E.T. *Chem. Commun*. 2004,*4*, 986-987.
[151] Rout, C.S.; Kulkarni, G.U.; Rao, C.N.R. *J. Phys.D. Appl. Phys*. 2007, *40*, 2777-2782.
[152] Height, M.J.; Madler, L.; Pratsinis, S.E. *Chem. Mater*. 2006, *18*, 572-578.
[153] Wang, Z.L.; Kong, X.Y.; Ding, Y.; Gao, P.; Hughes, W.L.; Yang, R.; Zhang, Y. *Adv. Funct. Mater* 2004, *14*, 943-956.
[154] Park, J.H.; Choi, Y.J.; Sohn, S.H.; Park, J.G. *J. Mater. Chem*. 2004, *14*, 35-36.
[155] Yang, Y.H.; Wang, C.X.; Wang, B.; Li, Z.Y.; Chen, J.; Chen, D.H.; Xu, N.S. *Appl. Phys. Lett*. 2005, *87*, 183109.
[156] Polarz, S.; Orlov, A.V.; Schuth, F.; Lu, A.H. *Chem. Err.J.* 2007, *13*, 592-597.
[157] Zhao, G.; Xu, J. J.; Chen, H. Y. *Anal. Biochem*. 2006, *350*, 145-150.
[158] George, P.; Hanania, G.I.H. *Biochem. J.* 1953, *55*, 236-243.
[159] Zhu, X. ; Yuri, I. ; Gan, X.; Suzuki, I.; Li, G. *Biosens. Bioelectron*. 2007, *22*, 1600-1604.
[160] Li, Y.F.; Liu, Z. M. ; Liu, Y. L.; Yang, Y. H.; Shen, G. L.; Yu, R.Q. *Anal. Biochem*. 2006, *349*, 33-40.
[161] Wei, A. ; Sun, X.W. ; Wang, J.X.; Lei, Y.; Cai, X.P.; Li, C.M.; Dong, Z.L.; Hung,W. *Appl. Phys. Let*t. 2006, *99*, 123902.
[162] Wang, J.X.; Sun, X.W.; Wei, A.; Lei, Y.; Cai, X.P.; Li, C.M.; Dong, Z.L. *Appl. Phys. Lett*. 2006, *88*, 233106.
[163] Dai, Z.; Shao, G.; Hong, J.; Bao, J.; Shen, J. *Biosens. Bioelectron*. 2009, *24*,1286-1291.
[164] Takahashi, H.; LI, B.; Sasaki, T.; Miyazaki, C.; kajino, T.; Inagaski, S. *Microporous Mesoporous Mater*, 2001, *45*, 755-762.
[165] Liu, S.; Ju, H.X. *Biosens. Bioelectron*. 2003, *19*, 177-183.
[166] Zhang, F.; Wang, X.; Ai, S.; Sun, Z.; Wan, Q.; Zhu, Z.; Xian, Y.; Jin, L.; Yamamoto, K. *Anal. Chim. Acta,* 2004, *519*, 155-160.
[167] Deng, Z.; Tian, Y.; Yin, X.; Rui, Q.; Liu, H.; Luo, Y. *Electrochem. Commun*. 2008, *10*, 818-820.
[168] Deng, Z.; Rui, Q.; Yin, X.; Liu, H.; Tian, Y. *Anal. Chem*. 2008, *80*, 5839-5846.

[169] Laviron, E. *J. Electroanal. Chem.*1979, *101*, 19-28.

[170] Singh, S.P.; Arya, PPandey, S.K.; Malhotra, B.D.; Saha, S.; Sreenivas, K.; Gupta, V. *Appl. Phys. Lett.* 2007, *91*, 063901.

[171] Solanki, P.R.; Kaushik, A.; Ansari, A.A.; Gumana, G.; Malhotra, B.D. *Appl. Phys. Lett.* 2008, *93*, 163903.

[172] Lobato, K.; Peter, L.M.; Wurfel, U. *J. Phys. Chem. B* 2006, *110*, 16201-16204.

[173] Yan, J.; Song, H.; Yang, S.; Yan, J.; Chen, X. *Electrochim.Acta* .2006, *53*, 6351-6355.

[174] DIDIMITRIJEVIC, N.M.; SAPONJIE, Z.V.; RABATIC, B.M.; RAJH, T. *J. AM. CHEM. SOC.* 2005,*127*, 1344-1345.

[175] Milsom, E.V.; Perrott, H.R.; Peter, L.M.; Marken, F. *Langmiur* 2005, *21*, 9482-9487.

[176] Topoglidis, E.; Lutz, T.; willis, R.L.; Barnett, C.J.; Cass, A.E. G.; Durrant, J.R. *Faraday Discuss.* 2000, *116*, 35- 46.

[177] Peng, X.; Chen, A. Adv. *Funct. Mater.* 2006, *16*, 1355-1362.

[178] Ou, H.H.; Lo, S.L. *Sep. Puef. Technol.* 2007, *58*, 179-191.

[179] Paddon, C.A.; Marken, F. *Electrochem. Commun.* 2004, *6*, 1249-1253.

[180] McKenzie, K.J.; Marken, F. *Langmuir.* 2003, *19*, 4327-4331.

[181] Milson, E.V.; Dash, H.A.; Jenkis, T.A.; Opallo, M.; Marken, F. *Bioelectrochem.* 2007, *70*, 221-227.

[182] Bonne, M.J.; Milson, E.V.; Helton, M.; Thielemans, W.; Wilkins, S.; Marken, F. *Electrochem. Commun.* 2007, *9*, 1985-1990.

[183] Zhang, Y.; He, P.; Hu, N. *Electrochim Acta.* 2004, *49*, 1981-1988.

[184] Zhang, T.; Tian, B.; Kong, J.; Yang, P.; Liu, B. *Anal. Chim. Acta.* 2003, *489*, 199-206.

[185] Song, M.; Zhang, R.; Wang, X. *Materials Lett.* 2006,*60*, 2143-2147.

[186] Liu, S. ; Chen, A. *Langmiur.* 2005, *21*, 8409-8413.

[187] Topoglidis, E. ; Campbell, C.J.; Cass, A.E.G.; Durrant, J.R. *Langmuir.* 2001,*17,* 7899-7906.

[188] Pankhurst, Q.A.; Connolly, J.; Jones, S.K.; Dobson, J. *J. Phys D Appl. Phys.* 2003, *36*, R161-R167.

[189] Mosbach, K.; Anderson, L. *Nature.* 1977, *270*, 259-261.

[190] Ito, A.; Shinkai, M.; Honda, H.; Kobayashi, T. *Cancer Gene Ther.* 2001, *8*, 649-654.

[191] Cheng, G.F.; Zhao, J.; Tu, Y.H.; He, P.G.; Fang, Y.Z. *Anal. Chim. Acta.* 2005, *533*, 1-16.

[192] Katz, E.; Weizmann, Y.; Willner, I. *J. Am. Chem. Soc.* 2005, *127*, 9191-9200.

[193] Liu, H.L.; Ko, S. P.; Wu, J.H.; Jung, M.H.; Min, J. H.; Lee, J. H.; An,B.H.; Kim, Y.K. *J. Magnetism Magnetic Mater.* 2007, *310*, e815-e817.

[194] Gupta, A.K.; Gupta, M. *Biomaterials.* 2005, *26*, 3995- 4021.

[195] Kim, S.H.; Kim, M.J.; Choa, Y.H. Mater. *Sci. Eng. A*, 2007, *449-451*, 386-388.

[196] Zhang, L.; Zhai, Y.; Gao, N.; Wen, D.; Dong, S. *Electrochem. Commun.* 2008, *10*, 1524-1526.

[197] Tanaka, T.; Matsunaga, T. *Anal. Chem.* 2000, *72*, 3518-3522.

[198] Li, Y.F.; Liu, Z.M.; Liu, Y.L.; Yang, Y.H.; Shen, G.L.; Yu, R.Q. *Anal. Biochem.* 2006, *349*, 33-40.

[199] Reetz, M.I.; Zonta, A.; Vijayakrishnan, V.; Schimossek, K. *J. Mol. Cata. A: Chem.* 1998, *134*, 251-258.

[200] Cao, D.; He, P.; Hu, N. *Analyst.* 2003, *128*, 1268-1274.

[201] Ma, Z.Y.; Guan, Y.P.; Liu, X.Q.; Liu, H.Z. *Langmuir.* 2005, *21*, 6987-6994.

[202] LI, D.; Teoh, W.Y.; Selomulya, C.; Woodward, R.C.; Amal, R.; Rosche, B. *Chem. Mater*. 2006, *18*, 6403-6413.
[203] Shaw, S.Y.; Chen, Y.; Ou, J.J.; Hu, L. *Enzyme Microb. Technol*. 2006, *39*, 1089-1095.
[204] Bai, S.; Guo, Z.; Lin, W.; Sun, Y. *Food Chem*. 2006, *96*, 1-7.
[205] Rossi, L.M.; Quach, A.D.; Rosenzweig, Z. *Anal. Bioana. Chem*. 2004, *380*, 606-613.
[206] Wang, W.; Deng, L.; Peng, Z.H.; Xiao, X. *Enzyme Microb. Technol*. 2007, *40*, 255-261.
[207] Li, G.Y.; Jiang, Y.R.; Huanmg, K.L.; Ding, P. Yao, L.L. *Colloids Surf. A: Physiochem. Eng. Aspects*. 2008, *320,* 11-18.
[208] Zhao, G.; Xu, J.J.; Chen, H. Y. *Electrochem. Commun*. 2006, *8*, 148-154.
[209] Xu, Q.; Bian, X.J.; Li, L.L.; Hu, X.Y.; Sun, M.; Chen, D.; Wang, Y. *Electrochem. Commun*. 2008, *10*, 995-999.
[210] Gong, J.; Lin, X. *Microchem. J*. 2003, *75*, 51-57.
[211] Nassar, A.E.F.; Bobbitt, J.M.; Stuart, J.O.; Rusling, J.F. *J.Am. Chem. Soc*. 1995, *117*, 10986-10993.
[212] Qiu, J.; Peng, H.; Liang, R. *Electrochem. Commun*. 2007, *9*, 2734-2738.
[213] Wang, S.; Tan, Y.; Zhao, D.; Liu, G. *Biosens. Bioelectron*. 2008, *23*, 1781-1787.
[214] Liu, Z.; Liu, B.; Kong, J.; Deng, *J. Anal. Chem*. 2000, *72*, 4707-4712.
[215] Qu, S.; Huang, F.; Chen, G.; Yu, S.; Kong, J. *Electrochem. Commun*. 2007, *9*, 2812-2816.
[216] Katz, E.; Willner, I. *Electrochem. Commun*. 2002, *4*, 201-204.
[217] Katz, E.; Willner, I. *J. Am. Chem. Soc*. 2002, *124*, 10290-10291.
[218] Katz, E.; Baron, R.; Wilner, I. *J. Am. Chem. Soc*. 2005, *127*, 4060-4070.
[219] Weizmann, Y.; Patolsky, F.; Katz, E.; Willner, I. *Chem. Biochem*. 2004, *5*, 943-948.
[220] E. Katz, L.S.H. Ichia, A.F. BucKMann, I. Willner, *Angew. Chem.Int. Ed*. 2002, *1*, 1343-1346.
[221] Hocevar, S.B.; Ogorevc, B.; Schachl, K.; Kalcher, K. *Electroanalysis*, 2004, *16*, 1711-1716.
[222] Schachl, K.; Alemu, H.; Kalcher, AK.; Jezkova, J.; Svancara, I.; Vytras, K. *Analyst*. 1997, 122, 985-989.
[223] Lima, F.H.B.; Calegaro, M.L.; Ticianelli, E.A. *J.Electroanal. Chem*. 2006, *590*, 152-160.
[224] Taba, Z.; Wang, J. *Electroanalysis*. 1991, *3*, 215-219.
[225] Turkusic, E.; Kalcher, J.; Kahrovic, E.; Beyene, N. W.; Moderegger, H.; Sofic, E.; Begic, S.; Kalcher, K. *Talanta*. 2005,*65*, 559-564.
[226] Beyene, N. W.; Kotzian, P.; Schachl. K.; Alemu, H.; Turkusic, E.; Copra, A.; Moderegger, H.; Svancara, I.; Vytras, K.; Kalcher, K. *Talanta*. 2004, *64*, 1151-1159.
[227] Yin, L.T.; Chou, J.C.; Chung, W.Y.; Sung, T.P.; Hsiung, K.P.; Hsiung, S.K. *Sens. Actuators B* 2001, *76*, 187-192.
[228] Yao, S.; Xu, J.; Wang, Y.; Chen, X.; Xu, Y.; Hu, S. *Anal. Chim. Acta*. 2006, *557*, 78-84.
[229] Dontsova, E.A.; Budashov, I.A.; Eremenko, A.V.; Kurochkin, I.N. *Nanobiotechnology in Russia*. 2008, *3*, 510-520.
[230] Yang, X.; Chen, X.; Zhang, X.; Yang, W.; Evans, D.G. *Sens. Actuators B*. 2008, *129*, 784-789.
[231] Han, X.; Jinling, W.; Xu, C.; WenSheng, Y. *Chin. Sci. Bullt*. 2008, *53*, 1152-1156.

[232] Yang, X.; Chen, X.; Zhang, X.; Yang, W.; Evans, D.G. *Sens. Actuators B*, 2008, *134*, 182-188.
[233] Ferreira, M.; Rubner, M. *Macromolecules*. 1995, *28*, 7107-7114.
[234] Lvov, Y.; Munge, B.; Giraldo, O.; Ichinose, I.; Suib, S.L.; Rusling, J.F. *Langmiur*. 2000, *16*, 8850-8857.
[235] Nakayama, M.; Tagashira, H. *Langmuir*, 2006, *22*, 3864-3869.
[236] Xu, J.J.; Feng, J.J.; Zhong, X.; Chen, H.Y. *Electroanalysis*, 2008,*20*, 507-512,
[237] Chen, J.; Zhang, W. D.; Ye, J.S. *Electrochem. Commun*. 2008, *10*, 1268-1271.
[238] Luo, X.L.; Xu, J.J.; Zhao, W.; Chen, H.Y. *Biosens. Bioelectron*. 2004, *19*, 1295-1300.
[239] Xu, J.J.; Zhao, W.; Luo, X. L.; Chen, H.Y. *Chem. Commun*. 2005, 792-794.
[240] Salimi, A. Roushani, M.; Haghighi, B.; Soltanian, S. *Biosens. Bioelectron*. 2006, *21* , 220-226.
[241] Kamal, H.; Elmaghraby, E.K.; Ali, S.A.; Abdel-Hady, K. *Thin Solid Films*. 2005, *483*, 330-339.
[242] Joudkazis, K. ; Juodkazyte, J.; Vilkauskaite, R. ; Jasulaitiene, V. *J. Solid State Electrochem*. 2008, *12*, 1469-1479
[243] You, T. ; Niwa, O. ; Chen, Z. Hayashi, K.; Tomita, M.; Hirono, S. *Anal. Chem*. 2003, *75*, 5191-5196.
[244] Xing, W.; Li, F.; Yan, Z.; Lu, G.Q. *J. power sources*, 2004, *134*, 324-330.
[245] Casella, I. G.; Cataldi, T.R.I.; Salvi, A.M.; Desimoni, E. *Anal. Chem*. 1993, *65*, 3143-3150.
[246] Shibili, S.M.A.; Beenakumari, K.S.; Suma, N.D. *Biosens. Bioelectron*. 2006, *22*, 633-638.
[247] Casella, I. G.; Gatta, M. *Anal. Chem*. 2000, *72*, 2969-2975.
[248] Salimi, A.; Roushani, M.; Soltanian, S.; Hallaj, R. *Anal. Chem*, 2007, *79*, 7431-7438.
[249] Salimi, A.; Roushani, M. *Electrochem. Commun*. 2005, *7*, 879-887.
[250] Salimi, A.; Roushani, M.; Hallaj, R. *Electrochem. Acta*. 2006, *51*, 1952-1959.
[251] Giovanelli, D. ; Lawrence, N. S.; Jiang, L.; Jones, T. G.J.; Compton, R.G. *Sens. Actuators B*. 2003, *88*, 320-328.
[252] Wolf, J.F.; Yeh, L.S.R.; Damjanovic, A. *Electrochim Acta*. 1981, *26*, 409-416.
[253] Salimi, A.; Sharifi, E.; NoorBakhash, A.; Soltanian, S. *Biosens. Bioelectron*. 2007, *22*, 3146-3153.
[254] Salimi, A.; Sharifi, E.; NoorBakhash, A.; Soltanian, S. *Electrochem. Commun*. 2006, *8*, 1499-1508.
[255] Salimi, A.; Sharifi, E.; NoorBakhash, A.; Soltanian, S. *Biophys.Chem*. 2007, *125*, 540-548.
[256] Tinoco, I.; Kauer, K.; Wang, G.C. *Physical Chemistry, Principals and applications in biological sciences, Printice Hall, Englewood Cliffs, NJ*. 1978, P 606.
[257] Zayats, M.; Katz, E.; Baron, R.; Willner, I. *J. Am. Chem. Soc*. 2005, *127*, 12400-12406.
[258] Moghaddam, A.B.; Ganjali, M.R.; Saboury, A.A.; Moosavi-Movahedi, A.A.; Norouzi, P. J.*Appl. Electrochem*. 2008, *38*, 1233-1239.
[259] Moghaddam, A.B.; Ganjali, M.R.; Dinarvand, R.; Saboury, A.A.; Razavi, T.; Moosavi-Movahedi, A.A.; Norouzi, P. *Biophys. Chem*. 2007, *129*, 259-268.
[260] Moghaddam, A.B.; Ganjali, M.R.; Dinarvand, R.; Razavi, T.; Saboury, A.A.; Moosavi-Movahedi, A.A.; Norouzi, P. *J. Electroanal. Chem*. 2008, *614*, 83-92

[261] Moghaddam, A.B.; Ganjali, M.R.; Dinarvand, R.; Ahadi, S.; Saboury, A.A. *Biphy.Chem.* 2008, *134*, 25-33.
[262] Li, C. ; Liu, Y. ; Li, L.; Du, Z. ; Xu, S.; Zhang, M. *Talanta.* 2008,*77*, 455-459.
[263] Kadam, L.D.; Pawar, S.H.; Patil, P.S. *Mater. Chem. Phys.* 2001, *68*, 280-282.
[264] Srinivasan, V.; Weidner, J.W. *J. Pow. Sources.* 2002, *108*, 15-20.
[265] Okabe, H.; Akimitsu, J.; Kubodera, T.; Matoba, M.; Kyomen, T.; Itoh, M. *Phys.B. Condensed Matter.* 2006, *378-380*, 863-864.
[266] Tyczkowski, J.; Kapica, R.; Lojewska, J. *Thin Solid Films.* 2007, *515*, 6590-6595.
[267] Longhi, M.; Formaro, L. *J. Electroanal. Chem.*1999, *464*, 149-157.
[268] Shinde, V.R.; Mahadik, S.B.; Gujar, T.P.; Lokhande, C.D. *Appl. Surf. Sci.* 2006, *252* , 7484-7492.
[269] Estrada, W.; Fantini, M.C.A.; Castro, S.C.D.; Fonseca, C.N.P.D.; Gorenstein, A. *J. Appl. Phys.* 1993, *74*, 5835-5841.
[270] Jiang, S.P.; Tseung, A.C.C. *J. Electrochem. Soc.* 1990, *137*, 764-769.
[271] Svegl, F.; Orel, B.; Svegl, I.G.; Kaucic, CV. *Electrochim. Acta.* 2000, *45*, 4359-4379.
[272] Casella, I.G.; Guascito, M.R. *J. Electroanal. Chem.* 1999, *476*, 54-63.
[273] Casella, I.G. *J. Electroanal. Chem.* 2002, *520*, 119-125.
[275] Salimi, A.; MamKhezri, H.; Hallaj, R.; Soltanian, S. *Sens. Actuators B.* 2008, *129*, 246-254.
[274] Alvarez, N.S.; Alvarez, P.S.; Castanon, M.J.L.; Ordieres, A.J.M.; Blanco, P. T. *Anal. Chem.* 2005, *77*, 4286-4289.
[275] Salimi, A.; Hallaj, R.; MamKhezri, H.; Hosaini, S.M.T. *J. Electroanal. Chem.* 2008, *619-620*, 31-38.
[276] Liu, S.; Dai, Z.; Chen, H.; Ju, H. *Biosens. Bioelectron.* 2004, *19*, 963-969.
[277] Yang, Y.; Wang, Z.; Yang, M.; Li, J.; Zheng, F.; Shen, G.; Yu, R. *Anal. Chim. Acta.* 2007, *584*, 268-274.
[278] Yang, P.; Zhao, D.; Margolese, D.I.; Chamelka, B.; Stucky, G. *Nature.* 1998, *396*, 512.
[279] Ye, B.; Trudeau, M.; Antonelli, D.M. *Adv. Mater.* 2001, *13*, 29-33.
[280] Xu, X.; Tian, B.; Kong, J.; Zhang, S.; Liu, B.; Zhao, D. *Adv. Mater.* 2003, *15*, 1932-1936.
[281] Xu, X.; Tian, B.; Zhang, S.; Kong, J.; Zhao, D.; Liu, B. *Anal. Chim. Acta.* 2004, *519*, 31-38.
[282] Santos, A.S.; Ferreire, R.S.; Kubota, L.T. J.*Electroanal. Chem.* 2003, *547*, 135-142.
[283] Feng, K. J.; Yang, Y. H.; Wang, Z.J.; Jiang, J.H.; Shen, G.L.; Yu, R. Q. *Talanta*, 2006, *70*, 561-565.
[284] Feng, J. J.; Xu, J. J.; Chen, H. Y. *Electrochem. Commun.* 2006, *8*, 77-82.
[285] Lu, X.; Wen, Z.; Li, J. *Biomaterials.* 2006, *27*, 5740-5747.
[286] Topoglidis, E.; Astuti, Y.; Duriaux, F.; Gratzel, M. ; Durrant, J.R. *Langmiur.* 2003, *19*, 6894-6900.
[287] Zhang, F.F.; Wang, X. L.; Li, C.X.; Li, X. H.; Wan, Q.; Xian, Y. Z.; Jin, L. T.; Yamamoto, K. *Anal. Bioanal. Chem.* 2005, *382*, 1368-1373.
[288] Park, J.Y.; Kim, Y. H.; Seong, A.; Yoo, Y. *Biotech. Bioprocess.Eng.* 2008, *13*, 431-435.

In: Nanostructured Materials for Electrochemical Biosensors ISBN: 978-1-60741-706-4
Editors: U. Yogeswaran; S. Kumar; S. Chen ©2009 Nova Science Publishers, Inc.

Chapter 7

RECENT ADVANCES IN NANO-STRUCTRURED METAL OXIDES BASED ELECTROCHEMICAL BIOSENSORS FOR CLINICAL DIAGNOSTICS

Anees A Ansari, Pratima R. Solanki, A. Kaushik, and B. D. Malhotra*

Department of Science and Technology Centre on Biomolcular Electronics, National Physical Laboratory, New Delhi 110012, India

ABSTRACT

Nanotechnology is playing an increasing important role in the development of biosensors. In recent years, electrochemical biosensors based on nanostructured metal oxides gained much attention in the field of health care for the management of various important analytes in a biological system. This article provides a comprehensive review of current research activities relating to nanostructured metal oxide based electrochemical biosensors. The unique properties of nanostructured metal oxides offer excellent prospects for interfacing biological recognition events with electronic signal transduction and for designing a new generation of bioelectronic devices. In this Chapter, we address various nanostructured metal oxides for fabrication of electrochemical biosensor and assembling procedures of these nanosensors. We discuss as to how these materials can be used for detection of various biological molecules and how such devices can be used to achive improved biosensing chrcateristics such as high sensitivity, selectivity and low detection limits.

*Corresponding author : bansi.malhotra@gmail.com, Phone 91-11-45609152 ; Fax: 91-11-45609310.

1. Introduction

Nanotechnology has recently become one of the most exciting forefront fields in material sciences. Nanotechnology is defined as the creation of functional materials, devices and systems through control of matter at the 1-100 nm scale [1-7]. A wide variety of metals and metal oxides nanoparticles, especially metal oxides nanoparticles with different properties have found wide applications in various fields of biomedical sciences [3-5]. Owing to their small size, metal oxide nanoparticles exhibit unique chemical, physical and electronic properties that are different from those of bulk materials, and can be used to construct novel and improved sensing devices; in particular, electrochemical sensors and biosensors [3,4]. The size and structure dependent nanomaterials offer excellent prospects for designing novel sensing systems with enhanced performance of desired bio-analytical assays [Fig. 1][6,7]. A large number of nanostructured metal oxides such as cerium oxide (CeO_2) [8,9], iron oxide (Fe_3O_4) [10-12], magnesium oxide (MnO_2) [13,14], niobium oxide (Nb_2O_5) [15], nickel oxide (NiO) [16], praseodymium oxide (Pr_2O_6) [17,18], tin oxide (SnO_2) [19,20], titanium oxide (TiO_2) [21-30], zinc oxide (ZnO) [31-41] and zirconium oxide (ZrO_2) [42-50] have been used for their application in electrochemical biosensors.

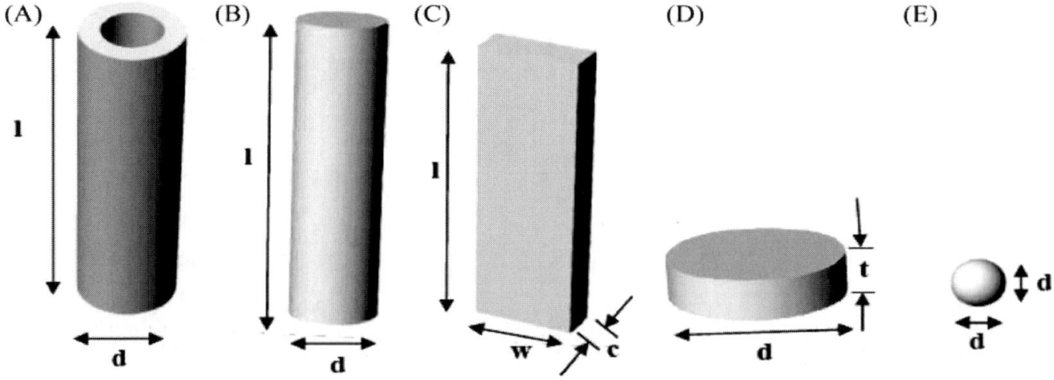

Figure 1. Various forms of nanostructures with typical dimensions. (A) Nanotube, l: length (greater than 1000 nm), d: diameter (less than 100 nm); (B) nanowire, l: length (greater than 1000 nm), d: diameter (less than 100 nm); (C) nanobelt, l: length (greater than 1000 nm), w: width (less than 500 nm), c: depth (less than 100 nm); (D) nanodiskette, t: thickness (less than 100 nm), d: diameter (generally between 500–1000 nm);(E) nanoparticles, d: diameter (order of few nanometers).

Electron transport properties of metal oxides nanoparticles are very important for electrical and electronic applications as well as for understanding the unique one-dimensional carrier transport mechanism. It has been noticed that the diameter of metal oxides nanoparticles, surface conditions, crystal structure and its quality i.e., chemical composition, crystallographic orientation along the film axis etc are important parameters that influence the electron transport mechanism. It is found that conductance of a nano-structure strongly depends on their crystalline structure. For example, in the case of perfect crystalline Si nanowires having four atoms per unit cell, generally three conductance channels are found [51]. One-or two-atom defect, either by addition or removal of one or two atoms may disrupt the number of such conductance channel and may cause variation in the conductance. It has been observed that change in the surface conditions of the nanowires can cause remarkable change in the transport behavior. This has been reported as change in the electrical conductivity that can be caused due to surface scattering phenomena of carriers in nanowires. This happens when the diameters of the nanowires are changed.

Electrochemical sensors offer several distinct advantages over others because of their rapid, accurate, quantitative and sensitive response as well as the simple and convenient operation. Thus, these nano-structured metal oxides have opened new opportunities for electrochemical biosensors. Different kinds of metal oxide nano-structures and different types of nano-structures of a given metal oxide can play different roles in different electrochemical sensing systems, such as enzymatic sensors, immunosensors and DNA sensors etc. Generally, metal oxide nano-structures have excellent conductivity and catalytic properties, which make them suitable for acting as "electronic wires" to enhance electron transfer between redox centers in proteins and electrode surfaces [3,5]. Besides this, metal oxide nanoparticles have high thermal stability, chemical inertness, non-toxicity, large surface-to-volume ratio, high surface reaction activity, biocompatibility and tunable electron transport properties due to quantum confinement effect that is strongly influenced by minor perturbations [5]. Because of their high surface-to-volume ratio and electrical properties of metal oxide nanoparticles are often used as labels or tracers for electrochemical analysis. The combination of biological molecules and nanostructured metal oxides play an important role in the development of nanoscale devices for future clinical diagnostics and electronic applications.

The goal of this chapter is to highlight application of advanced nanostructured metal oxides for electrochemical biosensors.

2. Preparation of Nanostructured Metal Oxides

Synthesis of one dimensional, two dimensional and three dimensional nanostructured metal oxides have attracted a great deal of interest for the past many years. Because of their size dependent catalytic and optoelectronic properties, they can be broadly tuned through size variation. Recently, extensive efforts have been made to synthesize one dimensional metal oxides nanostructures such as nanowires, nanobelts, nanotubes, nanorods, nanorings etc [Fig.2]. Various methods have been used in literature for development of nanostructured metal oxides of varying shape and sizes are as follows.

2.1. Electrochemical Deposition

During electrochemical deposition of metal oxides, metal hydroxides and metals, current are passed between an anode and cathode in a cell containing weakly alkaline electrolyte. The anion of the electrolyte is such that it does not form an insoluble salt with the metal anode. Metal ions issuing from the metal anode make contact with hydroxyl ions in solution and form finely divided oxides or hydroxides. The oxides or hydroxides are removed and chemically reduced to finely divided metal particles. The voltage necessary for carrying out the oxidation of the metal to metal ions is reduced through the use of an electrode as cathode, thereby reducing the cost of the process.

TiO_2 nanoparticles can be synthesized using electrochemical technique. Electrodeposition of TiO_2 film from $TiOSO_4+H_2O_2+HNO_3+KNO_3$ (pH 1.4, Eq. 1) solution involves indirect deposition of a gel of hydrous titanium oxo-hydrides (Eq.3), resulting from the reaction of titanium peroxo-sulfate (Eq.2) with hydroxide ions produced by nitrate electrochemical reduction [24].

$$NO_3^- + H_2O + 2e^- \rightarrow NO_2^- + 2OH^- \quad \text{(Eq.1)}$$

$$TiOSO_4 + H_2O_2 \rightarrow Ti\,(O_2)SO_4 + H_2O \quad \text{(Eq. 2)}$$

$$Ti(O_2)SO_4 + 2OH^- + (x + 1)H_2O \rightarrow TiO(OH)_2{\cdot}xH_2O_2 + SO_4^{2-} \quad \text{(Eq. 3)}$$

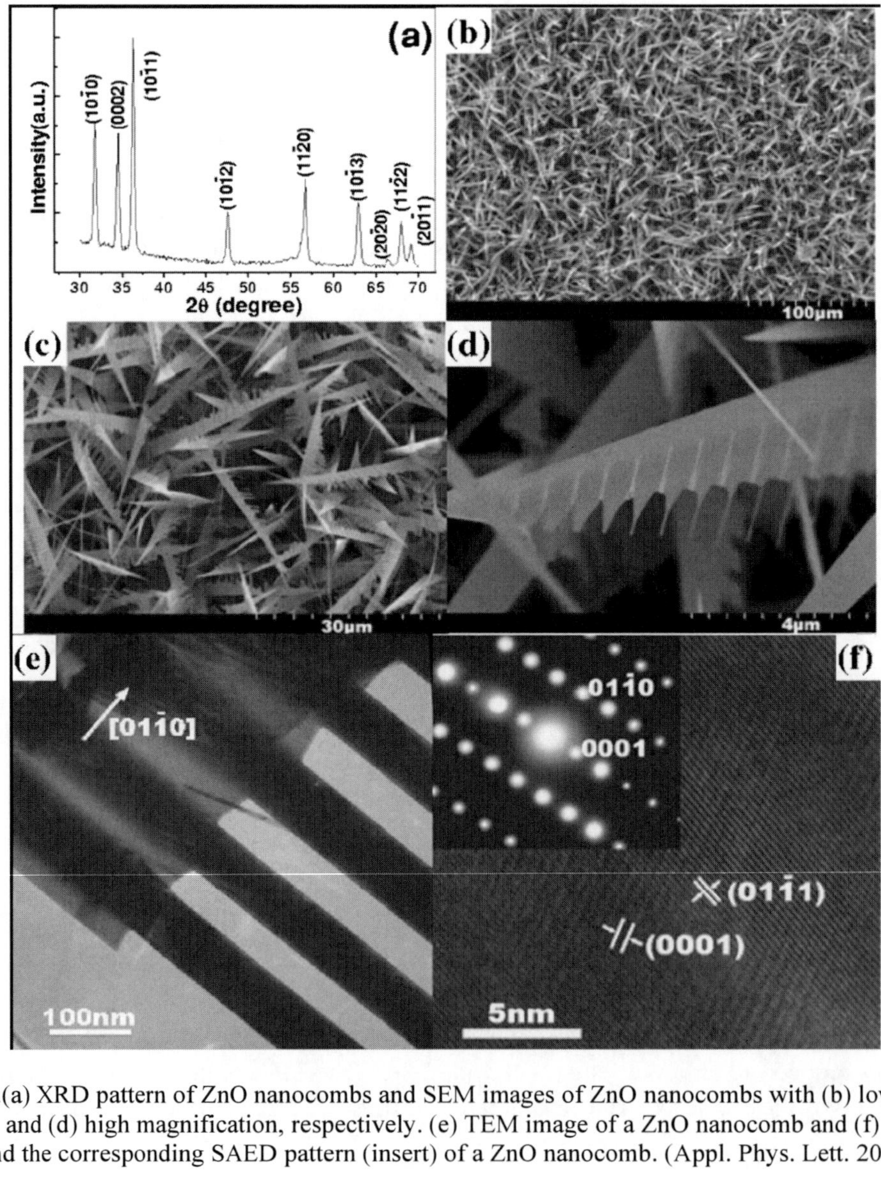

Figure 2.(a) XRD pattern of ZnO nanocombs and SEM images of ZnO nanocombs with (b) low, (c) medium, and (d) high magnification, respectively. (e) TEM image of a ZnO nanocomb and (f) HRTEM image and the corresponding SAED pattern (insert) of a ZnO nanocomb. (Appl. Phys. Lett. 2006, 88, 233106)

2.2. Electrophoretic Deposition (EPD)

The phenomenon of electrophoresis has been known since the beginning of the 19th century and it has found applications in traditional ceramics technology. EPD is essentially a two-step process: in the first step, charged particles suspended in a liquid migrate towards an electrode under the effect of an electric field (electrophoresis). In the second step, the particles deposit on the electrode forming a relatively dense and homogeneous compact or film. In general, EPD can be applied to any solid that is available in the form of a fine powder (<30 μm) or a colloidal suspension including metals and metal oxides.

2.3. Chemical Vapor Deposition (CVD) Method

The CVD technique involves decomposition of metal ions in presence of a catalyst. In this method, a catalyst is heated up to high temperature in a furnace with a flow of hydrocarbon gas through the tube reactor. The growth of a metal oxide (e.g In_2O_3) thin film is carried out in a horizontal CVD reactor (AIXTRON200). Trimethylindium (TMIn) and H_2O vapors are used as metal (indium) and oxygen precursors, respectively. The metal oxide (In_2O_3) thin films are synthesized on sapphire (0001) substrates by supplying TMIn and H_2O vapor with flow rates of 15 and 1160 μmol/min, respectively [5]. Highly textured In_2O_3 films are obtained at a substrate temperature of 600°C by using a 10 nm thick low-temperature (300°C) grown In_xO_y nucleation layer. Yu et al. have employed vapor deposition technique for fabrication of titania film on glassy carbon electrode via slow formation by titanium isopropoxide vapor at 25°C [25].

2.4. Rf Magnetron Sputtering Method

Rf sputtering film deposition can be performed by reactive magnetron sputtering in an argon (50%) and oxygen (50%) atmosphere (4×10^{-3} mbar) using a pure metal tungsten (W) target (99.999% purity) equipped with 12 holes that can be filled either with W or Fe insets. The substrate temperature is kept at 300°C, during the film deposition to promote the formation. Annealing is performed inside a furnace under a controlled flux of humid synthetic air at 500 °C for about 6 h. Temperature is slowly varied in order to avoid any possible stress or crack in the layers and to obtain in-depth oxidation. Singh et al. have developed ZnO thin film by rf magnetron sputtering technique on gold coated 7059 corning glass [35].

2.5. Sol-Gel Method

The sol-gel process is a wet-chemical technique (*Chemical Solution Deposition*) for the fabrication of *metal oxide* starting either from a chemical solution (sol short for solution) or colloidal particles (sol for nanoscale particle) to produce an integrated network (gel). Typical precursors are metal alkoxides and metal chlorides, which undergo *hydrolysis* and *polycondensation* reactions to form a *colloid* [a system composed of solid particles (size ranging from 1 nm to 1 μm) dispersed in a solvent]. The sol evolves towards the formation of an inorganic continuous network containing a liquid phase (*gel*). Formation of a metal oxide involves connecting the metal centers with oxo (M-O-M) or hydroxo (M-OH-M) bridges thereby generating metal-oxo or metal-hydroxo polymers in solution. The drying process serves to remove the liquid phase from the gel thus forming a porous material and then a thermal treatment (firing) may be performed in order to favor further polycondensation and enhance mechanical properties.

The precursor sol can either be deposited on a substrate to form a film (e.g. by dip-coating or spin-coating), cast into a suitable container with the desired shape (e.g. to obtain monolithic ceramics, glasses, fibers, membranes, *aerogels*), or used to synthesize powders (e.g. microspheres, nanospheres). The sol-gel approach is interesting in that it is a cheap and low-temperature technique that allows fine control on the product's chemical composition, as even small quantities of dopants, such as organic dyes and rare earth metals, can be introduced in the sol and end up in the final product finely dispersed. It can be used in *ceramics* manufacturing processes, as an *investment casting* material, or as a means of producing very *thin films* of metal *oxides* for various purposes. Sol-gel derived materials have diverse applications in optics, electronics, energy, space, (bio) sensors, medicine (e.g. controlled drug release) and separation (e.g. chromatography) technology. Many researchers have employed sol-gel technique for fabrication of nanostructured metal oxide films on solid substrates for sensing application [8,9].

2.6. Miscellaneous Methods

Nanostructured metal oxide film deposition can also be prepared by hydrothermal decomposition, film casting method (sonication of nanoparticles in aqueous solution (H_2O) or preparation of aqueous suspension of nanoparticles for spread on conducting glass plate) and nanosized metal nanoparticles prepared by controlled hydrolysis [16,18,19,21,26].

3. Characterization of Nanostructured Metal Oxides

X-ray diffraction technique is a non-destructive analytical technique that reveals information about *crystallographic* structure, chemical composition and physical properties of nanostructured materials. UV/Vis spectroscopy is routinely used in the *quantitative* determination of films of nanostructured metal oxides. The size, shape (nanocomb and nanorods etc,) and arrangement of the nanoparticles can be observed through transmission electron microscope (TEM) studies. Surface morphology of nanostructured metal oxides can be observed in atomic force microscopy (AFM) and scanning electron microscopy (SEM) studies.

5. Application of Nanostructured Metal Oxides for Electrochemical Biosensor

5.1. Zinc Oxide (ZnO)

ZnO is a versatile wide direct band gap (3.37 eV), n-type semiconductor material, that has attracted much attention for wide range of applications in biomedical sciences and material sciences. Some specific properties of nanostructured ZnO such as biocompatibility, non-toxicity and piezoelectricity(0.43C/cm^2), that allow transducers using either bulk acoustic waves (BAW) or surface acoustic waves (SAW) to measure changes in fundamental frequencies[32-35,52,53]. The higher piezoelectricity can enhance sensitivity of the electrode. Owing to its excellent film forming and adhesion ability, high surface area, strong adsorption capability (high isoelectric point, ~ 9.5), improved catalytic efficiency (oxygen storage capacity), better chemical stability, resistant against corrosion and oxidation, small grain size, which makes it highly promising for electrochemical biosensor applications [32-35].

Wei and his coworkers have prepared ZnO nanocomb on Au electrode by vapor phase depsotion method for glucose sensing [33]. They have shown that nanostructured composite exhibits high sensitivity (15.33μA/cm^{2}mM) with the linearity range from 0.02-4.5 mM (Fig.2). Further, these authors have grown ZnO nanorod using hydrothermal technique for fabrication of enzyme glucose biosensor. The biosensor shows linearity as 0.01-3.45 mM, and sensitivity as 23.1 μA cm^{-2} mM^{-1} with shelf life one week [32]. Zang et al. have constructed glucose biosensor based on ZnO nanowires as a platform to study their kinetic parameter such as Michaelis-Menten constant (K_m) [54]. These authors have, however, not examined the thermal stability, shelf life and response of the biosensor [55]. Zhao et al have immobilized glucose oxidase (GOx) onto Co doped ZnO (ZnO:Co) nanoclusters for glucose detection. This biosensor exhibits high K_m value 21.0mM, sensitivity as 13.3 μA/mA cm^2 with low detection limit (20 μM)[52]. Umar et al. have grown well-crystallized ZnO nanonails in a high density by thermal evaporation process used as supporting matrix for glucose estimation. The fabricated biosensor shows high sensitivity as 24.613 μA cm^{-2} mM^{-1} with response time less than 10s. Moreover, it shows linear range from 0.1-7.1 mM with a correlation coefficient (r^2= 0.9937) and detection limit of 5 μM [56]. A tetragonal pyramid-shaped porous ZnO (TPSP-ZnO) nanostructure has been for immobilization of GOx. They have shown that nanostructured composite matrix exhibits sensing characteristics such as linearity in the glucose concentration range from 0.05 to 8.2 mM with detection limit of 0.01 mM at an applied potential of -0.50 V [57].

Nanoporous ZnO film has recently been deposited on Au electrode by rf sputtering under high pressure and used it for cholesterol detection. A well preferred c-axis oriented ZnO film with porous surface morphology exhibits linearity as 25-400 mg/dl, response time of 15 s and stability of 75 days [35]. Khan et al. have been fabricated a nanocomposite film of ZnO nanoparticles containing chitosan (CH) for cholesterol estimation. This biosensor exhibits linearity from 5-300 mgdL^{-1} with detection limit of 5mg dl^{-1} and the value of K_m as 8.63 mgdL^{-1}[36]. Sol-gel derived ZnO film has been deposited on Pt electrode for development of an amperometric biosensor to determination of acetylcholine (ACh) and choline (Ch). The resulting biosensor shows linear response from 1.0 × 10^{-6} to 1.5 × 10^{-3} M to ACh with detection limit of 6.0 × 10^{-7} M and a linear response upto 1.6 × 10^{-3} M to Ch with detection limit of 5.0×10^{-7} M. These bioelectrodes possess stability upto 10 days [58]. Deng et al. have employed ZnO nanodisk electrode for superoxide anion determination. These nanodisk electrodes exhibit direct electron transfer of superoxide dismutase (SOD) indicating heterogeneous electron rate constant (17 ± 2 s^{-1}). The effect of common interfering species such as hydrogen peroxide, uric acid, ascorbic acid, and 3,4-dihydroxyphenylacetic acid have been monitored, resulting in negligible effect (<1%) at both +300 and 0 mV. They recorded 10% deviation of the current response of continuous measurements for 7 days [37]. Later these authors have reported a direct electron transfer mechanism of zinc–superoxide dismutase (Zn–SOD) onto a physical vapor deposited zinc oxide (ZnO) nanoparticles surface. SOD exhibits quasi-reversible electrochemical behavior in phosphate buffer solution (PBS, pH 7.25), with apparent formal potential of 195.2 ± 4.6 mV vs. [38].

ZnO nanoparticles dispersed CH composite films deposited onto glassy carbon electrode (GCE) have been used for immobilization of tyrosinase enzyme for phenol detection. This biosensor shows 95% of steady-state current within 10s, sensitivity as 182 μA $mmol^{-1}$ L with a detection limit of 5.0×10^{-8} mol/L, exhibits maximum response at 50°C and retains 91% current after about 20 days [39]. A sol-gel derived ZnO matrix has been used to immobilize tyrosinase for determination of phenol concentration from 1.5×10^{-7} to 4.0×10^{-5} mol L^{-1} with detection limit of 8.0×10^{-8} mol L^{-1} and sensitivity of 168 μA mmol L^{-1}. This biosensor shows 95% of steady-state current within 15s after 2 weeks [40]. Chen et al. have immobilized mushroom tyrosinase oxidase onto ZnO nanorods for the phenol and catechol detection. The linear concentration ranges have been obtained from 0.02 to 0.1 mM and 0.01 to 0.4 mM, for phenol and catechol, respectively. The apparent K_m has been estimated as 0.24 mM for phenol and 1.75 mM for catechol [59].

Zhang et al. have prepared ZnO nanorods to immobilize uricase enzyme for uric acid estimation. The linearity has been obtained for the uric acid concentration ranging from 5.0×10^{-6} to 1.0×10^{-3} mol L^{-1} and detection limit as 2.0×10^{-6} mol L^{-1} with high thermal stability up to 85°C. ZnO nanorods derived electrode retains enzyme bioactivity and could enhanced electron transfer between the enzyme and the electrode without using mediator. These nanorods resulting in enhanced uricase affinity towards uric acid. [60]. ZnO-CH nanobiocomposite film has been employed to immobilize urease (Urs) and glutamate dehydrogenase (GLDH) enzyme for urea detection. A wide linear range (5-100 mg/dL) has been achieved with detection limit of 3 mg/dL, response time of 10 s, reproducibility as 20 times and shelf-life of 3 months. This bioelectrode exhibits high value of K_m (4.92 mg/dL) indicating low affinity of enzyme with nanobiocomposite [34].

Amperometric hydrogen peroxide (H_2O_2) biosensor based on ZnO-multi walled carbon nanotubes (MWCNT) composite has been developed using horseradish peroxidase (HRP). This electrode exhibits H_2O_2 detection at low potential (-0.11 V) due to MWCNT facilitate improved electrochemical performance. This biosensor displays rapid response (<5 s), extended linear range, 9.9×10^{-7} to 2.9×10^{-3} mol/L with a correlation coefficient of 0.991 [61]. The electrocatalytic performance of hemoglobin (metallo-enzymes) immobilized onto nanosheet-ZnO microspheres has been obtained at -0.345 V (vs. Ag/AgCl) at buffer pH 7.0 for H_2O_2 detection. An apparent heterogeneous electron transfer rate constant (k_s) of 3.2 s^{-1} is observed for the ZnO. A wide linear range of 1-410 and 10-2700 μM has been achieved for H_2O_2 detection [41]. Yang et al have employed entrapment of HRP in a ZnO/CH composite matrix for development of H_2O_2 biosensor. The activity of the enzyme has been improved using hydroquinone mediator and glutaraldehyde as linker. This biosensor shows fast response (less than 10s), linearity as 5.0×10^{-6} to 2.0×10^{-3} mol/L with sensitivity of 43.8 μA /mM cm^{-2} [62]. Hydrothermally fabricated nanosized flower like ZnO matrix has been utilized to immobilize HRP for H_2O_2 determination. The fabricated bioelectrodes retains 78% response after 40 days [63]. Zhu et al have fabricated a H_2O_2 biosensor that exhibits linearity for H_2O_2 in the range of 1 x 10^{-7}- 8.0 x 10^{-4} M with detection limit $3x10^{-8}$ mol/L, and possess response 1.5s (Fig. 3) [64]. Electrochemically deposited ZnO film on glassy carbon electrode has been utilized for entrapment of myoglobin. The entrapped Mb results in direct electron transfer with the electrode and displays catalytic activity toward the reduction of hydrogen peroxide, nitrite and trichloroacetic acid [65].

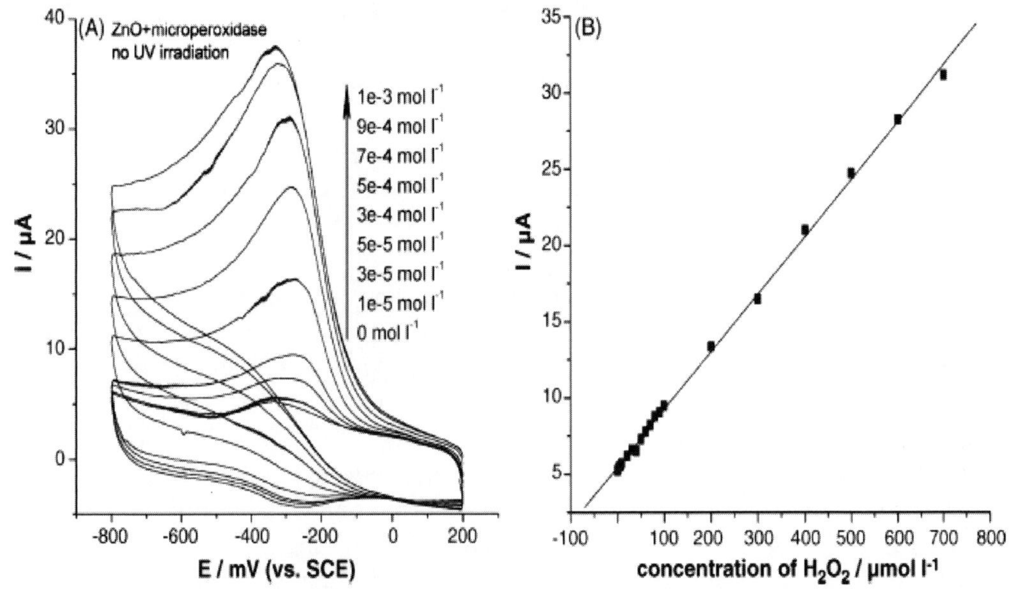

Figure 3. (A) Cyclic voltammograms of MP/ZnO NPs modified electrode after the addition of H_2O_2 in the test solution without UV irradiation. (B) The linear fitting program of the reduction peak current with the H_2O_2 concentration. (Biosensors and Bioelectronics 2007, 22, 1600).

Chitosan has been utilized along with hydrothermally prepared nano-ZnO nanoparticles for DNA hybridization detection. The detection limit is obtained as 1.09×10^{-11} mol L^{-1} of complementary target [66]. A MWNTs/nanoZnO/CH modified nanocomposite GCE electrode has been used for DNA immobilization via physisorption. This biosensor can effectively discriminate different DNA sequences related to PAT gene in the transgenic corn, with detection limit of 2.8×10^{-12} mol/L of target sequence [67]. In another report they have deposited ZnO nanoparticles, MWNTs and CH layer onto glassy carbon electrode to immobilize ssDNA probe. A remarkable synergistic effect of the ZnO nanoparticles and MWNTs has been achieved after ssDNA probe immobilization for fabrication of sensitive electrochemical DNA biosensor. The modified electrode shows a wide linear response for DNA hybridization detection. (1.0×10^{-11} to 1.0×10^{-6} mol/L) with detection limit of 2.8×10^{-12} mol/L [68].

5.2. Titanium Oxide (TiO_2)

TiO_2 has gained much interest for past ten years. In this context, research on the synthesis of nanosized TiO_2 materials and its application in catalytic industry and photo-cell have intensified. TiO_2 is an optically transparent semiconductor, being used to carry out direct electrochemistry of proteins such as hemoglobin (Hb) and cytochrome-c (Cyt-c) [26,21]. TiO_2 nanoparticles provide large surface area with pores of similar dimensions for immobilization of desired protein without loss of its structure and catalytic activity.

Cosnier et al. have dispersed mesoporous TiO_2 within polypyrrole matrix for electrochemical glucose detection. The thickness of the TiO_2 layer has been found to influence the performance of both H_2O_2 and glucose biosensor. The H_2O_2 biosensor exhibits shelf-life of 7 days with sensitivity of 4 mAM^{-1} cm^{-2} [69]. Porous nanocrystalline TiO_2 film with average nanoparticle size (5 nm) has been used for glucose oxidase immobilization. This biosensor has response time of 30s, sensitivity as 144 nA/mM and K_m as 6.08mM [70]. This sensor retains 80% of its initial activity after about 4 months [71]. Chen et al have utilized sol-gel-derived titanium oxide/copolymer composite matrix for determination of glucose concentration. The response time of the fabricated biosensor is 20 s, linearity upto 9 mM with sensitivity of 405 nA/mM. The fabricated biosensor is stable up to 1 month [72]. Viticoli et al. have been fabricated TiO_2 thin films on Si substrate and used it for immobilization of GOx and HRP. They have obtained linearity in the concentration range of 5.0 x 10^{-6} to 5.5 x 10^{-4} M for glucose and 1.0 x 10^{-6} to 2.0 x 10^{-4} M for H_2O_2, with response time as 7 s for glucose and 6 s for H_2O_2. The apparent K_m for GOx has been obtained as 7.5 mM and for HRP as K_m =1.0 mM [73]. In another report, GOx and HRP have been immobilized onto TiO_2 layer for development of glucose and H_2O_2 biosensor [74].

TiO_2 nanotubes have been directly grown on Au electrode to immobilize HRP for H_2O_2 detection. This biosensor exhibits linearity in the concentration range from 5×10^{-6} to 4×10^{-4} mol l^{-1} for estimation of H_2O_2 with detection limit of 2×10^{-6} moll^{-1} [75]. The modified TiO_2 nanotubes electrode has been used for co-adsorption of protein and thionine. Good stability and reproducibility have been achieved and electrochemical response is observed in the electrode potential range between -0.7 and 0.0 V. The amperometric response is highly linear in the concentration range of 1.1 x 10^{-5} -1.1 x 10^{-3} M with detection limit of 1.2 x 10^{-6} M. The shelf-life of TiO_2 nanotube modified Ti electrode is about 2 weeks [22]. HRP has been adsorbed on well-oriented TiO_2 nanotubes arrays, prepared by seed-growth mechanism for application to H_2O_2 detection. The value of the direct electron transfer (ET) constant (k_s) obtained as 3.82 s^{-1} indicates excellent electrocatalytic performance for H_2O_2 and apparent K_m is 1.9 mmol L^{-1}. This H_2O_2 biosensor has linearity from 5.0×10^{-7} mol L^{-1} to 1.0×10^{-5} mol L^{-1} [28]. A biosensor based on the HRP immobilized sol-gel titania/GCE electrode has been constructed for amperometric detection and quantitative determination of H_2O_2 in phosphate buffer solution. The resulting H_2O_2 biosensor shows response time below 30s and detection limit of 8 x 10^{-7} M. The observed thermal stability of electrode upto 55° C has been ascribed to reduced protein denaturation inside the sol-gel TiO_2 matrix [29]. The sol-gel porous titania matrix has been used for immobilization of HRP for H_2O_2 estimation. This bioelectrode displays linear response in the concentration range of 0.08-0.56mM with detection limit of 1.5μM and sensitivity as 61.5 μAmM^{-1}. After 90-days of storage period, the sensor retains 94% of its initial current response within 5s [29]. Vapor deposited TiO_2 film onto Au electrode has been utilized for amperometric H_2O_2 detection. Under optimized conditions, this biosensor is able to detect H_2O_2 with detection limit of 1.0 x 10^{-6} mol/L linearity in the concentration range of 2.2 x 10^{-6}- 6.0 x 10^{-4} mol/L. The fabricated biosensor retains 90% response after 60 days of use. This biosensor has been used for the determination of H_2O_2 concentration in real samples and has been found to yield satisfactory results [76]. Polymeric film containing of CMCS-GNPs/TiO_2-PTATB(3,4,9,10-perylenetetracarboxylic acid-toluidine blue and TiO_2 nanoparticles have been modified onto glassy carbon electrode by drop casting method to covalently immobilize hemoglobin as a model enzyme for the construction of H_2O_2 biosensor. This biosensor displays a linear response to H_2O_2 in the range from 1.4× 10^{-6} to 1.6× 10^{-3} M with limit of detection of 3.7× 10^{-7}M. The values of apparent K_m and the maximum current density (I_{max}) for the proposed biosensor have been estimated to be 0.62 mM and 211 μA/cm^2, respectively [77]. Khan et al have reported application of CH/TiO_2 dispersion deposited on ITO electrode as a new platform for covalent immobilization of HRP [78]. Electrochemically synthesized TiO_2 nanoparticles have been used for modification of a screen printed carbon electrode (SPE) to immobilize flavin adenine dinucleotide (FAD) for H_2O_2 detection. The value of sensitivity has been obtained as 1.86AM^{-1}. The linear range for H_2O_2 has been found from 0.15 × 10^{-6} to 3.0 × 10^{-3} M with the detection limit of 0.1 × 10^{-6} M [24]. The direct detection of H_2O_2 by electrocatalytic reduction of hemoglobin has been accomplished using carbonized TiO_2 nanotubes by amperometric technique. This biosensor demonstrates detection limit upto 0.92 μM, the value of apparent Michaelis-Menten constant as 87.5 μM. The TNT/C-Hb based H_2O_2 sensor shows low detection limit (0.92 μM), fast response time (3 s) and high dynamic response range (10^{-6} to 10^{-4} M) [79]. TiO_2 nanotube arrays co-adsorbed with HRP and thionin chloride (Th) have been investigated for detection of H_2O_2 using cyclic voltammetry. The TiO_2 nanotube arrays fabricated using potassium fluoride solution have been used for H_2O_2 detection in the range of 1 x 10^{-5}- 3 x 10^{-3}M at a potential of -600mV at pH 6.7. This bioelectrode retains 80% of its initial current response after one month of storage [80]. The HRP-TiO_2 bioelectrode has been demonstrated to show linearity of H_2O_2 concentration in the range of 7.5 x 10^{-6} - 1.23 x 10^{-4}M with detection limit of 2.5 x 10^{-6}M [81]. Zhang et al have constructed a sensitive amperometric H_2O_2 biosensor wherein myoglobin is immobilized on TiO_2/MWCNTs/GCE bioelectrode. MWCNT present at the biosensing surface facilitates electron transfer between the analyte and the electrode surface with the apparent K_m of 83.10 μmol/L for H_2O_2 detection [82]. The nanostructured titanium dioxide, deoxyribonucleic acid (DNA) and thionin (TN) as redox mediator have been electrochemically deposited on glassy carbon electrode (GCE). This biosensor shows excellent analytical performance for amperometric determination of H_2O_2, at reduced over potential (-0.2 V). The detection limit and linear range have been found to be as 0.05 mM and 0.05-22.3 mM, respectively. This biosensor has been used as an amperometric biosensor for the determination of H_2O_2 in real samples [83]. Liu et al. have developed sol-gel derived TiO_2/ITO electrode based photooxidized adsorbed ds-DNA. The methylene blue (MB) has been used to electrochemically monitor ds-DNA structure changes. This bioelectrode has been used for the evaluation of the antioxidant properties of glutathione and gallic acid [30].

Tavcar et al have used sol-gel derived CeO_2-TiO_2 film deposited onto indium-tin-oxide (ITO) glass for amperometric detection of counter ions (Li^+, Na^+, K^+, NH_4^+ and tetraethylammonium ions). The amperometric sensor has linearity over the range, 4 x 10^{-4} - 4.0 x 10^{-3} mol l^{-1} which is dependent on the Li^+ concentration and detection limit is 2 x 10^{-5} mol/L [84].

TiO_2 nanotubes composite electrode has been constructed for effective immobilization of cytochrome *c* and successful realization of its direct electrochemistry and electrocatalysis. The immobilized Cyt c/TiO_2 bioactive electrode exhibits favorable electrocatalytic activity toward the reduction of H_2O_2 with good stability and sensitivity. The linear range was obtained is 2×10^{-6} to 3.49×10^{-4} mol /L^{-1} with detection limit of 1.21×10^{-6} mol/L^{-1}. The fabricated biosensor retains 98.7% of the initial response after 30 days [27].

Sol-gel derived hybrid TiO_2 film deposited on glassy carbon electrode has been used to construct the phenol biosensor. The resulting biosensor is selective towards phenol with a linear range from $7.5 \times 10^{-8} - 6 \times 10^{-6}$ M with detection limit 1×10^{-8} and has response time as 10 s. The biosensor exhibits maximum response at 45 °C. The initial response current of the bioelectrode decreases to 95 % after 2 months [85].

Liu et al have developed TiO_2 nanotubes on glassy carbon electrode for development of electrochemical uric acid biosensor. This biosensor exhibits selective detection of analyte (dopamine) in the presence of ascorbate and uric acid at physiological pH, 7.4. The linearity for dopamine over the concentration range is 0.1-30 mM [23].

Khan et al have used TiO_2-chitosan nanocomposite film for an electrochemical immunoassay protocol. The concept has been demonstrated for a simultaneous immunoassay of rabbit-IgGs, bovine serum albumin protein, TiO_2-chitosan nanocomposite film and detection limit of 7.5 mM has been obtained [86].

5.3. Zirconium Oxide (ZrO_2)

Zirconia is a IV group element of the periodic table. It is thermally stable, chemical inert, non-toxic and has affinity for the groups containing oxygen. It is an ideal candidate of materials for immobilization of desired biomolecules. Zirconium oxide (ZrO_2) is very stable and biocompatible, has low isoelectric point (~ 4.15) and is suitable for adsorption of high IEP protein. Zirconia is a technologicals important material that has recently attracted considerable interest in electrochemical biosensors since its surface has both oxidizing and reducing properties, as well as acidic and basic properties. Liu et al have developed sol-gel derived ZrO_2-DNA modified glassy carbon electrode to investigate the effect of lanthanides concentration on its electron transfer behavior [87].

CH is a biopolymer that has been widely used as an effective dispersant of ZrO_2 nanoparticles and CNTs due to its adhesive nature. The resulting biocompatible nanocomposite of MWCNTs/nano-ZrO_2/chitosan has been utilized for covalent immobilization of ssDNA for DNA hybridization detection. The bioactive DNA electrode provides a linear response to DNA hybridization detection in the range of 1.49×10^{-10} to 9.32×10^{-8} mol L^{-1} with detection limit of 7.5×10^{-11} mol L^{-1}. The response has been found to be about 15minutes [42]. The advantage of zirconia (ZrO_2) and gold nanoparticles film modified glassy carbon electrode has been demonstrated by Zhang et al. to detect DNA hybridization through electrochemically and methylene blue has been used as an intercalator. The calibration plot is linear in the concentration range from 1.0×10^{-10} to 1.0×10^{-6} mol/L, and a detection limit of 3.1×10^{-11} mol/L [88]. In another approach, electrochemically deposited ZrO_2 film has been employed to electrochemically detect DNA hybridization. This sensor shows linearity of DNA concentration from 2.25×10^{-10} - 2.25×10^{-8} mol/l, with the detection limit of 1×10^{-10} mol/L [89].

Tong et al. have electro-chemically deposited zirconia composite film on Au electrode for determination of H_2O_2 concentration. The proposed biosensor exhibits response curve within the range from 3.5 μM and 10 mM with a detection limit of 0.8 μM. The bioelectrode loses 15% of initial response after one month [43]. Tong et al have electrodeposited zirconia doped with horseradish peroxidase film on Au plate for fabrication of H_2O_2 biosensor. The resulting biosensor (HRP-ZrO_2/Au electrode) shows a linear response to H_2O_2 over a concentration range from 0.02 to 9.45 mM with detection limit of 2 μM and apparent K_m has been found as 8.01 mM. This bioelectrode loses 14 % initial current response after 1 month [47]. Highly linear response (1-73 μM) is obtained for zirconia nanoparticles grafted collagen tri-helix scaffold on a graphite electrode and detection limit is 0.25μM. The optimized bioelectrode shows significantly better performance than other zirconium electrode in terms of sensitivity (0.26 $AM^{-1}cm^{-2}$), low K_m value (0.28mM), stability of about 2 months and response time as 5s [44]. Zong et al have utilized zirconia nanoparticles grafted collagen tri-helix scaffold to immobilize hemoglobin (Hb) for H_2O_2 detection. This biosensor shows improved characteristics such as linearity (0.8 to 132 μM), limit of detection (0.12 μM), fast response less than 5s and high sensitivity of 45.6 mA M^{-1} cm^{-2}. The modified bioelectrode retains 95% of initial current response after 2 months [45]. This research group has used it to immobilize myoglobin for H_2O_2 detection. The characteristics of this H_2O_2 biosensor include linearity as 1- 85μM, detection limit of 0.63μM, sensitivity as 97$mAM^{-1}cm^{-2}$, response time as 9 s and shelf life of about 50 days. The peak current of this bioelectrode decreases with increasing temperature up to 70°C [46]. And improvement in stability of the sol-gel deposited ZrO_2 matrix has been observed for H_2O_2 detection. The results indicate sensitivity of 111μAmM^{-1}, linearity over the concentration range from 2.5×10^{-7} to 1.5×10^{-4} $moll^{-1}$, detection limit of 1 x 10^{-7} mol/l, quick response of less than 10s and good stability over 3 months [48]. Further, hemoglobin has been immobilized onto nanometer-sized ZrO_2 modified pyrolytic graphite (PG) electrode for H_2O_2 detection. The proposed electrode shows high thermal stability up to 74°C and an electrocatalytic activity to the reduction of hydrogen peroxide (H_2O_2) without the aid of an electron mediator. The electrode shows linear response within the concentration range from 1.5 to 30.2 μM with a detection limit of 0.14 μM [49].

Several approaches have been developed for ZrO_2 based glucose biosensor. Yang et al. have utilized nanoporous ZrO_2/CH nanocomposite platform to fabricate the glucose biosensor. The electrode is obtained by deposition of a layer of ZrO_2/CH dispersion on glassy carbon electrode. The optimum configuration for biosensor allows fast response of less than 10s. The linear range obtained 1.25×10^{-5} to 9.5×10^{-3} M with a detection limit of 1.0×10^{-5} M and high sensitivity 0.028 μA mM^{-1}. After 45 days testing biosensor loses 60.4% of initial current response [50]. Kim et al. have used sol-gel derived zirconia/Nafion composite film on a platinized glassy carbon electrode for amperometric glucose biosensor. Results of these studies illustrate that the assembly of sol-gel derived zirconia/Nafion composite film provides interesting characteristics in terms of linearity (0.03-15.08mM), detection limit of 0.037mM, sensitivity of 3.4 μA/mM and quick response of 5s. It retains 90% of original activity for about 4 weeks. The K_m value for this glucose biosensor has been found to be 9.3mM [90].

Nanoporous ZrO_2/CH nanocomposite platform has been used to immobilize acetylcholinesterase for amperometric detection of pesticides in vegetable samples. A multilayer film of polyelectrolyte (chitosan/polystyrensulfonate) coated on the glassy carbon electrode exhibits linear response to acetylthiocholine within 9.90×10^{-6} to 2.03×10^{-3} M and

6.6×10^{-6} to 4.4×10^{-4} M for phoxim with a detection limit of 1.3×10^{-6} M, over a range of 1.0×10^{-8} to 5.9×10^{-7} M for malathion, and over a range of 8.6×10^{-6} to 5.2×10^{-4} M for dimethoate [50].

5.4. Iron Oxide (Fe_3O_4)

Magnetic nanoparticles have attracted increased interest for development of nanostructured materials for application to biotechnology and medicine. Magnetic nanoparticles as special biomolecule immobilizing carriers provide an alternative immobilization method for the construction of biosensors. The magnetic properties of nanoparticles such as Fe_2O_3, Fe_3O_4, etc. have been utilized for biomedical applications. Among the various iron oxide nanoparticles, Fe_3O_4 nanoparticles are the most commonly used magnetic materials because of their good biocompatibility, strong superparamagnetic property, low toxicity and easy preparation, ultra small size, high surface area and good dispersion in the analyte solution leading to rapid contact between the enzyme and its substrate and reduction of mass-transfer limitations [91,92].

Kouassi et al. have used magnetic nanoparticles of iron synthesized from thermal co-precipitation of ferric and ferrous chloride for the immobilization of cholesterol oxidase (ChOx). Their kinetic studies for free and bound enzyme have revealed that stability and activity of the enzyme are significantly improved upon binding with nanoparticles as the K_m value changes from 2.08 mM for free ChOx to 0.45 mM for immobilized cholesterol oxidase. Furthermore, the bound enzyme shows better tolerance to pH, temperature (25-70 ^oC) and substrate concentration. They have attributed these effects to the structural and conformational changes occurring in the enzyme on immobilization. The enzyme activity is well-preserved upon binding onto the nanoparticles when subjected to thermal and various pH conditions [10]. Rossi et al. have developed a nanometric glucose sensor by covalently attaching GOx enzyme onto the amino modified magnetic nanoparticles. The fabricated nanometric glucose sensor exhibits detection limit of 20 nM (Rossi et al. 2004). And a biosensor has been fabricated by drop coating of a ferricyanide–nano Fe_3O_4 mixture onto the surface of a screen-printed carbon electrode followed by the deposition of GOx (Lu and Chen 2006). The response time is 15 s with sensitivity of 1.74 mA/mM and linearity up to 33.3 mM [93].

Qiu et al. have prepared ferrocene-modified Fe_3O_4@SiO_2 magnetic nano-biomaterial as building blocks for construction of reagentless GOx based biosensors for glucose detection. Under optimal conditions, this glucose biosensor can detect glucose from 1×10^{-5} to 4×10^{-3} M, with the detection limit of 3.2 μM. When the biosensor is stored in dry at 4^oC, the biosensor retains 94% of its original sensitivity after four weeks [94]. The improved analytical performance of carbon nanotube (CNT)/nano-Fe_3O_4 composite has been observed for glucose detection, due to the ability of CNT to promote electron-transfer reactions, the high electrocatalytic behavior of CNT results in improved electrochemical performance of the biosensor [95]. Kaushik et al. have fabricated CH-Fe_3O_4 nanocomposite electrode for application to amperometric glucose biosensor. The modified glucose biosensor exhibits linearity as 10–400mg dL^{-1}, sensitivity as 9.3 μA/(mg $dLcm^2$) and shelf life of about 8 weeks [12]. Magnetic nanoparticles have been used for the development of a disposable glucose biosensor using screen printed carbon electrode. The sensitivity of the disposable glucose biosensor is observed to be 1.74 μAmM^{-1} with fast response time of 15s. This biosensor exhibits a selective determination of glucose at 10mV with linearity upto 33.3mM (Fig.4). In addition, polyaniline has been entrapped into the bulk CNT/Fe_3O_4 nanocomposite for application to electrochemical glucose biosensor [92]. The marked electrocatalytic activity toward hydrogen peroxide permits effective low-potential amperometric biosensing for glucose using polyaniline coated Fe_3O_4/CNT nanocomposite. The higher surface area and electrocatalytic effect of CNTs alongwith with magnetic properties of the iron nanoparticles can be used to manipulate and control the analytic signal in the presence of a specific substrate.

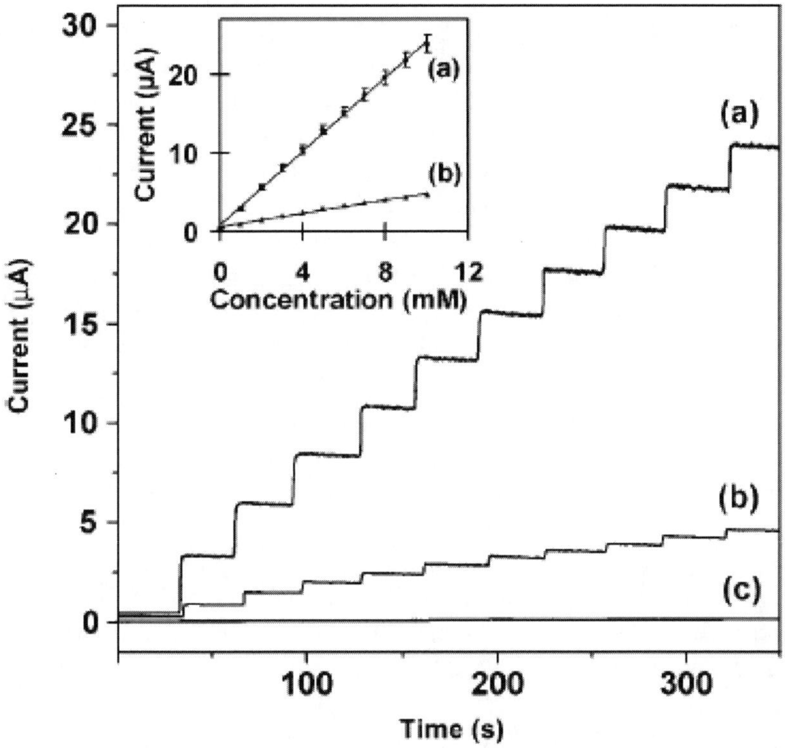

Figure 4. Amperometric response to the successive addition of 1 mM glucose at the potential of -0.1 V (vs. SCE) of the magnetic electrode loaded with PA–Fe_3O_4–CNT (a) and PA–Fe_3O_4 composite (b) with glucose oxidase immobilized and the bare electrode (c). Also shown (in the inset) are the plots of amperometric currents versus the concentrations of glucose at (a) and (b) (Small 2008, 4, 462).

The direct electron transfer of haemoglobin by immobilizing it on Fe_3O_4 nanoparticles multilayer film has recently been investigated [96]. These films have been constructed on several conductive bases (glassy carbon electrode, ITO glass, and Al foil) by first electrodeposition of CH/Fe_3O_4 thin films and then a layer-by-layer assembly using phytic acid and chitosan/Fe_3O_4. The response curve is found to be linear within the concentration range, 0.77-160 μmol/L. To enhance the sensitivity of the biosensor and minimize the problems of mediators, Cao et al. have investigated direct electron transfer rate between the immobilized hemoglobin onto layer-by-layer deposited Fe_3O_4 magnetic nanoparticles film on pyrolytic graphite electrode [97]. A remarkable feature and analytic advantage of the bienzyme electrode is the possibility to detect H_2O_2 at very low applied potential where the noise level and interference from other electro-oxidizable compounds are minimal. Another important characteristic of the monolayer bienzyme electrode shows possible existence of a direct electronic communication between HRP and the transducer surface because of the presence of nano-bridges, which guarantee the electron flow from the active enzyme center and the electrode surface. The biosensor exhibits rapid and sensitive response to the changes of H_2O_2 concentration and the reduction current increases steeply to reach a stable value. The amperometric response shows a linear relation with H_2O_2 concentration from 3.1 to 4.0 mM with a correlation coefficient of 0.998.The detection limit has been estimated to be 1.2 mM with a signal-to-noise ratio of 3. The biosensor when stored at 4^oC retains 95% of the initial response to H_2O_2 after about two weeks [98]. The studies on heme proteins (Mb, Hb and HRP) directly immobilized on Fe_3O_4 nanoparticles (Cao et al. 2003) represent a favorable microenvironment for the proteins to directly transfer electrons with electrodes. The proteins immobilized Fe_3O_4 PG electrode demonstrates excellent catalytic reactivity toward various substrates of biological or environmental significance, such as soluble oxygen, trichloroacetic acid (TCA), nitrite and hydrogen peroxide. Electrocatalytic reduction of these substrates at the three protein–Fe_3O_4 film electrode has been examined by CV. Highly linear response is obtained for hemoglobin, myoglobin and HRP, 0.4-11.9 mM, 2.6-16.3 mM and 3.1-18.2 mM with detection limit, 0.18 mM, 0.20 mM and 0.44 mM, respectively. The response current remains constant over 25 days [11]. Lin et al. have fabricated a CH-Fe_3O_4 nanocomposite modified glassy carbon electrode for determination of hydrogen peroxide (H_2O_2). The linearity range is obtained as 4-5 mM with detection limit 7.6 and 7.4 μmol/L and biosensor is stable up to 9 months [99]. Harbac et al. have fabricated carbon electrode modified by nanoscopic Fe_3O_4 particles based chemical sensor for estimation of H_2O_2 using amperometric technique [100]. In another approach Sljukic have utilized MWCNTs/magnetic nanocomposite platform for determination of H_2O_2 [91].

Ochratoxin-A (OTA), a mycotoxin produced in unstored food and beverages has recently been detected using CH-Fe_3O_4 nanobiocomposite modified indium-tin oxide (ITO) electrode [73]. This immunosensor shows a specific response to OTA detection in the range of 0.5 – 6 ng/dL with a detection limit of 0.5 ng dL^{-1}. The sensitivity of the bioelectrode has been found to be 36 μA/ng dL^{-1} cm^{-2} with response time of 18s [101].

Liao et al. have applied magnetic nanoparticles for development of a reagentless disposable amperometric ethanol biosensor. The electrochemical characteristics of modified electrode investigated by cyclic voltammetry, have been found as linearity (1-9.0 mM), sensitivity (0.61μAmM^{-1}) and response (20 s) [102].

5.5. Cerium Oxide (CeO_2)

Cerium (Ce) is a second element of lanthanides in periodic table. Cerium oxide (CeO_2) has a cubic fluorite-type structure with a lattice constant (a) of 0.5411 nm. CeO_2 thin films are highly attractive for electronic and electrochemical device applications as insulating buffer layers, ion-conducting layers, or ion-storage layers. Recently, a lot of interest has been generated in nano-structured cerium oxide for various electro-catalytic applications due to its ability to easily absorb and release oxygen. The ability to store oxygen is due to cerium's ability to change valence states and the presence of intrinsic O vacancies in the CeO_2 lattice. Nanostructured CeO_2 has unique electrocatalytic properties due to electron and phonon confinement and has thus received a great deal of attention as alternative matrix for biomolecules (enzymes, proteins and DNA) immobilization and to improve stability and sensitivity of biosensor. This matrix provides high surface area, high isoelectric point (IEP ~9.2) for higher enzyme loading and a biocompatible microenvironment helping enzyme to retain its bioactivity. A sol-gel nano-structured cerium oxide deposited on indium-tin-oxide substrate has been applied as a platform for cholesterol determination. Electrochemical response studies show linearity for cholesterol detection in the range of 10–400 mg/dL (Fig. 5.). The sensitivity of the modified electrode has been found to be about 2.08 mA (mgdL^{-1} cm^{-2}) with good storage and interference stability [8]. In another approach, these authors have employed sol-gel nanostructured CeO_2 film deposited on gold (Au) electrode for immobilization of GOx to detection of glucose. The storage stability has been tested by measuring the current response for the modified electrode stored dry at 4°C at different time intervals. The sensitivity obtained is 0.00287 μA/mg dL^{-1} cm^{-2} and detection limit has been found as 12.0 μM. The value of apparent K_m of GOx/CeO_2/Au bioelectrode has been found to be 13.55 μM [9].

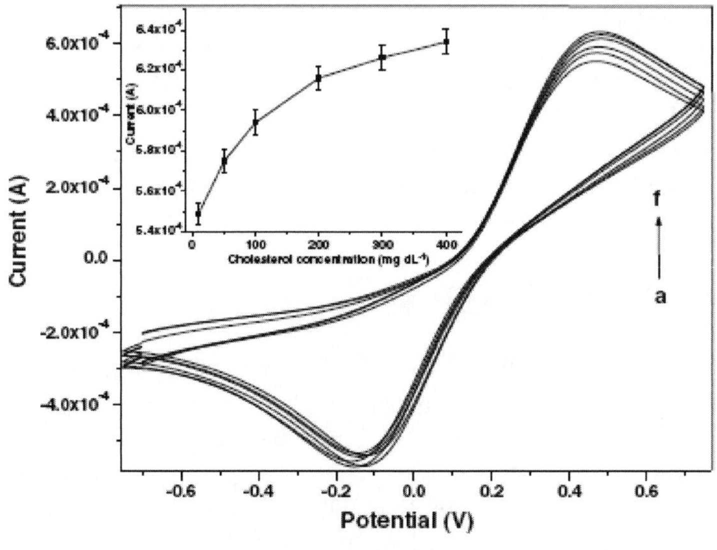

Figure 5. Electrochemical response of ChOx/NS-CeO2/ITO bioelectrode at different concentrations of cholesterol 10, 50, 100, 200, 300, and 400 mg/dL at scan rate of 50 mV/s.(Electrochem. Commun. 2008, 10, 1246)

CH containing CeO_2 nanoparticles films has been deposited on glassy carbon electrode for the single-stranded DNA (ssDNA) probe immobilization to detect DNA of colorectal cancer gene. The biosensor has high detection sensitivity, a relatively wide linear range from 1.59×10^{-11} to 1.16×10^{-7} mol L^{-1} and the ability to discriminate completely complementary target sequence and four-base-mismatched sequence. The maximum peak current observed at 45°C reveals highest hybridization efficiency of the bioelectrode [103].

5.6. Tin Oxide (SnO_2)

Tin oxide, such as rutile-type SnO_2 and tetragonal SnO structures have received a great deal of interest in the development of electrochemical biosensor. In practice, their large surface-to-volume ratio and relatively short diffusion length could enhance its electrochemical as well as kinetic properties. Because of its large band gap (3.6 eV), tin oxide is transparent in the visible-light region of the spectrum, and is thus useful as a conductive electrode and an antireflective coating. Topoglidis et al have reported that nanocrystalline SnO_2 films are more conductive than other metal oxides have an isoelectric point (IEP) of ~5 [19]. Some efforts have been made for the immobilization of cytochrome *c* (Cyt-*c*) and hemoglobin (Hb) onto nanoporous SnO_2 resulting in enhanced protein loadings. The values of electron-transfer rate constants for Cyt-*c*/SnO_2 and Hb/SnO_2 electrodes have been determined as 1 ± 0.03 and 0.53 ± 0.03 s^{-1}, respectively. The high protein loading and electrical conductivity of Hb/SnO_2 films allow it to be used for the electrochemical sensing of nitric oxide with a limit of detection of 1 μM.

Jia et al., [20] have employed sol-gel derived tin oxide film deposited on glassy carbon electrode to immobilize HRP for detection of H_2O_2. The linear concentration range of the fabricated biosensor is from 0.01 mM to 0.25 mM and K_m value has been estimated to be 0.166 mM.

An amperometric uric acid biosensor based on functionalized MWCNTs with SnO_2 nanoparticles has been developed by Zhang et al. This MWCNTs-SnO_2 electrode acts as an efficient promoter, and the system exhibits a linear dependence for the uric acid concentration over the range from 1.0×10^{-7} to 5.0×10^{-4} mol L^{-1}. This biosensor exhibits high sensitivity of the MWCNTs-SnO_2 modified enzyme electrode. This electrode has been used to monitor trace levels of uric acid in dialysate samples in rat striatum [104].

5.7. Mangnesium Dioxide (MnO_2)

Manganese dioxide (MnO_2) is a kind of attractive inorganic material and has been thoroughly investigated because of its important application in catalysis and as electrodes in lithium batteries. The MnO_2 nanoparticles modified electrodes show a bi-catalytic ability, i.e. the MnO_2 nanoparticles modified electrodes not only have catalytic oxidation ability to H_2O_2, but also have the catalytic reduction ability to H_2O_2. Yao et al. have reported a hydrogen peroxide amperometric sensor based on MnO_2 nanoparticles [105]. Amperometric response of H_2O_2 concentration has been obtained under optimal conditions within a concentration range of 1.2×10^{-7} - 2.0×10^{-3} M with low detection limit of 8.0×10^{-8}M. The proposed nanocomposite bioelectrode has sensitivity as 2.66×10^{5} μAM^{-1} cm^{-2} and shelf life of 10 days. This sensor has been used to measure H_2O_2 concentration in tooth paste and hair dye. Using sensors with injectable recognition elements (SIRE), trace concentration of glucose in urine samples can be estimated. The reactivity of H_2O_2 has been determined by immobilization of choline oxidase on electrochemically deposited MnO_2 nanoparticles modified glassy carbon electrode. This bioelectrode exhibits bi-direction electrocatalytic ability towards reduction/oxidation of H_2O_2. The results of square wave voltammetry experiments have revealed that the electrocatalytic reduction current increases linearly with increase of choline chloride concentration in the range of 1.0 x 10^{-5} – 2.1 x 10^{-3} M and no interference from ascorbic acid and uric acid is observed. This bioelectrode has shelf life of upto 2 months with good reproducibility and stability. It retains about 90% of its original response after one month, and 80% after two months [106].

A chitosan film containing MnO_2 nanoparticles has been electrochemically deposited on an electrode for amperometric detection of glucose. The influence of ascorbic acid on the response of modified glucose bioelectrode has been estimated. The effect of the content of MnO_2 nanoparticles and the deposition time on characteristics of the film, as well as the stability of the film during continuous exposure to ascorbic acid has been investigated. Glucose biosensors deposited with the film containing MnO_2 nanoparticles have been found to be suitable for determination of glucose in the presence of ascorbic acid [14].

An amperometric glucose biosensor based on GOx entrapped in mesoMnO_2 has been fabricated, in which mesoMnO_2 acts as a catalyst for the electrochemical oxidation of H_2O_2 produced by enzyme reaction. The results of transmission electron microscopy (TEM) studies show that the MnO_2 nanomaterial presents well-disordered porous structure and appropriate pore size suitable for the immobilization of GOx. The biosensor shows fast and sensitive current response to glucose in the linear range of 0.0009-2.73 mM. The response time ($t_{95\%}$) is less than 7 s. The sensitivity and detection limit are 24.2 μA cm^{-2} mM^{-1} and 1.8×10^{-7} M (S/N = 3), respectively [13]. The reproducibility obtained at the MnO_2 and glucose oxidase modified carbon fiber microelectrode glucose biosensor has been found to be reasonable with relative standard deviation of 11% (n = 5) for 5 mmol L^{-1} glucose solution. Authors have optimized and characterized several parameters such as deposition potential and time, concentration levels etc. The proposed microbiosensor has been employed as an amperometric glucose detector at pH 7.5 at an operating potential of + 0.58 V (vs. Ag/AgCl). Amperometric response is linear within the glucose concentration range from 1.5 to 15 mmol L^{-1}, and a limit of detection (S/N = 3) of 0.8 mmol L^{-1} [107].

Amperometric glucose biosensor based on electro-deposited MnO_2/MWNTs electrode has been reported by Chen et al. At an applied potential of +0.30 V, the MnO_2/MWNTs electrode gives a linear dependence (R = 0.995) for glucose concentration up to 28 mM with sensitivity of 33.19 μA mM^{-1}. In addition, interference from the oxidation of common interfering species such as ascorbic acid, dopamine, and uric acid has been investigated. [108].

A chitosan film containing MnO_2 nanoparticles has been electrodeposited as an external layer for the immobilization of lactate oxidase (LOD), which could effectively eliminate interference from ascorbic acid. The nanoscaled cobalt phthalocyanine (NanoCoPc) colloid is used as carrier for the immobilization of LOD. The electrode displays intrinsic electrocatalytic activity for the oxidation of H_2O_2, a product of enzymatic reaction. Under optimal conditions, the biosensor shows a wide linear response to lactate in the range of 0.020–4.0 mM, with high sensitivity (3.98 μA$cm^{-2}$$mM^{-1}$), as well as good reproducibility and long-term stability. The biosensor has been used for the estimation of lactate in real samples with an acceptable accuracy [109].

5.8. Niobium Oxide (Nb_2O_5)

Nanoporous niobium oxide (Nb_2O_5) or doped niobium oxide exhibits good photocatalytic and electronic properties and thus has potential applications for development of electronic and magnetic devices. Its electrical conductivity at potentials above the conduction band edge is expected to provide good possibility of nanoporous niobium oxide to promote direct electron transfer of redox proteins. Xu et al. first reported the biocapsulation of Cyt-c with mesoporous Nb_2O_5 films and its application to electrochemical studies including biomolecules immobilization. A highly ordered mesoporous niobium oxide fabricated by self-adjusted synthesis has been used as immobilization matrix for heme proteins including Cyt-c and HRP for their large surface areas, narrow pore size distributions and good biocompatibility. The midpoint redox potentials of adsorbed Cyt-c and HRP have been found as 14 and -122 mV, respectively. Furthermore, the immobilized HRP onto Nb_2O_5 derived electrode reveals good bioactivity. A Nb_2O_5 amperometric biosensor for detection of H_2O_2 in the range from 0.1 μM to 0.1 mM [110]. Santos et al [15] have reported a reagentless biosensor sensitive to H_2O_2 based on various dyes such as phenothiazine (methylene blue), phenoxazine (meldola's blue), phenazine (phenazine methosulfate) on silica gel modified with niobium oxide. HRP has been immobilized onto the graphite powder by cross-linking with glutaraldehyde and mixing it with one of the electron transfer mediators (dyes) adsorbed on niobium oxide. The results found using methylene blue dye shows a better operational stability (around 92% of the activity was maintained after 300 determinations). The biosensor shows good sensitivity (32.87 nA cm-2μmol -1 L) allowing hydrogen peroxide quantification at levels down to 0.52 × 10-6 mol L-1, an optimum response at pH 6.8 and at a potential of -50 mV and wide linear response range from 1 to 700 μmol L-1.

Lactate dehydrogenase (LDH) has been immobilized on silica gel coated with niobium oxide carbon paste electrode for the development of lactate biosensor. This biosensor shows good sensitivity allows lactate estimation upto 6.5 × 10-6 mol L^{-1}. Moreover, the biosensor shows linear range from 0.1 to 14 mmol L-1 for lactate. [111].

5.9. Miscellaneous Oxides

Recent rapid developments in biological analysis, medical diagnosis, pharmaceutical industry and environmental control have fueled the urgent need for recognition of particular DNA sequences from samples. It has been shown that hybridization of surface-immobilized single-stranded oligonucleotide on praseodymium oxide (evaluated as a biosensor surface for the first time) with complimentary strands in solution results in significant shift of electrical impedance curve. This shift is attributed to a change in electrical characteristics through modification of surface charge of the underlying modified praseodymium oxide upon hybridization with the complementary oligonucelotide strand. On the other hand, using a noncomplementary single strand in solution does not create an equivalent change in the impedance value. This result clearly suggests that a new and simple electrochemical technique based on the change in electrical properties of the modified praseodymium oxide semiconductor surface upon recognition and transduction of a biological event without using labeled species is revealed Shrestha et al. [17,18] .

Nickel oxide nanoparticles (NiO) have been used to fabricate a glucose biosensor wherein GOx and oxide nanoparticles are electrochemically co-deposited on a glassy carbon electrode [16]. NiO nanoparticles have shown strong adsorption to GOx, resulting in increased enzyme loading and improved biocompatibility. The electrode exhibits an apparent Michaelis–Menten constant of 2.7 mM and detection sensitivity of 446.2 nA/mM. In addition, this glucose biosensor shows fast amperometric response (3 s), detection limit of 24 μM and wide concentration range of 30 μM to 5 mM. This biosensor also exhibits good stability, reproducibility and long life time.

6. Conclusions and Future Prospects

The emergence of nanotechnology and nanomaterials including various new types of nanostructures such as nanowires, nanobelts, nanorods, nanotubes and nanodisks represent a powerful detection platform for construction of broad range of biosensors including electrochemical enzymatic biosensors, DNA biosensor, pH sensor, impedimetric biosensor and immunosensors. The unique physical, chemical and optical properties of nanostructured materials such as high surface area, strong adsorption capability, biocompatibility, non-toxicity, chemical and mechanical stability, isoelectric point, electrical conductivity, catalytic efficiency (oxygen storage capacity), and reduction in potential are likely to be helpful for the development of efficient electrochemical sensors and biosensors. For instance, biosensors with improved stability can be prepared using nanostructures as substrate for biomolecule immobilization, while electrochemical sensors or biosensors with enhanced sensitivity and selectivity can be developed as using catalytic properties of nanoparticles. Nanostructured metal oxides not only provide stability to biosensors but also improve the sensitivity, selectivity and improved detection limit of a desired biosensor. Given that most of the applications of nanostructured metal oxides till date are concerned with pushing the limits of detection, it is not yet clear as to how few molecules can be detected in a desired volume of solution. Nano-structured metal oxides based biosensors are inherently useful so long as the platforms are designed in such a way that the entire sample volume can be interrogated by the sensor. These overall properties provide additional benefits, which enable development of sensors made of multifunctional, structural materials. Such nano-structured based biosensors are likely to revolutionize the fields of clinical diagnostics, environmental monitoring, and security surveillance and for ensuring food safety etc.

References

[1] Murray, R. W. *Chem. Rev.* 2008, 108, 2688-2720.

[2] Wang, J. *Analyst* 2005, 130, 421-426.

[3] Wanekaya, A.K.; Chen, W.; Myung, N.V.; Mulchandani, A. *Electroanalysis* 2006, 18, 533-550.

[4] Luo, X.; Morrin, A.; Killard, A.J.; Smyth, M.R. *Electroanalysis* 2006, 18, 319-326.

[5] Huang, X.J.; Choi, Y.K. *Sens. Actuat. B* 2007, 122, 659-671.

[6] Valentini, F.; Palleschi, G. *Anal. Lett.* 2008, 41, 479-520.

[7] Pandey, P.; Dutta, M.; Malhotra, B.D. *Anal. Lett.* 2008, 41, 159-209.
[8] Ansari, A.A.; Kaushik, A.; Solanki, P.R.; Malhotra, B.D. *Electrochem. Commun.* 2008, 10, 1246-1249.
[9] Ansari, A.A.; Solanki, P.R.; Malhotra, B.D. *Appl. Phys. Lett.* 2008, 92, 263901-3.
[10] Kouassi, G. K.; Irudayaraj, J. *J. Nanobiotechnology* 2005, 3, 1-9.
[11] Cao, D. F.; He, P.L.; Hu, N. F. *Analyst* 2003, 128, 1268-1274.
[12] Kaushik, A.; Khan, R.; Solanki, P. R.; Pandey, P.; Alam, J.; Ahmad, S.; Malhotra, B. D. *Biosens. Bioelectron.* 2008, 24, 676-683.
[13] (13). Yu, J.; Zhao, T.; Zeng, B. *Electrochem. Commun.* 2008, 10, 1318-1321.
[14] Xu, J.-J. ; Luo, X.-L.; Du, Y.;, Chen, H.-Y. *Electrochem. Commun.* 2004, 6, 1169-1173.
[15] Santos, A. S.; Duran, N.; Kubota, L. T. *Electroanalysis* 2005, 17, 1103-1111.
[16] Salimi, A.; Sharifi, E.; Noorbakhsh, A.; Soltanian, S. *Biosens. Bioelectron.* 2007, 22, 3146-3153.
[17] Shrestha, S., Mills, C.E.; Lewington, J.; Tsang, S.C. *J. Phys. Chem. B* 2006, 110, 25633-25637.
[18] Shrestha, S.; Yeung, C.M.Y.; Mills, C.E.; Lewington, J.; Tsang, S.C. *Angew. Chem. Intern. Ed.* 2007, 46, 3855-3860.
[19] Topoglidis, E.; Astuti, Y.; Duriaux, F.; Gratzel, M.; Durrant, J. R. *Langmuir*, 2003, 19, 6894-6900.
[20] Jia, N.-Q.; Xu, J.; Sun, M.-H.; Jiang, Z.-Y. *Anal. Lett.* 2005, 38, 1237-1248.
[21] Topoglidis, E.; Cass, A. E. G. ; Oregan, B.; Durrant, J. R. *J. Electroanal. Chem.* 2001, 517, 20-27.
[22] Liu, S.; Chen, A. *Langmuir* 2005, 21, 8409-8413.
[23] Liu, A.; Wei, M.; Honma, I.; Zhou, H. *Adv. Funct. Mater.* 2006, 16, 371-376.
[24] Kumar, S. A.; Lo, P. H.; Chen, S. M. *Nanotechnology* 2008, 19, 255501-255508.
[25] Yu, J.; Ju, H. *Anal. Chem.* 2002, 74, 3579-3583.
[26] Topoglidis, E.; Campbell, C. J.; Cass, A. E. G. ; Durrant, J. R. *Langmuir*, 2001, 17, 7899-7906.
[27] Zhao, G. ; Lei, Y.; Zhang, Y.; Li, H.; Liu, M. *J. Phys. Chem. C* 2008, 112, 14786-14795.
[28] Wu, F.; Xu, J.; Tian, Y.; Hu, Z.; Wang, L.; Xian, Y.; Jin, L. *Biosens. Bioelectron.* 2008, 24, 198-203.
[29] Xu, X.; Zhao, J.; Jiang, D.; Kong, J.; Liu, B.; Deng, J. *Anal. Bioanal. Chem.* 2002, 374, 1261-1266.
[30] Liu, J.; Roussel, C.; Lagger, G.; Tacchini, P.; Girault, H.H. *Anal. Chem.* 2005, 77, 7687-7694.
[31] Kumar, S.A.; Chen, S.-M. *Anal. Lett.* 2008, 41, 141-158.
[32] Wang, J. X.; Sun, X. W.; Wei, A.; Lei, Y.; Cai, X. P.; Li, C. M.; Dong, Z. L. *Appl. Phys. Lett.* 2006, 88, 233106-3.
[33] Wei, A.; Sun, X.W.; Wang, J.X.; Lei, Y.; Cai, X.P.; Li, C.M.; Dong, Z.L.; Huang, W. *Appl. Phys. Lett.* 2006, 89, 123902-3.
[34] Solanki, P. R.; Kaushik, A.; Ansari, A. A.; Sumana, G.; Malhotra, B. D. *Appl. Phys. Lett.* 2008, 93, 163903-3.
[35] Singh, S.P.; Arya, S.K.; Pandey, P.; Malhotra, B.D.; Saha, S.; Sreenivas, K.; Gupta, V. *Appl. Phys. Lett.* 2007, 91, 063901-3.

[36] Khan, R.; Kaushik, A.; Solanki, P. R.; Ansari, A. A.; Pandey, M. K.; Malhotra, B.D.; *Anal. Chim. Acta* 2008, 616, 207-213.
[37] Deng, Z.; Rui, Q.; Yin, X.; Liu, H.; Tian, Y. *Anal. Chem.* 2008, 80, 5839-5846.
[38] Deng, Z.; Tian, Y.; Yin, X.; Rui, Q.; Liu, H.; Luo, Y. *Electrochem. Commun.* 2008, 10, 818-820.
[39] Li, Y.-F.; Liu, Z.-M.; Liu, Y.-L.; Yang, Y.-H.; Shen, G.-L.; Yu, R.-Q. *Anal. Biochem.* 2006, 349, 33-40.
[40] Liu, Z.; Liu, Y.; Yang, H.; Yang, Y.; Shen, G.; Yu, R. *Electroanalysis* 2005, 17, 1065-1070.
[41] Lu, X.; Zhang, H.; Ni, Y.; Zhang, Q.; Chen, J. *Biosens. Bioelectron.* 2008, 24, 93-98.
[42] Yang, Y.; Wang, Z.; Yang, M.; Li, J.; Zheng, F.; Shen, G.; Yu, R. *Anal. Chim. Acta* 2007, 584, 268-274.
[43] Tong, Z.; Yuan, R.; Chai, Y.; Chen, S.; Xie, Y. *Biotechn. Lett.* 2007, 29, 791-795.
[44] Zong, S.; Cao, Y.; Zhou, Y.; Ju, H. *Langmuir* 2006, 22, 8915-8919.
[45] Zong, S.; Cao, Y.; Zhou, Y.; Ju, H. *Anal. Chim. Acta* 2007, 582, 361-366.
[46] Zong, S.; Cao, Y.; Zhou, Y.; Ju, H. *Biosens. Bioelectron.* 2007, 22, 1776-1782.
[47] Tong, Z.; Yuan, R. ; Chai, Y.; Xie, Y.; Chen, S. *J. of Biotechnology* 2007, 128, 567-575.
[48] Liu, B.; Cao, Y.; Chen, D.; Kong, J.; Deng, J. *Anal. Chim. Acta* 2003, 478, 59-66.
[49] Liu, S.; Dai, Z.; Chen, H.; Ju, H. *Biosens. Bioelectron.* 2004, 19, 963-969.
[50] Yang, Y.; Yang, H.; Yang, M.; Liu, Y.; Shen, G.; Yu, R. *Anal. Chim. Acta* 2004, 525, 213-220.
[51] Zhao, J.; Buia, C.; Han, J.; Lu, J.P. *Nanotechnology* 2003, *14*, 501-504.
[52] Zhao, Z.W.; Chen, X.J.; Tay, B.K.; Chen, J.S.; Han, Z.J.; Khor, K.A. *Biosens. Bioelectron.* 2007, 23, 135-139.
[53] Krishnamoorthy, S.; Bei, T.; Zoumakis E.; Chrousos, G.P.; Illiadis, A. A. *Biosens. Bioelectron.* 2006, 22, 707-714.
[54] Zang, J.; Li, C.M.; Cui, X.; Wang, J.; Sun, X.; Dong, H.; Sun, C.Q. *Electroanalysis* 2007, 19, 1008-1014.
[55] Zhang, C.L.; Liu, M.C.; Li, P.; Xian, Y.Z.; Cheng, Y.X.; Zhang, F.F.; Wang, X.L.; Jin, L.T. *Chin. J. Chem.* 2005, 23, 144 -148.
[56] Umar, A.; Rahman, M.M.; Kim, S.H.; Hahn, Y.B. *J. Nanosci. Nanotech.* 2008, 8, 3216-3221.
[57] Dai, Z.; Shao, G.; Hong, J.; Bao, J.; Shen, J. *Biosens. Bioelectron.* 2008 *Article in Press*
[58] Yang, M.; Yang, Y.; Yang, Y.; Shen, G.; Yu, R. *Anal. Chim. Acta* 2005, 530, 205-211.
[59] Chen, L.; Gu, B.; Zhu, G.; Wu, Y.; Liu, S.; Xu, C. *J. of Electroanal. Chem.* 2008, 617, 7-13.
[60] Zhang, F.; Wang, X.; Ai, S.; Sun, Z.; Wan, Q.; Zhu, Z.; Xian, Y.; Yamamoto, K. *Anal. Chim. Acta* 2004, 519,155-160.
[61] Bai, H.P.; Lu, X.X.; Yang, G.M.; Yang, Y.H. *Chin. Chem. Lett.* 2008, 19, 314-318.
[62] Yang, Y.H.; Yang, M.H.; Jiang, J.H.; Shen, G.L.; Yu, R.Q. *Chin. Chem. Lett.* 2005, 16, 951-954.
[63] Liu, Y. L.; Yang, Y. H.; Yang, H. F.; Liu, Z. M.; Shen, G. L.; Yu, R. Q. *J. of Inorg. Biochem.* 2005, 99, 2046-2053.

[64] Zhu, X.; Yuri, I.; Gan, X.; Suzuki, I.; Li, G. *Biosens. and Bioelectron.* 2007, 22, 1600-1604.
[65] Zhao, G.; Xu, J.-J.; Chen, H.-Y. *Anal. Biochem.* 2006, 350, 145-150.
[66] Liu, Z.-M.; Liu, Y.-L.; Shen, G.-L.; Yu, R.-Q. *Anal. Lett.* 2008, 41, 1083-1095.
[67] Zhang, W.; Yang, T.; Huang, D.M.; Jiao, K. *Chin. Chem. Lett.* 2008, 19, 589-591.
[68] Zhang, W.; Yang, T.; Huang, D.; Jiao, K.; Li, G. *J. of Memb. Sci.* 2008, 325, 245-251.
[69] Cosnier, S.; Senillou, A.; Grätzel, M.; Comte, P.; Vlachopoulos, N.; Jaffrezic Renault, N.; Martelet, C. *J. of Electroanal. Chem.* 1999, 469, 176-181.
[70] Li, Q.; Luo, G.; Feng, J.; Zhou, Q.; Zhang, L.; Zhu, Y. *Electroanalysis* 2001, 13, 413-416.
[71] Choi, H. N.; Kim, M. A.; Lee, W.Y. *Anal. Chim. Acta* 2005, 537, 179-187.
[72] Chen, X.; Dong, S. *Biosens. Bioelectron.* 2003, 18, 999-1004.
[73] Viticoli, M.; Curulli, A.; Cusma, A.; Kaciulis, S.; Nunziante, S.; Pandolfi, L.; Valentini, F.; Padeletti, G. *Mater. Sci. Engin. C* 2006, 26, 947-951.
[74] Oliveira, E.M.; Beyer, S.; Heinze, J. *Bioelectrochemistry* 2007, 71, 186-191.
[75] Kafi, A.K.M.; Wu, G.; Chen, A. *Biosens.and Bioelectron.* 2008, 24, 566-571.
[76] Gan, N.; Yu, Y.-F.; Wang, Z.-Y.; Ge, C.-X.; Xu, W.-M. *Chin. J. Sensors and Actuators* 2007, 20, 262-266.
[77] Li, W.; Yuan, R.; Chai, Y.; Hong, C.; Zhuo, Y. *J. Electrochem. Soc.* 2008, 155, F97-F103.
[78] Khan, R.; Dhayal, M. *Electrochem. Commun.* 2008, 10, 263-267.
[79] Guo, C.; Hu, F.; Li, C.M.; Shen, P.K. *Biosens. Bioelectron.* 2008, 24, 819-824.
[80] Xiao, P.; Garcia, B. B.; Guo, Q.; Liu, D.; Cao, G. *Electrochem. Commun.* 2008, 9, 2441-2447.
[81] Zhang, Y.; He, P.; Hu, N. *Electrochem. Acta* 2004, 49, 1981-1988.
[82] Zhang, L.; Tian, D.B.; Zhu, J.J. *Chinese Chemical Letters* 2008, 19, 965-968.
[83] Lo, P.-H.; Kumar, S.A.; Chen, S.-M. *Coll. and Surf. B: Biointerfaces* 2008, 66, 266-273.
[84] (84). Tavčar, G.; Kalcher, K.; Ogorevc, B. *Analyst* 1997, 122, 371-375.
[85] Zhang, T.; Tian, B.; Kong, J.; Yang, P.; Liu, B. *Anal. Chim. Acta* 2003, 489, 199-206.
[86] Khan, R.; Dhayal, M. *Electrochem. Commun.* 2008, 10, 492-495.
[87] Liu, S. Q.; Xu, J. J.; Chen, H. Y. *Bioelectrochemistry* 2002, 57,149-154.
[88] Zhang, W.; Yang, T.; Jiang, C.; Jiao, K. *Appl. Surf. Sci.* 2008, 254, 4750-4756.
[89] Zhu, N.; Zhang, A.; Wang, Q.; He, P.; Fang Y. *Anal. Chim. Acta* 2004, 510, 163-168.
[90] Kim, H. J.; Yoon, S. H.; Choi, H. N.; Lyu, Y. K.; Lee, W. Y. *Bull. Korean Chem. Soc.* 2006, 27, 65-70.
[91] Sljukic, B.; Banks, C. E.; Compton, R. G. *Nano Lett.* 2006, 6, 1556-1558.
[92] Liu, Z.; Wang, J.; Xie, D.; Chen, G. *Small* 2008, 4, 462-466.
[93] Rossi, L.M.; Quach, A.D.; Rosenzweig, Z. *Anal. Bioanal. Chemistry* 2004, 380, 606-613.
[94] Qiu, J.; Peng, H.; Liang, R. *Electrochemistry Commun.* 2007, 9, 2734-2738.
[95] Qu, S.; Wang, J.; Kong, J.; Yang, P.; Chen, G. *Talanta* 2007, 71,1096-1102.
[96] Zhao, G.; Xu, J. J.; Chen, H. Y. *Electrochem. Commun.* 2006, 8,148-154.
[97] D.; Hu, N. *Biophys. Chem.* 2006, 121, 209-217.
[98] Zhang, H. L.; Zou, X. Z.; Lai, G. S.; Han, D. Y.; Wanga, F.; *Electroanalysis* 2007, 19 1869-1874.

[99] Lin, M. S.; Leu, H. J. *Electroanalysis* 2005, 17, 2068-2073.
[100] Hrbac, J.; Halouzka, V.; Zboril, R.; Papadopoulos, K.; Triantis, T. *Electroanalysis* 2007, 19, 1850-1854.
[101] Kaushik, A.; Solanki, P. R.; Ansari, A. A.; J.; Ahmad, S.; Malhotra, B. D. *Electrochem. Commun.* 2008, 10, 1364-1368.
[102] Liao, M. H. ; Guo, J. C.; Chen, W. C. *J. Magn. Magnetic Mater.* 2006, 304, e421-e423.
[103] Feng, K.-J.; Yang, Y.-H.; Wang, Z.-J.; Jiang, J.-H.; Shen, G.-L.; Yu, R.-Q. *Talanta* 2006, 70, 561-565.
[104] Zhang, F.-F.; Wang, X.-L.; Li, C.-X.; Li, X.-H.; Wan, Q.;, Xian, Y.-Z.; Jin, L.-T.; Yamamoto, K. *Anal. Bioanal. Chem.* 2005, 382, 1368-1373.
[105] Yao, S.; Xu, J.; Wang, Y.; Chen, X.; Xu, Y.; Hu, S. *Anal. Chim. Acta* 2006, 557, 78-84.
[106] Bai, Y.-H.; Du, Y.; Xu, J.-J.; Chen, H.-Y. *Electrochem. Commun.* 2007, 9, 2611-2616.
[107] Hocevar, S.B.; Ogorevc, B.; Schachl, K.; Kalcher, K. *Electroanalysis* 2004,16, 1711-1716.
[108] Chen, J.; Zhang, W.-D.; Ye, J.-S. *Electrochem. Commun.* 2008,10,1268-1271.
[109] Wang, K.; Xu, J.-J.; Chen, H.-Y. *Sens. Actuat. B* 2006, 114, 1052-1058.
[110] Xu, X.; Tian, B.; Zhang, S.; Kong, J.; Zhao, D.; Liu, B. *Anal. Chim. Acta* 2004, 519, 31-38.
[111] Pereira, A.C.; Macedo, D.V.; Santos, A.S.; Kubota,L.T. *Electroanalysis* 2006, 18 1208-1214.

In: Nanostructured Materials for Electrochemical Biosensors ISBN: 978-1-60741-706-4
Editors: U. Yogeswaran; S. Kumar; S. Chen ©2009 Nova Science Publishers, Inc.

Chapter 8

CONSTRUCTION OF NANO-ARRAY ELECTRODE MATERIAL FOR AMPEROMETRIC DETECTION APPLICATION

Yibing Xie*
School of Chemistry and Chemical Engineering, Southeast University, China

ABSTRACT

The electrochemical biosensor with a well-aligned nanotube array structure has been developed for amperometric detection and quantitative determination on the basis of bioelectrocatalysis mechanism. The independent and free-standing titania nanotube array has been successfully fabricated through an electrochemical anodization process of titanium sheet precursor in a fluoride-containing electrolyte, which can act well as a suitable electrode material for the biosensor application due to its high surface area and superior biocompatibility. In view of a more feasible loading of enyzme probes in accessible tubular channels, nanotube morphologies have been promoted by expanding tube diameter from 60 to 110 nm and increasing tube length from 520 nm to above 920 nm when anodization process at voltage of 20 V in acidic aqueous electrolyte has been adjusted into that at 60 V in neutral ethylene glycol/glycerol electrolyte. The functionalization modification of the titania nanotube array has been sequentially achieved by filling highly-bioactive glucose oxidases into as-formed nanotubes and then electropolymerizing pyrrole monomer into conductive polypyrrole for an interfacial immobilization of these bioactive enzymes. Morphology & microstructure characterization, electrochemical properties and bioelectrocatalytic reactivities of composite electrodes have been fully investigated. Electrochemical impedance spectroscopy has been employed to investigate the electrical conductivity and capacitance analysis. The direct amperometric detection of hydrogen peroxide through a direct electro-reduction reaction can be well fulfilled on bare titania nanotube array with a detection limit up to 2.0×10^{-4} mM for ordinary nanotubes and 2.2×10^{-4} mM for long nanotubes. A nano-array biosensor based on the glucose oxidase-titania/titanium composite electrodes have been assembled in a conventional three-electrode system for amperometric detection and quantitative determination of glucose concentration in a pH

* Corresponding author. Tel: +86-25-52090620; E-mail address: ybxie@seu.edu.cn (Y.B. Xie)

6.8 phosphate buffer solution at a potentiostatic condition of -0.4 V vs. the saturated calomel electrode. The glucose oxidase biosensor with a well-constructed nanotube array structure show an excellent performance with a high detection sensitivity of 45.5 μA mM^{-1} cm^{-2}, a fast responding time of 5.6 s and a very low detection limit of 2.0×10^{-3} mM. A good operational reliability has also been achieved with a relative standard deviation below 3.0 %. Such a well-designed biosensor with a desired nanotube array structure can consequentially contribute to the potential application of molecule detection and quantitative determination.

Keywords: Biosensor; Titania nanotube array; Hydrogen peroxide; Amperometric detection

1. INTRODUCTION

The electrochemical biosensor is a device for the amperometric detection of an analyte that combines a biological component with a functional transducer or detector. It consists of three parts: 1. The sensitive biological element that includes biological materials (eg. tissue, microorganisms, organelles, cell receptors, enzymes, antibodies, nucleic acids, etc), a biologically derived material or biomimic. 2. The transducer or detector element that works in an electrochemical, physicochemical, optical or piezoelectric way to transform the signal resulting from the interaction of the analyte with the biological element into another signal that can be more easily measured and quantified. 3. The associated electronics or signal processors that are primarily responsible for the display of the results in a user-friendly way. Usually, the bioelectrocatalysis process of various biosensors involves a highly specific recognition or interaction of enzyeme-substrate, antibody-antigen, lectin-glycoprotein and hormone-receptor [1]. In particular, the enzymatic biocatalysis exhibits a very high specificity because each protein enzyme exclusively catalyzes its corresponding substrate only. Any change of interactions can be detected as a shift in the electric current response, yielding a direct electrical signal related to the electrochemical reaction. The bioelectrocatalytic system allows the sensitive detection of affinity-based interactions between complementary molecule pairs [2]. Corresponding amperometric biosensors contribute many convenient and potential applications in the area of biomedical diagnosis as well as environmental analysis [3-5]. In general, all these biosensing configurations should be constructed on well-structured electrode materials as a sensing matrix. Effective immobilization of enzymes with an original bioactivity is another key point. These factors ultimately influence the interaction effectiveness as well as sensitivity in a continuous and credible testing application. Therefore, electrode materials with a tailored architecture are highly desired to act as a biosensing matrix. In general, the micro- or nano-structured semiconductor oxides have been often used as a supporting matrix for bioactive modification to form the functionalized electrode materials. Several metal oxides multiporous films, such as titanium oxide (TiO_2), zinc oxide (ZnO) and niobium oxide (Nb_2O_5), have been investigated in the respect of protein electrode interactions [6, 7]. Recently, titania nanotubes in a powdery form have been synthesized by using the template-based synthesis route or hydrothermal reaction method, and surface modification is also fulfilled by coating or even filling approaches [8, 9]. However, it is still unlikely to assemble these powdery nanotubes to form a well-aligned array structure on substrates in a large scale. To date, multiporous semiconductor films supported on indium-tin oxide (ITO) or fluorine-doped tin oxide (FTO) conductive glass, glassy carbon or noble metal platinum/gold disk are widely used as the supporting matrix of the working electrode, which can be fabricated by a sol dip-coating process. Such sorts of superficially coated oxide film electrodes are then modified by different biological probes to form the functionalized modules, which are finally applied to construct various micro-devices [10, 11]. Traditional biosensors usually use these porous oxide film electrodes as the interactive matrix for compound detection and quantitative determination. The microstructure of these oxide layers mostly affects the interfacial adsorption of biological probes [12, 13]. Unfortunately, the randomly-aligned structure decreases its effective interaction area of metal oxide film. The surface-adsorbed enzymes are also likely to desquamate from the coating film to lessen its bioactivity after a continuous utilization. Additionally, a high electrical resistance due to the weak bonding between semiconductor film and its substrate also inhibits interfacial electron transfer process during electrochemical interaction. These defects evidently restrain its sensing application.

This chapter presents a new three-dimensional electrode material of TiO_2/Ti with highly-ordered and self-organized nanotube array structure to act as a supporting matrix. Each tube channel with independent single-wall structure can provide individual nano-spaced reaction chamber. Both TiO_2 and Ti are good biocompatible materials, which exhibit a superior bioaffinity for immobilization of bio-probes as well as accumulation of these detected compounds on TiO_2 surface [14]. As the electrode substrate of biosensors, TiO_2/Ti nanotube array has a much higher surface area-to-volume ratio, stronger micromechanical bonding strength and a better electron transfer channel than the conventional TiO_2/conductive glass film electrode formed by surface coating process. Accordingly, the novel nano-array biosensor is developed by employing the oxidase enzyme-modified TiO_2/Ti nanotube array as a functional electrode material. A bioelectrocatalytic redox system is established for amperometeric detection and concentration measurement.

The most widespread biosensor is the blood glucose biosensor, in which the glucose oxidase (GOD) enzyme can catalyze and break down glucose to conduct a specific enzymatic reaction. It uses two electrons to electrochemically reduce the flavin adenine dinucleotide (FAD, a component of the GOD enzyme) to the reduced state of flavin adenine dinucleotide (FADH2). This in turn is oxidized into FAD by accepting two electrons from the electrode for a reversal redox reaction in a number of steps. At the same time, the biocatalysis process between GOD and glucose can cause a concomitant release of hydrogen peroxide (H_2O_2), which enables to trigger an electrochemical oxidation or reduction reaction on TiO_2/Ti electrode. The responsive current intensity mostly reflects the interfacial electron transfer amount on the enzyme-functionalized TiO_2/Ti nanotube array electrode. The quantitative relationship can be associated between amperometric current and compound concentration in a certain range, which provides a fundamental theory principle for this biosensing application. In this case, the electrode is the transducer and the enzyme is the biologically active component. The resulting current is a measure of the glucose concentration. The amperometric detection mechanism of GOD-modified TiO_2 biosensor can be schematically shown below [15].

Glucose + GOD-flavin adenine dinucleotide (FAD) $\rightarrow$ Gluconolactone + GOD-reduced state of FAD ($FADH_2$)

$O_2 + GOD\text{-}FADH_2 \rightarrow H_2O_2 + GOD\text{-}FAD$

$H_2O_2 + 2e^-(TiO_2) \rightarrow 2OH^-$ or $H_2O_2 - 2e^-(TiO_2) \rightarrow 2H^+ + O_2$

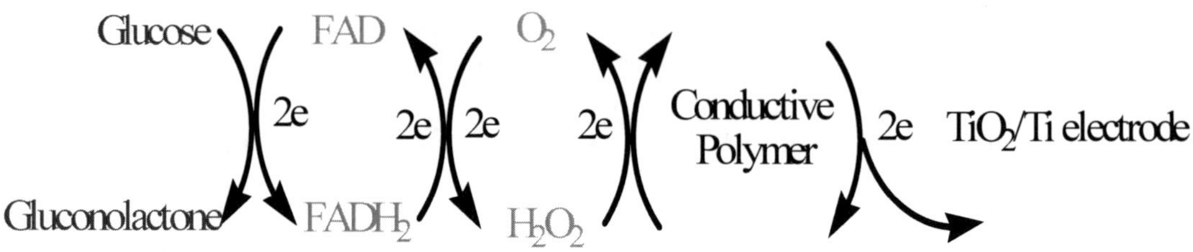

As a universal molecule detection method, it is much desired to develop a sensitive biosensor based on a specific bioelectrocatalysis reaction using enzymes-modified functional electrode. The highly-ordered nanotubular configuration could contribute a superior sensing performance in the area of the concentration measurement [16]. In this chapter, the well-aligned TiO_2/Ti nanotube array with free-standing and independent structure will be fabricated through an electrochemical anodization route. Fully tailored TiO_2/Ti acts as a good biocompatible substrate for GOD enzyme modification. Such a functionalized GOD–TiO_2/Ti electrode is ultimately applied to make a nano-array biosensor for amperometric detection and concentration determination of H_2O_2 and glucose. Noticeably, a serial of biosensors with a similar nanotube array structure could also be constructed on the principle of biomolecules pair interaction of antigen-antibody interaction or supramolecular recognition. The novel nano-array biosensor with a nanotubular configuration could promote a high performance in the area of the amperometric detection of various compounds.

2. Experimental Section

2.1. Materials

Titanium sheet (Ti, > 99.6 % purity, thickness 0.20 mm) was purchased from Goodfellow Cambridge Ltd. Biological enzyme of Glucose Oxidase (GOD, 2000-10000 units/g solid, from Aspergillus niger without any added oxygen), D-(+) glucose (Glu, anhydrous, >99.8% purity), pyrrole monomer (Py, > 99.0% purity), organic solvent of ethylene glycol (EG, >99.0% purity) and glycerol (GL, >99.0% purity) were regent grade and purchased from Sigma-Aldrich Company. All other chemical reagents such as hydrogen peroxide (H_2O_2, 30 wt.%), hydrofluoric acid (HF, 40 wt.%), ammonium fluoride (NH_4F, >96 % purity), phosphoric acid (H_3PO_4, >80 % purity), and so on, were analytical grade and purchased from Fluka Chemical Corporation. Doubly distilled water was used throughout the whole experiments in this research work. Electrochemical measurements were carried out in a 0.1 M phosphate buffed saline (PBS) solution with pH 6.8.

2.2. Preparation of Nanotube Array Biosensor

Firstly, the TiO_2 ordinary nanotube array was fabricated by a potentiostatic anodization process at 20 V in 0.15 M hydrofluoric acid and 0.5 M phosphoric acid aqueous solution, which was directly grown on Ti metal sheet. Alternatively, the enlarged titania nanotube array had also been fabricated by an adjusted electrochemical synthesis at 60 V in a neutral ethylene glycol/glycerol electrolyte with 0.3 wt.% ammonium fluoride and 3.0 wt.% water. An annealing process at 450°C for 2 h was followed to crystallize TiO_2 nanotubes from amorphous to anatase phase. GOD–TiO_2/Ti nanotube array electrode was then prepared by a coupling encapsulation process. Under a nitrogen-purging condition, TiO_2/Ti nanotube electrode substrate was immersed in 50 g L^{-1} GOD, 0.1 M phosphate buffer solution for 12 hours at 4°C. For a purpose of a better surface immobilization of enzyme molecules, a biocompatible conductive polymer was introduced into this system to improve interfacial connection between GOD enzymes and TiO_2/Ti substrate, where the electropolymerization process was conducted in 2.0 mM pyrrole monomer at 0.8 V for 20 min. As a result, the functionalizing process of TiO_2 nanotube array was achieved by filling GOD inside nanotubular channels to form a compacted enzyme layer with inherent biocatalytic reactivity. Sufficiently rinsing treatment was followed to keep an ultra thin adsorption layer on the inner surface of TiO_2 tubules so that more functional groups of GOD enzymes would keep a high bioelectrocatalysis activity when contacting with glucoses. Finally, the nano-array biosensor could be constructed in an electrochemical testing system assembled with as-prepared GOD–TiO_2/Ti functional electrode and controlled by an electrochemical workstation in the 0.1 M PBS electrolyte.

2.3. Characterization and Analytical Methods

Field emission scanning electron microscopy (FESEM, JEOL JSM-6335F), high resolution transmission electron microscopy (HRTEM, JEOL-2010F) and atomic force microscopy (AFM, Nanoscope DI-3100) were used to investigate surface morphology and microstructure. Electrochemical impedance spectrometry experiments were conducted in a conventional three-electrode system on the electrochemical workstation (IM6ex, ZAHNER-elektrik GmbH & Co. KG, Germany). Linear sweep voltammetry experiments were applied to evaluate electrochemical behaviors of bare TiO_2/Ti substrate and GOD–TiO_2/Ti nano-array electrode. A time-based amperometeric response was used for a quantitative determination of the detected compound.

2.4. Experimental Setup and Procedures

The electrochemical sensing system was set up in a cylindrical quartz cell equipped with a standard three-electrode configuration and controlled by an electrochemical workstation (CHI 660C, CH Instruments Co., Ltd. USA). Both bare TiO_2/Ti and functional GOD–TiO_2/Ti nanotube array were used as the working electrodes with an effective reaction area of 2.0 cm^2. A standard Hg/Hg_2Cl_2 saturated calomel electrode (SCE) was used as a reference electrode and Pt foil was used as a counter electrode. Standard calibration curve (responsive current intensity in a function of compound concentration) was initially conducted for a direct determination of H_2O_2 based on TiO_2/Ti and indirect determination of glucose based on GOD–TiO_2/Ti in PBS solution under a constant potential. Quantitative determination of glucose was achieved through an amperometric detection method on the basis of electrochemical reduction reaction of H_2O_2, which was preferentially generated by inherent ligase chain reaction between GOD enzyme and glucose compound. In order to keep its original bioactivity of GOD enzyme, the whole electrochemical process was carried out in 50 mL, 0.1 M PBS electrolyte aerated with 25 ml min^{-1} oxygen gas. The electrochemical measurement system is schematically shown in Fig. 1.

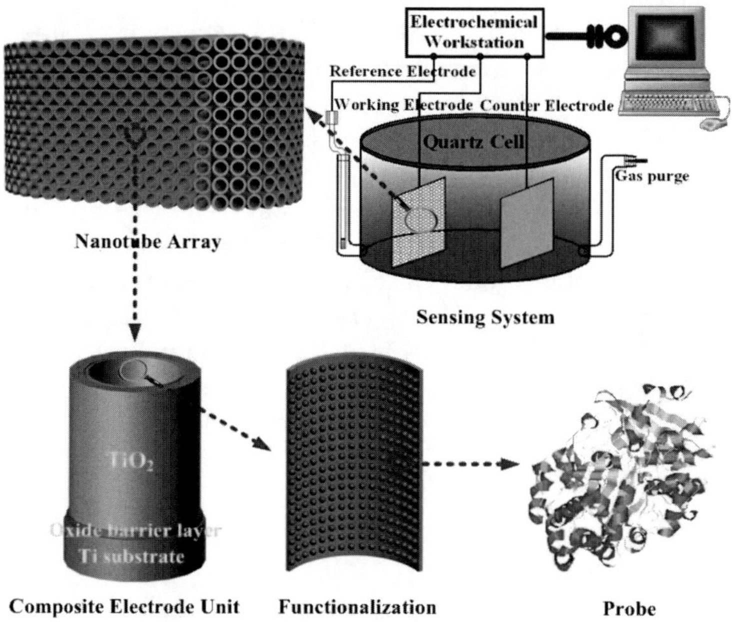

Figure 1. Schematic diagram of bioelectrocatalytic detection system.

3. RESULT

3.1. Microstructural Characterization

The morphology and structure of TiO_2/Ti electrode substrates have been fully investigated by FESEM and HRTEM characterization and their images are shown in Fig. 2 and 3. FESEM image of the surface layer shows that highly-ordered and vertically-aligned TiO_2 nanotube array can be well fabricated by an anodization process in aqueous HF-H_3PO_4 electrolyte. These independent TiO_2 nanotubes can directly grow on titanium sheet with a free-standing structure and a regular arrangement. Each tube has the length of 520 nm, wall thickness of 15 nm and the inner diameter of approx 60 nm on average (see Fig. 2 A and B). These uniform tubes have a unique open-mouth structure on the top of titania layer while each nanotube has a closed bottom due to the presence of oxide barrier layer with a thickness of tens of nanometer. For the purpose of a more feasible loading modification in these accessible tubular channels, nanotube morphologies have been further promoted by expanding tube diameter and length. Herein, the ethylene glycol and glycerol has been additionally introduced into reaction electrolyte in order to form the desired nanotube array with an enlarged pore size. Accordingly, the interior diameter has increased from normal 60 nm up to 110 nm, which can benefit a more uniform embedment of enzymes inside these magnified tubular channels and more feasible mass transfer in the sensing/biosensing process. At the same time, the tube length has also increased from 520 nm for ordinary nanotubes up to 920 nm for long nanotubes, which can provide more effective channels for the loading modification of enzymes (see Fig. 2C and D). Furthermore, the plane-view HRTEM image of TiO_2 ordinary nanotubes shows that the series of interfacial fringes with a circle-like shape are clearly exposed on the surface layer of TiO_2. The dispersive patches with a bright color are assigned to the open mouth of nanotubes and the cirques with a dark color are ascribed to nanotube walls. The corresponding FESEM image can clearly demonstrate these fine structures of TiO_2 nanotube array, which has been observed in above HRTEM image. So, the HRTEM characterization result is in agreement with that of the corresponding FESEM analysis (see Fig. 3A and B). Furthermore, the magnification view of nanotube walls along its axial direction reveals these well-arranged intercrystalline planes, which is corresponding to the characteristic crystal lattice {101} plane of anatase TiO_2 with the interplanar spacing of $d_{\{101\}} = 0.36 \pm 0.01$ nm (see Fig. 3C). This fact indicates that the well-defined nanotube array with a nanocrystalline structure of anodic TiO_2 has been completely formed.

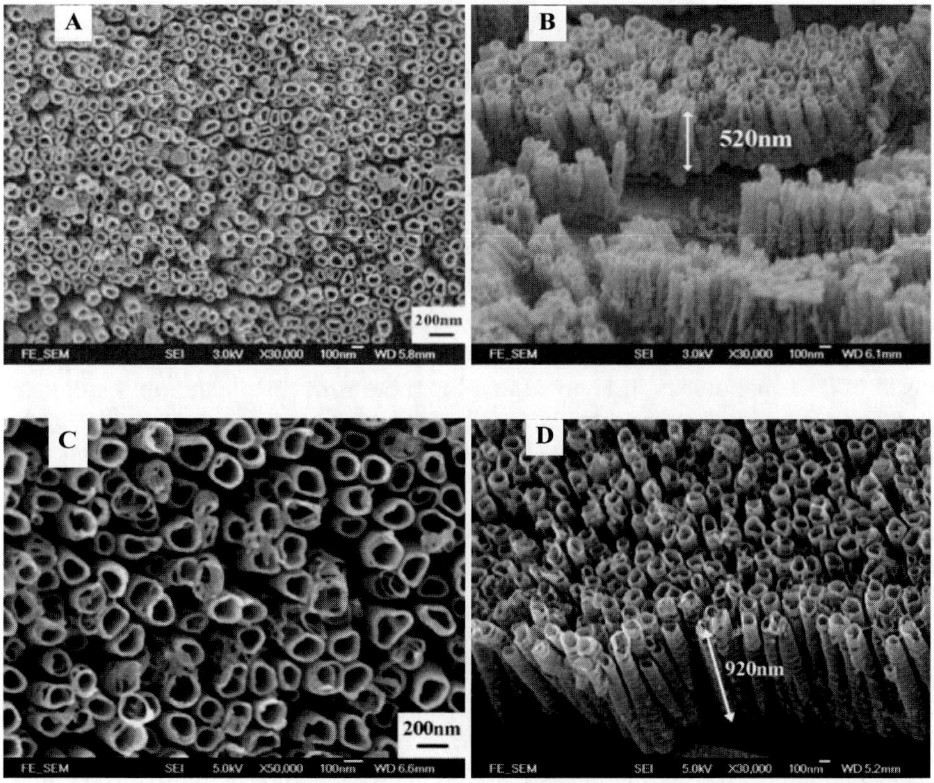

Figure 2. (A) Top view and (B) cross-sectional view of FESEM images of TiO2 nanotube array prepared in HF-H3PO4 aqueous electrolyte; (C) Top view and (D) cross-sectional view of FESEM images of TiO2 nanotube array prepared in NH4F-H3PO4 EG/GL organic electrolyte.

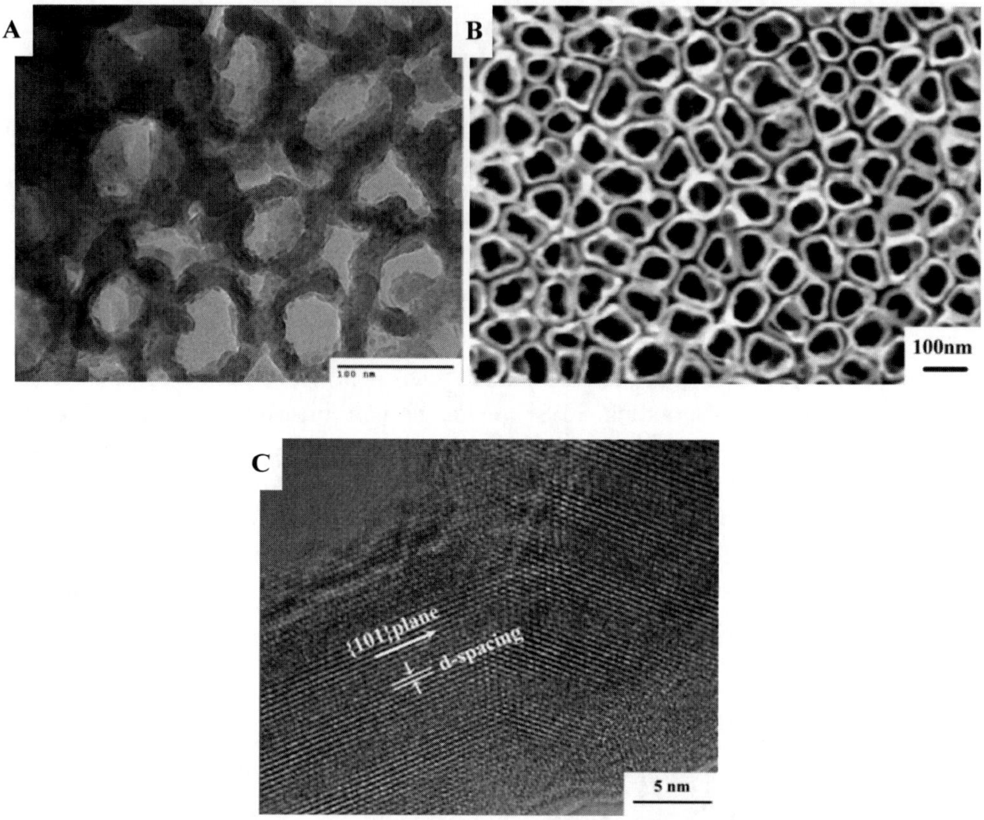

Figure 3. (A) Plane view of HRTEM image and (B) corresponding FESEM image of the same TiO2 nanotube array; (C) enlarged view of HRTEM image of TiO2 single nanotube wall.

In view of enzymes modified TiO_2 ordinary nanotube array, GOD molecules unevenly aggregate on the surface of nanotube mouths and partially disperse inside nanotube channels. High interface intension of nanotube walls is most likely responsible for the uneven distribution of GOD. The electroplymerization of pyrrole is applied for GOD deposition on the sidewall of TiO_2 nanotubes. It is noted that top mouths of most nanotubes still keep open. As a result, GOD enzymes trapped in polypyrrole (PPy) film tend to deposit primarily on the tube mouse and then disperse along the sidewalls. Total thickness of GOD-TiO_2 is approx 560 um, which is similar to the size of 520 nm for initial bare TiO_2 ordinary nanotubes (see Fig. 4A and B). The corresponding AFM image shows the deposition positions on TiO_2 surface are obviously higher than that of its original nanotube mouths, which is ascribed to the aggregation effect of GOD enzymes. All these GOD deposition areas keep a uniform shape and similar height (see Fig. 5). Tube pores can be mostly preserved, which is in agreement with the result of above FESEM observation.

In this chapter, an ordinary nanotube array with a tube diameter of 60 nm and tube length of 520 can be fabricated at a cell voltage of 20 V in hydrofluoric acid aqueous solution. A long titania nanotube array with pore size of 110 nm and tube length of 920 nm can be prepared by an adjusted electrochemical synthesis route in ammonium fluoride/ethylene glycol/glycerol electrolyte with a much lower water content below 3.0 wt.%, but a neutral pH value above 6.0 and a higher voltage up to 60 V. In the enzyme modification process, TiO_2

nanotubes should be able to provide a large channel spaces to fill glucose oxidase holoenzyme, whose three-dimension size is approximate 70Å×55Å×80Å [17]. The nanotubes fabricated in aqueous electrolyte at a low voltage usually have a low aspect-ratio below 10 and a small pore size below 60 nm [18]. In general, the surface intension energy of nanotubes can be highly diminished by increasing tubule diameter. Considering a more matchable dimension between nanotubes and enzymes, the amplified TiO_2 nanotubes with a higher aspect-ratio and bigger pore size have been synthesized by means of anodization at a higher voltage in an organic electrolyte. Such a desired microstructure can contribute a more feasible loading of enzymes and also favor charge-transfer, mass-transfer and interfacial reaction in these nano-spaced channels.

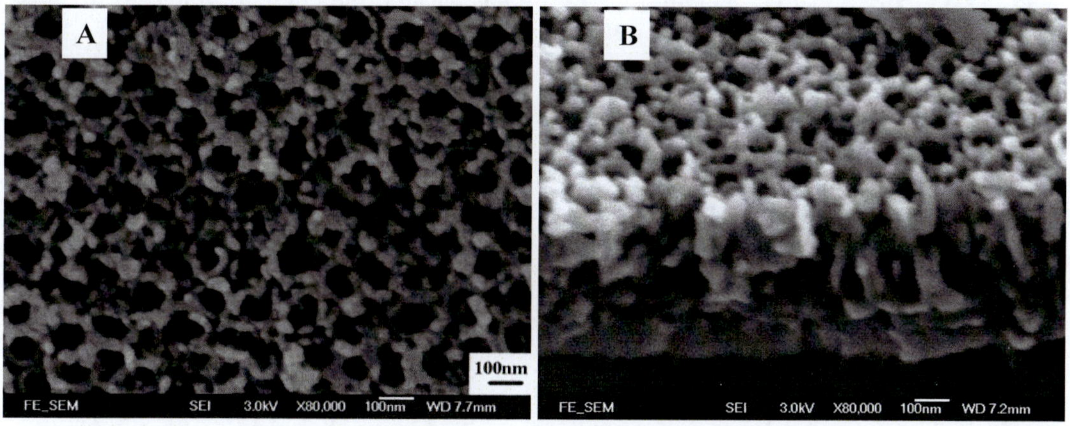

Figure 4. (A) Top view and (B) cross-sectional view of SEM images of GOD–TiO_2/Ti ordinary nanotube array electrode.

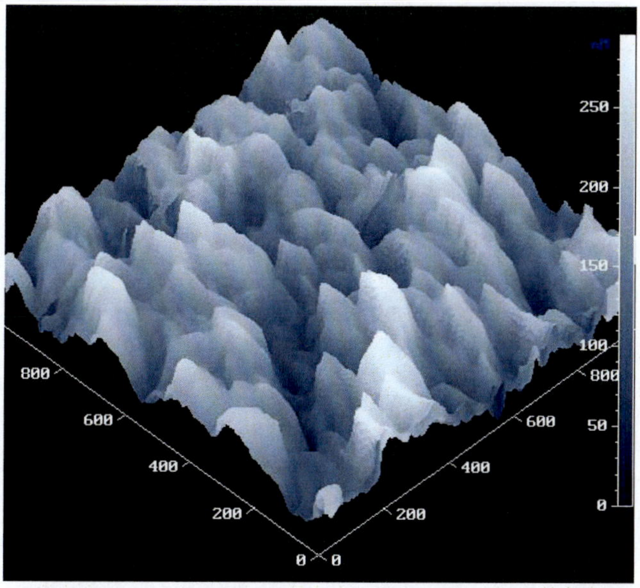

Figure 5. AFM image of GOD–TiO_2/Ti nanotube array electrode.

3.2. Electrochemical Properties

The interfacial reactivity of functional electrodes can mostly influence the amperometric detection signal in the bioelectrocatalytic process. Herein, the electrochemical impedance spectroscopy (EIS) has been applied to investigate the interfacial charge transfer or mass transfer process of bare TiO_2/Ti substrates and GOD–TiO_2/Ti composite electrodes. The EIS measurements over a frequency from 100000 to 0.01 Hz are carried out in a conventional three-electrode system under a sinusoidal perturbation of ± 5 mV and a constant potential of -0.4 V.

The complex impedance in terms of the applied frequency has been investigated for TiO_2/Ti ordinary and long nanotubes. It is found that that the complex impedances quickly decrease when the working frequency continuously rises from 0.03 to 40 Hz for this ordinary nanotube array and from 0.56 to 315 Hz for the long nanotube array. Then both of them gradually approach to a steady value in a medium and high frequency range. Comparatively, the complex impedance value has increased from 9.5 Ω for ordinary nanotubes up to 12.6 Ω for long nanotubes at a high frequency range. So, TiO_2/Ti long nanotubes exhibit higher impedance than ordinary ones in the whole testing frequency range although both of them exhibits a very similar variation law. Such a difference is more obvious at a low frequency range below 100 Hz (see Fig. 6A). The impedance response mostly reflects the efficiency of interfacial electron transfer. Lower impedance means more feasible charge transfer for the working electrodes.

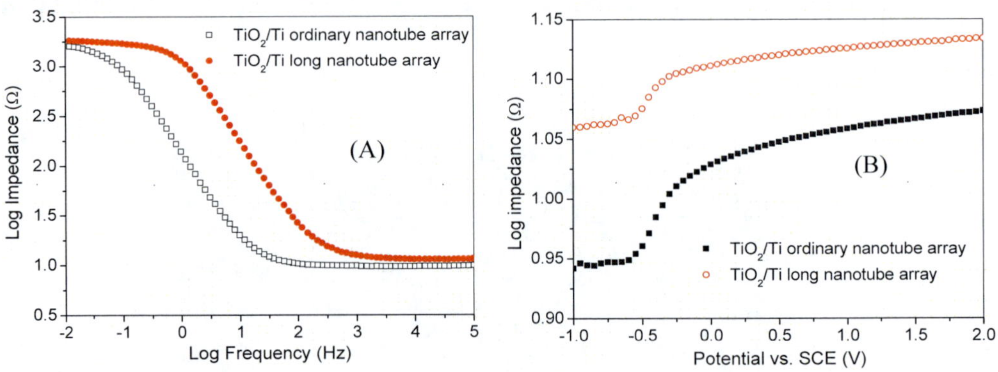

Figure 6. Complex impedance curves depending on (A) the applied frequency at a constant potential of -0.40 V vs. SCE and (B) the applied potential at a constant frequency of 1000 Hz for TiO_2/Ti ordinary and long nanotube array.

The complex impedance in terms of the applied electrode potential has been also investigated for two sorts of TiO_2/Ti nanotube composites. The complex impedance response at a medium frequency of 1000 Hz is particularly important, which usually corresponds to the characteristic frequency of molecular interaction [19]. Herein, both complex impedances continuously decrease till to appear a sharp descent when the electrode potential is swept from positive to negative direction, which is regarded as the typical characteristic of n-type semiconductor of TiO_2. The critical electrode potential, corresponding to the significant variation of complex impedances, is determined as the range of -0.6 ~ -0.1 V for both TiO_2/Ti nanotube array electrodes (see Fig. 6B). Significantly, the complex impedance value of

TiO_2/Ti long nanotubes arising from the charge-transfer resistance is obviously higher than that of ordinary nanotubes under the same electrode potential during the electrochemical process, which is due to the thicker titania oxide layer of the long nanotube electrode. So, the electrode potential is able to considerably affect the complex impedance response. In our detection measurement, the applied potential of the working electrode is controlled at -0.4 V vs. SCE, which is very sensitive to the impedance variation during the whole electrochemical process.

Additionally, the Nyquist impedance plots of two TiO_2/Ti nanotube electrodes have been investigated, where the EIS experimental data are denoted as individual symbols and the fitting curves are shown as solid lines. The corresponding equivalent circuit has been proposed to calculate the simulated impedance elements in the electrochemical process (see Fig. 7A and B). In general, the complex impedance is composed of a charge transfer resistance in series with a mass transfer impedance containing linear and nonlinear diffusion terms. The corresponding curves usually present a semicircle-like characteristic in its complex plane when the electrode impedance is predominantly determined by the charge transfer resistance in a kinetics-controlled process [20]. In equivalent circuit, *Rs denotes* the uncompensated electrolyte solution *resistance.* The parallel combination of $R_{TiO2/Ti}$ and C is associated with the electrical resistance and capacitance of the TiO_2/Ti nanotube electrodes. The parallel combination of impedance elements is associated with the interfacial charge transfer resistance ($R_{TiO2/Ti\text{-}E}$) and the constant phase element (CPE), which is defined by CPE-T and CPE-P. Therefore, the difference of charge transfer resistance can be figured out by quantitatively comparing these electrochemical elements. The simulation parameters of equivalent circuits of TiO_2/Ti ordinary and long nanotube array electrodes are listed in Table 1. Obviously, the semicircle-like shape in the corresponding Nyquist impedance plots indicates that a kinetics-controlled electrochemical behavior must have predominantly occurred on both TiO_2/Ti electrodes in above electrochemical process. According to the fitting results, CPE-P is determined as 0.92 and 0.95 for two types of TiO_2/Ti electrodes, whose values are approximately close to 1.0. Thus, the CPE-T obtained herein is similar to a capacitor. Additionally, the similar resistance value of $R_{TiO2/Ti}$ is obtained for both nanotube array electrodes, which is determined as approx 634 for TiO_2/Ti ordinary nanotubes and 529 Ω for the long nanotubes respectively. Such a result is mainly ascribed to the similar thickness of titania barrier layer located between TiO_2 nanotubes and Ti matrix for both samples. Additionally, the n-type semiconductor characteristic of TiO_2 contributes the low electrical resistance value of $R_{TiO2/Ti}$ at a negative potential of -0.4 V vs. SEC. However, the high resistance value of $R_{TiO2/Ti\text{-}E}$ is obtained up to 4498 Ω for ordinary nanotube array and even 7911 Ω for the long one, respectively. Such a resistance response of this impedance element is mostly dependent on active surface area since the charge transfer is a predominant process than the mass transfer. It is believed that the promotion of interfacial charge-transfer is more effective by decreasing nanotube diameter rather than by increasing nanotube length. The simulated values of charge flow resistance, interfacial charge transfer resistance and the electrochemical capacitance are highly related to the effective surface area and interfacial reactivity of TiO_2/Ti nanotube electrodes. In general, the overall impedance response results from dominant resistances of charge flow across TiO_2/Ti & TiO_2/electrolyte interfaces, subordinate resistances of electrolyte solution and Ti matrix, and capacitances of TiO_2 surface layer & Helmholtz double layer [21, 22]. Although the enlarged long nanotube structure can benefit the loading modification of big biological molecules, the smaller nanotube structure can provide a more effective surface area that benefits the electron-diffusion transportation at tube walls. The lower resistance and capacitance results in a better charge transfer for this TiO_2/Ti ordinary nanotubes electrode. The apparent complex impedance value can approximately reflect the total efficiency of primary electron transfer and subordinate mass transfer in the electrochemical process.

Table 1. Simulation parameters of equivalent circuits of TiO_2/Ti ordinary and long nanotube array electrodes.

TiO_2/Ti electrode	Rs (Ω)	C (mF)	$R_{TiO2/Ti}$ (Ω)	CPE-T	CPE-P	$R_{TiO2/Ti-E}$ (Ω)
ordinary nanotube array	3.1	0.93	634	0.000292	0.9588	4498
long nanotube array	10.2	2.81	529	0.000324	0.9139	7911

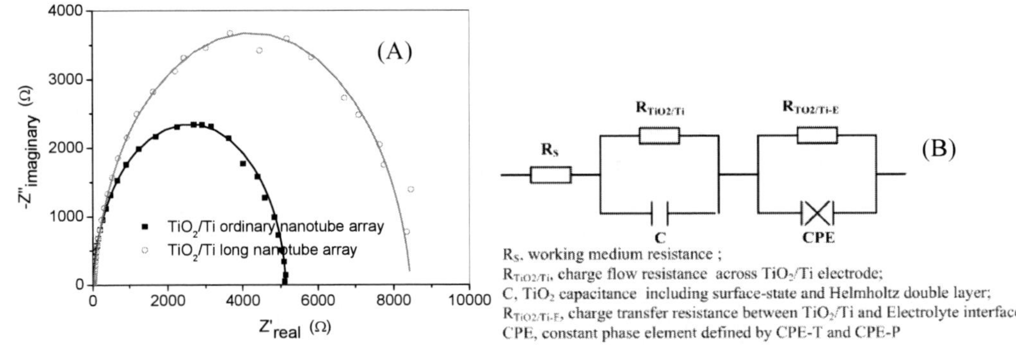

Figure 7. (A) Nyquist plots of TiO_2/Ti ordinary and long nanotube array and (B) their corresponding equivalent circuit.

Usually, the working potential can greatly influence the electro-reduction reaction of H_2O_2 on the surface of the working electrode. Linear sweep voltammetry (LSV) is applied to examine electrochemical behaviors of bare TiO_2/Ti substrate and GOD–TiO_2/Ti nanotube array electrode in PBS electrolyte. LSV experimental results are shown in Fig. 8. In the absence of H_2O_2, the peak of a direct electro-reduction reaction begins to appear when the negative potential is below -0.43 V for bare TiO_2/Ti electrode, which is mostly due to hydrogen generation by water decomposition reaction ($2H_2O + 2e^- \rightarrow H_2 + 2OH^-$) (see curve a). However, in the presence of H_2O_2, the rapid generation of a strong reductive peak has been observed when the negative potential is only below -0.20 V, which is mainly due to electrochemical reduction reaction of H_2O_2 on TiO_2 ($H_2O_2 + 2e^-(TiO_2) \rightarrow 2OH^-$) (see curve b). The intensity of such an electro-reduction current mostly depends on H_2O_2 concentration as well as the applied potential. This electrochemical reduction peak could be intensively enhanced when a more negative potential is applied on TiO_2/Ti electrode. It means that the electro-reduction reaction of H_2O_2 is very accessible on the surface of TiO_2 nanotube array at a certain potential range. Once this TiO_2/Ti electrode is controlled at a potentiostatic condition, the amperometric signal intensity is only a function of H_2O_2 concentration.

The bioelectrocatalytic performance of GOD–TiO_2/Ti functional electrode with an ordinary nanotube array structure has been intensively investigated. The strong electro-reduction peak begins to emerge when the negative potential is below -0.21 V for GOD–TiO_2/Ti in the presence of glucose. This critical electrochemical potential is less negative a bit than that in the absence of glucose (see curves c, d). LSV experiment result in Fig. 8 reveals that the critical reaction potential of glucose on GOD–TiO_2/Ti electrode agrees well with that of H_2O_2 on bare TiO_2/Ti electrode. Actually, GOD catalyzes the aerobic electro-oxidation reaction of glucose to release a concomitant product of H_2O_2 in oxygen-saturated PBS electrolyte. This intermediate product of H_2O_2 then triggers an electro-reduction reaction once the working potential is controlled below this critical reduction potential. Such a bioelectrocatalytic process is accompanied by an instant generation of current signal. Therefore, the quantitative determination of glucose as well as H_2O_2 compounds becomes very feasible when the amperometric response of GOD–TiO_2/Ti electrode is initially calibrated. Furthermore, the electrochemical reduction current observed at the critical potential of -0.21 V is quite low in the absence of any glucose. So, the influence of this electrochemical noise can be neglected when comparing with the detection current in the presence of glucose. In the case of the constant potential, the responding current intensity mostly depends upon glucose concentration in the electrolyte solution. This detecting approach of amperometric response becomes very credible according to above enzymic biocatalysis & electrochemical reduction reactions on the surface of GOD–TiO_2/Ti electrode.

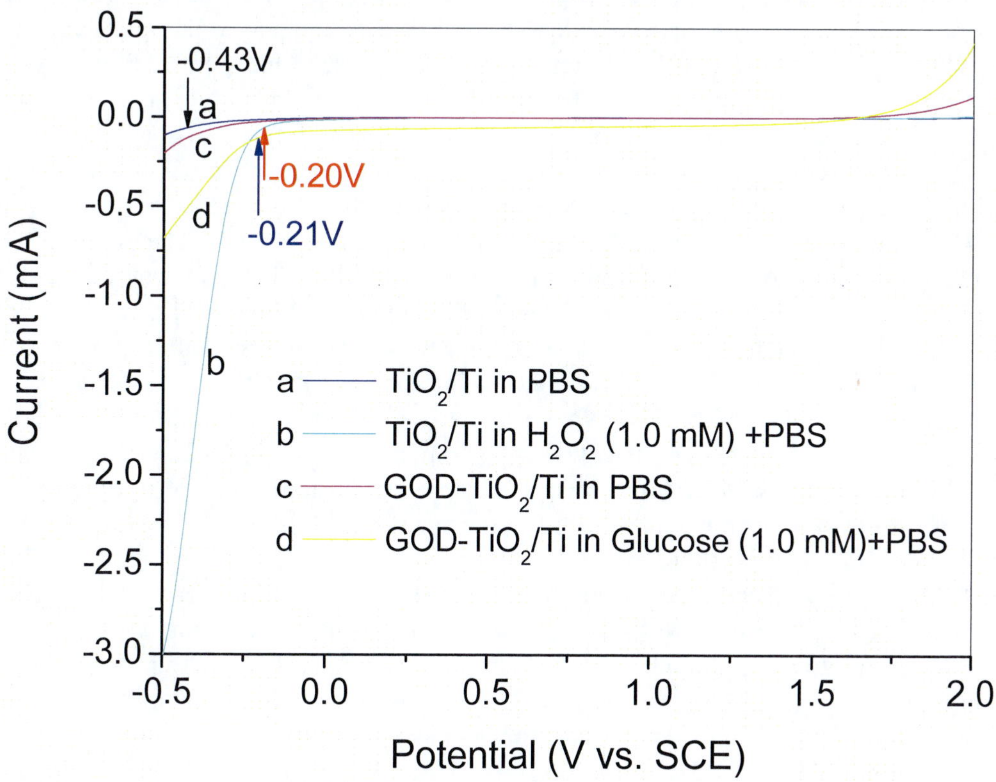

Figure 8. Linear sweep voltammetry curves of bare TiO_2/Ti and GOD–TiO_2/Ti nanotube array electrodes.

3.3. Detection Application

The optimization of the working electrode potential has been carried out to achieve a high performance for glucose detection. Fig. 9 shows the responsive current curves depending on interaction time under different potentiostatic conditions for GOD–TiO_2/Ti electrode. Obviously, the reduction current is improved along with reinforcing cathodic potential. However, the responsive time of cathodic current up to a steady value is also prolonged from 0.5 to 6.4 s when the working potential is reinforced from -0.1 to -0.6 V (see Fig. 9A). These corresponding changes can well obey the laws of exponential decay for responsive time (t) and exponential growth for steady current (I) in a function of the applied potential (P). Both experimental results and fitting curves are shown in Fig. 9B. On the one hand, the increase of the cathodic potentials on the working electrode can effectively promote the steady current intensity, which can accordingly intensify the detective signal. On the other hand, the corresponding delay of responsive time weakens the sensitivity of this nano-array biosensor in the cause of the detection application. Actually, the response time mostly depends upon the interfacial reactivity of this functional electrode, which is quite related to its configuration, microstructure and the working potential. A short response time usually means a high effectiveness for a high-performance biosensor. Considering both the responsive time of steady current and amplification effect of amperometric signal on the base of this transducer, it is reasonable that the optimized working potential is determined to the range of -0.40 ~ -0.50 V vs. SCE (see Fig. 9B). Herein, the working electrode potential is accordingly controlled at a constant value of -0.40 V vs. SCE for the sensing applications, at which the hydrogen evolution process is also minimized on the surface of TiO_2. As a result, the rapid responsive time of 2.1 s is quite acceptable for the measurement practices; meanwhile the amperometric signal intensity can also keep high enough to fulfill a quite low detection limit.

On the base of electrochemical reduction response, amperometric detection of H_2O_2 has been carried out on bare TiO_2/Ti nanotube array electrode in PBS electrolyte. Responsive current curves depending on different H_2O_2 concentration are shown in Fig. 10A for ordinary TiO_2/Ti ordinary nanotubes. When the H_2O_2 concentration is increased from 0.1 to 2.0 mM, the steady current intensity is accordingly reinforced up to -1418 μA. Meanwhile, the responsive time is also prolonged from 0.3 to 5.4 s. A standard calibration curve is obtained for a quantitative measurement of H_2O_2 concentration using this TiO_2/Ti electrode substrate (see Fig. 10B). The electrochemical response curve demonstrates a good linear relationship between steady current (I_{H2O2}, μA) and H_2O_2 concentration (C_{H2O2}, mM) in the full range of 0.1 ~ 2.0 mM. The regression equation of the fitting curve is $I_{H2O2} = -24.9514 - 716.8776 \times C_{H2O2}$ with a correlation coefficient of 0.9988. The relative standard derivations are approximately below 1.0 % for five independent measurements of a constant H_2O_2 concentration by applying this TiO_2/Ti nanotube array electrode. Additionally, a more accurate fitting result can be well achieved in the case of a low concentration range below 0.01 mM H_2O_2. Accordingly regarding this initial linear part of the calibration plot, the detection limit of H_2O_2 is determined as 2.0×10^{-4} mM for bare TiO_2/Ti ordinary nanotube array electrode at a signal-to-noise of 3. Similarly, such a detection limit of H_2O_2 is determined as 2.2×10^{-4} mM for TiO_2/Ti long nanotube array electrode.

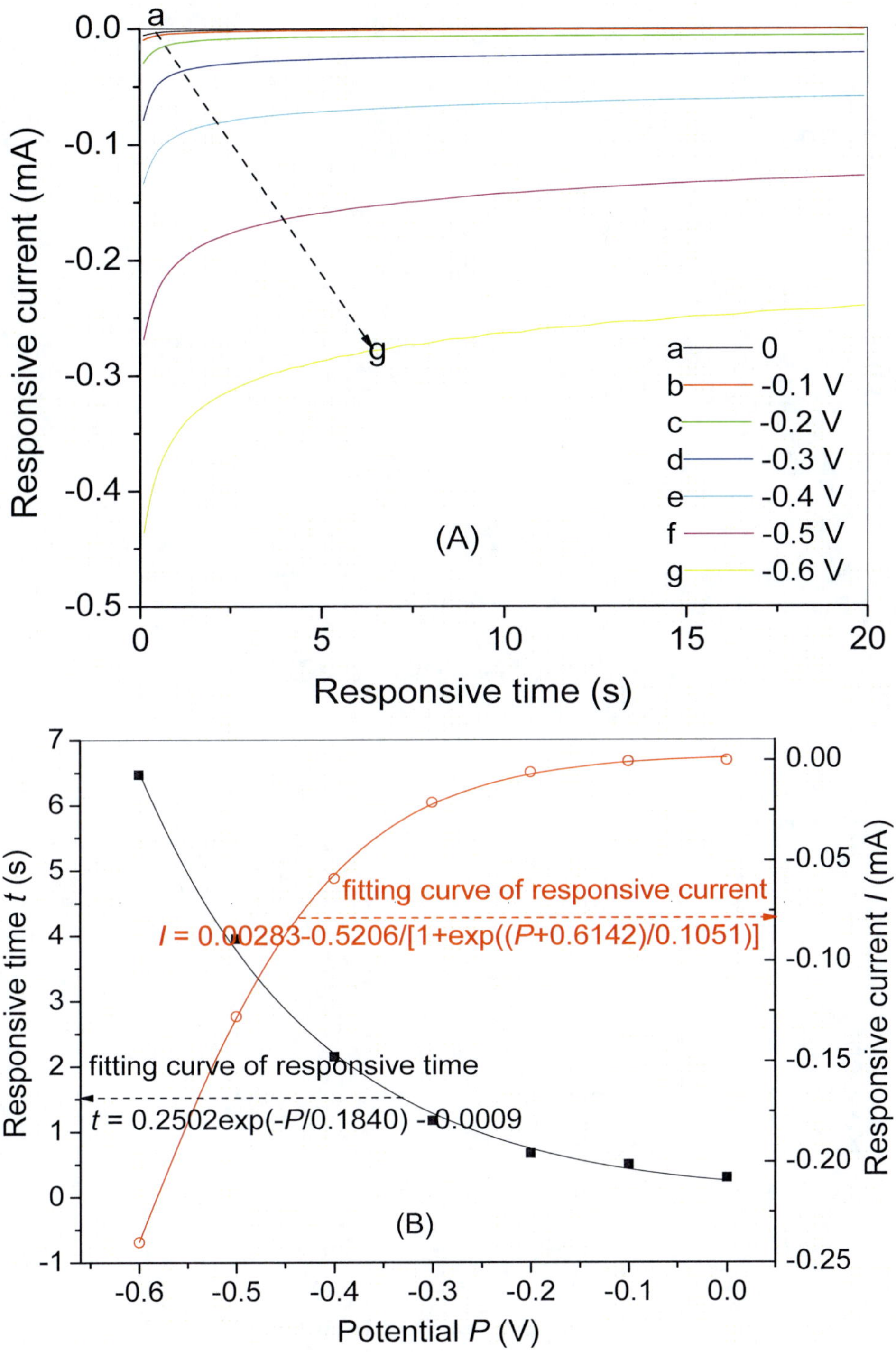

Figure 9. (A) Responsive current-time curves of GOD–TiO_2/Ti electrode under different potentiostatic condition and (B) responsive time and steady current in terms of applied cathode potential (flow rate of O_2 gas, 25 mL min^{-1}; glucose concentration, 0.4 mM).

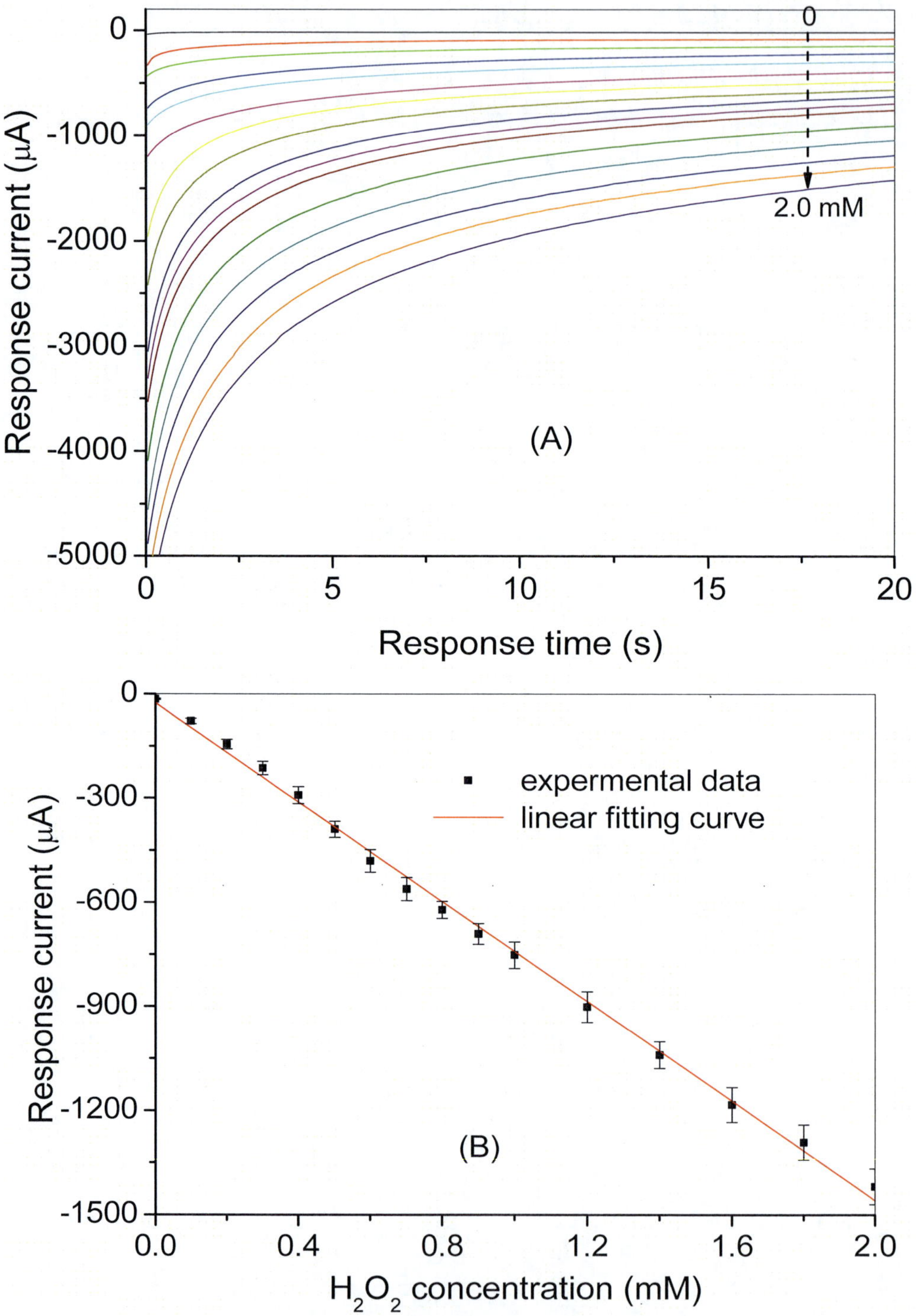

Figure 10. (A) Responsive current curves and (B) standard calibration plot of pure TiO_2/Ti nanotube array electrode for amperometric detection of H_2O_2.

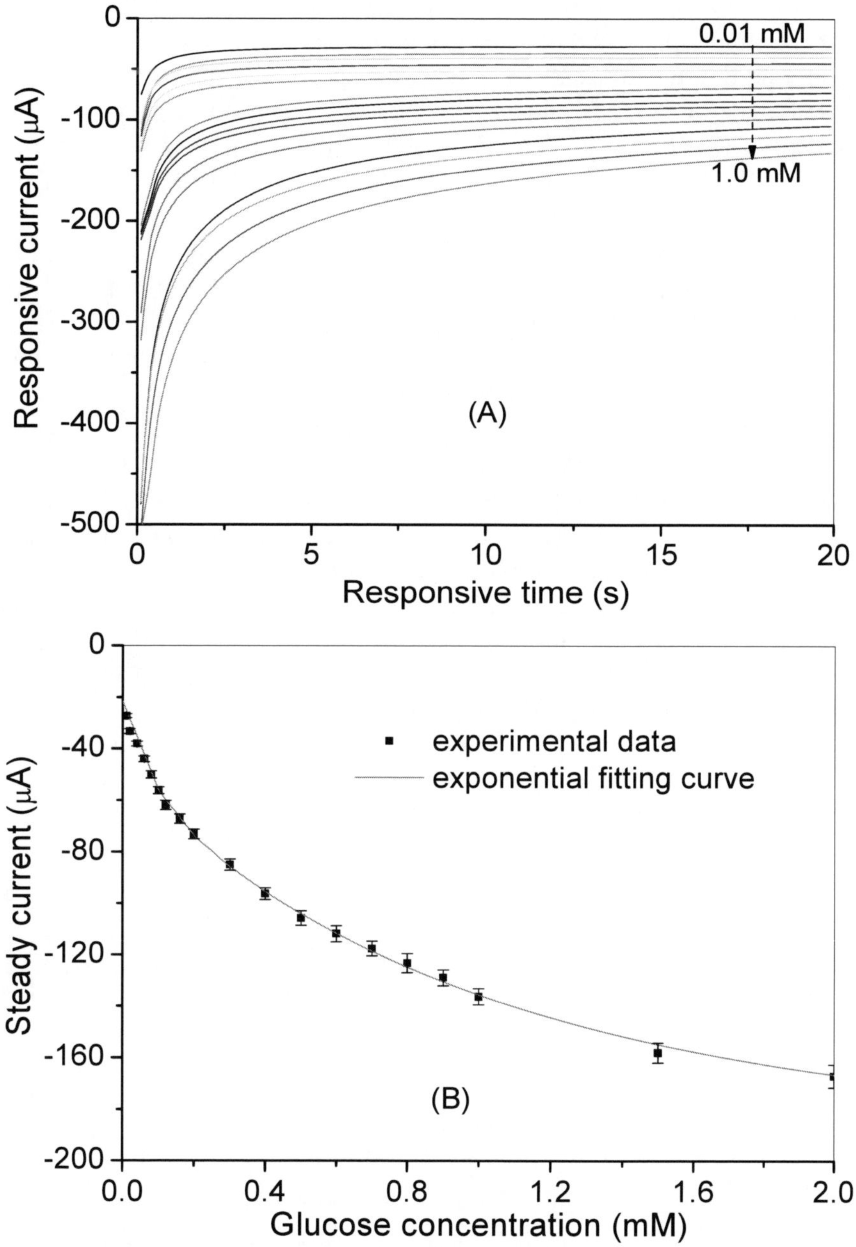

Figure 11. (A) Responsive current curves and (B) standard calibration plot of GOD–TiO_2/Ti nanotube array electrode for amperometric detection of glucose (working potential, constant at -0.40 V vs. SCE; electrolyte, 0.1 M PBS).

Amperometric detection of glucose has been carried out in PBS electrolyte based on the bioelectrocatalysis mechanism for GOD–TiO_2/Ti ordinary nanotube array electrode. Both enzymic biocatalysis and electro-reduction reactions can proceed satisfactorily when the working potential is fixed at -0.40 V vs. SCE. Fig. 11A shows that in the presence of glucose, the current signal is generated quickly and then reaches to a steady value. When glucose concentration increases from 0.01 to 1.0 mM, the steady current is quantitatively promoted from -27.2 to -136.2 μA. At the same time, the responsive time is accordingly prolonged from 1.1 to 5.6 s. Furthermore, Fig. 11B reveals that a nonlinear dependent relationship is obtained in the full concentration range of 0.01 - 1.0 mM between the steady current ($I_{glucose}$, μA) and the glucose concentration ($C_{glucose}$, mM), which well obeys the law of the first-ordered exponential decay. The regression equation of the fitting curve is $I_{glucose} = 148.4\times\exp(-C_{glucose}/0.781) - 181.3$ with a correlation coefficient of 0.9906. Especially regarding amperometric detection in the low concentration range below 0.01 mM glucose, a good linear relationship can be achieved for concentration determination of glucose. According to this initial linear part of the calibration plot, the detection limit of glucose is determined as 2.0×10^{-3} mM for GOD–TiO_2/Ti nanotube array biosensor at a signal-to-noise of 3. The relative standard deviations (RSD) are below 3.0 % in four successive measurements of glucose concentration. Especially, a reproducible current response with RSD of 2.3 % (n=4) is observed for the constant 1.0 mM glucose. Detection sensitivity of GOD–TiO_2/Ti nanotubular electrode is 45.5 μA mM^{-1} cm^{-2}, which is obviously better than these previously reported TiO_2/ITO film electrodes [23, 24]. Therefore, the bioelectrocatalysis application of GOD–TiO_2/Ti nanotube array electrode becomes very feasible for quantitative determination of glucose. Additionally, the enzymic biocatalysis reaction of between GOD and glucose is much slower than electrochemical reduction reaction of H_2O_2 on the surface of TiO_2/Ti electrode. As a result, the steady time has been obviously prolonged for indirect detection of glucose by using GOD–TiO_2/Ti in comparison with direct detection of H_2O_2 by using bare TiO_2/Ti nanotube array electrode in the case of the same current response (see Fig. 12).

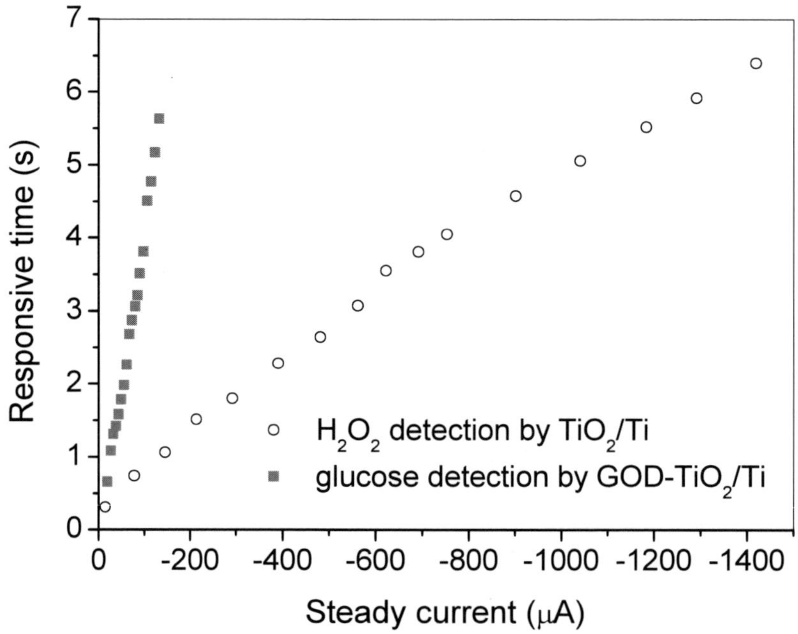

Figure 12. Responsive time in terms of steady current for direct detection of H_2O_2 by TiO_2/Ti and indirect detection of glucose by GOD–TiO_2/Ti electrode.

Fig. 10B and 11B only show the whole changing law in a wide concentration range up to 2.0 mM. The detection limit is usually located in a low concentration range, which only can be determined through the initial linear part of the calibration plot. Fig. 13 shows the amperometric detection experimental data and the fitting curves of both hydrogen peroxide and glucose at a low concentration range below 0.01 mM. Actually, the electrochemical measurement is initially conducted in a pure 0.1 M phosphate buffer solution of pH 6.8 under the same working potential as that of amperometeric detection of hydrogen peroxide and glucose compounds. The obtained current response, including -2.9 μA for pure TiO_2/Ti nanotube array electrode and -4.6 μA for GOD–TiO_2/Ti nanotube array electrode, can be regarded as the noise current. Especially in the low concentration range below 0.01 mM for hydrogen peroxide or glucose, a good linear relationship can be well achieved between amperometric signal intensity and compound concentration. Accordingly, the detection limit can be obtained from calculation results according to the regression equations at 3σ (signal-to-noise ratio=3), where σ is the detection noise without any presence of hydrogen peroxide or glucose. Therefore, the detection limit of H_2O_2 is determined as 2.0×10^{-4} mM for bare TiO_2/Ti ordinary nanotube array at a signal-to-noise of 3. Comparatively, the detection limit of glucose is determined as 2.0×10^{-3} mM for GOD–TiO_2/Ti ordinary nanotube array biosensor at a signal-to-noise of 3. Such a result indicates that indirect biocatalysis & electro-reduction process is still less sensitive than the direct electro-reduction process in the sensing application of nano-array electrode materials.

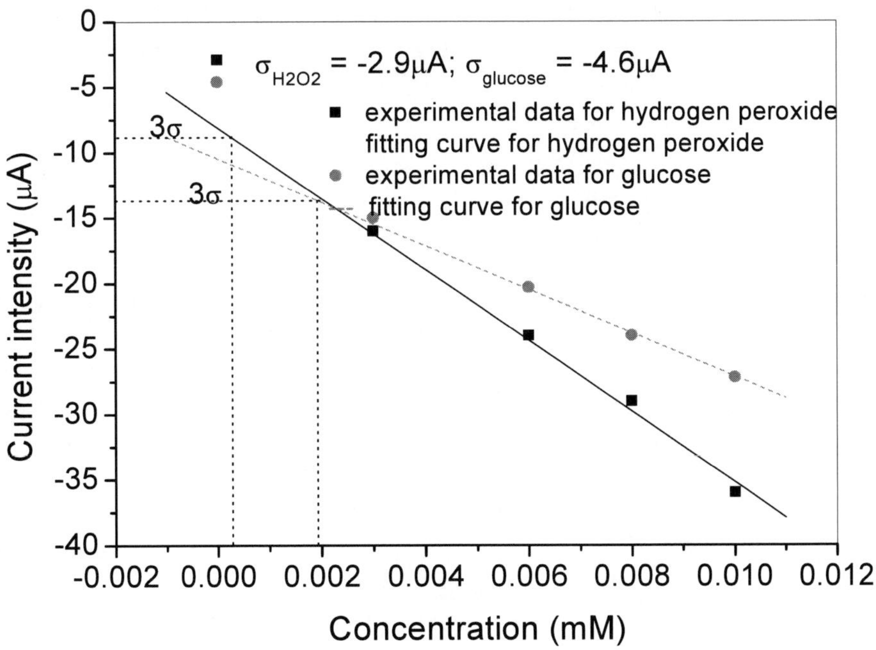

Figure 13. Amperometric detection experimental data and fitting curves of hydrogen peroxide and glucose at a low concentration range below 0.01 mM.

The nano-array biosensor based on GOD–TiO_2/Ti nanotube array electrode exhibits the reinforced current response in a bioelectrocatalysis and electro-reduction process, which can promote amperometric detection of glucose concentration with a high sensitivity and a low detection limit. In particular, such a nano-array biosensor based on GOD–TiO_2/Ti nanotube array electrode can be potentially used for a better detection of somatic blood glucose for diabetic patients. We believe that a serial of biosensors with these nanotube array structured electrode materials can also be constructed on the principle of biomolecules pair interaction of antigen-antibody interaction or supramolecular recognition. More sensitive, inexpensive, noninvasive bioanalytical micro-devices may be achieved for quantitative measurement of various molecules through further intensive investigation. Other practical applications, such as biomedical diagnosis and environmental testing operation can be likely fulfilled for a rapid and effective detection of infections, disease markers and even environmental pollutants.

4. Conclusion

TiO_2/Ti electrode substrates with a designed nanotube array structure have been synthesized for an amperometric detection application. TiO_2/Ti ordinary nanotube array electrode can provide a high interactive surface areas and very feasible electron-transfer interfaces by introducing the well-aligned small nanotube structure, which can ultimately promote the amperometric response for the concentration determination of hydrogen peroxide. On the basis of enzyme biocatalysis and electro-reduction reaction on GOD–TiO_2/Ti nanotube array electrode under a potentiostatic condition, the nano-array biosensor application has been achieved by using an electrochemical workstation for amperometeric detection of glucoses. This biosensor exhibits a very high sensitivity and low detection limit for the corresponding determination of the glucose concentration. Such kind of enzyme-titania/titanium nanotube array electrode can also contribute to other potential prospects in biomedical diagnosis and even environmental analysis.

Acknowledgment

The work was supported by National Natural Science Foundation of China (20871029), Research Fund for the Doctoral Program of Higher Education of China (200802861071), Program for New Century Excellent Talents in University (NCET-08-0119), Southeast University and Hong Kong Polytechnic University.

References

[1] DeGrado, W. F. *Nature,* 2003, 423(6936), 132-133.
[2] Lojou, E.; Bianco, P. *J. Electroceram.,* 2006, 16(1), 79-91.
[3] Yemini, M.; Reches, M.; Gazit, E.; Rishpon, J. *Anal. Chem.,* 2005, 77(16), 5155-5159.
[4] Akyilmaz, E.; Sezginturk, M. K.; Dinckaya, E. *Talanta,* 2003, 61(2), 73-79.
[5] Dzyadevych, S. V.; Anh, T. M.; Soldatkin, A. P.; Chien, N. D.; Jaffrezic-Renault, N.; Chovelon, J. M. *Bioelectrochemistry,* 2002, 55(1-2), 79-81.
[6] Zhang, F. F.; Wang, X. L.; Ai, S. Y.; Sun, Z. D.; Wan, Q.; Zhu, Z. Q.; Xian, Y. Z.; Jin, L. T.; Yamamoto, K. *Anal. Chim. Acta,* 2004, 519(2), 155-160.
[7] Xu, X.; Tian, B. Z.; Kong, J. L.; Zhang, S.; Liu, B. H.; Zhao, D. Y. *Adv. Mater.,* 2003, 15(22), 1932-1936.

[8] Lee, S.; Jeon, C.; Park, Y. *Chem. Mat.,* 2004, 16(22), 4292-4295.

[9] Tian, Z. R. R.; Voigt, J. A.; Liu, J.; McKenzie, B.; Xu, H. F. *J. Am. Chem. Soc.,* 2003, 125(41), 12384-12385.

[10] Topoglidis, E.; Cass, A. E. G.; O'Regan, B.; Durrant, J. R. *J. Electroanal. Chem.,* 2001, 517(1-2), 20-27.

[11] Yang, Y. H.; Yang, H. F.; Yang, M. H.; Liu, Y. L.; Shen, G. L.; Yu, R. Q. *Anal. Chim. Acta,* 2004, 525(2), 213-220.

[12] Kenausis, G. L.; Voros, J.; Elbert, D. L.; Huang, N. P.; Hofer, R.; Ruiz-Taylor, L.; Textor, M.; Hubbell, J. A.; Spencer, N. D. *J. Phys. Chem. B,* 2000, 104(14), 3298-3309.

[13] Reimhult, E.; Hook, F.; Kasemo, B. *J. Chem. Phys.,* 2002, 117(16), 7401-7404.

[14] Oh, S. H.; Finones, R. R.; Daraio, C.; Chen, L. H.; Jin, S. H. *Biomaterials,* 2005, 26(24), 4938-4943.

[15] Wilkins, E.; Atanasov, P. *Med. Eng. Phys.,* 1996, 18(4), 273-288.

[16] Xie, Y. B.; Zhou, L. M.; Huang, H. T. *Biosensors & Bioelectronics,* 2007, 22(12), 2812-2818.

[17] Hecht, H. J.; Schomburg, D.; Kalisz, H.; Schmid, R. D. *Biosens. Bioelectron.,* 1993, 8(3-4), 197-203.

[18] Xie, Y. B. *Electrochim. Acta,* 2006, 51(17), 3399-3406.

[19] Abidian, M. R.; Kim, D. H.; Martin, D. C. *Adv. Mater.,* 2006, 18(4), 405-409.

[20] Marsh, J.; Gorse, D. *Electrochim. Acta,* 1998, 43(7), 659-670.

[21] Yuan, S.; Hu, S. S. *Electrochim. Acta,* 2004, 49(25), 4287-4293.

[22] Mantzila, A. G.; Prodromidis, M. I. *Electrochim. Acta,* 2006, 51(17), 3537-3542.

[23] Cosnier, S.; Senillou, A.; Gratzel, M.; Comte, P.; Vlachopoulos, N.; Renault, N. J.; Martelet, C. *J. Electroanal. Chem.,* 1999, 469(2), 176-181.

[24] Li, Q. W.; Luo, G. A.; Feng, J.; Zhou, Q.; Zhang, L.; Zhu, Y. F. *Electroanalysis,* 2001, 13(5), 413-416.

In: Nanostructured Materials for Electrochemical Biosensors ISBN: 978-1-60741-706-4
Editors: U. Yogeswaran; S. Kumar; S. Chen ©2009 Nova Science Publishers, Inc.

Chapter 9

ANODIC TiO_2: FABRICATION, CURRENT APPLICATIONS AND FUTURE PERSPECTIVES

Haitao Huang,* Guoge Zhang, Haichao Liang and Limin Zhou†
The Hong Kong Polytechnic University,
Hung Hom, Kowloon, China

ABSTRACT

Although nanostructured alumina was successfully fabricated by electrochemical anodization decades ago, it is only until recently that the electrochemically anodized TiO_2 begins to attract more and more research interest and is now becoming an emerging area of a wide range of important applications, such as, gas sensing, self cleaning, antifogging, water purification, anticorrosion, solar cell, lithium batteries, electrochemical supercapacitors, photo cleavage of water, antibacterial coating, and the improvement of biocompatibility, etc. This is due fundamentally to the fact that TiO_2 is a semiconductor with reactivity or photoreactivity closely related to its defect structure. A variety of attractive functional properties of TiO_2 are the result of its unique electronic band structure which can also be easily tuned by defects. In this article we will give a detailed review on recent progress in the fabrication of anodic TiO_2 nanostructure, the control of its morphology by varying anodization conditions, and the microstructure related properties. We will also review the recent research efforts in various practical applications of anodic TiO_2 with dopants or modifications. Potential future applications of anodic TiO_2 with highly ordered nanostructures are also suggested.

* Department of Applied Physics and Materials Research Center, The Hong Kong Polytechnic University, Hung Hom, Kowloon, China. Email address: aphhuang@polyu.edu.hk
† Department of Mechanical Engineering, The Hong Kong Polytechnic University, Hung Hom, Kowloon, China. Email address: melmzhou@inet.polyu.edu.hk

INTRODUCTION

Nowadays, nanomaterials are of particular research interest due to its fundamental and technical importance in various areas. The existence of broken chemical bonds at the surface of a material brings about completely different physical and chemical properties on the surfaces as compared to that of the bulk and hence results in many attractive size-dependent properties as the surface-to-volume ratio is varied with the size of materials [1-12].

As one of the important functional materials, semiconducting titania (TiO_2) has stimulated significant research activities to be used as a photocatalyst since the pioneering work by Fujishima *et al.* [13]. Their work marked the beginning of a new era in heterogeneous photocatalysis. Some of the applications include the use of TiO_2 in solar cell [14], photodegradation of organics present in polluted water and air [15], gas sensing [16], electrochromic devices [17], photochromic devices [18], self-cleaning by wettability tailoring [19], photocleavage of water [13], and improvement of biocompatibility [20].

Over the past two decades, enormous progress has been achieved in the synthesis, characterization and device applications of nanostructured TiO_2. Among the various types of nanostructured TiO_2, the quasi-one-dimensional nanostructure has attracted particular attention. This chapter will give a comprehensive review on the synthesis of this quasi-one-dimensional TiO_2 nanostructure by electrochemical anodization method, the characterization of its properties, and its potential for applications.

SYNTHESIS OF TITANIA NANOSTRUCTURES

There exist a variety of methods to synthesize quasi-one-dimensional nanostructured materials, which include but not limited to vapor phase growth, template-assisted synthesis, sol-gel deposition, surfactant-assisted growth, sonochemical method, hydrothermal method, and electrochemical deposition [21]. Among the various methods, the electrochemical anodization method is one of the simplest and cheapest methods to synthesize ordered quasi-one-dimensional nanostructure.

The electrochemical anodization method to synthesize nanostructured metal oxide has been known for more than 50 years [22]. However, it was only until quite recently that highly ordered Al_2O_3 nanostructure was obtained by anodization [23]. Thereafter, self-assembled anodic TiO_2 nanostructure with a certain degree of ordering became a hot area of research partly due to the attractive properties of TiO_2, which are promising for various applications.

Different Morphologies of Anodic TiO_2

So far the self-organized anodic TiO_2 has been synthesized by halide ions containing solution, either aqueous or non-aqueous. The overall reactions for anodic oxidation of titanium can be represented as

$$2H_2O \rightarrow O_2 + 4H^+ + 4e \qquad (1)$$

$$Ti + O_2 \rightarrow TiO_2 \quad (2)$$

In the earlier days, the anodization of titanium was carried out mainly using diluted HF as the electrolyte [24], in some cases with the addition of other acids such as H_2SO_4 [25], HNO_3, H_3BO_3 [26], acetic acid [27], and H_3PO_4 [28]. The resulting solution has generally a low pH value (<3) and a high chemical dissolution speed for titania according to the following equation,

$$TiO_2 + 6F^- + 4H^+ \rightarrow TiF_6^{2-} + 2H_2O \quad (3)$$

The ability of the electrolyte to dissolve TiO_2 as soluble $[TiF_6]^{2-}$ complex is necessary to produce tubular structure [29]. On the other hand, the high rate of chemical dissolution of TiO_2 is also the factor that limits the length of titania nanotubes to only a few hundred nanometers [24-28]. Fig. 1(a) shows the scanning electron microscopy (SEM) image of a well-ordered TiO_2 nanotubular array structure produced in an electrolyte made of HF(0.15M)-H_3PO_4(0.5M) and anodized under 20 V for 40 min [28]. The nanotube array was with an average diameter of 60 nm and length of 540 nm. The average thickness of the wall of nanotubes is about 15 nm.

Fig. 1(b) shows the bottom view of the peeled off TiO_2 layer from metallic substrate [24]. It is apparent that the nanotubes are closed on the bottom. The closed bottom corresponds to the so-called barrier layer, a thin oxide layer separating the nanotubes from the metallic substrate. It is evident from the cross-section SEM image that the tube wall showed periodic ring structures, the origin of which was not explained by the author. The regularly spaced rings are suggested to be related to the anodization current oscillations accompanied by pH burst [30]. The local acidification leads to a temporarily increased dissolution rate and results in the variations of the tube walls' thickness. However, it was pointed out that, even if no current oscillation was detected, rings at the tube sidewalls were still observed [31].

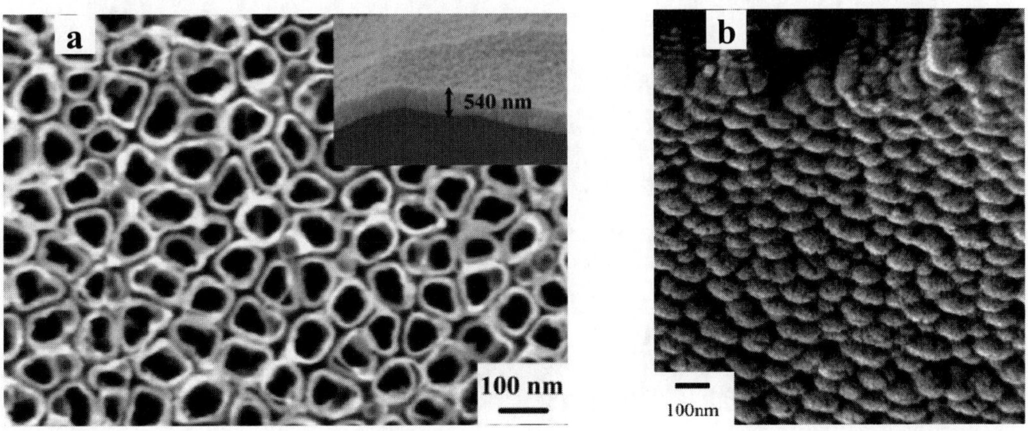

Figure 1. SEM images of titania nanotubes synthesized by anodization: (a) top view [28], (b) bottom view [24]. The inset of (a) shows the cross-section image.

To achieve longer TiO_2 nanotubes, fluorine ion containing salts were used in the electrolyte to replace HF [29, 32] and the pH value was adjusted to control the dissolution speed of titania. The thickness of TiO_2 nanotube is the result of an equilibrium between the electrochemical formation of TiO_2 at the tube bottom and the chemical dissolution of the tube mouth. Increasing pH value decreases the chemical dissolution rate, and apparently prolongs the time needed to reach the equilibrium. As a result, substantially longer TiO_2 nanotube over 2 μm was reported as shown in Fig. 2 [32]. It is also noted that by increasing pH values, the hydrolysis content increases, resulting in a significant amount of hydrous titanic oxide precipitated on the nanotube surface. Consequently, electrolyte with lower pH value forms shorter but clean nanotubes, whereas the one with higher pH value results in longer nanotubes and unwanted precipitates [29]. The best range pH value for the formation of relatively longer TiO_2 nanotubes is between 3 and 5. An increase in the length of these nanotubes not only enhances the effective surface area but also reduces failures in devices such as high temperature sensors, where the electrode material can diffuse and come into contact with the unanodized part of the titanium substrate.

A common feature of these TiO_2 nanotubes fabricated using aqueous electrolyte is the considerable variation of the thickness of side walls (Fig. 2). To tackle this problem, highly viscous electrolyte such as glycerol was used to decrease the diffusion constant and suppress the local concentration fluctuations [30]. Although the anodization potential was not changed, the current density was much lower than that in pure aqueous electrolyte. This is in line with a diffusion controlled process. Such an anodization process was very stable and the resulting TiO_2 nanotubes were smooth over their entire length as shown in Fig. 3 [30]. Only minimal variations (2 nm) in thickness can be determined from the TEM image (Fig. 3 (c)).

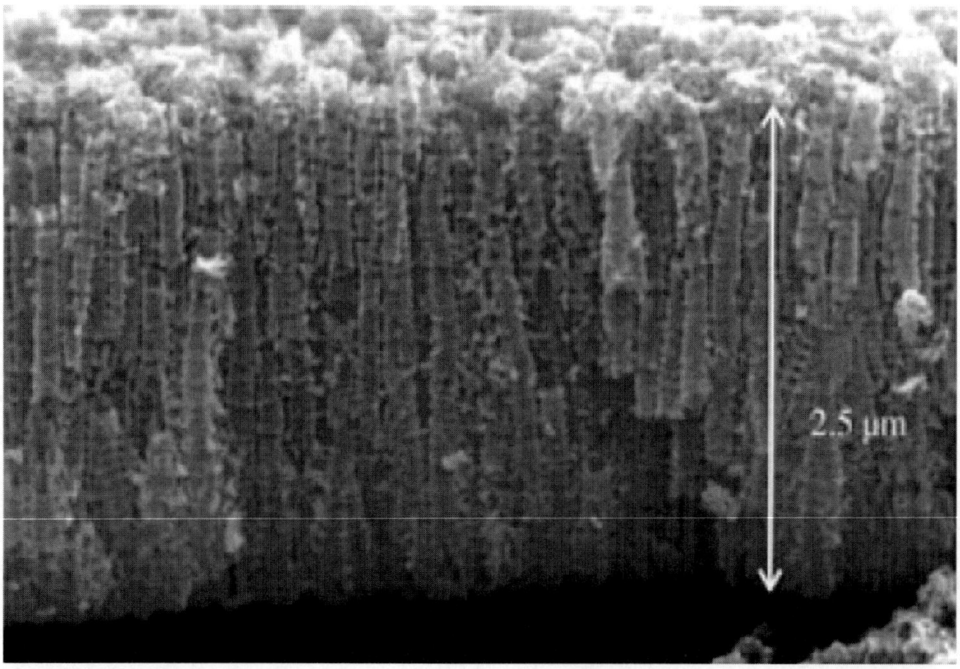

Figure 2. SEM cross section image of TiO_2 nanotubes. The anodization was conducted under 20 V in 1 M $(NH_4)_2SO_4$ + 0.5 wt.% NH_4F using a potential sweep from open-circuit potential to 20 V with a sweep rate 0.1 V/s [32].

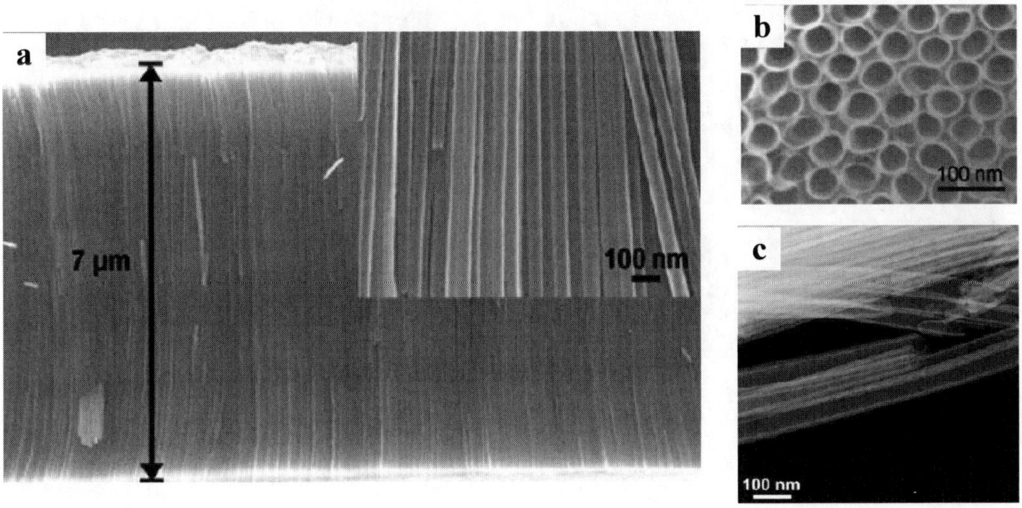

Figure 3. SEM Images of smooth TiO_2 nanotube: (a) cross section image, the inset shows the magnified part; (b) top view; and (c) TEM image. The samples were anodized in glycerol with 0.5 wt.% NH_4F at 20 V for 13 h [30].

Other organic electrolytes such as ethylene glycol, dimethyl sulfoxide, formamide, and N-methylformamide have also been used to fabricate smooth and long TiO_2 nanotubes [33-36], among which ethylene glycol shows the best result. The potentiostatic anodization of titanium in the mixture of NH_4F, ethylene glycol and small amounts of water dramatically increases the nanotubes growth rate, which is the result of faster high field ionic conduction through the barrier layer. Due to the negligible chemical dissolution of anodic TiO_2 in this electrolyte, significantly longer TiO_2 nanotubues up to a thickness of 720 μm was reported [36].

Although TiO_2 nanotubes formed with organic electrolyte are better ordered than those fabricated with water based solution, they are still randomly distributed with irregular shape of the tube mouth. Through the use of well organized concave dimples left on titanium substrate from previous anodization as the template for subsequent anodization, hexagonal close packed nanoporous TiO_2 was developed (Fig. 4 (a)) [37]. Apart from producing the ordered template, another key factor to achieving the highly ordered porous structure is the proper voltage ramp rate at the final anodization step. If the voltage ramps up too slow, the distance between neighboring pore nucleation sites is smaller than that of the dimples left by the previous anodization step and more than one pore can be developed on each dimple, forming the irregular porous structure as shown in Fig. 4 (b). The highly ordered structure shown in Fig. 4 (a) was localized and the ordered domain size was about 1 to 2 μm. Such a structure was achieved by the anodization of as-received titanium foil without any heat treatment. Because the defects of the ordered pores usually appear at the grain boundaries, surface irregularities, and the stress concentrated sites, it is expected that the self-organization can be further improved by surface polishing, stress relief annealing and/or using titanium foils with larger grains just as what has been done in the anodization of aluminum.

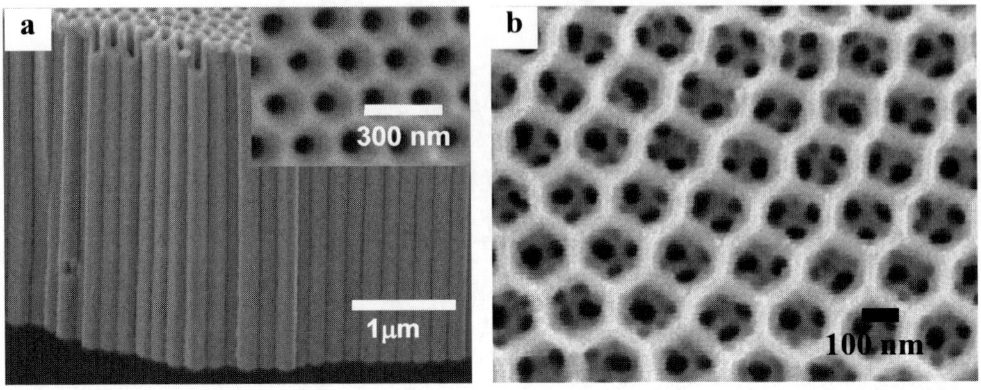

Figure 4. SEM images of (a) highly ordered, and (b) irregular nanoporous anodic TiO_2. Both samples were anodized with a three-step anodization under 60 V in an electrolyte of ethylene glycol added with 0.25 wt.% NH_4F. The anodization voltage ramp rate was 60 V/s for (a) and 0.1 V/s for (b) in the final step anodization [37].

Besides conventional nanotubes, other nanostructured anodic TiO_2 was also reported. TiO_2 nanowires (Fig. 5) were developed under specific anodization condition [38]. Like bamboo splitting, the nanowires originated from the vertical splitting of nanotubes, which was caused by the electric field induced longitudinal flow of ions. A small addition of water is essential for the formation of nanowires and the amount of water required decreases with increasing applied potential.

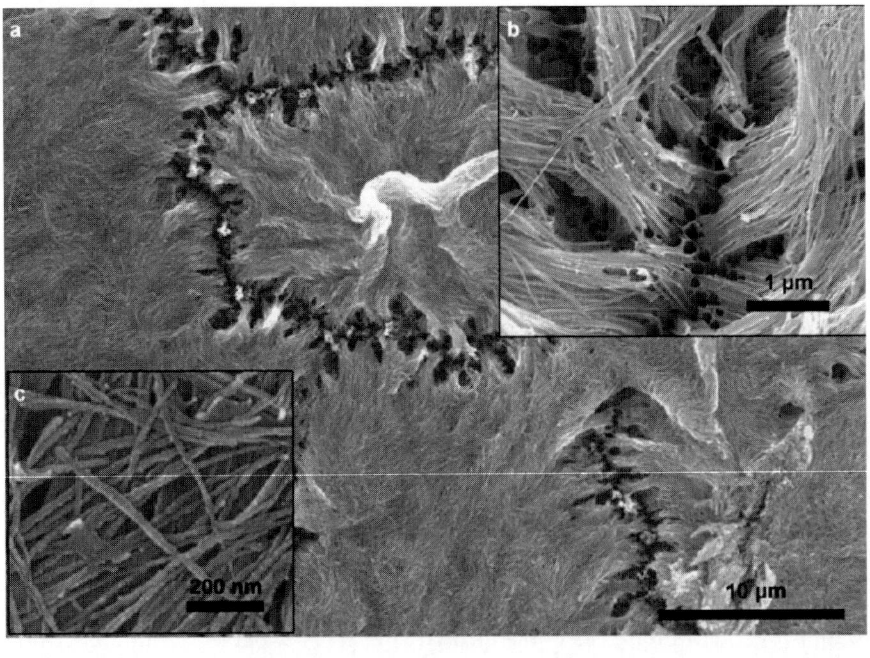

Figure5. SEM images of TiO_2 nanowires prepared by anodization of titanium foils at 80 V in ethylene glycol containing 0.25 wt.% NH_4F for 5h: (a) overview of nanowires on the entire TiO_2 nanotube arrays, (b) nanowires results from the splitting of porous nanotubes, and (c) enlarged view of nanowires with a diameter of a few tens of nanometers [38].

Two dimensional nanolace sheets can be obtained with alternating anodization potentials. Fig. 6 shows such nanolace sheets formed by extended anodization with a sequence of 50 s at 120 V and 600 s at 0V [39]. "Aged" solution (ethylene glycol with the addition of 0.2 M HF and 0.12 M H_2O_2 after anodization at 120 V for 24 h) was used as the electrolyte. TiO_2 nanotubes and compact oxide layer were formed repeatedly, and bamboo-type structure was produced when the voltage was alternated between the two formation voltages. After subjected to an extended anodization, the thinnest part of the tube wall which was formed at higher voltage was etched away and the reinforced compact part was left behind. When more and more such "bamboo rings" were etched out and stacked on each other, two dimensional nanolace structure was achieved.

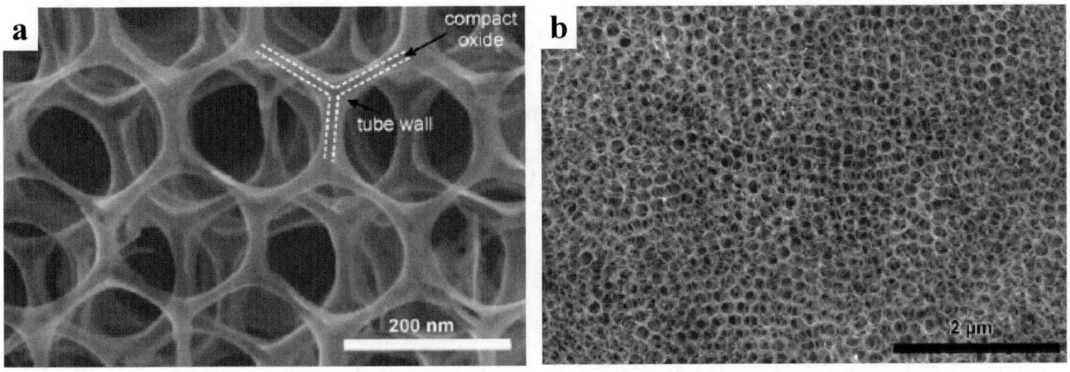

Figure 6. TiO_2 nanolace sheets. (a) Detailed view with indication of original tube walls and compact oxide formed by voltage alternating. (b) Morphology of nanolace over a larger area [39].

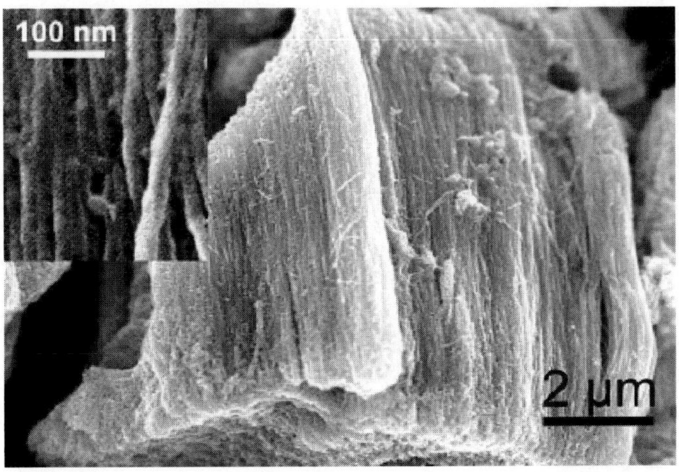

Figure 7. SEM image of nanotube bundles anodized in 0.5 M oxalic acid with 0.3 M NH_4Cl under 13 V for 80 seconds. The inset shows the small diameter of these nanotubes [41].

Fluorine ion was once believed to be the necessary element for producing nanostructured anodic TiO_2. Addition of other halide such as bromide and chloride initiated only pitting and no nanopores were observed during anodization [40]. Recently, nanostructured anodic TiO_2

was synthesized by using electrolyte containing chlorine or bromine ions [41-45]. The process of chlorine based nanotube formation was very rapid and the tube diameter was significantly small [41]. After only 80 seconds' anodization, bundles of nanotubes up to several tens of micrometers can be observed (Fig. 7). This is in sharp contrast to fluorine ion based anodization, where several hours are needed to produce nanotubes of micrometer scale length. However, the chlorine based nanotubes is less ordered than fluorine based nanotubes. The diameter of nanotubes appears to be relatively independent on the anodization voltage, and the electrochemical conditions under which the tubes are produced are more stringent, resulting in less tunable dimensions. Further studies are needed to widen the processing window of the chlorine or bromine based anodic nanostructured TiO_2.

Influence of Electrochemical Conditions

In anodization with fluorine ion containing electrolyte, the nanostructure of anodic TiO_2 is readily controlled by the electrochemical conditions, such as electrolyte composition, potential sweep rate, potential, temperature, time and pH value. TiO_2 nanotube could be produced only within certain voltage range depending on the electrolyte composition. At low anodizing voltage, the anodic TiO_2 was of sponge-like morphology. At high anodizing voltage, the nanotube structure was lost and a randomly porous structure was formed [24]. The diameter of nanotubes was found to be proportional to the potential applied but was independent of the anodization time [29]. Fluorine ion concentration of the electrolyte was another parameter remarkably affecting the nanotube diameter, with higher concentration resulting in larger diameter. The difference in the pH value of electrolyte also led to significant variations in the diameter of nanotubes [46].

Similar to the diameter of nanotubes, the tube length was also reported linearly dependent on anodization potential in an electrolyte containing HF and H_3PO_4 [47]. The thickness of the nanotube walls can be changed by changing the anodization temperature, with lower temperature resulting in thicker walls [27]. When aqueous electrolyte with low pH value was used, TiO_2 nanotube length was found to be independent on the anodization time with a maximum length of a few hundred nanometers [20-23, 28, 46]. Due to the significantly reduced chemical etching rate of anodic TiO_2 in organic electrolyte, nanotube length can be increased with extended anodization time [33-36].

Generally, the anodization of Ti is carried out under magnetic stirring in order to reduce the double layer thickness at the oxide/electrolyte interface, and to facilitate uniform electrolyte composition distribution over the Ti substrate. Ultrasonic bath was occasionally utilized to replace stirring for quicker mass flow through anodic TiO_2 nanotubes [48]. The formation rate of the TiO_2 nanotubes by this sonoelectrochemical method was reported to be almost twice as fast as that of the magnetic stirring method.

Cation was found to be the key parameter influencing both the nanotube growth rate and length [49]. With increasing cation size, the interfacial oxide layer was getting thinner. Ionic transport was facilitated and the nanotube growth was enhanced. The thinnest nanotubes ever reported was 5 nm, which was obtained in an electrolyte containing 0.5 M tetrabutylammonium fluoride in formamide with 5% water (Fig. 8).

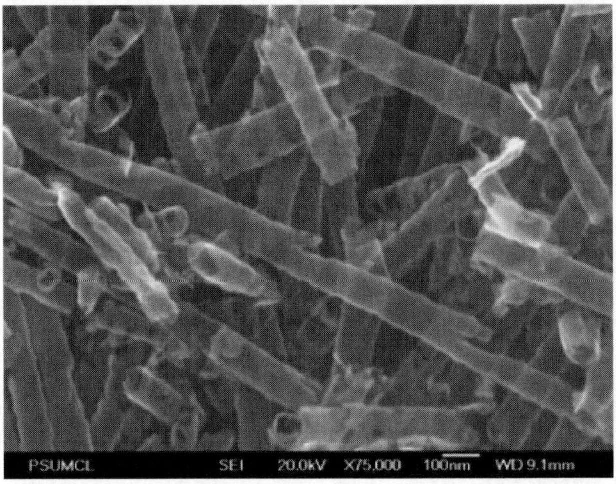

Figure 8. FESEM image of nanotubes formed in 0.5 M solution of Bu_4NF in formamide electrolyte containing 5% water [49].

Under certain anodization conditions, such as the use of fluoride containing ethylene glycol as the electrolyte, the content of water had a significant influence on the morphology of anodic TiO_2 [50]. The addition of a minimum amount of 0.18 wt.% water was required to form well ordered TiO_2 nanotubular arrays, while high water content (>0.5 wt.%) showed increased amount of ridges on the circumference of the nanotubes.

Tapered, conical shaped TiO_2 nanotubes were fabricated through the variation of anodization voltage [51]. The linearly increasing voltage (10 V to 23 V) resulted in a linearly increasing nanotube diameter as shown in Fig. 9. However, when the voltage was linearly decreased from 23 to 10 V, irrespective of the sweep rate, the resulting tubes were straight with the pore diameter equal to the one achieved at a constant voltage anodization at 10V.

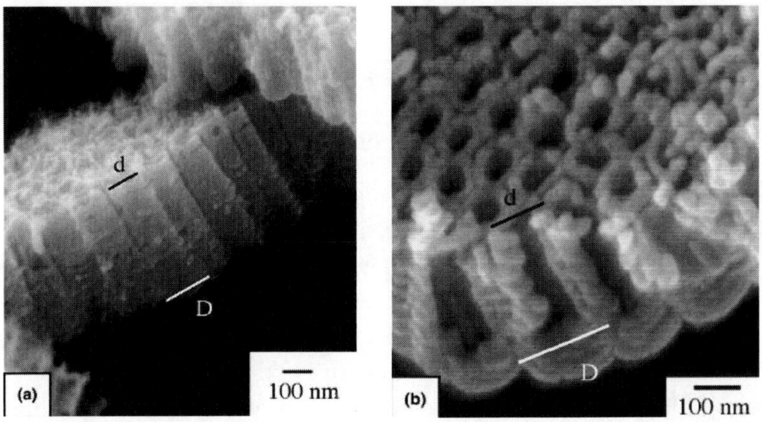

Figure 9. Cross-sectional SEM images of tapered TiO_2 nanotubes obtained by using a time-varying anodization voltage. *d* and D denote the diameter of apex and cone base, respectively. (a) Nanotubes obtained using a voltage ramp rate of 0.43 V/min from 10 to 23 V and then hold at 23 V for 10 min. (b) Nanotubes obtained by initial anodization at 10 V for 20 min, followed by the linearly increasing voltage at a rate of 1.0 V/min up to 23 V, and finally a constant voltage at 23 V for 2 min [51].

Closely stacked double layer of TiO_2 nanotubes have also been reported. Such architecture was obtained by a two-step anodization [52]. The short nanotube layer was formed in the first anodization with acidic electrolyte containing hydrofluoric acid and the second longer layer directly underneath the first one was then developed using a different electrolyte, a mixture of glycerol and NH_4F. Due to the significantly different tube diameters developed in these two electrolytes (100 nm vs 40 nm, Fig. 10), branched TiO_2 nanostructure was resulted as schematically shown in Fig. 11. The second nanotube layer was preferentially grown from the bottom of the first layer. Although the space between nanotubes of the first layer was also filled with electrolyte, no branching of the nanotubes can be observed in the first layer.

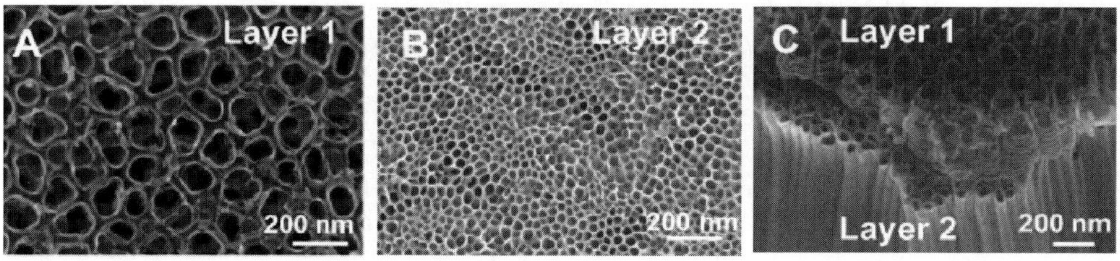

Figure 10. Top-view SEM images of (a) the first and (b) the second layer TiO_2 nanotubes. (c) is the interface between the first and second layers. The first layer was produced in 1 M H_2SO_4 + 0.16 M HF at 20 V for 2h. The second layer was produced in glycerol with 0.27 M NH_4F at 20 V for 16 h [52].

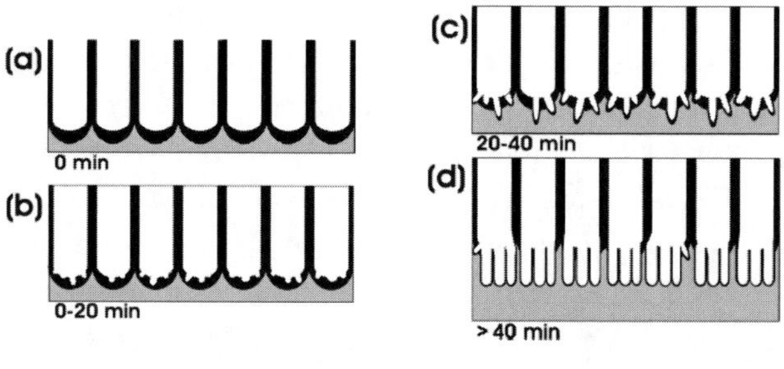

Figure 11. Schematic drawing showing four consecutive steps in the formation of the second nanotube layer during the second anodization step [52].

Potential sweep rate was shown to have a significant influence on the initiation and growth of anodic TiO_2 [53]. The higher the sweep rates, the higher the current densities. Even after an extended anodization of 2 h, the current density of a sample anodized with a high voltage ramp rate did not drop to the values obtained with a lower ramp rate. The composition of barrier layer, particularly the OH^-/O ratio, is dependent on the sweeping rate and so does the morphology of anodic TiO_2. With 1 M $(NH_4)_2SO_4$ + 5 wt% NH_4F as the electrolyte, very irregular and cross-linked porous layers were obtained at a sweep rate higher than 1 V/s.

Cathode material also shows certain effects on the morphology of anodic TiO_2. Nanotubes with different tube diameters and lengths can be obtained with different cathode materials under the same anodization conditions. The appearance of surface precipitates was dependent on cathode materials. The difference in overpotential for cathode materials was suggested to be the cause for different morphologies [54]. Some materials such as Fe, Co, Pd and C showed promising results to replace the conventional expensive Pt cathode. The incorporation of dissolved cathode ions into the anodic TiO_2 gave rise to the possibility of in situ band gap engineering of the nanotubes.

Mechanism of the Formation of Anodic TiO_2

Titanium anodization bears lots of similarity to the anodization of its sister material – aluminum. Both anodic films have approximately cylindrical pores extending from the top surface to the barrier layer. The barrier layer is convex, matching the concave dimples left on the metal substrate. Generally, each nanotube is located within an anodic cell. Cells have the tendency to be self-organized and form an ordered structure as the anodization goes on. Field-assisted oxidation and dissolution are also the key processes for the fabrication of anodic TiO_2. However, comparing to the anodization of aluminum, the chemical dissolution of anodic material is relatively high for titanium anodization. This brings to a slightly different formation mechanism for anodic TiO_2. There are four key processes for the fabrication of anodic TiO_2 nanostructure [51]: (1) Oxidation of Ti surface layer due to the interaction between Ti and oxygen containing ions (such as O^{2-} or OH^-). After the formation of an initial oxide layer, these anions can further migrate through the oxide layer to react with Ti at the Ti/TiO_2 interface. (2) Migration of Ti ions (Ti^{4+}) to the electrolyte from the Ti/TiO_2 interface under an electric field. (3) Field assisted dissolution of anodic TiO_2 at the oxide/electrolyte interface which is resulted from then weakening of Ti-O bonds by the applied electric field. (4) Chemical dissolution of anodic TiO_2 by the electrolyte. A mechanism of the formation of anodic TiO_2 nanotubes was proposed based on the above four processes and schematically shown in Fig. 12 [51, 53].

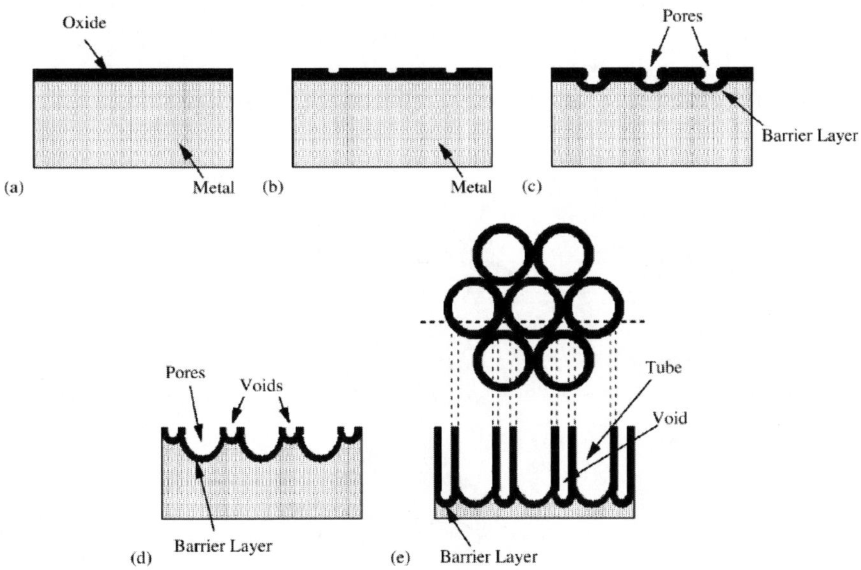

Figure 12. Schematic diagram of the evolution of an anodic TiO_2 nanotube array: (a) Formation of a compact oxide layer. (b) Formation of pits due to the dissolution and breakdown of the barrier oxide film. (c) The barrier layer at the bottom of the pits is relatively thin and this leads to the enhanced electric field assisted dissolution of TiO_2, which results in further pore growth. (d) Voids formed in the inter-pores region. (e) Fully developed nanotube array with a corresponding top view [51].

PROPERTIES OF TITANIA NANOSTRUCTURES

Semiconducting TiO_2 is a good photocatalyst. When it is excited by a photon with an energy higher than its bandgap, electron-hole pairs are generated at the valence and conduction bands, respectively, where holes are good oxidants (+1.0 ~ 3.5V) and electrons are good reductants (+0.5 ~ 1.5V) [55]. Actually, the bottom of conduction band is the reduction potential of photogenerated electrons and the energy level at the top of valence band determines the oxidizing ability of photo-induced holes. From a thermodynamic point of view, surface absorbed radicals can be reduced photocatalytically by conduction band electrons if they have redox potentials which are more positive than the flat band potential of the conduction band, or can be oxidized by valance band holes if they have redox potentials more negative than the flat band potential of the valence band. In fact, pH value also has an effect on shifting the Fermi level of a semiconductor. For TiO_2, the position of the Fermi level, as determined by the flat band potential, shifts with the pH value because the adsorption of excess H^+ or OH^- produces a potential drop. This shift, given by $E_F = E_F(pH = 0) - 0.059pH$ at 25°C, results in a greater reducing power for conduction band electrons as the pH value increases [56].

TiO_2 exists in three distinct polymorphs: rutile, anatase and brookite. Their structures are shown in Fig. 13. Rutile is the most stable structure while the others are metastable. Other forms are irreversibly converted to rutile when heated to temperatures between 700 and 920°C [57]. The stability of anatase can be increased by doping of 0.1% of certain anion. Rutile has a bandgap energy of 3.02 eV (411nm) while the bandgap in anatase is 3.2eV (384nm). Rutile has a better visible light response and anatase has a better photocatalytic activity. The structures of both rutile and anatase are tetragonal while brookite is orthorhombic. All of them can be described in terms of chains of TiO_6 octahedra, while the structural difference in rutile, anatase and brookite is due to the manner in which these octahedra bond to each other. The octahedron possesses a body centered Ti^{4+} ion surrounded by six O^{2-} ions. The Ti – Ti distance is greater and Ti – O distance is shorter in anatase than those in rutile.

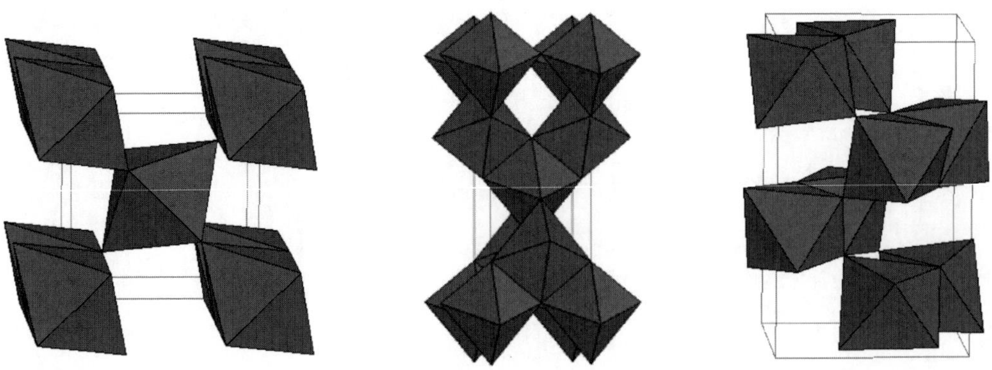

Figure 13. Structure of TiO_2 in rutile, anatase, and brookite phases (left to right). Only the oxygen octahedra are shown. Ti^{4+} ions are inside the oxygen octahedra.

The photocatalytic efficiency of TiO_2 depends on the photons received and the transit time for the charge to diffuse to the surface. Therefore, minimizing the particle size is a method to increase the efficiency. The decrease in particle size also results in an increased surface area, which further enhances the photocatalytic activity since the redox reaction takes place on the materials surface. However, when the size of TiO_2 goes to the nano-range, the quantum size effect (bandgap enlargement) and the particle agglomeration become significant. Therefore, there exists an optimal particle size for photocatalytic redox reaction. The electrochemical anodic TiO_2 provides such a choice since the size of nanotubes is tunable by using different anodization conditions. Moreover, the nanostructure obtained by anodization is stable even after heat treatment at 450°C, which releases the problem of particle agglomeration. Hence the electrochemical anodic TiO_2 is a better photocatalyst of choice than TiO_2 in other forms (powders or thin films).

APPLICATIONS

The properties of functional materials are strongly dependent on their microstructure. Anodic TiO_2 nanotubes have good mechanical adhesion strength and electronic conductivity. Particular advantages of regular tube arrays are the large surface area and the defined geometry. The defined geometry results in special diffusion paths not only for entering the tubular depth (e.g., reactants to be transported to the tube bottom) but also for species to be transported through the tube wall (e.g., electrons, holes and ions). Therefore, nanotubular TiO_2 is expected to have great potential applications in electronics, optics, catalysis, energy storage/conversion, and biomedicine, etc.

Water Purification

Anodic TiO_2 as a photocatalyst can be applied in water purification under UV or visible light irradiation. Quan *et al.* reported the environmental application of anodic TiO_2 layer (average tube diameter of ~60 nm and tube length of ~400 nm) as a photoelectrode [58], where pentachlorophenol in aqueous solution can be degraded under UV irradiation. A significant synergistic effect was observed in photoelectrochemical process. However, the effects of nanotube structures, crystallinity, tube diameter, tube length, and wall thickness on the photocatalytic activity were ignored in their report.

Lai *et al.* and Liang *et al.* investigated the effects of morphologies and structures on the photocatalytic activity of TiO_2 with details [59, 60]. It was observed that the morphology, crystal structure, and nanotube structure (including tube length, diameter, and wall thickness) have a significant influence on the photocatalytic activity of TiO_2 nanotubes. Liang *et al.* further compared the photocatalytic activity of anodic TiO_2 nanotube films and traditional sol-gel processed TiO_2 films [61, 62]. Two experiments were conducted under the same conditions with an initial 2,3-DCP concentration of 20 mg L^{-1} and initial pH of 5.3. The results showed that the photocatalytic degradation of 2,3-dichlorophenol using TiO_2 nanotube films was 2.6 times faster than that using traditional TiO_2 films. It is well known that when TiO_2 semiconductor is irradiated by UV light, electrons and holes are generated, but could recombine immediately. To increase the lifetime of electron-hole pairs, they need to be either trapped in some metal-stable states or migrate to the semiconductor surface separately. The nanotube array architecture of the anodic TiO_2 film with a wall thickness of 28 nm ensures that the holes are never generated far from the semiconductor–electrolyte interface because the wall thickness is much less than the minority carrier diffusion length of $L_p \approx 100$ nm in TiO_2 [63], thus the separation of charge carrier takes place efficiently. In addition, the hollow feature of nanotubes enables the electrolyte species to permeate the entire internal and external surfaces. Paulose *et al.* suggested that this could cause the holes to reach the electrolyte surface through diffusion [64], which takes place on a time scale of picoseconds, and finally also reduce the bulk recombination of electron-hole pairs.

Recently, Zhang et al. investigated the degradation of azo dye, methyl orange in aqueous solution with sonophotoelectrocatalytic process [65], where TiO_2 nanotubes were used as electrode in photoelectrocatalytic (PEC), sonophotoelectrocatalytic (SPEC) processes or as photocatalyst in photocatalytic (PC), sonophotocatalytic (SPC) processes. Experimental results showed that under the optimized experimental conditions, the rate constants of decolorization of dye were 0.0732 min^{-1} for SPEC process; 0.0523 min^{-1} for PEC process, 0.0073 min^{-1} for SPC process and 0.0035 min^{-1} for PC process, respectively. The rate constants indicate that there exist a synergistic effect in the ultrasonic, electro-assisted and photocatalytic processes.

To make TiO_2 nanotubes photocatalytic active under visible light, several different surface modifications have been proposed and employed. However, there were quite limited reports on the application in water purification because these visible-induced photocatalysts used in water system should be nontoxic, non-photocorrosible, highly photochemical stable and highly effective. Recently, Liang and Li developed a visible-induced photocatalyst with polymer sensitized-TiO_2 nanotube arrays for the degradation of organic pollutants in water [66]. When polymer (polythiophene) was deposited with a suitable amount on/in TiO_2 nanotubes, the obtained composites showed a strong photoresponse in the visible region at 500 nm and a significant photocatalytic activity under visible light irradiation. Interestingly, they also found that side-chains of polythiophene could influence the photocatalytic activity of TiO_2 nanotubes significantly in an order from high to low as poly3-methylthiophene ≈ polythiophene > polythiophenecarboxylic acid > poly3-hexylthiophene. The results may provide useful information for further development of some effective polymer-semiconductor catalysts for pollutant degradation under sunlight irradiation for water and wastewater treatment.

In summary, the immobilized TiO_2 nanotube film used as a photocatalyst for the removal of organic and inorganic contaminants in water has earned much attention. The ordered and interconnected nanotube architecture offers the potential for improved electron transport leading to higher photo-efficiency. A variety of TiO_2 nanotubes are in various stages of research and development, each possessing unique functionality, and the system of TiO_2 nanotubes combined with other advanced oxidation technologies is potentially applicable to the remediation of industrial effluents, groundwater, surface water and drinking water.

Water Splitting to Produce Hydrogen

Hydrogen produced from water using solar light is a clean, renewable, and sustainable energy source, which will be a critical breakthrough with respect to the rising concern of environmental pollution caused by the use of fossil fuels. Intensive efforts have been made to achieve this goal for the last 30 years. Its technique relies on the using of a light sensitive material to harness the power of the sunlight to split water into oxygen and hydrogen gases. TiO_2 has been frequently studied for water splitting and has shown promising results. Particularly, TiO_2 nanotube arrays have several advantages for the production of hydrogen. For example, (1) due to light scattering within a porous structure, incident photons are more effectively absorbed than on a flat electrode; (2) the architecture of TiO_2 nanotube array results in a large specific surface area in close proximity to the electrolyte, thus enabling photogenerated holes to be diffusively transported to oxidizable species in the electrolyte; (3) typical structure size of TiO_2 nanotube array, i.e., half of the tube wall thickness, is generally less than 20 nm, which is below the retrieval length of crystalline TiO_2 powders [67]. Hence bulk recombination is greatly suppressed and the quantum yield is enhanced.

Grimes and co-workers reported the photocleavage of water with highly ordered TiO_2 nanotube arrays under UV irradiation [27]. They found that the nanotube wall thickness is a key parameter influencing the magnitude of the photoanodic response and the overall efficiency of the water-splitting reaction. For TiO_2 nanotubes with 22 nm inner pore diameter and 34 nm wall thickness, upon UV (320-400 nm) illumination at an intensity of 100 mW/cm^2, hydrogen can be generated at a normalized power-time rate of 960 μmol/hW (24 mL/hW) with an overall conversion efficiency of 6.8%. They claimed that this hydrogen generation rate is the highest reported for a titania-based photoelectrochemical cell.

They further developed highly efficient, easily fabricated materials for the solar generation of hydrogen by water photoelectrolysis. Here, they modified the bandgap of TiO_2 by in-situ doping or surface modifications [64, 68] so that the resulted nanotubes become photocatalytically active to visible light.

Also, Yin *et al.* fabricated a core/sheath heterostructured CdS/TiO_2 nanotube array electrode by ac deposition of CdS to anodic TiO_2 nanotube arrays and used it in photoelectrochemical water-splitting [69]. They claimed that the core/sheath heterostructured CdS/TiO_2 nanotube electrode plays a critical role in the photoelectrochemical splitting of water under solar irradiation. Firstly, CdS, having a bandgap of 2.4 eV, made the composite electrode more responsive to the visible spectrum. Secondly, the core/sheath structure of CdS/TiO_2 increased the total absorption of solar light and improved charge separation by increasing contact area between CdS and TiO_2. Thirdly, the columnar structure of TiO_2 nanotubes facilitated electron transport to the back conductor. The maximum photocurrent density was obtained when the nanotube length was 2.5 μm.

In practice, improving the quantum efficiency for photocatalytic water splitting for solar H_2 production is still a key research challenge. Reported quantum efficiencies to date are relatively modest. Besides developing new materials absorbing more visible light, increasing the photogeneration and utilization of the charge carriers is of particular interest. Mohapatra *et al.* has reported a double-sided TiO_2 nanotube arrays for high volume hydrogen generation by water splitting [70]. These double-sided $TiO_2/Ti/TiO_2$ materials are used as both photoanode (carbon-doped titania nanotubes) and cathode (Pt nanoparticles dispersed on TiO_2 nanotubes; $PtTiO_2/Ti/PtTiO_2$) in a specially designed photoelectrochemical cell to generate hydrogen. The experimental results showed that the double-sided TiO_2 nanotube photoanode with a surface area of 16 cm^2 possesses good photoactivity to generate a high volume of hydrogen (38 mL/h) under the illumination of solar spectrum on both sides of the photoanode. This approach can be used for large-scale hydrogen generation using renewable energy sources.

Solar Cells

In the field of photovoltaics, dye-sensitized solar cells (DSSCs) have been investigated extensively as potential alternatives to conventional silicon solar cells because it is a relatively low-cost solar cell technology by using wide-bandgap nanocrystalline TiO_2 sensitized with sensitizing dyes. For example, Adachi *et al.* has fabricated DSSCs with electrodes composed of 4 μm-thick disordered single crystalline TiO_2 nanotubes (10 nm in diameter and 30-300 nm in length) using molecular assemblies to obtain an efficiency of 4.88% [71]. By using ruthenium complexes through novel molecular design, Nazeeruddin *et al.* and Chiba *et al.* have reported an efficiency over 11% [72], which is far below that of silicon solar cells with efficiency up to 24.7% [73]. Therefore, an enhancement of DSSCs efficiency is required for this technology to become commercially viable.

The slow percolation of electrons through a random polycrystalline network and the poor absorption of low energy photons by available dyes are two of the major factors limiting further improvement in the photoconversion efficiency achievable using nanocrystalline dye-sensitized solar cells. There are at least two obvious reasons to use TiO_2 nanotube array as the photoelectrode. Firstly, the large surface area of the hollow nanotubes enables efficient light harvesting, maximizing the amount of photogenerated charges. Secondly, electron transport along nanotubes is enhanced due to reduced scattering at grain boundaries or structural disorders as compared to polycrystalline electrodes. An ordered and strongly interconnected nanoscale photoanode architecture offers the potential for improved electron transport leading to higher photoefficiency [74].

However, recent work shows that the anodic TiO_2 nanotube-DSSCs have a poorer light-to-electricity conversion efficiency than that of the nanoparticle type. For example, Macák *et al.* reported an incident photon-to-photocurrent efficiency ($IPCE_{max}$) of 3.3% when using dye (N3)-sensitized anodic TiO_2 nanotubes (540 nm in length) as photoelectrodes [75]. Grimes and co-workers compared the efficiency of front-side illuminated and back-side illuminated nanotube-array DSSCs that were sensitized by a self-assembled monolayer of dye N719 [76]. The front-side illuminated DSSCs showed an efficiency of 4.7% although the transparent nanotube-array negative electrode is only 360 nm thick. The back-side illuminated DSSCs showed a solar conversion efficiency of only 4.4%. The photoconversion efficiency can be increased to 6.9% if very long nanotube arrays, up to 220 μm-length were used in back-side illuminated dye-sensitized solar cells [77].

Comparison between the nanoparticle and nanotube-array DSSCs indicates that more efforts must be under way to improve the photoconversion efficiency of nanotube-array DSSCs. To improve the efficiency of TiO_2 nanotube-array based DSSCs, it is necessary to find optimum device architectures that enhance light absorption by controlling the dye aggregation on nanotubular TiO_2 electrodes and by determining appropriate dimensions of the nanotube structure that leads to higher surface area for more dye coverage. In fact, voltage-decay measurements indicate that the highly ordered TiO_2 nanotube arrays, in comparison to nanoparticle systems, have superior electron lifetimes and provide excellent pathways for electron percolation [74]. The researchers suggested that remarkable photoconversion efficiency may be obtained, possibly to the ideal limit of ~31% for a single photosystem scheme, with optimum of the nanotube-array length.

Chemical Sensors

Chemical sensors are of critical importance for industrial process control, medical diagnosis, and ensuring of a safe environment. For example, hydrogen sensors have been widely used in the chemical, petroleum and semiconductor industries. They have also been used as diagnostic tools to monitor certain types of bacterial infections in infants. Since hydrogen is flammable and explosive, sensors are needed to detect hydrogen leakage. However, one problem often found in hydrogen sensors is that those sensors often become contaminated or poisoned, which eventualy limit their lifetime and genarate false signals. Typically, the more sensitive the sensor, the more susceptible to contamination it is [78]. A sensor should be able to self-clean and recover from environmental insult.

Grimes and co-workers have reported a self-cleaning, room-temperature TiO_2-nanotube hydrogen gas sensor [78] as schmatically shown in Fig. 14. The hydrogen sensor comprises an array of 22-nm inner-diameter TiO_2 nanotubes 200 nm in length coated with a 12-nm palladium layer. This sensor can be self-cleaned with exposure to UV light and fully recovered to its initial properties after being contaminated by either motor oil and/or stearic acid. The response to hydrogen of the sensor is dramatic, with a 3-order-of-magnitude change in electrical resistance upon exposure to 1000 ppm hydrogen at 25 °C. Further improvement on the sensor was made by coating TiO_2 with Pd and Pt so that it could selectively detect H_2 [79]. Sensor made by this method had a wide dynamic range for H_2 concentration from less than 20 to 1000 ppm and had a room temperature 90% response time of approximately 10 to 20 s. The electrical resistance of the TiO_2 nanotubes was changed by almost 7 orders of magnitude upon exposure to 1000 ppm H_2.

Besides the use in hydrogen sensors, anodic TiO_2 nanotube arrays have also attracted great interest in their sensing behavior for other gases, such as oxygen, carbon monoxide, carbon dioxide and even ammonia. Recently, the demands for oxygen sensors are rapidly increasing. Oxygen concentration is one of the most widely used parameters in many fields, such as the controlling of the air/fuel mixture in automobile engines [80]. Lu *et al.* has investigated the oxygen sensing properties of amorphous and anatase TiO_2 nanotube arrays at low temperatures over a wide range of oxygen concentrations [81]. The as-prepared amorphous TiO_2 nanotubes show remarkable recoverable responses to oxygen at a low temperature of 50 °C. At 100 °C the sensing properties (sensitivity, recovery, linear correlation with oxygen concentration and response range) are the best and the lowest detectable concentration is 200 ppm. These results demonstrated that amorphous TiO_2 nanotubes can be very promising candidates for oxygen sensors, particularly at low temperatures.

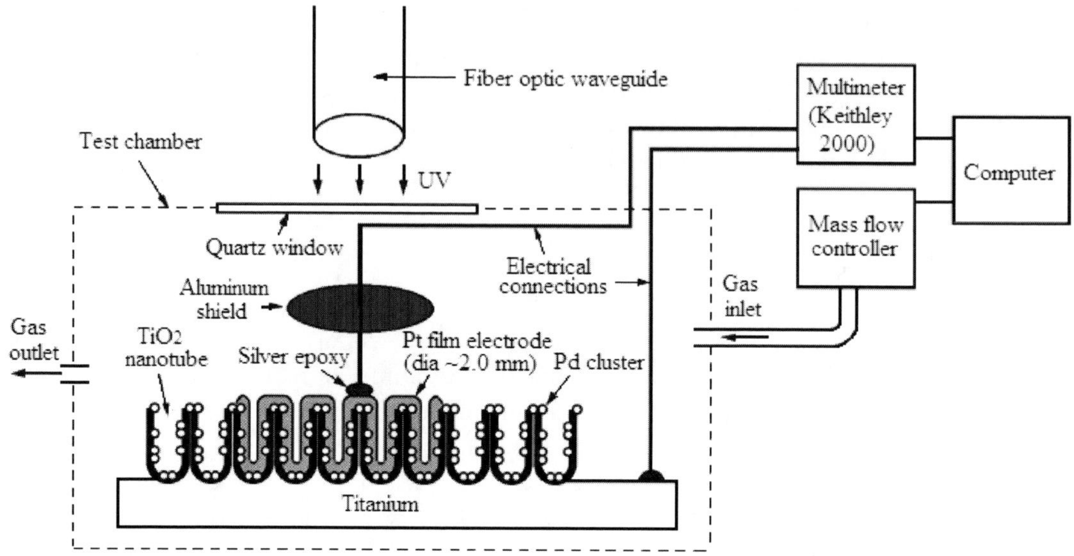

Figure 14. Schematic diagram of experimental set up used for investigating the self-cleaning capability of the TiO_2-based room temperature hydrogen gas sensor [79].

TiO_2 nanotube array based sensors have also been used for chemical oxygen demand (COD) determination. COD is frequently used as an important index for controlling the operation of wastewater treatment plants, wastewater effluent monitoring, and taxation of wastewater pollution. Zheng *et al.* have found that TiO_2 nanotube array sensors exhibit good accuracy, stability, and reproducibility in the determination of COD [82]. Coupled with the potential for rapid analysis and minimization of secondary pollution, the nanotube sensors might be practical devices for online monitoring and controlling of environmental pollutants.

Biomedical Applications

Due to their good mechanical properties and biochemical compatibility, anodic TiO_2 nanotube arrays start to receive great attention in biomedical applications, such as, apatite growth, cell interactions, and biosensing, etc.

TiO_2 nanotubes have been thought to be a novel material for improving bioactivity of titanium [83]. To evaluate the potential use of such nanotube layer as a coating for biomedical implants, Tsuchiya *et al.* have examined the growth of hydroxyapatite on TiO_2 nanotube layers upon exposure to a simulated body fluid (SBF) [84]. In their experiment, the nanotube layers (with a tube diameter of 100 nm and a length of 2 μm) significantly enhanced apatite formation. While by contrast, on a flat TiO_2 compact layer, no apatite was formed even after 14 days soaking in SBF. Interestingly, the apatite coverage of the nanotube layer was dependent on the nanotube length, which was attributed to a different surface roughness of the nanotubes influencing the nucleation of hydroxyapatite precipitation.

Recently, Oh *et al.* have investigated the effects of incorporated chemical species in the anodic TiO_2 nanotube layer on the formation of bioactive apatite in biological fluid [85]. They have found that the ions incorporated on the anodic TiO_2 surface acted as preferential nucleation sites for calcium phosphate by interaction with Ca^{2+} ion in the biological fluid. The anodic oxide films formed at higher additive content demonstrated a higher precipitation capability of the bioactive Ca–P compounds. Furthermore, Ma *et al.* have proved that the precalcification (Pre-Ca) procedure can be effective to accelerate the precipitation of hydroxyapatite on the TiO_2 nanotubes, thus improving their bioactivity [83].

Recently, cell interactions with TiO_2 nanotubes have been studied and results have shown that cell adhesion, proliferation and migration are all dependent on the diameter of nanotubes [86]. Clearly, geometries with a spacing of approximately 15 nm were most stimulating for cell growth and differentiation, whereas nanotube diameters greater than 100 nm led to a dramatically reduced cellular activity and a high extent of programmed cell death.

The interaction of biomaterials with adjacent host tissues has been reported to be directly related to surface properties like morphology, contact angle and surface energy, which can cause a significant change in cell adhesion, proliferation, and differentiation in vitro [87, 88]. In general, low contact angle and high surface energy are beneficial to bone cell attachment and proliferation on surfaces of TiO_2 nanotube arrays. The use of anodic TiO_2 nanotube layers for the photocatalytic killing of cancer cells has also been investigated [89]. Upon low dose of UV irradiation, the cancer cells cultured on the nanotube layer reduced their shape and size and a significant amount of the dead cells was found.

Recently, by embedding glucose oxidases inside TiO_2 nanotube channels and electropolymerizing pyrrole for interfacial immobilization we have constructed a biosensor for amperometric detection and quantitative determination of glucose in a phosphate buffer solution (pH 6.8) under a potentiostatic condition (−0.4V versus SCE) [90]. Promising results are obtained with a response time below 5.6 s and a detection limit of 2.0×10^{-3} mM.

Future Perspectives

Other applications of anodic TiO_2 nanotubes involve power storage devices. Lithium-ion batteries have emerged as power sources for modern electronics because of their high specific energy and no memory effect [91]. TiO_2 nanotubes are found to be very promising as electrodes in lithium-ion battery because of their high capacity, low cost, and harmless property. However, the low lithium ion (Li^+) insertion and poor electronic conductivity of TiO_2 nanotubes are still the main obstacles for their application. Conductive fillers are frequently added to lithium-ion battery electrode to construct conductive network and to compensate for the low electronic conductivity of active electrode material like $LiMn_2O_4$ [92]. The conductive network can also increase the battery power and fast charge–discharge performance. To improve the electronic conductivity and charge–discharge capacity, Fang *et al.* have loaded Ag nanoparticles onto TiO_2 nanotubes and a good electrochemical performance of Li-ion batteries has been achieved [93].

Recently, we have explored the use of anodic TiO_2 nanotube layers as electrodes for electrochemical capacitors [94]. Nickel oxide was incorporated into the TiO_2 nanotubes, with nickel-to-titanium atom ratio being 9.6 at% and 36.4 at%, respectively, for redox capacitance application. The experimental results showed that the corresponding specific redox capacitance was 26 and 85 mF/cm^2 with highly reversible charge–discharge stability, respectively. The superior redox capacitance achieved was thought to be resulted from the highly accessible reaction sites of NiO inside TiO_2 nanotube arrays.

Anti-fogging applications of TiO_2 nanotube layers have also been exploited recently. TiO_2 itself is a hydrophilic material. Roughening the surface of TiO_2 nanotubes may cause it to become superhydrophilic because of the reduced contact area between the water and solid surface. Chen *et al.* have demonstrated that anodic TiO_2 nanotubes display a superhydrophilic property such that water drops spread out quickly over the tube surface [95]. In contrast, the contact angle decreases to zero after UV radiation was applied on the surface for several minutes. Therefore, the ordered TiO_2 nanotube arrays with a great surface area exhibit a superhydrophilic nature and can act as a promising material for anit-fogging applications.

A potential application of TiO_2 nanotubes is photochromic switching. By depositing noble metal (e.g. Ag) nanoparticles on the TiO_2 nanotubes, a material that shows considerable photochromic contrast can be created [96]. The applications of TiO_2 nanotubes can significantly be expanded, if secondary material can be uniformly deposited into the tubes. This is a key step towards magnetic nanotube materials, solid junction solar cells, water splitting, or biomedical release systems.

CONCLUSION

In this chapter we have given a comprehensive review on the recent progress in the synthesis and applications of electrochemical anodic TiO_2 nanostructures. Due to the multifunational properties of TiO_2 itself, anodic TiO_2 nanostructures are attracting more and more research attention. There are still plenty of rooms to play with the anodic TiO_2 nanostructures if judged from the current performance of the materials and what is the expected from the materials and their nanostructures.

ACKNOWLEDGMENT

This work has been supported by the Research Grants Council of the Hong Kong Special Administrative Region, China (Project No.: PolyU5166/05E) and the Hong Kong Polytechnic University (Projects No.: A-PA6A, G-YE50, G-YG85, and G-YE68).

REFERENCES

[1] Huang, H.; Yang, Y. *Comp. Sci. Tech.* 2008, *68*, 2948-2953.
[2] Zhang, Y.; Ke, S.; Huang, H.; Zhao, L.; Yu, L.; Chan, H. L. W. *Appl. Phys. Lett.* 2008, *92*, 052910.
[3] Zhang, Y.; Li, Y.; Li, G.; Huang, H.; Chan, H. L. W.; Daoud, W. A.; Xin, J. H.; Li, L. *Chem. Mater.* 2007, *19*, 1939-1945.
[4] Hu, Y.; Tan, O. K.; Pan, J. S.; Huang, H.; Cao, W. *Sensors & Actuators B* 2005, *108*, 244-249.
[5] Pan, L. K.; Huang, H.; Sun, C. Q. *J. Appl. Phys.* 2003, *94*, 2695-2697.

[6] Sun, C. Q.; Wang, Y.; Tay, B. K.; Li, S.; Huang, H.; Zhang, Y. B. *J. Phys. Chem. B* 2002, *106*, 10701-10705.
[7] Sun, C. Q.; Chen, T. P.; Tay, B. K.; Li, S.; Huang, H.; Zhang, Y. B.; Pan, L. K.; Lau, S. P.; Sun, X. W. *J. Phys. D: Appl. Phys.* 2001, *34*, 3470-3479.
[8] Sun, C. Q.; Sun, X. W.; Tay, B. K.; Lau, S. P.; Huang, H.; Li, S. *J. Phys. D: Appl. Phys.* 2001, *34*, 2359-2362.
[9] Huang, H.; Sun, C. Q.; Tianshu, Z.; Hing, P. *Phys. Rev. B* 2001, *63*, 184112.
[10] Ye, H.; Sun, C. Q.; Huang, H.; Hing, P. *Appl. Phys. Lett.* 2001, *78*, 1826-1828.
[11] Huang, H.; Sun, C. Q.; Hing, P. *J. Phys.: Condens. Matter* 2000, *12*, L127-L132.
[12] Sun, C. Q.; Sun, X. W.; Gong, H. Q.; Huang, H.; Ye, H.; Jin, D.; Hing, P. *J. Phys.: Condens. Matter* 1999, ***11***, L547-L550.
[13] Fujishima, A.; Honda, K. *Nature* 1972, *238*, 37-38.
[14] O'Regan, B.; Gratzel, M. *Nature* 1991, *353*, 737-740.
[15] Hoffmann, M. R.; Martin, S. T.; Choi, W.; Bahnemann, D. W. *Chem. Rev.* 1995, *95*, 69-96.
[16] Varghese, O. K.; Gong, D.; Paulose, M.; Ong, K. G.; Grimes, C. A. *Sensors and Actuators B* 2003, *93*, 338-344.
[17] Ghicov, A.; Tsuchiya, H.; Hahn, R.; Macak, J. M.; Munoz, A. G. *Electrochem. Commun.* 2006, *8*, 528-532.
[18] Iuchi, K.-i.; Ohko, Y.; Tatsuma, T.; Fujishima, A. *Chem. Mater.* 2004, *16*, 1165-1167.
[19] Balaur, E.; Macak, J. M.; Taveira, L.; Schmuki, P. *Electrochem. Commun.* 2005, *7*, 1066-1070.
[20] Oh, S. H.; Finones, R. R.; Daraio, C.; Chen, L. H.; Jin S. *Biomaterials* 2005, *26*, 4938-4943.
[21] Lu, J. G.; Chang, P.; Fan, Z. *Mater. Sci. Eng. R* 2006, *52*, 49-91.
[22] Keller, F.; Hunter, M. S.; Robinson, D. L. *J. Electrochem. Soc.* 1953, *100*, 411-419.
[23] Masuda, H.; Fukuda, K. *Science* 1995, *268*, 1466-1468.
[24] Gong, D.; Grimes, C. A.; Varghese, O. K.; Hu, W.; Singh, R. S.; Chen, Z.; Dickey, E. C. *J. Mater. Res.* 2001, *16,* 3331-3334.
[25] Beranek, R.; Hildebrand, H.; Schmuki, P. *Electrochem. Solid-State Lett.* 2003, *6,* B12-B14.
[26] Ruan, C.; Paulose, M.; Varghese, O. K.; Grimes, C. A. *Sol. Energy Mater. Sol. Cells* 2006, *90,* 1283-1295.
[27] Mor, G. K.; Shankar, K.; Paulose, M.; Varghese, O. K.; Grimes, C. A. *Nano Lett.* 2005, *5,* 191-195.
[28] Xie, Y.; Zhou, L. M.; Huang, H. *Mater. Lett.* 2006, *60,* 3558-3560.
[29] Cai, Q.; Paulose, M.; Varghese, O. K.; Grimes, C. A. *J. Mater. Res.* 2005, *20,* 230-236.
[30] Macák, J. M.; Tsuchiya, H.; Taveira, L.; Aldabergerova, S.; Schmuki, P. *Angew. Chem., Int. Ed.* 2005, *44,* 7463-7465.
[31] Tsuchiya, H.; Macak, J. M.; Taveira, L.; Balaur, E.; Ghicov, A.; Sirotna, K.; Schmuki, P. *Electrochem. Commun.* 2005, *7,* 576-580.
[32] Macák, J. M.; Tsuchiya, H.; Schmuki, P. *Angew. Chem., Int. Ed.* 2005, *44,* 2100-2102.
[33] Macák, J. M.; Schmuki, P. *Electrochim. Acta* 2006, *52,* 1258-1264.
[34] Paulose, M.; Shankar, K.; Yoriya, S.; Prakasam, H. E.; Varghese, O. K.; Mor, G. K.; Latempa, T. A.; Fitzgerald, A.; Grimes, C. A. *J. Phys. Chem. B* 2006, *110,* 16179-16184.

[35] Albu, S. P.; Ghicov, A.; Macak, J. M.; Schmuki, P. *Phys. Stat. Sol. (RRL)* 2007, *1,* R65-R67.
[36] Prakasam, H. E.; Shankar, K.; Paulose, M.; Varghese, O. K.; Grimes, C. A. *J. Phys. Chem. C* 2007, *111,* 7235-7241.
[37] Zhang, G.; Huang, H.; Zhang, Y.; Chan, H. L. W.; Zhou, L. *Electrochem. Commun.* 2007, *9,* 2854-2858.
[38] Lim, J. H.; Choi, J. *Small* 2007, *3,* 1504-1507.
[39] Albu, S. P.; Kim, D.; Schmuki, P. *Angew. Chem. Int. Ed.* 2008, *47,* 1916-1919.
[40] Raja, K. S.; Misra, M.; Paramguru, K. *Electrochim. Acta* 2005, *51,* 154-165.
[41] Richter, C.; Wu, Z.; Panaitescu, E.; Willey, R. J.; Menon, L. *Adv. Mater.* 2007, *19,* 946-948.
[42] Nguyen, Q. A.; Bhargava, Y. V.; Devine, T. M. *Electrochem. Commun.* 2008, *10,* 471-475.
[43] Allam, N. K.; Grimes, C. A. *J. Phys. Chem. C* 2007, *111,* 13028-13032.
[44] Allam, N. K.; Shankar, K.; Grimes, C. A. *J. Mater. Chem.* 2008, *18,* 2341-2348.
[45] Hahn, R.; Macak, J. M.; Schmuki, P. *Electrochem. Commun.* 2007, *9,* 947-952.
[46] Ghicov, A.; Tsuchiya, H.; Macak, J. M.; Schmuki, P. *Electrochem. Commun.* 2005, *7,* 505-509.
[47] Bauer, S.; Kleber, S.; Schmuki, P. *Electrochem. Commun.* 2006, *8,* 1321-1325.
[48] Mohapatra, S. K.; Misra, M.; Mahajan, V. K.; Raja, K. S. *J. Catal.* 2007, *246,* 362-369.
[49] Shankar, K.; Mor, G. K.; Fitzgerald, A.; Grimes, C. A. *J. Phys. Chem. C* 2007, *111,* 21-26.
[50] Raja, K. S.; Gandhi, T.; Misra, M. *Electrochem. Commun.* 2007, *9,* 1069-1076.
[51] Mor, G. K.; Varghese, O. K.; Paulose, M.; Mukherjee, N.; Grimes, C. A. *J. Mater. Res.* 2003, *18,* 2588-2593.
[52] Macák, J. M.; Albu, S.; Kim, D. H.; Paramasivam, I.; Aldabergerova, S.; Schmuki, P. *Electrochem. Solid-State Lett.* 2007, *10,* K28-K31.
[53] Taveira, L. V.; Macak, J. M.; Tsuchiya, H.; Dick, L. F. P.; Schmuki, P. *J. Electrochem. Soc.* 2005, *152,* B405-B410.
[54] Allam, N. K.; Grimes, C. A. *Sol. Energy Mater. Sol. Cells* 2008, *92,* 1468-1475.
[55] Serpone, N. *J. Photochem. Photobio. A* 1997, *104*, 1-12.
[56] Ward, M. D.; White, J. R.; Bard, A. J. *J. Am. Chem. Soc.* 1983, *105*, 27-31.
[57] Grant, F. A. *Rev. Mod. Phys.* 1959, *31*, 646-674.
[58] Quan, X.; Yang, S.G.; Ruan, X. L.; Zhao, D. M. *Environ. Sci. Technol.* 2005, *39*, 3770-3775.
[59] Lai, Y. K.; Sun, L.; Chen, Y. C.; Zhuang, H. F.; Lin, C. J.; Chin, J. W. *J. Electrochem. Soc.* 2006, *153*, D123-127.
[60] Liang, H. C.; Li, X. Z. *J. Hazard Mater.* 2008, doi:10.1016/j.jhazmat.2008.06.033.
[61] Liang, H. C.; Li, X. Z.; Yang, Y. H.; Sze, K. H. *Chemosphere.* 2008, *73*, 805-812.
[62] Yu, J. G.; Zhao, X. J.; Zhao, Q. N. *Mater. Chem. Phys.* 2001, *69*, 25-29.
[63] Hamnett, A. *Faraday Discuss. Chem. Soc.* 1980, *70*, 127-134.
[64] Paulose, M.; Mor, G. K.; Varghese, O. K.; Shankar, K.; Grimes, C. A. *J. Photochem. Photobiol. A* 2006, *178*, 8-15.
[65] Zhang, Z. H.; Yuan, Y.; Liang, L. H.; Fang, Y. J.; Cheng, Y. X.; Ding, H. C.; Shi, G. Y.; Jin, L. T. *Ultrason. Sonochem.* 2008, *15*, 370-375.
[66] Liang, H. C.; Li, X. Z. *Appl. Catal. B* 2008, doi: 10.1016/j.apcatb.2008.07.015.

[67] Lubberhuizen, W. H.; Vanmaekelbergh, D.; Van Faassen, E. *J. Porous Mater.* 2000, *7*, 147-152.
[68] Mor, G. K.; Varghese, O. K.; Paulose, M.; Shankar, K.; Grimes, C. A. *Sol. Energ. Mater. Sol. Cells.* 2006, *90*, 2011–2075.
[69] Yin, Y. X.; Jin, Z. G.; Hou, F. *Nanotechnology* 2007, *18*, 495608.
[70] Mohapatra, S. K.; Mahajan, V. K.; Misra, M. *Nanotechnology* 2007, *18*, 445705.
[71] Adachi, M.; Murata, Y.; Okada, I.; Yoshikawa, S. *J. Electrochem. Soc.* 2003, *150*, G488-493.
[72] Nazeeruddin, M. K.; Angelis, F. D.; Fantacci, S.; Selloni, A.; Viscardi, G.; Liska, P.; Ito, S.; Takeru, B.; Grätzel, M. *J. Am. Chem. Soc.* 2005, *127*, 16835-16847.
[73] Frank, A. J.; Kopidakis, N.; van de Lagemaat, J. *Coord. Chem. Rev.* 2004, *248*, 1165-1179.
[74] Mor, G. K.; Shankar, K.; Paulose, M.; Varghese, O. K.; Grimes, C. A. *Nano Lett.* 2006, *6*, 215-218.
[75] Macák, J. M.; Tsuchiya, H.; Ghicov, A.; Schmuki, P. *Electrochem. Commun.* 2005, *7*, 1133–1137.
[76] Paulose, M.; Shankar, K.; Varghese, O. K.; Mor, G. K.; Grimes, C. A. *J. Phys. D: Appl. Phys.* 2006, *39*, 2498–2503.
[77] Shankar, K.; Mor, G. K.; Prakasam, H. E.; Yoriya, S.; Paulose, M.; Varghese, O. K.; Grimes, C. A. *Nanotechnology* 2007, *18*, 065707.
[78] Mor, G. K.; Varghese, O. K.; Paulose, M.; Grimes, C. A. *Sensor Lett.* 2003, *1*, 42-46.
[79] Varghese, O. K.; Mor, G .K.; Grimes, C. A.; Paulose, M.; Mukherjee, N. *J. Nanosci. Nanotechnol.* 2004, *4*, 733-737.
[80] Wu, M. T.; Yao, X.; Yuan, Z. H.; Sun, H. T.; Wu, W. C.; Chen, Q. H.; Xu, G. Y. *Sensor Actuat. B* 1993, *14*, 491.
[81] Lu, H. F.; Li, F.; Liu, G.; Chen, Z. G.; Wang, D. W.; Fang, H. T.; Lu, G. Q.; Jiang, Z. H.; Cheng, H. M. *Nanotechnology* 2008, *19*, 405504.
[82] Zheng, Q.; Zhou, B. X.; Bai, J.; Li, L. H.; Jin, Z. J.; Zhang, J. L.; Li, J. H.; Liu, Y. B.; Cai, W. M.; Zhu, X. Y. *Adv. Mater.* 2008, *20*, 1044-1049.
[83] Ma, Q. Q.; Li, M. H.; Hu, Z. Y.; Chen, Q.; Hu, W. Y. *Mater. Lett.* 2008, *62*, 3035–3038.
[84] Tsuchiya, H.; Macák, J. M.; Müller, L.; Kunze, J.; Müller, F.; Greil, P.; Virtanen, S.; Schmuki, P. *J. Biomed. Mater. Res.* 2006, *77*, 534-541.
[85] Oh, H. J.; Lee, J. H.; Kim, Y. J.; Suh, S. J.; Lee, J. H.; Chi, C. S. *Mater. Chem. Phys.* 2008, *109*, 10-14.
[86] Park, J.; Bauer, S.; Von der Mark, K.; Schmuki, P. *Nano Lett.* 2007, *7*, 1686-1691.
[87] Das, K.; Bose, S.; Bandyopadhyay, A. *J. Biomed. Mater. Res.* 2008, doi: 10.1002/jbm.a.32088.
[88] Das, K.; Bandyopadhyay, A.; Bose, S. *J. Am. Ceram. Soc.* 2008, *91*, 2808-2814.
[89] Kalbacova, M.; Macák, J. M.; Schmidt-Stein, F.; Mierke, C. T.; Schmuki, P. *Phys. Stat. Sol.* 2008, *2*, 194-196.
[90] Xie, Y. B.; Zhou, L.; Huang, H. *Biosens. Bioelectron.* 2007, *22*, 2812-2818.
[91] Son, J. T.; Park, K. S.; Kim, H. G.; Chung, H. T. *J. Power Sources* 2004, *126*, 182-185.
[92] Huang, S. H.; Wen, Z. Y.; Yang, X. L.; Gua, Z. H.; Xu, X. H. *J. Power Sources* 2005, *148*, 72-77.
[93] Fang, D.; Huang, K. L.; Liu, S. Q.; Li, Z. J. *J. Alloys Comp.* 2008, *464*, L5-9.

[94] Xie, Y.; Zhou, L.; Huang, C.; Huang, H.; Lu, J. *Electrochim. Acta* 2008, *53*, 3643-3649.
[95] Chen, C. C.; Lin, J. S.; Diau, E. G.; Liu, T. F. *Appl. Phys. A* 2008, *92*, 615-620.
[96] Paramasivam, I.; Macák, J. M.; Ghicov, A.; Schmuki, P. *Chem. Phys. Lett.* 2007, *445*, 233-237.

In: Nanostructured Materials for Electrochemical Biosensors ISBN: 978-1-60741-706-4
Editors: U. Yogeswaran; S. Kumar; S. Chen ©2009 Nova Science Publishers, Inc.

Chapter 10

ACETYLCHOLINESTERASE - NANOMATERIALS HYBRID SENSORS FOR THE DETECTION OF ORGANOPHOSPHOROUS AND CARBAMATE PESTICIDES

Periasamy Arun Prakash , Umasankar Yogeswaran, and Shen-Ming Chen*

National Taipei University of Technology, Taipei, Taiwan.

ABSTRACT

In the past decades, development of electrochemical enzyme sensors is of much interest, since they posse's great compatibility, good stability with much low cost of production. This review majorly focuses on nanomaterial based acetylcholinesterase (AChE) sensors which belongs to the category of pesticide sensors in which the enzyme AChE is immobilized either onto glassy carbon, screen printed carbon, gold or graphite electrode surfaces. The enzyme activity is majorly affected by the traces of organophosphorus (OP) and carbamate (CA) pesticides existing in the environment. Detection of these pesticides in trace amounts is essential and it is achieved efficiently by the use of AChE sensors. These pesticide compounds are detected quantitatively by measure of AChE inhibition activity. This is usually carried out by measuring the electrooxidation current of thiocholine generated by the AChE catalyzed hydrolysis of acetylthiocholine (ATCh). In few sensors, residual activity of the enzyme is compared with the initial activity. The working electrode surface shows a dramatic enhancement with lowest detection limit of pesticides when modified with carbon nano tubes (CNTs), gold nano particles, silica nano particles and sol-gel matrix respectively.

Keywords: acetylcholinesterase, electrochemical sensors, organophosphate, carbamate, pesticide, thiocholine, acetylthiocholine, nano materials

---

* Fax: +886 2270 25238; Tel: +886 2270 17147, E-mail: smchen78@ms15.hinet.net

1. INTRODUCTION

Acetylcholinesterase (AChE) is an important enzyme present in the neuromuscular junctions of central nervous system of human beings. It converts the neurotransmitter acetylcholine into inactive choline and acetic acid and thus facilitates the proper functioning of muscular system [1]. However, this major function of AChE is inhibited by organophosphorus (OP) and carbamate (CA) pesticides present in the environment [2]. OP compounds have their extensive applications in agriculture, medicine, industry and chemical warfare agents. [3]. On the other hand, CA compounds are increasingly used instead of organochlorine and organophosphorous pesticides due to their lower environmental persistence. Moreoever, OP and CA undergo both reversible and irreversible reaction with the active site of AChE, which blocks the nervous transmission impulse. This may be due to the reason that OP compounds have much tendency to form stable complex with AChE and inhibits the enzyme phosphorylation and enzyme activity [4]. This overall leads to the accumulation of choline in the muscular tissues and eventually paves way to severe muscular paralysis. Consequently, more attention has been paid to develop highly precise instruments to monitor trace quantity of OP and CA compounds in the environment. Though liquid chromatography was employed in the past for pesticide determination [5], nevertheless it consumes more time and requires expensive equipment, highly trained personnel, complicated sample pretreatments and is not suitable for field conditions.

Alternatively, electrochemical enzyme sensors possess high sensitivity, long term stability, short time response, simple and low cost detection capabilities for biological binding events [6]. These properties have made electrochemical enzyme sensors extremely suitable for sensitive pesticide determination. In such enzyme based sensors, detection is based on the irreversible inhibition of AChE activity by OP and CA pesticides [7]. The degree of inhibition has been calculated by comparing the residual activity of the enzyme with the initial activity [4]. However, the enzyme immobilization techniques remain to be rather complicated and involve complex matrices [8]. The enzyme incorporated into certain mediator modified matrices also exhibit less stability [9]. Further, the reproducibility of the sensors after pesticide inhibition was poor in few AChE sensors. Thus in order to improve the stability of the immobilized enzyme, to achieve precise trace pesticide detection, AChE has been immobilized onto several nanomaterial matrices including carbon nanotubes (CNTs), gold nano particles (AuNPs) and silica nanoparticles, respectively. Those nanomaterial incorporated sensors exhibit excellent stability with very high sensitivity and even nM detection of pesticides like Malathion, carbofuran in real samples could be achieved with high accuracy. Interestingly in the recent years many nanomaterial based pesticide sensors were reported in the literature [10-20]. However, until now no one has presented a review on nanomaterial based pesticide sensors. In this chapter we have summarized the nanomaterial based pesticide sensors developed in the recent years for the selective determination of OP and CA pesticides.

2. Pesticide Sensors for OP and CA Detection

In the following section we discuss in detail about pesticide sensors type, different electrode materials used, various electrochemical techniques employed, advantages and limitations in measurements.

2.1. Mediator Free Screen Printed Electrode Based AChE Sensors

In this section, we discuss about the screen printed electrode (SPE) based AChE sensors for the selective determination of OP and CA pesticides. In the past decades, several attempts were made by the researchers to develop SPE based pesticide sensors, where the enzyme AChE was immobilized either directly onto the electrode or above other matrices incorporated SPE surfaces. Both approaches resulted in the good, rapid detection of OP and CA pesticides. Earlier, Hart et al. employed AChE/SPE to detect OP and CA pesticides [21]. They measured the enzyme activity from the rate of hydrolysis of acetylthiocholine iodide. Three polymers such as hydroxyethyl cellulose, dimethylaminoethyl methacrylate, and polyethyleneimine were used as enzyme immobilization matrices. Initially, electrodes were exposed to drops of water or pesticide solution, dried and their activity was screened after 24 h. They found that, when the enzyme matrix was hydroxyethyl cellulose, electrode activity inhibited both by water as well as by pesticides. While with co-polymer matrix, a significant response towards pesticides alone was observed. Further, the long-term storage stability of electrodes was highest when the enzyme matrix consisted of the co-polymer. The electrodes retained their activity for nearly one year. In contrast, the electrodes made of hydroxyethyl cellulose or polyethyleneimine possess less stability.

2.2. Mediator Modified Screen Printed Electrode Based AChE Sensors

Hernandez et al. developed a mediator modified AChE sensor with SPE and for the detection of OP and CA pesticides in river water samples [22]. The SPE surface was modified with a mediator, tetracyanoquinodimethane (TCNQ). In the absence of this mediator, the direct oxidation of thiocholine requires higher working potential (upto 680 mV). However, this working potential has been considerably lowered in the presences of mediator. In prior to each experiment, the SPE surface was coated either with 2 μl of a solution of 0.1 mM of TCNQ in acetonitrile or with 2 μl of a suspension containing 5 μl of 1 mM TCNQ solution in acetonitrile and 50 μl NF. The modified SPE was stored overnight at room temperature, in the presence of desiccant and used. The detection of OP and CA was based on the measurement of the degree of inhibition of AChE. About 50 μl of river water samples were added to 1 ml of 0.1 M PBS pH 7.5 with AChE (1 U ml^{-1}) and incubated for 10 min. Then 20 μl of the 0.5 mM acetylthiocholine (ATCh) solution was added. After 5 min, 100 μl of this solution was directly dropped on the surface of the modified SPE. The oxidation peak current obtained in DPV measurements was calculated as (I_2) and later it was compared with the oxidation current obtained without pesticide (I_1).

The percentage of inhibition (I %) was calculated using the following formula:

$$I\% = 100[(I_1 - I_2)/ I_1] \quad (1)$$

The scan speed, the pulse amplitude in DPV was optimized and an inhibition calibration curve was obtained using carbofuran as reference pesticide. The linear range was observed to be 1 nM to 1 μM. A lowest detection limit of 9 nM has been achieved using this AChE immobilized tetracyanoquinodimethane (TCNQ)/NF modified SPE. In the case of carbofuran contaminated water samples, the detection limit was observed to be 20 nM and the developed sensor has a good analytical performance in comparison with the results obtained by standard methods using gas chromatography coupled to a Finningan Mat 800 ion trap detector mass spectrometer (GC-ITDMS).

Suprun et al. also carried out a similar approach to immobilize AChE on SPE, but using prussian blue (PB) as mediator and glutaraldehyde as cross-linking agent [9]. Prior to modification, the SPE was pre-activated by polarization at 1.7 V vs. Ag/AgCl for 3 min. Then 5 μl of 0.1 M $K_3Fe(CN)_6$ in 0.01 M HCl were mixed with 5 μl of $FeCl_3$ solution of the same concentration and placed onto the working area of the electrodes. After 10 min, the pretreated SPE was washed with HCl and dried at 100°C for 90 min. AChE was immobilized onto this PB modified electrode by cross-linking with glutaraldehyde. In order to increase the stability of the working electrode, 2 μl of 0.1% nafion (NF) was casted onto the electrode surface and dried. Then a mixture with equal volumes of 0.2 U μl^{-1} AChE, 1% BSA, 1% glutaraldehyde and 0.1% NF were dropped above NF modified SPE, dried and used. CV results show that, PB modified electrodes show a pair of well defined redox couples at 0.2 V, in the presence and absence of AChE. This indicates the redox reaction of PB at the modified SPE. However, the redox peak height of PB found to decrease with the addition of thiocholine. The apparent value of Michaelis-Menten constant (K_m) app was calculated to be 0.84 ± 0.44 mmol l^{-1} for AChE immobilized electrode and for NF additional layer it has been observed to be 0.84 ± 2.0 mmol l^{-1}. However, this value corresponds to the value obtained with PB sensors for enzyme free conditions 0.4 ± 0.12 mmol l^{-1}. Moreover, this AChE/PB modified SPE detects pesticides like Aldicarb, Paraoxon and Parathion-Methyl with limits of detection 30, 10 and 5 ppb, respectively (incubation 10 min). All these pesticides showed strong inhibition towards AChE activity. In order to reduce the matrix interferences, the electrolysis of the grape juice with Al anode and evaporation of ethanol were experienced. However, these procedures decreased the sensitivity of pesticide detection and stability of the sample tested. The detection limit calculated after the electrolysis of diluted juice with Al anode was equal to 0.1 ppm for Parathion-Methyl and 1 ppm for Aldicarb. Thus after electrolysis, the AChE activity of spiked juice decreased to 20-30%. Blank and spiked samples of juices under fermentation were tested and the results show that no spontaneous reactivation of inhibited AChE was observed during the measurement conditions. Thus in PB presence the modified SPE showed improved response towards the detection of pesticides. Further, the working potential of thiocholine oxidation has been considerably decreased in the presence of PB.

2.3. Amperometric AChE Pesticide Sensors

This following section discusses in detail about the amperometric, flow injection analysis (FIA) accompanied AChE sensors for the determination of OP and CA pesticides. With such amperometric sensors lowest detection limit can be achieved with higher sensitivity. Khayyami et al. earlier developed a new type of amperometric sensor using reticulated vitreous carbon (RVC) alone or in the form of composite material composed of RVC and superporous agarose as working electrode [8]. This composite material possesses high electrical conductivity, high mechanical rigidity, large surface area and low pressure to liquid flow. 5 μM of Meldola's blue was used as mediator to lower the working potential. Moreover, the signals from unwanted electroactive compounds at those potentials can be avoided. In this study the enzyme AChE was immobilized either directly on the RVC surface or above the composite electrode surface containing superporous agarose gel structure. The schematic representation of a typical AChE biosensor used in this study is shown in Fig.1.

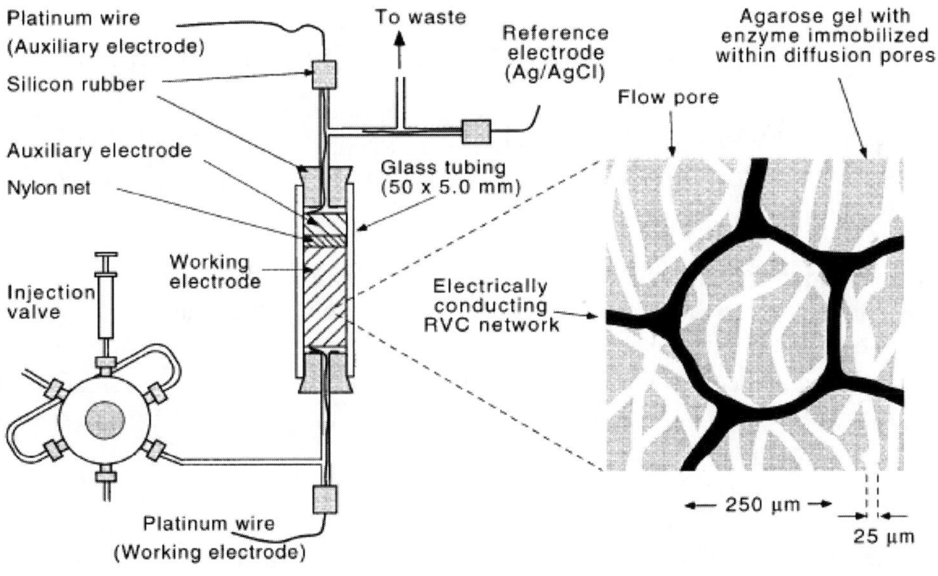

Figure 1. Schematic representation of Biosensor design used. The working electrode: reticulated vitreous carbon (RVC) coated with immobilized AChE / reticulated vitreous carbon together with superporous agarose gel (RVC-agarose composite), containing immobilized AChE. The magnified part shows the principle structure of the RVC-agarose composite. The electrode was operated in a FLA arrangement. The transporting buffer contained the mediator Meldola Blue. When the electrode was used for pesticide determination the transporting buffer also contained the substrate ATCh. (Reproduced with permission from M. Khayyami et al. Talanta 1998, 45, 557–563).

The flow rate was maintained as 1 ml min^{-1} since high flow rate resulted in decrease in the current of acetyl choline hydrolysis reaction. The results show that, the composite electrode showed good stability even after 1 month period when 250 samples were injected on each occasion. After some time, the response gradually diminished, although very slow rate was employed. However, after 1 month the response was still 60% of the original. Further 60 % of the composite material was composed of agarose gel and thus provides an ample volume for attachment of immobilized AChE (1.5 mg of enzyme). If it is assumed that known surface area of RVC (67 cm^2 cm^{-3}) was completely covered by AChE molecules, then by geometrical calculations, maximum binding capacity could be calculated as 0.01 mg of enzyme, i.e. less than 1% of the value ascribed to the RVC composite. The composite electrode showed a linear response up to 1 mM of ATCh. One disadvantage of using the composite gel electrode was that the response peaks become slightly broader, about 50% broader than in the absence of agarose. This may be due to the comparatively slow diffusion of thiocholine and Meldola Blue within the agarose gel. By using this composite electrode 1 nM of paraoxon in the sample, could be detected. The detection limit was 0.5 nM for a signal to noise ratio of 3.

Similarly, Neufeld et al. reported the fabrication of rapid amperometric micro flow injection electrochemical biosensor for the detection of highly toxic OP compound, 2, 2-dichlorovinyl phosphate (DDVP) [4]. Here, the detection was done by monitoring the inhibition of enzymatic reaction by DDVP. The reduction of $[Fe(CN)_6]^{-3}$ to $[Fe(CN)_6]^{-4}$ followed by the reaction with thiocholine in the working solution generates sharp, rapid and reproducible electric signals. The net reaction is explained in (2) and (3).

$$(CH3)_3N + CH_2CH_2S\text{-}OCH_3 + H_2O \rightarrow 2\ (CH_3)_3N\text{+ } CH_2CH_2SH + CH_3COOH \quad (2)$$

$$2(CH_3)_3N + CH_2CH_2SH + 2\ [Fe\ (CN)_3]^3 \rightarrow (CH_3)N + CH_2CH_2S\text{-}CH_2CH_2N + (CH_3)_3$$
$$+2[Fe(CN)_3]^{4-} \quad (3)$$

Immunodyne disc membrane of 6 mm in diameter was used as enzyme immobilization matrix. AChE was dissolved in 0.1 M PBS pH 7.5 to obtain a final concentration of 0.1 mg ml^{-1}. About 5 µl of the enzyme solution was applied onto the nylon membranes and air dried. The modified membranes were then transferred to 0.1 M PBS pH 7.5 containing 0.1 M glycine (blocking agent). This glycine blocks the remaining unbound groups. Finally, the membranes were thoroughly washed with 0.1 M PBS, pH 7.5 and stored at 4°C. During FIA analysis, the flow rate was maintained at 100 µl min^{-1} at an applied potential of 0.3 V. Here, the initial enzyme activity was recorded by injecting 5 µl of ATCh and then inhibitor activity was recorded by injecting 5 µl of DDVP and the flow system was stopped at different incubation times between 1 and 30 min. At a flow rate of 100 µl min^{-1}, 5 µl of ATCh was again injected and residual activity of the inhibited enzyme was thus measured. The degree of inhibition was calculated from the ratio between the enzymatic activity before and after adding the inhibitor. Further studies reveal that, the residual activity of the enzyme could be influenced by the inhibitor exposure time. The results show that AChE activity decreased on increase in exposure time. Even a small amount of DDVP caused an apparent inhibition after 9 min. The degree of inhibition was directly proportional to the inhibitor concentration and incubation time. With higher concentration and longer incubation time, the inhibition efficiency gets greatly increased. Although the amperometric response is clear in this approach, the system has several disadvantages. Every time the working solution must be replaced with a fresh one, and the electrodes should be washed thoroughly. Moreover, the measurement is slow (20 min). These difficulties could be overcome by employing flow injection system. Furthermore, micro flow injection system allows the use of very small volumes.

3. Role of Nanomaterials in Electrochemical Sensors

The SPE used in sec 2.1, 2.2 is rather inexpensive, easy to prepare, less cost effective. Similarly, the amperometric sensors discussed in sec 2.3 possess good sensitivity. However, nM detection has been achieved only in limited cases. Moreover, the enzyme immobilization procedures, the immobilization matrix remains rather complicated and less interaction between the enzyme and the matrix is often noticed. This in turn leads to the low stability of the immobilized enzyme. However, these limitations were successfully overcome by the researchers in recent years by using nanomaterial matrices. Nanomaterials possess certain unique properties like high mechanical strength, good conductivity and large surface area. With miniaturized size nanomaterials are free of internal dislocations and thus widely employed in the electrode modification and electrochemical sensor development. Many reviews discuss about the distinct properties of various nanomaterials, their applications in electrochemical sensor development. Earlier, Haick reported in detail about main concepts and approaches related to the use of molecularly modified metal nano particles in chemical sensors [23]. Interestingly, Punera et al. has reported about the main techniques and methods employed with nanoscale materials for the construction of electrochemical biosensors [24]. Gou et al have reported the recent advances in the synthesis and electrochemical applications of AuNPs [25]. The most common biosensors strategies in both label based metal nanoparticles and label-free (CNT-FET) devices has been reported by Kerman et al. [26]. All these reviews displayed the reality that nanomaterial implementation has led to the development of highly sensitive electrochemical devices. However, the development of more sensitive and novel electrochemical biosensors is rather challenging and it can be achieved only if nanoparticles with unique shapes like tripod, tetrapod, core-shell or hollow nano particles synthesized.

Other than metal nano particles, carbon nano tubes (CNTs) are widely used in sensor design and development. CNTs possess distinctive properties like excellent electrical conductivity, high mechanical strength and good stability, thus extensively used in the development of electrochemical biosensors, organic solar cells, transistors and photovoltaic devices [27-31]. The incorporation of CNTs onto the electrode surface results in the enhanced electron transfer rate and the electrode surface is free of fouling [32]. AChE immobilized onto CNTs modified surfaces exhibit enhanced catalytic activity. As a result of large working surface area available on CNTs, the electrocatalytic activity gets greatly enhanced at the edge-plane-like graphite site of the CNT ends. Thus the presence of CNT layer often leads to a greatly improved anodic detection of enzymatically generated thiocholine at lower oxidation over potential (0.1 V) with higher sensitivity [11]. Recently, Vairavapandian et al. has reviewed the various strategies followed in the preparation and modification of CNTs for catalytic applications in sensors. They conclude that incorporation of metal nanoparticles into CNTs matrices lead to enhanced catalytic behavior [33]. Furthermore, broad range of environmental applications of carbon based nanomaterials including environmental sensors development have been presented as review by Mauter et al [34]. To know more about the electroanalytical applications of CNTs, the readers may refer these reviews in the literature [35-36].

4. Nanomaterial Based Pesticide Sensors

4.1. CNT Based Pesticide Sensors

As discussed in sec 3, CNTs have been extensively used to develop pesticide sensors with higher sensitivity and longer stability. In this section we discuss about the design and the development of CNT based pesticide sensors. Joshi et al. reported the detection of OP compounds at a disposable biosensor with AChE-functionalized acid purified multi-wall carbon nanotubes (MCNTs) modified SPE [10]. The degree of inhibition of AChE by OP compounds was determined by measuring the electro oxidation current of the thiocholine generated by the AChE catalyzed hydrolysis of ATCh. The large surface area and electro-catalytic activity of MWCNTs lowered the over potential for thiocholine oxidation to + 0.2 V. Further, mediators were not used in this case and enzyme immobilization was done by physical adsorption.

The electrode preparation, the enzyme immobilization procedure was described as follows. About two mg of acid treated MWCNTs was ultrasonicated in 1 μL of N, N dimethylformamide (DMF) until a black suspension was obtained. About 15 μl of this MWCNTs suspension was casted on the working area of SPE surface and dried in an oven at 80 °C for 30 min. About 10 μl of AChE solution (0.132 U) was dropped on the MWCNTs modified electrode surface and dried at room temperature under a current of air and used. Hydrodynamic voltammetric studies results shows that significant response was observed at MWCNT-SPE towards 2mM thiocholine, whereas the response was poor at the unmodified electrode (Fig. 2). The linear response of the MWCNT-SPE modified sensor was found to be between 5 μM - 430 μM (r^2 = 0.999) with a sensitivity of 6.018 mA/M. In contrast, the response of AChE/SPE modified electrode was only 5 % and thus this result further reveals the contribution of MWCNTs in improving the sensitivity.

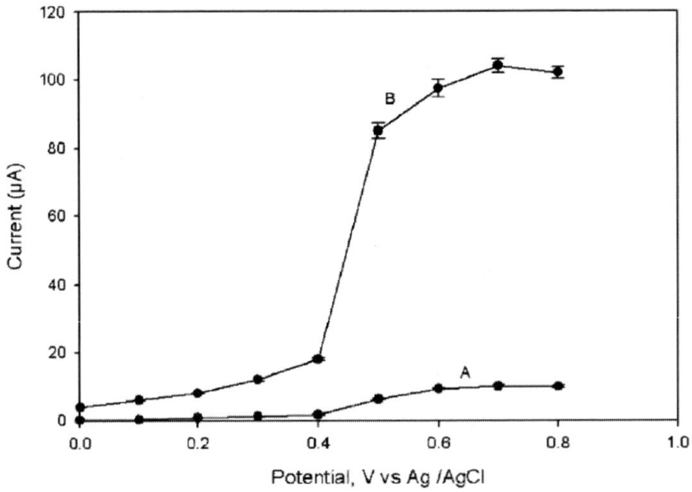

Figure 2. Hydrodynamic voltammogram for 2 mM thiocholine at A) Unmodified SPE and B) MWCNT modified SPE. Measurement conditions: 50 mM phosphate buffer containing 0.1 M KCl, pH 7.4 (Reproduced with permission from Joshi et al. Electroanalysis 2005, 17, 54-58).

From the slope of the plot of current vs. (current/concentration of ATCh), the K_m app for AChE was determined to be 0.66 mM. This biosensor also showed good precision and operational stability for the measurement of ATCh. The relative inhibition of AChE activity was calculated as a function of paraoxon concentration. . The linearity was observed up to 6.9 nM (slope, 14.36%/nM; correlation coefficient, 0.9859) to 6.9 nM and the limit of detection of 0.5 nM (0.145 ppb). Moreover, the detection limit for methyl parathion using the present sensor could be expected to be 1.65 nM. Real sample analysis results were in good agreement (90%), which demonstrates the validity of this MWCNTs-SPE modified biosensor to a practical problem.

Liu et al. reported a highly sensitive flow injection amperometric biosensor for OP compounds and nerve agents based on self-assembled AChE on MWCNTs modified glassy carbon electrode (GCE) [12]. The self assembly of AChE on MWCNTs modified GCE was done by the following procedure. About 20 μl of negatively charged acid treated MWCNTs solution was dropped on to the GCE surface and dried at room temperature. Then, AChE (0.2 U ml^{-1}) was immobilized on this negatively charged MWCNTs surface followed by alternative assembling of cationic poly (diallyldimethylammonium chloride) (PDDA) layer and an AChE layer.

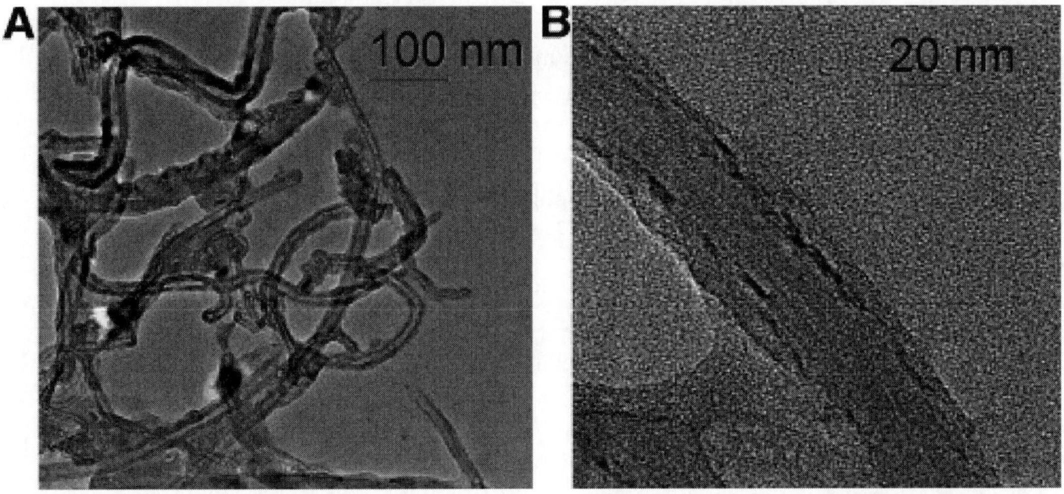

Figure 3. TEM images of PDDA/AChE/PDDA/CNT hybrid material at low (A) and high magnification (B) (Reproduced with permission from Liu et al. Anal. Chem. 2006, 78, 835-843).

This results in a sandwich-like structure of PDDA/AChE/PDDA on the MWCNTs surface, which provides a favorable microenvironment to the immobilized AChE. Transmission electron microscopy (TEM) results confirm the formation of layer-by-layer nanostructures on carboxyl-functionalized MWCNTs (Fig. 3).

Fourier transform infrared reflectance spectrum (FTIR) results indicate that AChE was immobilized successfully on the MWCNT/PDDA surface. CV results show that electrooxidation of thiocholine occurs at a much lower oxidation potential +0.55 V at MWCNT/GCE and the electrooxidation current is ten times higher than that of bare GCE. In addition, amperometric results show that the response of thiocholine at MWCNT/GCE was 200 times more than that of bare GCE. This significant enhancement in the anodic oxidation current of the enzymatic product thiocholine can be attributed to the fast electron transfer and big working surface area of CNTs. MWCNT/GCE showed a Linear response towards thiocholine in the concentration range of 2 x10^{-5} M to 2 x 10^{-3} M with a LOD of 5 μM to a signal to noise ratio of 3. The apparent Michaelis-Menten constant (Km) app was estimated to be 1.75 mM using the Lineweaver-Burk plot of 1/I versus 1/[ATCh]. FIA results show that PDDA/AChE/PDDA/CNT/GCE exhibits good reproducibility and stability with no surface fouling effect and thus this sensor is effectively applied to monitor OP compounds like paraoxon. Moreover, the relative inhibition of AChE activity increased with the concentration of paraoxon in the range 10^{-13} to 10^{-7} and it was linear with -log [paraoxon] at the concentration range 1 x 10^{-12} to 1 x 10^{-8} M with a detection limit of 4 x 10^{-13} M. Inhibition studies show that, no decrease in the activity of enzyme was observed after 1 week of continuous use of the biosensor, whereas a decrease of 15% of the activity of enzyme was observed after 3 weeks testing. This shows the good stability of this self assembled MWCNTs modified sensor.

Du et al. reported a sensitive, fast and stable amperometric sensor for quantitative determination of OP insecticide, triazophos [14]. Where, AChE was immobilized on MWNTs–chitosan (MC) composite matrix. Prior to enzyme immobilization, GCE surface was activated by applying a potential of +1.75 V for 300 s and scanned in the potential range +0.3 to +1.25V and +0.3 to −1.3V until a steady-state curve was obtained. This pretreated GCE surface was coated with 2.0 μl of MWCNTs, chitosan and glutaraldehyde mixture, followed by coating 4 μl of AChE solution, dried and used. CV results show that the oxidation peak of thiocholine occurs at +0.66V with much higher peak height at AChE/MC/GCE than at AChE/CS/GCE without MWCNTs. This shows that MWCNTs presence lowers the oxidation potential of thiocholine at the MC composite electrode. CV studies were also carried out to study the inhibition activity of triazophos at the composite electrode. The results show that, the peak currents decreased at the composite electrode with increase in triazophos concentration (Fig. 4).

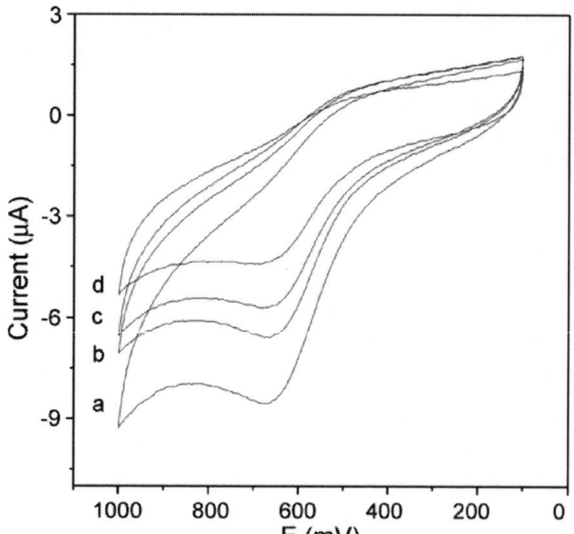

Figure 4. CVs of AChE-MC/GCE in pH 7.0 PBS containing 0.4mM ATCl after incubation in 0 μM (a), 1.5 μM (b), 3.5 μM (c) and 5.2 μM and (d) triazophos solution with 10 min (Reproduced with permission from Du et al. Sensors and Actuators B 2007, 127, 531–535).

The inhibition of triazophos was proportional to its concentration in two ranges, from 0.03 to 7.8 μM and 7.8 to 32 μM, with correlation coefficients of 0.09966 and 0.9960, respectively. The calibration sensitivity was 6.78, 0.87% μM^{-1} and the detection limit was 0.01 μM, respectively. AFM results show the surface morphological differences between the various films and confirm the presence of AChE in the composite film (Fig. 5).

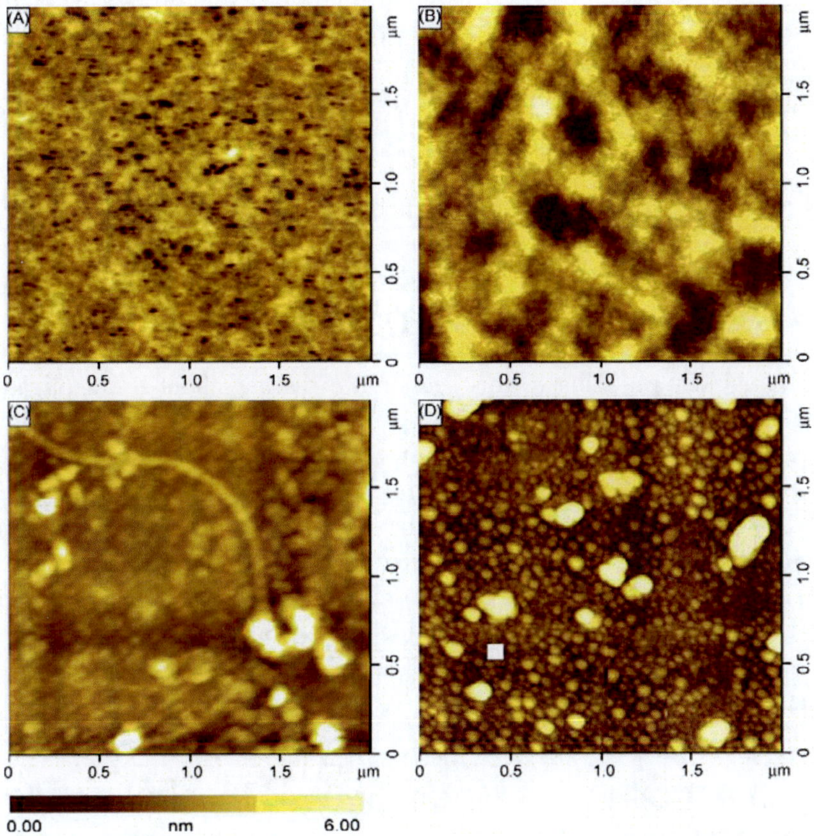

Figure 5. AFM images of bare surface (A), chitosan film (B), MC composite (C) and AChE immobilized on MC (D). (Reproduced with permission from Du et al. Sensors and Actuators B 2007, 127, 531–535).

Du et al. also reported a rapid sensitive determination of triazophos at AChE incorporated silica solgel (SiSG)–MWCNTs matrix [15]. The sol–gel matrix provided a biocompatible microenvironment around the enzyme and efficiently prevented leakage of the enzyme from the film. CV results show that the MWCNTs presence in the composite matrix promoted the electron transfer and increased the sensitivity of the sensor towards triazophos detection. Further, with increase in MWCNTs amount, anodic peak current gets increased and it reaches maximum at 20 % (V_{MWCNTs}/V). Thermal stability studies show that no loss of enzyme activity occurred in the temperature range 20 – 50 °C. This indicates the excellent activity of the enzyme in this temperature range without any denaturation. Enzyme inhibition studies shows that up to 12 min, with increase in immersion time the composite electrode displayed a decrease in peak current, which shows the significant enzyme inhibition activity by triazophos. However, after 12 min the peak current gets stabilized which indicates that binding interactions with active target groups in the enzyme reached saturation. The maximum value of inhibition of triazophos was not 100%, which is attributable to the binding equilibrium between pesticide and binding sites in the enzyme. Under optimum experimental conditions, the inhibition of triazophos was proportional to its concentration from 0.02 μM to 1 μM and from 5 μM to 30 μM, with correlation coefficients of 0.9957 and 0.9986, respectively. Furthermore, the determination of triazophos in garlic samples showed acceptable accuracy at this AChE-MWCNTs-SiSG/GCE. Fabrication reproducibility of the sensor was also good and stability was acceptable. Thus the sensor is a promising new tool for OP pesticide analysis.

4.2. Gold Nanoparticle Based Pesticide Sensors

As mentioned in the previous section, the response, the stability and the enzyme activity found greatly enhanced at the MWCNT platform. Other than CNTs, AuNPs also possess some unique properties and recent years it has been widely employed in the biosensors to immobilize biomolecules. Thus in this section we discuss about the application of AuNP matrix for the immobilization of AChE for pesticide sensor development. With the use of AuNPs, the efficiency and the stability of the pesticide sensor gets greatly amplified. Moreover, the nanoparticles matrix offers much friendly environment for the immobilized enzyme and thus the catalytic activity of the enzyme got greatly amplified. Interestingly, Shulga et al. applied AChE immobilized colloidal AuNPs sensor for the nM determination of carbofuran, a CA pesticide [16]. The enzyme-modified electrode sensor was also utilized for the sensitive electrochemical detection of thiocholine from the enzyme catalyzed hydrolysis of acetylthiocholine chloride (ATCl). The fabrication and the enzyme catalyzed reaction at the AuNPs coated electrode surface is shown in Fig. 6.

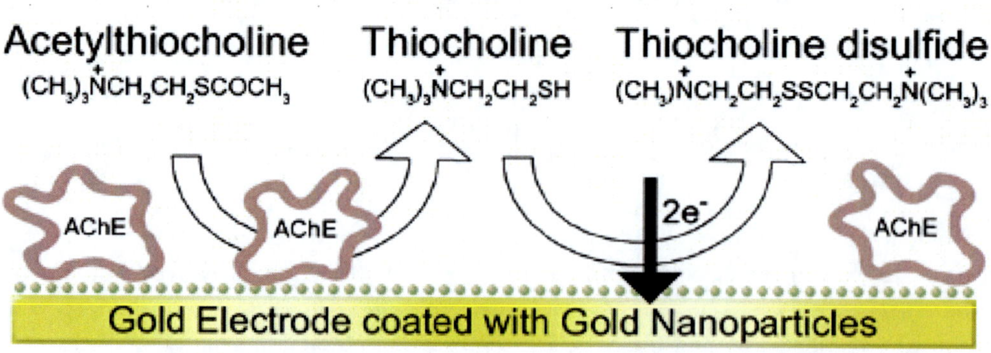

Figure 6. Schematic representation of the enzymatic reaction at the AuNPs coated AChE electrode. (Reproduced with permission from Shulga et al Electrochem. Commun. 2007, 9, 935–940).

AuNPs were electrodeposited onto a clean gold electrode surface by electrodeposition method. Where, the gold electrode was twice cycled in the potential range + 1.1 V to 0 V in deoxygenated solution containing 0.77 mM $HAUCl_4$ in 0.5 M H_2SO_4 at 10 mV s^{-1} scan rate. This AuNPs modified electrode was then immersed into a 300 μl solution of 0.1 M phosphate buffer (PBS) pH 8, containing 60 μg of AChE for 24 h at 4 °C. Finally this AChE modified electrode was removed from the enzyme solution and soaked in PBS for 5 min prior to use. AFM results show that the surface roughness increased to 67 nm for nanoparticles modified electrode and the particle size and the morphology of the surface were greatly influenced by deposition scan rate, solution stirring rate and the number of cycles. (Km) app value is 0.18 ± 0.02 mM for immobilized AChE and 0.051 ± 0.012 mM for AChE in bulk solution. This result shows that (Km) app value found to be increased by a factor of 3.5 for immobilized enzyme, integrity of the enzyme in immobilized condition. CV results show that, the irreversible oxidation of thiocholine takes place at + 0.66 V, only in the presence of AuNPs. Amperometric response of AuNP/AChE towards ATCl and the AChE inhibitor carbofuran addition has been shown in Fig. 7.

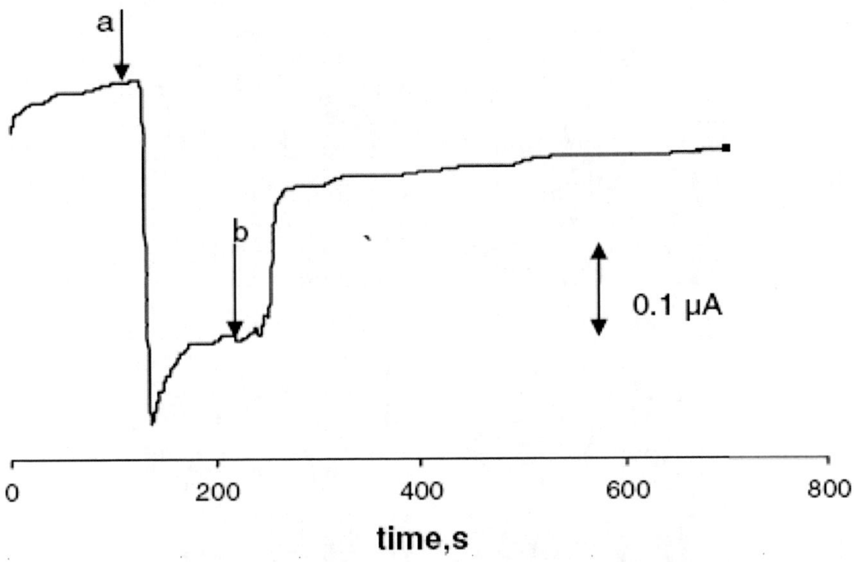

Figure 7. Amperometric response of the AuNP/AChE electrode (a) after injection of 10 μL of a 20 mM ATCl solution, and (b) after injection of 20 μL of 1 mM carbofuran. The final concentrations of ATCl and carbofuran were 66.4 and 6.6 μM, respectively. The arrows denote the time of injection. (Reproduced with permission from Du et al. A. Shulga et al. Electrochem. Commun. 2007, 9, 935–940).

Fig.7 shows that AUNP/AChE shows a significant response towards the addition of 10 μl of 20 mM ATCl. The dramatic decrease in the signal (55% inhibition efficiency) towards the addition of 20 μl of 1mM carbofuran is shown in b. The detection limit was observed to be 33 nM with a linear range of 10-135 nM.

Recently, Du et al. reported an AChE electrochemical sensor based on enzyme-induced growth of gold nanoparticles (AuNPs) without the addition of any gold nano-seeds [17]. They have successfully used $[Fe(CN)_6]^{3-/4-}$ as a probe to indicate the process of electron transfer across the interface and also analyze the enzyme inhibitor quantitatively. Initially, cleaned gold electrode was coated with 0.5 % (w/v) chitosan solution and AChE was later immobilized onto this chitosan modified gold electrode. CV results show that, AuNPs presence increases the peak current and decreases the peak separation. This confirms the presence of AuNPs on the chitosan modified electrode surface. However, the peak current of

AChE/CS/Au modified electrode in growth solution (0.02 % $HAuCl_4$ and 3 mM ATCl) increased with incubation time and decreased after 10 min. This may be attributed to the reason that congregated AuNP clusters might have blocked the electron transfer. Similarly, CV and AFM results together showed that the nanoparticle size is greatly influenced by ATCl concentration. With increase in ATCl concentration, the nanoparticles size gets increased and results in the aggregation of NPs, surface roughness (Fig. 8). Moreover, increase in inhibitor concentration decreased the activity of AChE. AChE activity was thus greatly inhibited by Malathion in the concentration range 0.1 - 500 ng ml^{-1} (R=0.9989) with a detection limit of 0.03 ng ml^{-1}. This developed AChE/NP/Chi sensor showed good preciscion and reprodubility with a RSD value of 3.3% for five replicate measurements. This clearly demonstrates the applicability of this AuNPs sensor towards pesticide determination.

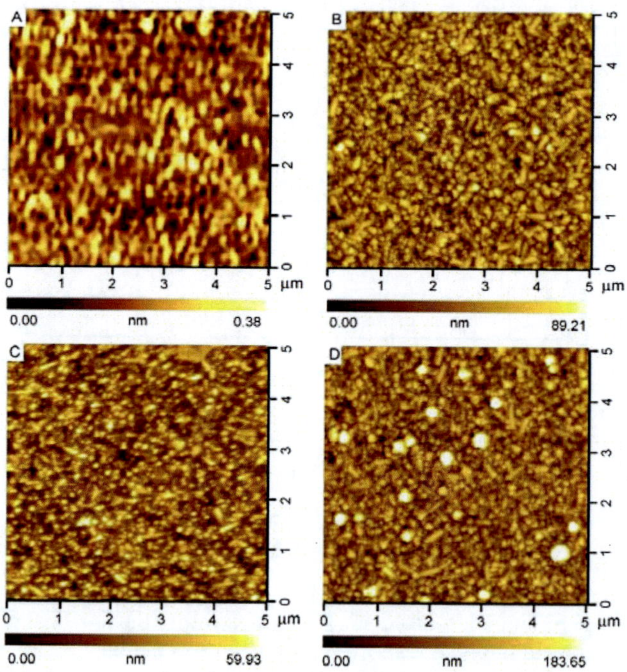

Figure 8. AFM images of (A) bare Au substrate and the different AuNPs surfaces after incubation of AChE-CS/Au in growth solution containing (B) 1.2, (C) 3.0 and (D) 4.8mM ATCl. (Reproduced with permission from Dua et al. A. *Sens. Actuators B* 2007, 127, 317–322).

Other than AUNPs, Quantum dots have also been employed in the development of pesticide sensors. Li et al. have synthesized Poly (N-vinyl-2-pyrrolione) (PVP)-capped CdS quantum dots (QCdS-PVP) from $CdCl_2$ and Na_2S in the presence of PVP [37]. AChE was immobilized onto this QCdS-PVP matrix incorporated GCE surface. The resulting GCE/ QCdS-PVP/AChE sensor was used for the detection of OP pesticides, such as trichlorfon. The enzyme immobilization procedure was described as follows. About 3 ml of QCdS-PVP was deposited on the surface of the GCE and dried in air. Then 3 ml of 0.5 mg ml^{-1} AChE along with 2.5% GA was deposited on the surface of the QCdS-PVP modified GCE and dried for 1 h at room temperature. TEM results show that, the QCdS-PVP particles were homogeneously distributed and they possess an average size of 2-4 nm (Fig. 9).

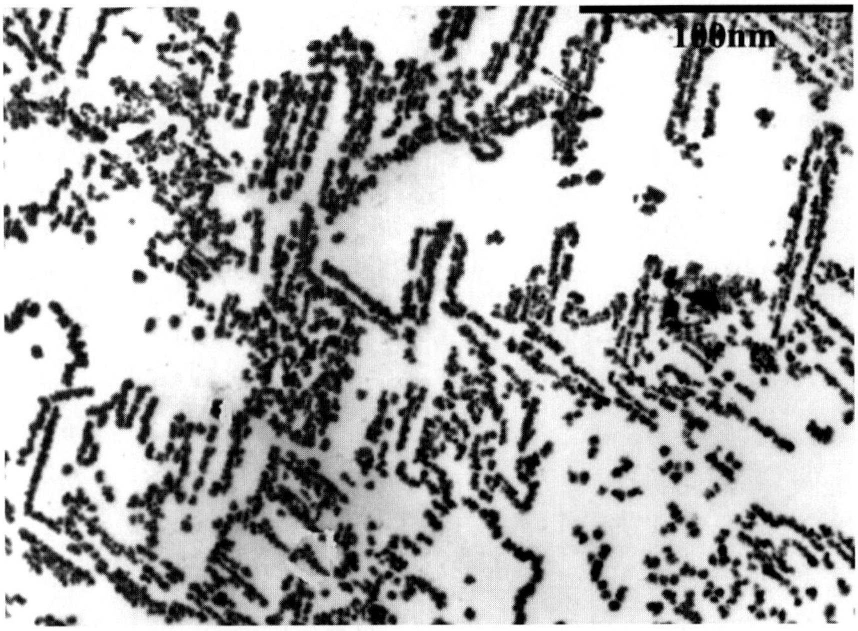

Figure 9. TEM image of QCdS-PVP (Reproduced with permission from Li *et al Electroanalysis* 2006, 18, 2163 – 2167).

CV results show that, a well defined oxidation peak was observed at +0.60 V for GCE/QCdS-PVP/AChE. This confirms the catalytic ability of this sensor towards thiocholine oxidation. The pH results show that the sensor exhibits stable response towards ATCl at neutral pH. Amperometric studies reveal that the QCdS-PVP/AChE sensor showed a good response to ATCl in the linear range 2.0 x 10^{-5} M to 7.0 x 10^{-4} M with the linear regression equation I = 0.0724 + 0.0917. The correlation coefficient was 0.9983 and detection limit was 5 x10^{-6} M for S/N=3. From the inhibition plot it was obvious that the relative inhibition of AChE activity increased with the concentration of trichlorfon in the range 1x10^{-8} to 2x10^{-6} M (2.5 to 515 ppb) and is linear with log [trichlorfon] at the concentration range from 1x10^{-7} M to 2x10^{-6} M (25 to 515 ppb) with a detection limit of 12 ppb (4.8 x 10^{-8} M). Moreover, this QCdS-PVP/AChE sensor showed good reproducibility and it can be regenerated simply by buffer dipping for a limited inhibition.

SUMMARY

In recent years, the risks of human health care and the environment rouse to critical level with the excessive use of unwanted amounts of certain pesticides in agriculture. OP and CA compounds are widely employed in agriculture to control many pests and thus used for many direct benefits. Though OP compounds holds the advantage of easy degradation in environment, their excess use inhibits the enzyme AChE activity and results in respiratory, myocardial and neuromuscular transmission impairment [38]. Thus the low level detection of these pesticides in real samples is essential which intentionally depends on high precise instruments. In contrast, electrochemical sensors have unique ability to bind for specific target molecules and achieve their detection with very high accuracy. Despite extensive progress in biosensor research, few AChE sensors find their real sample applications with limited accuracy. The advances in nanotechnology together with the beneficial properties of nanomaterials have opened new horizons for the electrochemical sensor development. Upon the implementation of nanomaterials including CNTs, AuNps, quantum dots in electrochemical sensors, dramatic enhancement in the electrocatalytic activity with very high sensitivity and stability towards pesticide detection has been achieved. Moreover, most nanomaterial matrices displayed a stable environment for the immobilized enzyme and assist to maintain their activity on long storage. In addition, paramount nM detection limit has been achieved for real samples containing Malathion and carbofuran. This robustly illustrates the inherent ability of this nanomaterial based pesticide sensors.

REFERENCES

[1] Stoytcheva, M.; Sharkova, V.; Magnin, J. P. *Electroanalysis* 1998, 10, 994 - 98.

[2] Pandey, P. C.; Upadhyay, S.; Pathak, H. C.; Pandy, C. M. D.; Tiwari, I. *Sensor. Actuator. B*, 2000, 62, 109–116.

[3] Shi, M.; Xu, J.; Zhang, S.; Liu, B.; Kong, J. *Talanta* 2006, 68, 2006.

[4] Neufeld, T.; Eshkenazi, I.; Cohen, E.; Rishpon, J. *Biosens. & Bioelectron.* 2000, 15, 323–329.

[5] Corcia, A. D.; Marchetti, M.; *Anal. Chem.* 1991, 63, 580–585.

[6] Bakker, E.; Qin, Y. *Anal. Chem.*, 2006, 78, 3965-3984.

[7] Anitha, K.; Mohan, S. V.; Reddy, S. J. *Biosens. & Bioelectron.* 2004, 20, 848–856.

[8] Khayyami, M.; Pita, M. T. P.; Garcia, N. P.; Johansson, G.; Danielsson, B.; Larsson, P.O. *Talanta*, 1998, 45, 557–563.

[9] Suprun, E.; Evtugyn, G.; Budnikov, H.; Ricci, F.; Moscone, D.; Palleschi, G. *Anal Bioanal Chem.* 2005, 383, 597–604.

[10] Joshi, K. A.; Tang, J.; Haddon, R.; Joseph, W.; Chen, W.; Mulchandani, A. *Electroanalysis* 2005, 17, 54 - 58.

[11] Liu, G.; Riechers, S. L.; Mellen, M. C.; Lin, Y. *Electrochem. Commun.* 2005, 7, 1163-1169.

[12] Liu, G.; Lin, Y. *Anal. Chem.* 2006, 78, 835-843.

[13] Du, D.; Huang, X.; Cai, J.; Zhang, A.; Ding, J.; Chen, S. *Anal. Bioanal. Chem.* 2007, 387, 1059–1065.

[14] Du, D.; Huang, X.; Cai, J.; Zhang, A. *Sens. & Actuators B*, 2007, 127, 531–535.

[15] Du, D.; Cai, J.; Song, D.; Zhang, A. *J. Appl. Electrochem.* 37, 2007, 893–898.

[16] Shulga, O.; Kirchhoff, J. R. *Electrochem. Commun.* 2007, 9, 935–940.

[17] Du, D.; Ding, J. Cai, J. Zhang, A. *Sens. Actuators B* 2007, 127, 317–322.

[18] Du, D.; Chen, S.; Cai, J.; Zhang, A. *Biosens. & Bioelectron.* 2007, 23, 130–134.

[19] Luckarift, H.R.; Greenwald, R.; Bergin, M. H.; Spain, J. C.; Johnson, G. R. *Biosens. & Bioelectron.* 2007, 23, 400–406.

[20] Du, D.; Chen, S.; Cai, J.; Zhang, A. *Talanta* 2008, 74, 766–772.

[21] Hart, A. L.; Collier, W. A. *Sens. Actuators B* 1998, 53, 111–115.

[22] Hernandez, S.; Palchetti, I.; Mascini, M. Intern. *J. Environ. Anal. Chem.* 2000, 78, 263-278.

[23] Haick, H.; *J. Phys. D. Appl. Phys.* 2007, 40, 7173–7186.
[24] Pumera, M.; Sanchez, S. Ichinose, I.; Tang, J. *Sens. Actuators B* 2007, 123, 1195–1205.
[25] Guo, S.; Wang, E. *Anal. Chim. Acta* 2007, 598, 181–192.
[26] Kerman, K.; Saito, M.; Yamamura, S.; Takamura, Y.; Tamiya, E, *Trends in Anal.Chem.* 2008, 27, 585-592.
[27] Breton, Y.; Desarmot, G.; Salvetat, J. P.; Delpeux , S.; Sinturel, C.; Beguin, F.; Bonnamy, S. *Carbon*, 2004, 42, 1027–1030.
[28] Xu, Z.; Wang, L.; Zheng, Q. *Small* 2008, 4, 733–737.
[29] Hobara, R.; Yoshimoto, S.; Ikuno, T.; Katayama, M.; Yamauchi, N.; Wongwiriyapan1, W.; Honda, S. I.; Matsuda, I.; Hasegawa, S.; Kenjiro, O. *Jap. J. Appl.Phys.* 2004, 43, 1081–1084.
[30] Ulbricht, R.; Lee, S.; Jiang, X.; Inoue, K.; Zhang, M.; Fang, S.; Baughman, R. H.;Zakhidov, A. A. *Solar Energy Materials & Solar Cells*, 2007, 91, 416–419.
[31] Allen, B.L.; Kichambare, P. D.; Star, A. *Adv. Mater.* 2007, 19, 1439–1451
[32] Kachoosangi, R. T.; Musameh, M. M.; Yousef, I. A.; Yousef, J. M.; Kanan, S. M.; Xiao, L.; Davies, S. G.; Russell, A.; Compton, R. G. *Anal. Chem.* 2009, 81, 435–442.
[33] Vairavapandian, D.; Vichchulada, P.; Lay, M. D. *Anal. Chim. Acta* 2008, 62, 6119–129.
[34] Mauter, M.; Elimelech, M.; *Environ. Sci. Technol.*, 2008, 42, 5843-5859.
[35] Valentini, F.; Palleschi, G. *Anal. Lett.* 2008, 41, 479–520.
[36] Agui, L.; Sedeno, P. L.; Pingarron, J. M. *Anal. Chim. Acta* 2008, 622, 11–47.
[37] Li, X. H.; Xie, Z.; Min, H.; Li, C.; Liu, M. Xian, Y.; Jin, L. *Electroanalysis* 2006, 18, 2163– 2167.
[38] Darko, G.; Akoto, O. *Food & Chem. Toxicol.* 2008, 46, 3703–3706.

In: Nanostructured Materials for Electrochemical Biosensors ISBN: 978-1-60741-706-4
Editors: U. Yogeswaran; S. Kumar; S. Chen ©2009 Nova Science Publishers, Inc.

Chapter 11

NOVEL MESOPOROUS SILICAS AS ELECTROCHEMICAL BIOSENSORS

***Jian-Shan Ye**[*1]**, Xue-Ling Li**[1] **and Fwu-Shan Sheu**[†2]*
[1] South China University of Technology, P. R. China
[2] National University of Singapore, Singapore, Singapore

ABSTRACT

Mesoporous silicas (MPS) have been widely used as electrode modifier for electrochemical biosensors due to their attractive properties such as unique structure and high pore volume containing large number of widely accessible active centers, tailored pore size for different biomolecules, and good biocompatibility. These properties have been intelligently combined to improve the response and sensitivity of the resulting modified electrodes and to design novel electrochemical biosensor for electrocatalytic reaction and detection. This up-to-date review summarizes the recent progresses made in the electrochemical biosensors by application of MPS modified electrodes and introduces advantages (for examples, their novel structure, functionalized by different organic or inorganic groups with different pore size that can simultaneously fit with different proteins etc) of some novel MPS that have been synthesized in literature. The outlook and successful realization for the development of MPS in electrochemical biosensors requires proper control of their chemical and physical properties and surface functionalization.

Keywords: Mesoporous silica; Enzyme; Redox protein; Modified electrode; Biosensor

INTRODUCTION

Nanostructured silica-based materials have been widely used in chemical industries for many decades. They have been extensively exploited in electrochemistry for several advanced

* Corresponding author. Tel: 86-20-8711 3241, Fax: 86-20-8711 2901, e-mail: jsye@scut.edu.cn
† Corresponding author. Tel: 65-6516 2857, Fax: 65-6779 2486, elesfs@nus.edu.sg

applications, including electroanalysis and sensors [1-10], electrocatalysis [11], spectroelectrochemical devices [12], solid electrolytes and power sources [13-14]. However, the majority of these applications use natural or synthetic zeolites, with structural repeats on 1–2 nm scale, and pore sizes less than 1 nm. Consequently, they are not suitable hosts for biomacromolecules such as proteins or enzymes. The use of zeolites in biotechnology is therefore rather limited. In contrast, mesoporous silica (MPS) is a subclass of nanostructured porous silica. Since they were first synthesized in 1992 by a group of scientists in the Mobil Oil Corporation [15], these materials were originally envisaged as large pore zeolite equivalents and offered more scope for biotechnology applications. Compared with smaller size of zeolites, MPS is much favorable in electrochemistry study due to their unique morphology. According to the IUPAC definition, pores with diameters between 2 and 50 nm are termed as mesopores. Mesoporous materials are further characterized by high specific surface areas (up to *ca.* 1500 m^2 g^{-1}) and pore volumes (up to *ca.* 1.5 cm^3 g^{-1}), which renders them ideal candidates as hosts for biomolecules. Moreover, surfactant micelles are used to produce small cation directing agents and to induce silica polymerization at the surface of large templates. This give rise to a novel class of solids made of well-defined and uniform channels regularly arranged in the space with controlled particle size and pore size, various morphology (hexagonal, cubic, lamellar, wormlike), gathering both sieving properties (with much larger pores than mesoporous materials) and surface chemistry very similar to those of non-ordered silica gels. Due to its unique structure and high porosity, controllable pore size (2-30 nm) and good biocompatibility which provide a possibility to immobilize large biomolecules, MPS attracts tremendous interest especially in biosensors. Many reviews of the application of MPS in electrochemical analysis have been published [14, 16-20], herein, this chapter will briefly summarize some intrinsic features about MPS and emphasize on the recent development of the MPS application in electrochemical biosensors.

DISCUSSION

2.1 The Synthesis of MPS

MPS is typically obtained by introducing supramolecular aggregates of ionic surfactants (long-chain alkyltrimethylammonium halides) as structure-directing agents (SDAs). These SDAs, in the form of a lyotropic liquid-crystalline phase, lead to the assembly of an ordered mesostructured composite during the condensation of the silica precursors under optimal conditions. The mesoporous materials are then obtained by subsequent removal of the surfactant by extraction or calcination. Two different mechanisms are involved in the formation process of these composite materials: 1) in true liquid-crystal templating (TLCT), the concentration of the surfactant is so high that under the prevailing conditions (temperature, pH) a lyotropic liquid-crystalline phase is formed without requiring the presence of the precursor, inorganic framework materials (normally tetraethyl- (TEOS) or tetramethylorthosilica (TMOS)) [21]; 2) it is also possible that this phase forms even at lower concentration of surfactant molecules, for example, when there is cooperative self assembly of the SDA and the already added inorganic species, in which case a liquid-crystal phase with hexagonal, cubic, or laminar arrangement can develop [22]. In the meantime, the original approach has been extended by a number of variations, for example, by use of tri-block copolymer templates under acidic conditions by which the so-called SBA silica phases may be synthesized. The syntheses of ordered mesoporous solids described above are classified as endotemplate methods ("soft-matter templating"). In exotemplate methods ("nanocasting"), a porous solid is used as the template in place of the surfactant. Thus, this method is also known as "hard-matter templating". The hollow spaces that provide the exotemplate framework are filled with an inorganic precursor, which is then transformed under suitable conditions. In this way, the pore system of the template is copied as a "negative image". After removal of the now-filled exotemplate framework, the incorporated material is obtained with a large specific surface area. Examples of periodic porous solids employed as exotemplates are ordered mesoporous silica phases (e.g., MCM-48 and SBA-15 types). This replication method was used for the first time by Ryoo et al., [23] for the synthesis of mesoporous carbon (CMK-1). The resulting material is highly porous (pore volume $>$0.7 mL g^{-1}) and exhibits high specific surface areas (500-1500 m^2 g^{-1}). Tunability of pore sizes can be achieved during the synthesis and processing of the porous solid, but pore openings remain fixed thereafter. One recent example of pore tailoring in ordered silicas with cage-like mesoporous structures (e.g., FDU-1, SBA-16) was provided by Jaroniec and co-workers, who adjusted cage openings by post-synthesis surface modification and synthesis temperature selection [24]. The techniques are also applicable to mesoporous channel structures [25]. Anwander and Wiedenmeyer achieved pore size control in high-quality cubic mesoporous silica, MCM-48, by utilizing Gemini surfactants and controlling reaction temperatures and pH values [26]. The synthesis scheme is shown in Fig 1. Up to now, there are still no uniform nomenclature rules to reach a universal classification of MPS.

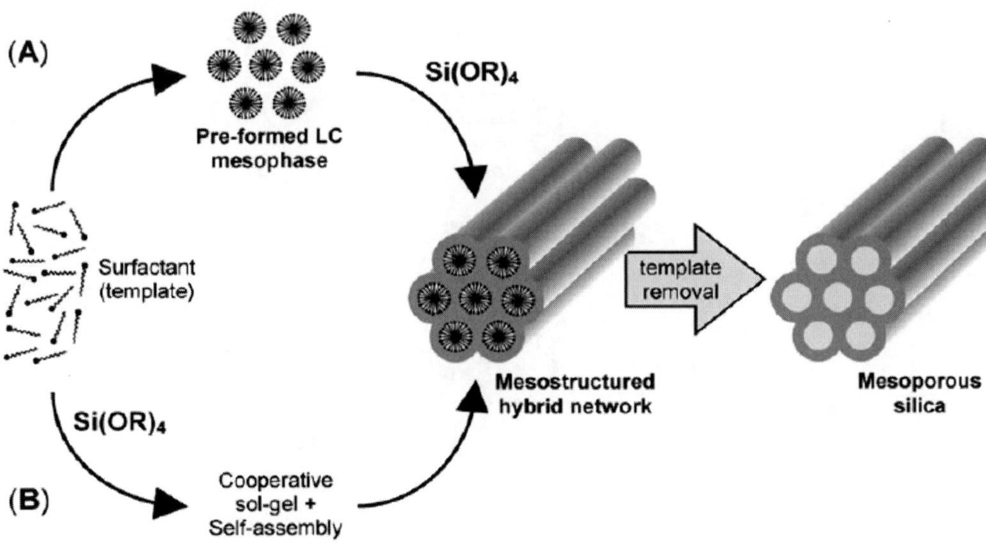

Figure 1. Schematic pathway for preparing surfactant-templated mesoporous silicas, illustrating a formation mechanism based on preformed liquid crystal (LC) mesophase (route A) or a cooperative process (route B). Reprinted from [20], Copyright (2008) WILEY-VCH Verlag GmbH&Co.

2.2 The Application of MPS in Electrochemical Biosensors

2.2.1 Functionalized MPS for Protein Immobilization

The application of MPS in biosensor has received more and more attention in the past few years. It was reported that functionalized mesoporous silica nanomaterials have good biocompatibility to be internalized by animal and plant cells without posing any cytotoxicity issue *in vitro* [27-29]. These findings may generate new types of drug/gene delivery and biosensor, particularly in the development of electrochemical biosensors. We will mainly discuss the advancements in morphology control and surface functionalization of MPS for proteins immobilization and the recent developments of proteins encapsulated MPS biosensors.

Before realizing the application of bio-molecules encapsulated MPS in electrochemical biosensors, a great deal of work needs to be carried out on investigating how to encapsulate protein/enzyme stably on the exterior or interior of the MPS. MPS can be functionalized either by doping or by covalent binding of organic groups. Doping relies on the introduction of reactants, biomolecules or organic polymers, as driven by weak interactions between the inorganic matrix and the organic moieties. More interesting is the durable immobilization via covalent and non-hydrolysable Si-C bonds. This can be achieved by three methods: 1) post-synthesis grafting with organosilane reagents; 2) direct functionalization by co-condensation of silicon alkoxides and organosilane reagents in the presence of a template (One-pot synthesis); and 3) the resort to bridge silesquioxanes $(RO)_3Si-R'-Si(OR)_3$ precursors that are co-condensed with a silicon alkoxide in the presence of a template to form periodic mesoporous hybrid materials containing the organofunctional groups inside the mesopore walls [30]. The synthesis scheme is shown in Fig 2.

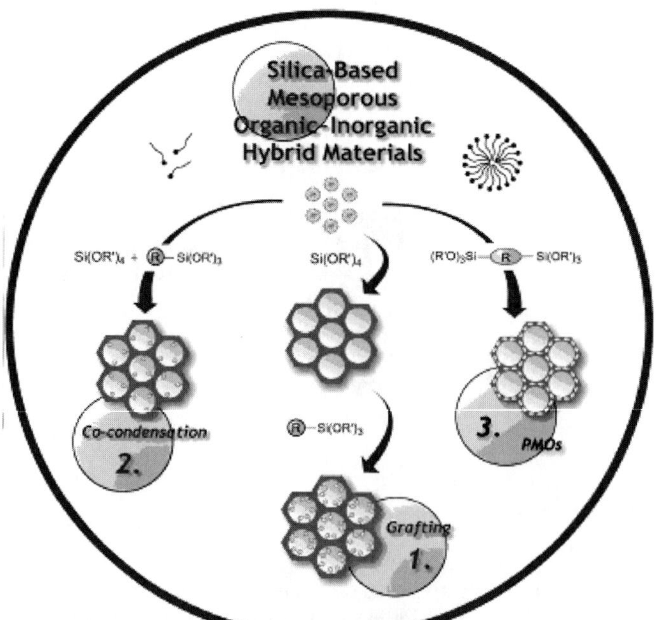

Figure 2. The scheme shows MPS organic functionalization in three strategies. Reprinted from [30], Copyright (2006), WILEY-VCH Verlag GmbH&Co.

The achievements of functionalized MPS for protein/enzymes immobilization have been reviewed by Hartmann [31], and Yiu and Wright [32]. Generally, the immobilization of enzyme/protein to the surface of the pore walls or interior of the pore involves physical adsorption or actual chemical bonding. Although in the latter case there is always the risk of partial or total denaturation and hence a considerable decrease in activity, in this connection, it is expected that strengthening the chemical bonding force by functionalized different groups on the MPS avoids the leaching of enzymes out of MPS pore. Unmodified MCM-41/48 and SBA-15 phases [33], as well as carboxylic acid, aminopropyl-, thiol, cyano-, and chloride functional groups were modified on the surface of SBA-15 have been used by Yiu et al., [34] for the immobilization of trypsin. The resulting supported enzyme catalysts were shown to be active and stable catalysts for the hydrolysis of *N*-α-benzoyl- DL-arginine-4-nitroanilide (BAPNA). The solids prepared by supporting the enzyme on thiol-functionalized SBA-15 prepared by in situ synthesis were found to be the most promising and recyclable. Ma et al., [35] studied the activity of porcine pancreas lipase immobilized on the surface of MCM-41 samples by virtue of the hydrogen bonding interactions between the abundant weakly acidic hydroxyl groups of the support and the enzyme. The activity of the immobilized enzyme fell off rapidly when reused, owing to the leaching of enzyme out from the pores, while MPS was functionalized with vinyl-, the activity remained constant over five cycles of re-usage indicated that the grafting of vinyl- had led to the enzyme being immobilized inside a “mesoporous reactor” from which leaching of the enzyme was prevented without inhibiting access to the substrate and release of the products. *Mucor javanicus* lipase was immobilized in the channel system of SBA-15 at different pH values (pH 5-8) [36]. The loading and hydrolysis activity were the highest at pH 6. Chemical adsorption was achieved by functionalization of the support medium with glutardialdehyde (pentaldial). Besides, Takahashi et al., [37] discussed the effect of different pore size and surfactant of MPS on enzyme immobilization. Enzymes were selectively adsorbed to FSM-16 and MCM-41 prepared with a cationic surfactant, whose pore sizes were over the molecular diameters of the enzymes, and were not adsorbed significantly to SBA-15 prepared with a non-ionic surfactant. The higher adsorption to FSM-16 or MCM-41 rather than on SBA-15 may be due to the ionic characteristics of the mesopore, which would be consistent with the observed larger adsorption capacity to the cationic pigment rather than the anionic pigment of these materials. Horseradish peroxidase (HRP) and subtilisin, immobilized in FSM-16 showed the best stability and peak catalytic activity in an organic solvent when the average mesopore size just exceeded the molecular diameters of the enzymes. Also, the immobilization of conalbumin [38], cytochrome *c* [39], subtilisin [40], (chloro-) peroxidase [37, 40] and lysozyme [41] in SBA-15 has been reported. As results of these basic achievements of protein/enzymes immobilized MPS, the study of the protein/enzymes-MPS biosensors has been developed very fast.

2.2.2 The Development of Proteins/Enzymes Encapsulated MPS Biosensors

Owing to the capability of controlled sizes of MPS to tailor different enzymes and/or proteins, MPS is considered to be ideal host for immobilizing biomolecules. Some MPS, such as MSU (Michigan State University) [42], SBA-15 (Santa Barbara Amorphous) [43-46], FSM (folded sheet mesoporous) [47-48], MCM (Mobil Composition of Matter) [49] or other hexagonal mesoporous silicas [50-51], have been successfully used to enhance the direct electron transfer rate and the catalysis toward target molecules. Encapsulation of enzymes and other proteins in ordered MPS has attracted increasing attention over the past few years and this field has been reviewed by Kim et al., [52], and some part by Walcarius [16, 18, 20]. A huge amounts of work directly point out that direct electron transfer of cytochrome c [53, 54], hemoglobin (Hb) [37, 39-40, 44-45, 49-50], myoglobin (Mb) [48, 55] and glucose oxidase (GOD) [44, 49, 56-58] can occur by encapsulation of enzymes in MPS particles. The well-defined voltametric responses indicate that proteins immobilized within the MPS particles retain their biological activity. Additionally, MPS-based biosensors are more sensitive for detection and have a longer life. For example, the immobilized heme protein exhibits enhanced response towards the catalytic reduction of hydrogen peroxide (H_2O_2) compared with that of the MPS-free heme protein electrode. The versatility of the MPS-modified electrode was also applied to the design of bienzymatic systems, as illustrated for HRP, light harvesting protein and Mb [47].

The protein/enzymes-MPS electrodes are usually fabricated by doping the suspension of protein/enzymes and MPS (mix both solutions for certain period of time with or without stirring) on the substrate electrode and dry in ambient condition [46, 48, 58], or firstly doping the suspension of MPS on the substrate surface to form a MPS thin film or deposit the MPS thin film on the substrate directly, then dip the electrode in the protein solution for several hours [43] for the absorption of protein into the mesopores. However, this approach usually led to poorly stable deposits. To enhance the mechanical stability of the MPS deposition layers, an additional polymeric coating with ensured sufficient robustness for handling can be added. Nafion [49] chitosan [51] sol-gel [45, 50, 54] are used for this purpose. Beside the bilayer arrangement of MPS particles covered with a polymer, single composite layers made of MPS particles dispersed into a polymeric matrix could also be prepared as thin films on the electrode surfaces. The organic agents referred above can be dissolved in the suspension containing the particulate material, resulting in encapsulation of the MPS particles within the interpenetrated polymer chains upon solvent evaporation. Note that the binder can interfere with the electrochemical behavior because the as prepared MPS is not a continuous thin film.

Another pathway to fabricate enzymes encapsulated MPS electrode is the layer-by-layer (LbL) method. LbL assembly of proteins and/or enzymes with polyelectrolyte is a novel method for protein film fabrication that emerged over the past decade [59-66]. LbL has been established as a new procedure for studying redox proteins with electrochemical technology. The principle of the LbL assembly is based on alternative adsorption of oppositely charged species from the solutions by electrostatic interaction between them. Compared with casting method, the LbL assembly technology develops a "molecular architecture" with precise control of the composition, the number of layers, and the thickness of films at a molecular or nanometer level. Moreover, the LbL method is simple and suitable to a variety of substrate matrix with different shapes. Since the PI of MPS is below 2, the charge of protein can be modulated by the change of pH, and proteins and/or MPS can be absorbed LbL. After LbL absorption, proteins in these films retain their near native structures and electroactivities. Thus, LbL method is extensively used in studies of the direct electrochemistry of proteins [55, 60, 67-68]. The LbL absorption scheme is shown in Fig 3.

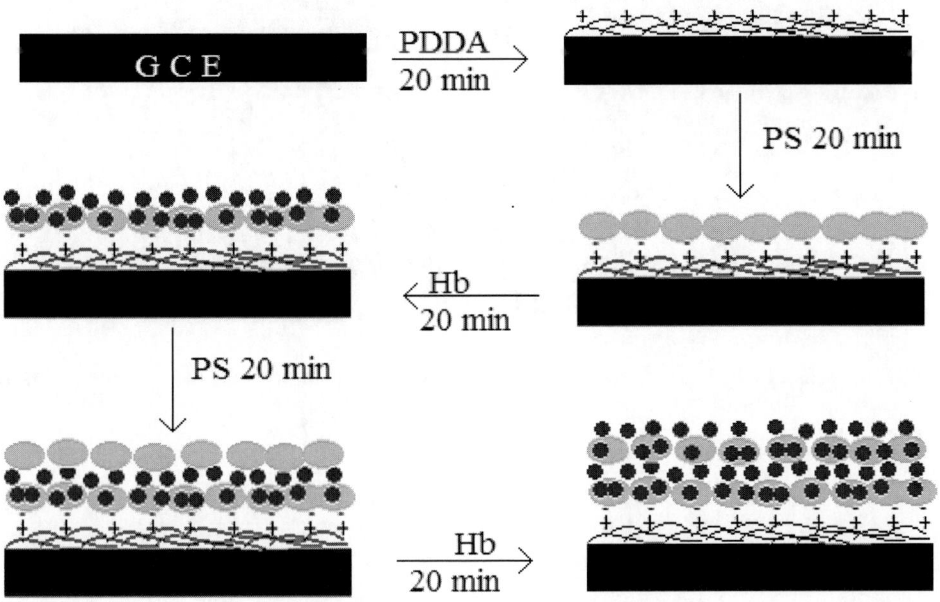

Figure 3. The absorption process of Hb in MPS via LbL method.

As MPS is nonconductive, this disadvantage may reduce its electrochemical response while applied in electrochemical analysis. With circumvent to dop metal nanoparcticles to improve its poor conductivity, Sun et al., [44] successfully synthesized gold nanoparticles-mesoporous silica (GNPs-MPS) composite as a GOD immobilization matrix for amperometric glucose biosensor. GNPs-SBA-15 was formed from $AuCl_4^-$ adsorbed H_2N-SBA-15 by $NaBH_4$ reduction. The TEM images are illustrated in Fig.4. The biosensors exhibits an excellent electrocatalytic response to glucose with a fast response time less than 7 s and a linear range of 0.02-14 mM, high sensitivity of 6.1 μA $mM^{-1}cm^{-2}$, as well as good long-term stability and reproducibility. These advantages could be ascribed to excellent conductivity and good biocompatibility of GNPs-MPS. Xian et al., [43] also used the same method to gain Au-SBA-15 composites for the encapsulation of Hb with satisfied results. The Hb/Au-SBA-15 electrode displayed good electrocatalytic reduction for H_2O_2 with a detection limit of 1.0 μM, about 3 times as low as that for the Hb/SBA-15. Furthermore, Liu et al., [45] got a lower detection limit (2.3×10^{-9} M) for the detection of H_2O_2 by using an Hb/SBA-15/silica sol sensor. The different sensitivity may be ascribed to the different pore properties of SBA-15 type MPS and other different experimental conditions. Palladium (Pd) nanoparticles have been successfully encapsulated into the channels of modified SBA-15 *in situ* via a facile, ethylene glycol (EG)-assisted sonochemical method also in Liu's laboratory [46]. The Hb/Pd/SBA-15 sensor showed an excellent response to the reduction of H_2O_2, and the linear range for the determination of H_2O_2 was from 1.8 to 119.3 μM with a detection limit of 0.8 μM and enhanced the direct electron transfer between Hb and the electrode surface. An illustration is shown in Fig 5.

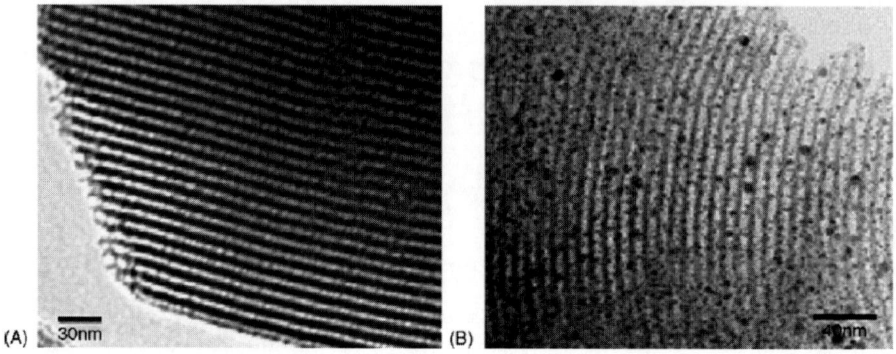

Figure 4. TEM images of (A) SBA-15 and (B) GNPs-SBA-15. Reprinted from [44], Copyright (2007), Elsevier.

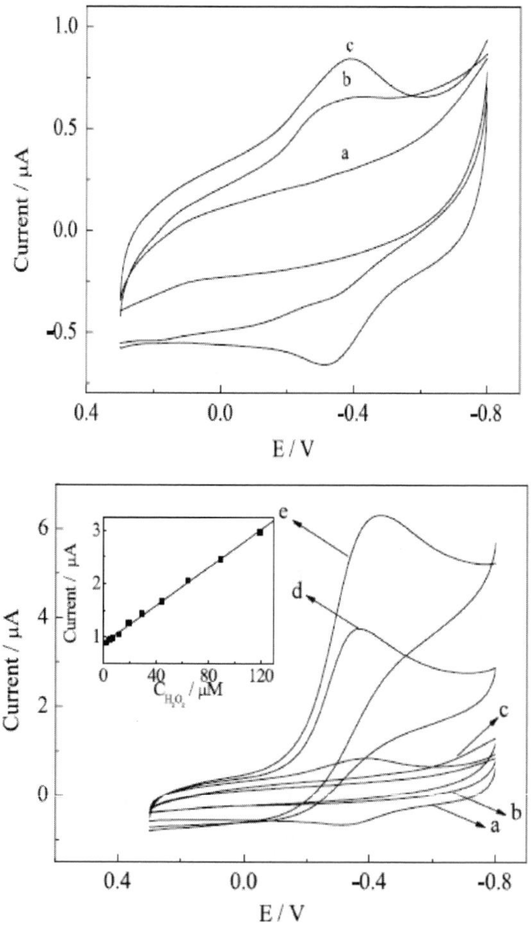

Figure 5. CVs of (a) Pd/SBA-15/GCE, (b) Hb/SBA-15/GCE, and (c) Hb/Pd/SBA-15/GCE in 0.1 M PBS pH 7.0 (left); CVs of Hb/Pd/SBA-15/GCE (a, d, e) and Pd/SBA-15/GCE (b, c) in 0.1 M PBS and pH 7.0 containing no H_2O_2 ((a) and (b), 0.18 mM H_2O_2 (d) and 0.38 mM H_2O_2 ((c) and (e), respectively (right). Inset: plot of the catalytic current versus H_2O_2 concentration. Scan rate: 100 mV s^{-1}. Reprinted from [46], Copyright (2008), IOP Publishing Ltd.

To obtain excellent electrochemical properties and better biocompatibility, novel mesoporous silica materials should be designed and synthesized. Wu et al., [69] have designed a novel mesocellular silica-carbon nanocomposite foam (MSCF) combining the properties of MPS and mesoporous carbon. The as-prepared MSCF has a highly ordered mesostructure, good biocompatibility, favorable conductivity and hydrophilicity, large surface area and a narrow pore-size distribution (the structure is shown in Fig 6). For practical purposes, the mesopore size can be controlled by changing the pore size of the MSF template. Furthermore, the hydrophilicity and conductivity of the material can be changed by adjusting the relative amounts of carbon and silica, thereby enabling the immobilization and biosensing of different proteins. Using GOD as a model, GOD/MSCF electrode shows direct electrochemistry with a fast electron transfer rate ($14.0 \pm 1.7\ s^{-1}$), a linear response to glucose concentrations ranging from 50 μM to 5.0 mM with a detection limit of 34 μM at an applied potential of -0.4 V. The biosensor shows good stability and selectivity and is able to exclude interference from AA and UA species that always coexists with glucose in real samples. Zhang et al., [51] designed a bimodal MPS for proteins encapsulated biosensors, that is, there were two different pore sizes in bimodal MPS, whose large pores with 10-40 nm provided favorable conditions for protein immobilization and small pores with 2-3 nm avoided the mass-transfer limitation

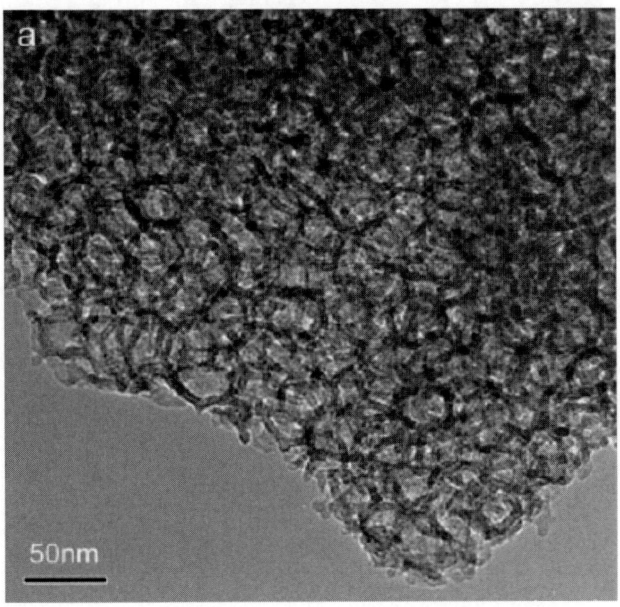

Figure 6. TEM image of MCSF. Reprinted from [69], Copyright (2008) WILEY-VCH Verlag GmbH&Co.

Up to now there is still not much research on the mechanism of how the MPS enhance the catalysis of proteins and how the direct electron transfer occur while the proteins encapsulated in the MPS pore. The mechanism is not clear. Besides, as this chapter referred above, many scientists found that the protein/enzymes encapsulated on normal MPS surface and in the pore were not stable and lots of endeavor was devoted to solve this problem [34-38]. Abundant of work is currently carrying out on the study of the electrochemical application of the protein/enzymes encapsulated MPS sensors, however, surprisingly nearly no literature discuss about the leaching problem. There are two issues to be addressed for the future work: one is the utility of Nafion, chitosan or other polymer as binder to make the composite more stable on the substrate surface and avoid the leaching of enzymes; the other is although the study of protein/enzymes encapsulated MPS in electrochemical biosensors is still very young but scientists have to pay much attention to the leaching problem.

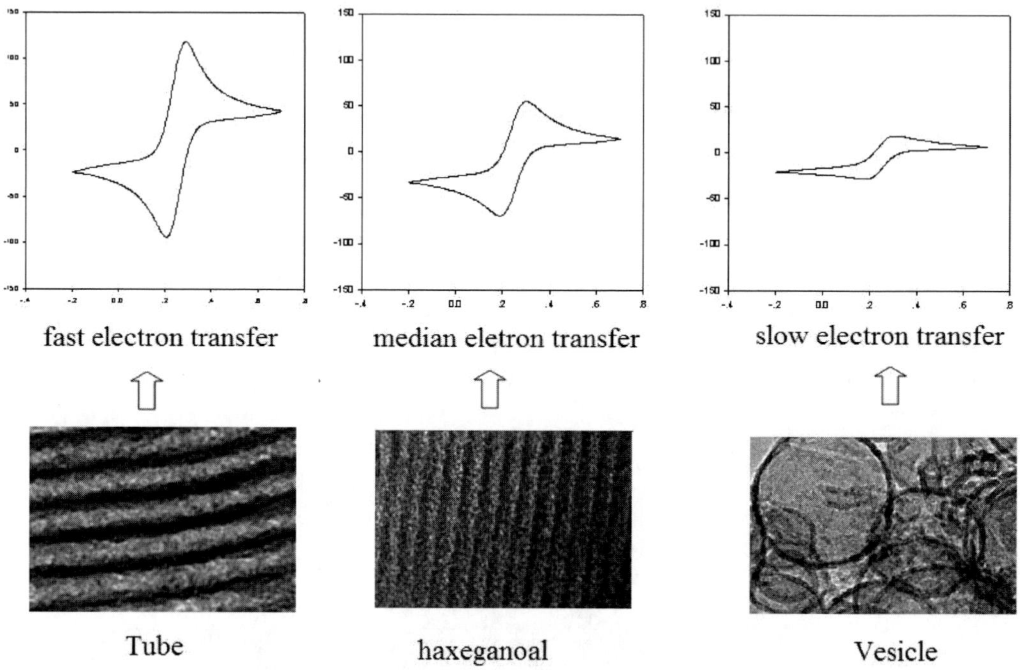

Figure 7. Cyclic voltammograms of three different structures of MPS modified carbon nanotubes paste electrodes in 5 mM $K_3[Fe(CN)_6]$ and 0.5 M KCl, scan rate: 50 mV s^{-1} (unpublished data from author's laboratory).

Another problem which needs to be answered is how the pore size and morphology of various MPS affects the electrochemical properties of the guest protein/enzymes? It is reported that different structure of mesoporous silica can affect the diffusion rate, the trend of increasing permeability with respect to the mesostructure type was as the following: 2D hexagonal and rhombohedral$<$3D hexagonal$<$orthorhombic and cubic mesostructure [17]. An illustration for different diffusion rate with different structure of MPS is given on Fig 7. It has also been demonstrated that the different structure and pore size can affect the absorption and the stability of enzyme immobilization [37, 70]. However, what about its effect on electrochemical properties? Vamvakaki and Chaniotakis [71] studied the stability and operational lifetimes of GOD and HRP immobilized in mesoporous silica beads with different pore sizes. He pointed out that the size matching between pore size and the molecule diameter of the enzymes was very important to achieve high enzymatic activity and prevented the enzyme from leaching. We have been studying the direct electrochemistry of Hb encapsulated in different morphology and pore size of MPS via LbL method aiming to find out some rules that can be used to guide the MPS synthesis for protein immobilization. The different electrochemical property of three kinds of Hb encapsulated in porous silica (Tube: 16 nm, Meso: 13 nm, Vesicle: 100 nm) to the reduction of H_2O_2 is shown in Fig.8. The results indicate that attractive and unusual electrochemical response of the redox biomolecules at the MPS-based biosensors can be attributed to the unique structure and size of porous silica.

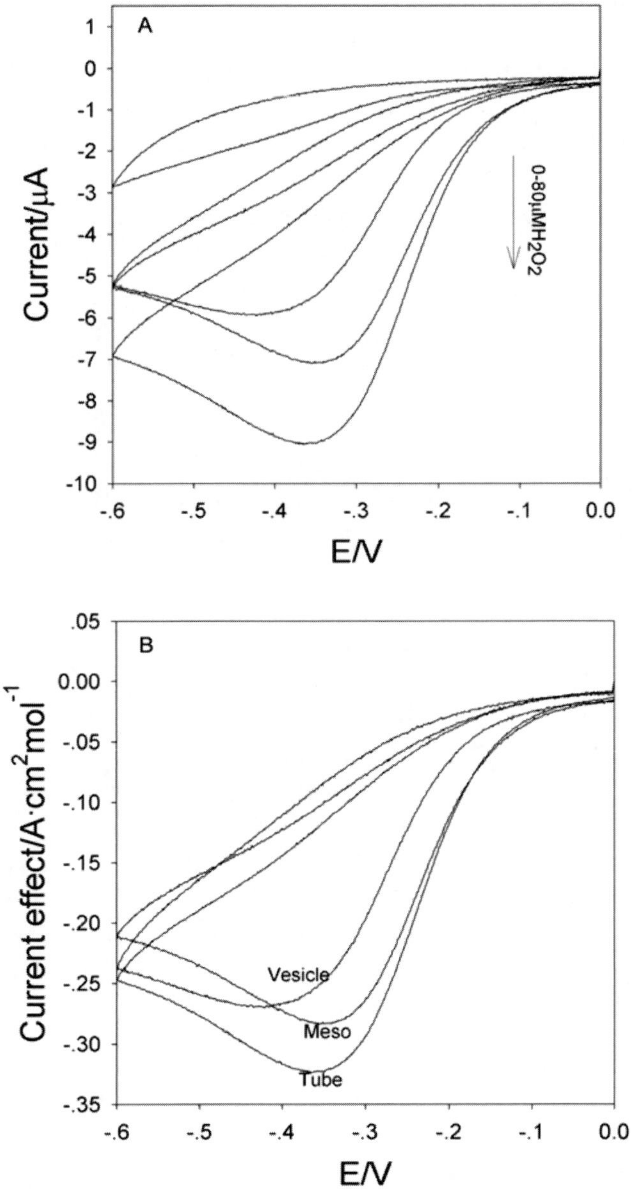

Figure 8. (A) Cyclic voltammograms of $(Hb/tube)_2$/PDDA/GCE in pH 7.4 PBS at 50 mV/s with 0 (dotted line), 20, 40, 60 80 μM H_2O_2 from up to down; (B) Cyclic voltammograms of meso, tube, or vesicle-based electrode in pH 7.4 PBS with 80 μM H_2O_2 vs. surface coverage (unpublished data from author's laboratory).

CONCLUSION

The application of MPS in electrochemical biosensors attracts much attention and has gained some achievements. A great amount of MPS have been designed with different morphology and different sizes to tailor different biomolecules which have different three dimension structure in order to improve the electrocatalytic ability and experimental life time. Besides, more and more organic groups have been functionalized onto the MPS which can improve the electrochemical properties of the biomolecules and the stability between MPS and biomolecules. These efforts circumvent the disadvantages of MPS and enlarge their applications. Many protein-MPS electrochemical biosensors (e.g., Hb、GOD、HRP -MPS biosensors) have been successfully fabricated with low detection limit, long life time and good reproducibility. However, the study of MPS is still not consummate; many problems need to be explored: for examples, how the pore size and structure affect the electrochemical properties of protein/enzymes encapsulated MPS biosensors? What is the mechanism of the interaction between MPS host and guest protein? In addition, many areas in biosensors are still unexplored with the use of mesoporous silica materials, including the immobilization of antibodies, DNA and RNA, lipids and carbohydrates. Therefore, the application of mesoporous silica will pace a promising future by cross-fertilization of ideas among various branches of sciences. It seems likely that the further insight concerning the mesoporous silica principle of novel biosensors will come from collaborations of investigators from diverse background and disciplines.

REFERENCES

[1] Walcarius, A. *Electroanalysis* 1996, *8*, 971-986.
[2] Walcarius, A. *Anal. Chim. Acta* 1999, *384*, 1-16.
[3] Alber, K. S.; Cox, J. A. *Mikrochim. Acta* 1997, *127*, 131-147.
[4] Lin, J.; Brown, C. W. *Trends Anal. Chem.* 1997, *16*, 200-211.
[5] Collinson, M. M. *Mikrochim. Acta* 1998, *129*, 149-165.
[6] Walcarius, A. *Electroanalysis* 1998, *10*, 1217-1235.
[7] Walcarius, A. *Electroanalysis* 2001, *13*, 701-718.
[8] Rabinovich, L.; Lev, O. *Electroanalysis* 2001, *13*, 265-275.
[9] Collinson, M. M. *Trends Anal. Chem.* 2002, *21*, 30-38.
[10] Navratilova, Z.; Kula, P. *Electroanalysis* 2003, *15*, 837-846.
[11] Rolison, D. R.; Bessel, C. A. *Acc. Chem. Res.* 2000, *33*, 737-744.
[12] Ross, S. E.; Shi, Y.; Seliskar, C. J.; Heineman, W. R. *Electrochim. Acta* 2003, *48*, 3313-3323.
[13] Lev, O.; Wu, Z.; Bharathi, S.; Glezer, V.; Modestov, A.; Gun, J.; Rabinovich, L.; Sampath, S. *Chem. Mater.* 1997, *9*, 2354-2375.
[14] Walcarius, A. *Chem. Mater.* 2001, *13*, 3351-3372.
[15] Kresge, C. T.; Leonowicz, M. E.; Roth, W. J.; Vartuli, J. C.; Beck, J. S. *Nature* 1992, *352*, 710-712.
[16] Walcarius, A. *C. R. Chimie* 2005, *8*, 693–712.

[17] Etienne, M.; Quach, A.; Grosso, D.; Nicole, L.; Sanchez, C.; Walcarius, A. *Chem. Mater.* 2007, *19*, 844-856.
[18] Walcarius, A.; Kuhn, A. *Trends Anal. Chem*. 2008, *27*, 593-603.
[19] Ganesan, V.; Walcarius, A. *Mater. Sci. Eng. B* 2008, *149*, 123–132.
[20] Walcarius, A. *Electroanalysis* 2008, *20*, 711 – 738.
[21] Attard, G. S.; Glyde, J. C.; GVltner, C. G. *Nature* 1995, *378*, 366 –368.
[22] Monnier, A.; SchEth, F.; Huo, Q.; Kumar, D.; Margolese, D.; Maxwell, R. S.; Stucky, G.; Krishnamurty, M.; Petroff, P.; Firouzi, A.; Janicke, M.; Chmelka, B. *Science* 1993, *261*, 1299 – 1303.
[23] Ryoo, R.; Joo, S. H.; Jun, S. *J. Phys. Chem. B* 1999, *103*, 7743 –7746.
[24] Kruk, M.; Antochshuk, V.; Matos, J. R.; Mercuri, L. P.; Jaroniec, M. *J.Am.Chem.Soc.* 2002, *124*, 768–769.
[25] Beck, J. S.; VartUli, J. C.; Roth,W. J.; Leonowicz, M. E.; Kresge, C. T.; Schmitt,K. D.; Chu,C. T-W.; Olson, D. H.; Sheppard, E. W.; McCullen, S. B.; Higgins,J. B.; Schlenker, J. L. *J. Am.Chem.Soc*. 1992, *114*, 10834–10843.
[26] Widenmeyer, M.; Anwander, R. *Chem. Mater.* 2002, *14*, 1827-1831.
[27] Slowing, I. I.; Trewyn, B. G.; Giri, S.; Lin. V. S. Y. *Adv. Funct. Mater.* 2007, *17*, 1225–1236.
[28] Trewyn, B. G.; Giri, S.; Slowing, I. I.; Lin. V. S. Y. *Chem. Commun*. 2007, 3236–3245.
[29] Trewyn, B. G.; Nieweg, J. A.; Zhao, Y.; Lin, V. S. Y. *Chem. Eng. J.* 2008, *13*, 23–29.
[30] Hoffmann, F.; Cornelius, M.; Morell, J.; Froba, M. *Angew. Chem. Int. Ed.* 2006, *45*, 3216 – 3251.
[31] Hartmann, M. *Chem. Mater.* 2005, *17*, 4577-4593.
[32] Yiu, H. H. P.; Wright, P. A. *J. Mater. Chem.* 2005, *15*, 3690–3700.
[33] Yiu, H. H. P.; Wright, P. A.; Botting, N. P. *Microporous. Mesoporous. Mater.* 2001, *44-45*, 763-768.
[34] Yiu, H. H. P.; Wright, P. A.; Botting, N. P. *J. Mol. Catal. B* 2001, *15*, 81 – 92.
[35] Ma, H.; He, J.; Evans, D. G.; Duan, X.; *J. Mol. Catal. B* 2004, *30*, 209 – 217.
[36] Salis, A.; Meloni, D.; Ligas, S.; Casula, M. F.; Monduzzi, M.; Solinas, V.; Dumitriu, E. *Langmuir* 2005, *21*, 5511 – 5516.
[37] Takahashi, H.; Li, B.; Sasaki, T.; Miyazaki, C.; Kajino, T.; Inagaki, S. *Microporous Mesoporous Mater*. 2001, *44–45*, 755 –762.
[38] Han, Y. J.; Stucky, G. D.; Butler, A. *J. Am. Chem. Soc.* 1999, *121*, 9897–9898.
[39] Kriel, L. W.; Jimenez, V. L.; Balkus Jr, K. J. *J. Mol. Catal. B* 2000, *10*, 453–469.
[40] Han, Y. J.; Watson, J. T.; Stucky, G. D.; Butler, A. *J. Mol. Catal. B* 2002, *17*, 1–8.
[41] Vinu, A.; Murugesan, V.; Hartmann, M. *J. Phys. Chem. B* 2004, *108*, 7323 – 7330.
[42] Sun, Z. Y.; Li, Y. Q.; Zhou, T. S.; Liu, Y.; Shi, G. Y.; Jin, L. T. *Talanta* 2008, *74*, 1692–1698.
[43] Xian, Y.; Zhou, L. H.; Wu, F. H.; Ling, Y.; Jin, L. T. *Electrochem. Commun*. 2007, 9, 142–148.
[44] Bai, Y.; Yang, H.; Yang, W. W.; Li, Y. C.; Sun, Ch. Q. *Sensor Actuat. B* 2007, *124*, 179–186
[45] Liu, Y. G.; Xu, Q.; Feng, X. M.; Zhu, J. J.; Hou, W. H. *Anal. Bioanal. Chem*. 2007, *387*, 1553–1559.
[46] Liu, Y. G.; Zhang, J. J.; Hou, W. H.; Zhu, J. J. *Nanotechnology* 2008, *19*, 135707/1-135707/8.

[47] Fukushima, Y.; Kajino, T.; Itoh, T. *Current Nanoscience* 2006, *2*, 211-218.
[48] Itoh, T.; Ishii, R.; Ebina, T.; Hanaoka, T.; Ikeda, T.; Urabe, Y.; Fukushima, Y.; Mizukami, F. *Biotech. Bioeng.* 2007, *97*, 200-205.
[49] Dai, Z. H.; Ni, J.; Huang, X. H.; Lu, G. F.; Bao, J. C. *Bioelectrochemistry* 2007, *70*, 250–256.
[50] Dai, Z. H.; Liu, S. Q.; Ju, H. X.; Chen, H. Y. *Biosens. Bioelectron.* 2004, *19*, 861–867.
[51] Zhang, Li.; Zhang, Q.; Li, J. H. *Electrochem. Commun,* 2007, *9*, 1530–1535.
[52] Kim, J.; Grate, J. W.; Wang, P. *Chem. Eng. Sci.* 2006, *61*, 1017 – 1026.
[53] Kriel, L.W.; Jimenez, V. L.; Jr, K. J. B. *J. Mol. Catal. B* 2000, *10*, 453-469.
[54] Zhang, X.; Wang, J.; Wu, W.; Qian, S.; Man, Y. *Electrochem. Commun.* 2007, *9*, 2098-2104.
[55] Wang, L. W.; Hu, N. F. *Bioelectrochemistry* 2001, *53*, 205–212.
[56] Nadzhafova, O.; Etienne, M.; Walcarius, A. *Electrochem. Commun.* 2007, *9*, 1189–1195.
[57] Yao, K.; Zhu, Y. H.; Wang, P.; Yang, X. L.; Cheng, P. Zh.; Lu, H. *Mater. Sci. Eng. C* 2007, *27*, 736–740.
[58] Dai, Z. H.; Fang, M.; Bao, J. Ch.; Wang. H. SH.; Lu, T. H.; *Analy. Chim. Acta* 2007, *591*, 195–199.
[59] Lvov, Y.; Caruso, F.; *Anal. Chem.* 2001, *73*, 4212-4217.
[60] Lvov, Y.; Munge, B.; Giraldo, O.; Ichinose, I.; Suib, S. L.; Rusling, J. F. *Langmuir* 2000, *16*, 8850-8857.
[61] Zhou, Y. L.; Li, Z.; Hu, N. F.; Zeng, Y. H.; Rusling, J. F. *Langmuir* 2002, *18*, 8573-8579.
[62] He, P. L.; Hu, N. F.; Rusling, J. F. *Langmuir* 2004, *20*, 722-729.
[63] He, P. L.; Hu, N. F. *Electroanalysis* 2004, *16*, 1122-1131.
[64] Lvov, Y. M; Lu, Z. Q.; Schenkman, J. B.; Zu, X. L.; Rusling, J. F. *J. Am. Chem. Soc.* 1998, *120*, 4073-4080.
[65] Ma, H. Y.; Hu, N. F.; Rusling, J. F. *Langmuir* 2000, *16*, 4969-4975.
[66] He, P. L.; Hu, N. F.; Zhou, G. *Biomacromolecules* 2002, *3*, 139-146.
[67] Yao, K.; Zhu, Y. H.; Wang, P.; Yang, X. L.; Cheng, P. Zh.; Lu, H. *Mater. Sci. Eng. C* 2007, *27*, 736–740.
[68] Jin, Y. D.; Shao, Y.; Dong, S. J. *Langmuir* 2003, *19*, 4771-4777.
[69] Wu, S.; Ju, H. X.; Liu, Y. *Adv. Funct. Mater.* 2007, *17*, 585–592.
[70] Takahashi, H.; Li, B.; Sasaki, T.; Miyazaki, C.; Kajino, T.; Inagaki, S. *Chem. Mater.* 2000, *12*, 3301-3305.
[71] Vamvakaki, V.; Chaniotakis, N. A.; *Biosens. Bioelectron.* 2007, *22*, 2650–2655.

In: Nanostructured Materials for Electrochemical Biosensors ISBN: 978-1-60741-706-4
Editors: U. Yogeswaran; S. Kumar; S. Chen ©2009 Nova Science Publishers, Inc.

Chapter 12

ELECTROCHEMICAL DETECTION OF NEUROTRANSMITTERS AT STRUCTURALLY SMALL ELECTRODES

Shaneel Chandra and Danny K.Y.Wong*
Department of Chemistry and Biomolecular Sciences, Macquarie University, Sydney, NSW 2109, Australia

ABSTRACT

Electroanalytical chemistry has been widely applied to the study of neurochemical systems. This feasibility stems from the ease of oxidative detection of many neurotransmitters, the small dimensions of electrodes and their inherent fast response time.

Dopamine is a neurotransmitter that has long been of interest to both chemists and neuroscientists. For instance, a loss of dopamine-containing neurons or its transmission is related to a number of illnesses and conditions including Parkinson's disease and schizophrenia. It is therefore of interest to perform quantitative and qualitative determination of dopamine in the extracellular fluid in animals in order to gain an understanding of the neurotransmission processes. Such a study will also aid in correlating neurochemistry with behaviour.

Among the electroanalytical techniques, fast-scan cyclic voltammetry is often used to detect dopamine *in vivo*. Detection of dopamine is further enhanced when fast-scan cyclic voltammetry is conducted at probes with a micrometer-dimension. A review of common materials and techniques for fabricating physically small electrodes is therefore presented in this chapter. Unfortunately, detecting dopamine at naked electrodes is challenging partly because of overlapping oxidation signals from interferents of high concentrations in the brain. Furthermore, electrode fouling caused by adsorption of biological molecules is another common problem encountered in detecting dopamine *in vivo*. In this chapter, a number of approaches including electrode surface modification and diamond electrodes used to minimize these shortcomings have also been reviewed.

1. INTRODUCTION

Electroanalytical chemistry has been widely applied to the study of neurochemical systems. The outcomes of such a study are expected to contribute to a better understanding of many aspects of neurotransmission, for example, neural circuitry and neural substrates of compulsive drug use[1]. This feasibility partly stems from the ease of oxidative detection of many neurotransmitters including dopamine, acetylcholine, norepinephrine, serotonin, glutamic acid and γ–aminobutyric acid. The structures of these molecules are shown in Figure 1. In addition, the development of structurally small electrodes has made *in vivo* detection neurotransmitters possible in biological microenvironments[1-3]. In this respect, the small dimension of such electrodes permits minimal tissue damage upon implantation and, of equal importance, permits very careful selection of the region of tissue where measurements can be performed. Moreover, the inherent fast response time of structurally small electrodes makes it feasible to follow biochemical events frequently taking place on a ms time scale (e.g. neuronal firing).

Various electrode materials have been reported for use in constructing structurally small electrodes of different geometries and sizes[4-7]. Common electrode materials, both modified and otherwise, include metals such as tungsten and aluminium, gold nanoparticle-deposited aluminum, various forms of carbon e.g. doped diamond, nanocrystalline diamond, pyrolyzed carbon, carbon fibers, and gold nanoparticles deposited on glassy carbon.

A common problem encountered during *in vivo* detection of neurotransmitters is the adsorption of high molecular weight proteins, lipids, and peptides present in biological matrices on an electrode surface. Formation of these layers leads to electrode fouling which distorts the voltammetric signal and suppresses the sensitivity of the electrode. Considerable research effort has been devoted to addressing electrode fouling problems. Approaches ranging from fast scan voltammetry[8], immobilizing a protective organic film on the electrode surface[9], completely altering the surface termination[10], fabricating nanocrystalline diamond coated electrodes[11] or doped diamond electrodes[12], to gold electrodes modified with gold nanorods and gold nanoparticles have been developed[13]. Apart from overcoming fouling, these methods have also demonstrated other advantages such as wider potential windows, greater durability, increased robustness and enhanced sensitivity.

In this chapter, we aim to review the techniques used in developing structurally small electrodes of different geometries, which were then applied to the detection of neurotransmitters. We will also pay special emphasis on the strategies used to minimize electrode fouling during electrochemical detection of neurotransmitters at these electrodes. A comparison of these methods and possible future directions in the development of structurally small electrodes for detection of neurotransmitters will also be presented.

* Email: danny.wong@mq.edu.au

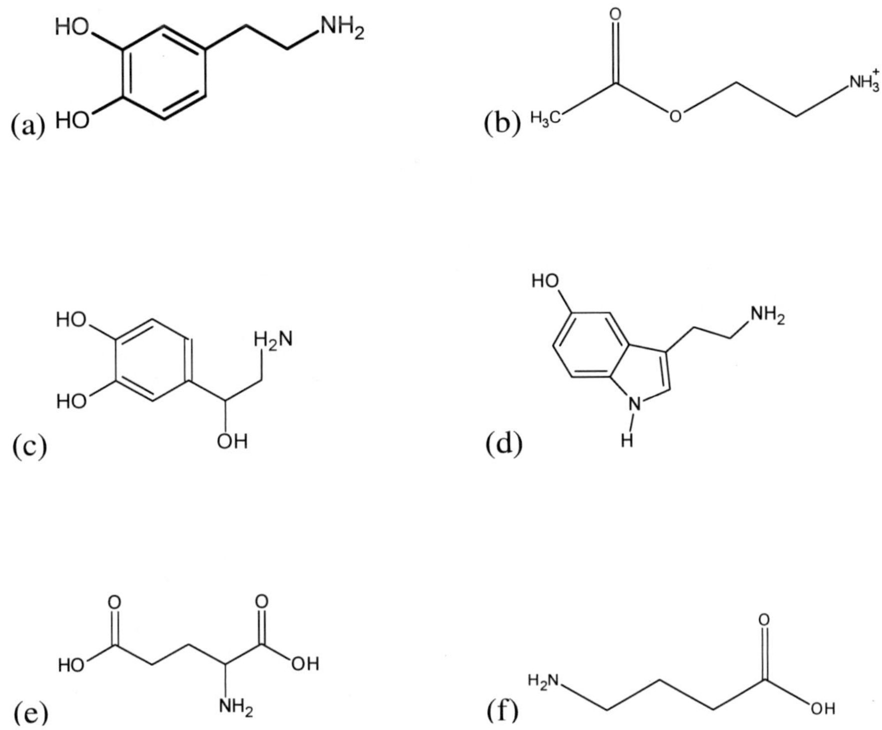

Figure 1. Common neurotransmitters: (a) dopamine; (b) acetylcholine; (c) norepinephrine; (d) serotonin; (e) glutamic acid; (f) γ–aminobutyric acid.

2. NEUROTRANSMITTERS AND THEIR DYNAMICS

In the mammalian brain, neuronal networks process vast amounts of information received from a subject's environment through the senses. Much of the signaling within the brain uses small molecules called neurotransmitters as messengers between neurons. During neuronal communication, neurotransmitters are released from the axon end of a neuron, usually followed by uptake of the released neurotransmitter by receptors on an adjacent neuron (i.e. the dendrites). The process of uptake involves interaction between the released neurotransmitters with membrane-bound proteins called transporters, which transport the extracellular neurotransmitter back into the cell. The remaining neurotransmitters can diffuse out of the neuronal region and be subsequently metabolized[2]. The processing in the brain networks eventually manifests as animal behavior. The brain is a challenging environment for chemical sensing because low concentration of analytes must be detected in the presence of interferences with yet minimal tissue damage. To conduct meaningful measurements, the properties of the analytical sensor and the general characteristics of the biological system must be understood.

Catecholamines is a group of biogenic monoamine neurotransmitters containing a nucleus of catechol, which is the aromatic portion comprising of a benzene ring with two adjacent hydroxyl groups and an aliphatic side chain of ethylamine or one of its derivatives. The immunomodulatory functions of catecholamines acting as chemical messengers transporting information between cells have been long documented[3]. Between cells, catecholamines act as chemical messengers that transport information[7]. This has been an area of interest to researchers as is evidenced by numerous publications in literature aimed at understanding catecholamine and quinone electrochemistry[14-17].

Among the catecholamines, dopamine has long been of interest to both chemists and neuroscientists. It is one of the most important neurotransmitters and is ubiquitous in the mammalian central nervous system[5]. It modulates many aspects of brain circuitry in a major system of the brain including the extra pyramidal and mesolimbic system, as well as the hypothalamic pituitary axis[6]. It also plays a crucial role in the functioning of the central nervous, cardiovascular, renal and hormonal systems[4]. A loss of dopamine containing neurons or its transmission is also related to a number of illnesses and conditions including Parkinson's disease, schizophrenia, motivational habit, reward mechanisms and the regulation of motor functions and in the function of the central nervous, hormonal and cardiovascular system[5,18,19]. It is therefore of interest to measure dopamine in the extracellular fluid in animals to order to monitor neurotransmission processes and correlate neurochemistry with behavior[19].

3. Measurement of Dopamine Concentrations

The dynamics of the release and uptake of dopamine into brain extracellular space are currently under intense investigation[20-22]. Dopamine is a well-known extrasynaptic messenger that functions *via* volume transmission, escaping from the synaptic cleft to bind to extrasynaptic receptors and transporters. High sensitivity, chemical selectivity, and fast temporal resolution are all desirable characteristics in detecting neurotransmitters *in vivo*. In practice, it is difficult to achieve all of these with one method.

Two techniques that have evolved to accomplish this are microdialysis and electrochemistry[5]. For measurements of basal concentration, microdialysis techniques with superb chemical specificity and sensitivity are often employed. However, the main limitations to microdialysis are spatial resolution due to the large probe size (≥200 μm), resulting in significant damage to the region of the probe insertion and poor temporal resolution of 5–20 min per sample[23,24]. On the other hand, electrochemical techniques are well suited for the measurement of transient changes in concentration. Such techniques are concerned with the interplay between electricity and chemistry, namely the measurement of electrical quantities such as current, potential or charge, and their relationship to chemical parameters[23,25]. Electroanalytical techniques have been widely developed and, more recently, applied to the investigation of neurochemical systems, leading to a better understanding of neurotransmission through the detection of several compounds including acetylcholine, dopamine, norepinephrine, serotonin, γ–aminobutyric acid, and glutamic acid[26]. They provide a platform for the construction of sensors of the concentration fluctuations of easily oxidised neurotransmitters in the extracellular fluid of the brain[25]. An overview of the development of analytical chemistry demonstrates that electrochemical sensors represent the most rapidly growing class of chemical sensors[27,28].

4. Applications of Electroanalytical Chemistry to Study of Neurochemical Systems

For the detection of dopamine, controlled-potential (potentiostatic) techniques, which are concerned with the study of charge transfer processes at the electrode-solution interface, are favored due to a number of advantages. These include high sensitivity, selectivity towards electroactive species, wide linear range, portability and low cost of instrumentation, speciation capability and a wide range of electrodes which allow assays of unusual environments[29].

Although multiple electrochemical techniques exist, those used in freely moving animals are chronoamperometry, differential normal-pulse voltammetry, and fast-scan cyclic voltammetry. Excellent comparisons between these can be found in literature, particularly Troyer *et al.*[5,7,30] and Robinson *et al.*[8] and therefore will not be diskussed here.

Fast-scan cyclic voltammetry has been used extensively to investigate the rapid events associated with neurotransmission *in vivo* and *in vitro*. It is a valuable preclinical tool to evaluate both drug mechanisms and animal models of disease associated with dopaminergic transmission. Relative to other available techniques, fast-scan cyclic voltammetry offers several advantages including real time measurements of dopamine concentration on a subsecond timescale, quantification of the increases and decreases in dopamine concentrations in the nM to μM range, and positive identification of dopamine *via* the cyclic voltammograms. Detection of dopamine is further enhanced when fast-scan cyclic voltammetry is conducted at probes with a micrometer-dimension that give fine spatial resolution with minimal tissue damage[31].

Additionally, electroanalytical techniques coupled with microelectrodes offer further advantages such as enhanced current densities due to the hemispheric diffusion field around the electrodes, a lack of sensitivity to solution flow, reduced double-layer charging effects and the ability to be used in highly resistive media as the ohmic drop is small[32]. Further, the small size of microelectrodes *in vivo* imparts only minimal physical damage in living tissues while implanting into the specimen, as well as permitting a careful selection of the neural region to be investigated[33].

5. Ultramicroelectrode Geometries

As low concentrations of dopamine are released and rapidly cleared from the extracellular space, the sensing electrodes must be sensitive, and selective and respond quickly[6]. For *in vivo* detection of neurotransmitters such as dopamine, physically small electrodes are advantageous due to their small size and high sensitivity to catecholamines[34]. There are currently no electrodes small enough to measure dopamine concentrations within the approximately 100-nm synapse, but considerable developments are being made in minimizing electrode size to approach synapses as closely as possible and also to minimize tissue damage[35]. In addition, as there are other electroactive species present at a much higher concentration than dopmaine in the extracellular medium, chemical selectivity on the electrode is absolutely essential. Furthermore, because dopamine conveys information on a subsecond time scale, fast temporal response is needed to follow these changes[34]. Electrochemical methods using ultramicroelectrodes have been proven to be rapid, simple and sensitive in the determination of dopamine[35]. In general, ultramicroelectrodes are defined as electrodes with a characteristic length that is less than 20 μm. For example, this can be an electrode with μm length in one dimension and with mm length in another dimension.

Electrodes of different materials have been miniaturised in many geometric shapes with the common characteristic that the electrode is significantly smaller than the diffusion layer at the electrode surface for ordinary voltammetric time scales (e.g. 1-10 s)[36]. According to Koichi[37], if the characteristic length of a small electrode, such as an ultramicroelectrode, is made infinitesimally small, it tends to adopt the geometry of either a point, a line, or a plane. On this basis, ultramicroelectrodes can generally be classified into a point electrode, a line electrode, and a plane electrode.

A point electrode resembles a spot. It adopts a spherical-shaped concentration profile and potential distribution in the solution. As a result, such electrodes easily achieve a steady state and yield a steady-state current. This current is expected to be proportional to the characteristic length (radius) of the electrode. A typical point electrode is a disk electrode inlaid on an insulating plane. On the other hand, an ultrathin ring electrode shares characteristics of the point electrode and the line electrode. It appears as a point from a position distal from the electrode, but it resembles a curved line upon closer inspection. It exhibits a steady-state current because of the feature of the point electrode. Next, a plane electrode of interest is a microarray electrode, which is composed of point electrodes and line electrodes on a planar insulator. It is versatile in functionality by designing the geometrical arrangement. A mode of mass transport depends on whether elementary electrodes are a point or a line electrode.

In the following sections, different geometries of electrodes will be discussed, and categorized as point or line electrodes. Most of these are based on carbon. This is often due to its broad potential window, low background current, rich surface chemistry, low cost, chemical inertness and suitability for various sensing and detection applications. While all common carbon electrodes share the basic structure of a six-member aromatic ring and sp^2 bonding, they differ in the relative density of the edge and basal planes at their surfaces. The edge orientation tends to be more reactive than the basal plane towards electron transfer and adsorption. As a result, materials with different edge to basal plane ratios display different electron transfer kinetics for a given redox analyte[38].

5.1. Disk-Shaped Point Electrodes

In general, a disk electrode consists of a short cylindrical rod of the electrode material embedded in a tightly fitting tube of an insulating material (e.g. Teflon). Electrical contact is made at the rear end. Disk-shaped nanometer-sized electrodes are often used because they are relatively simple and can attain true steady-state current. Another approach to fabricate nanometer sized disk electrodes is the glass-sealed approach[34], in which a metal wire is sealed into a glass pipette before it is pulled into a nanometer-sized tip with the help of a laser pipette puller. Finally, the tip covered with glass is exposed either by etching away or by micropolishing a small portion of glass insulator. Similarly, Wong and Xu[35] fabricated ultrasmall carbon disk electrodes constructed by pyrolyzing methane gas at a pressure of approximately 900 kPa in pulled quartz capillaries. This was found to be sufficient to form a carbon deposit at the tip of the capillary. Electrical contact to the carbon deposit was accomplished with mercury and a nichrome wire. The electrodes were estimated to exhibit structural diameters of 500–1000 nm with a fabrication success rate of 85%. Favorable stability was also observed by having current deterioration of 10% over a period of 5 days. More recently, disk microelectrode fabrication has been extended to dual-disk electrodes. This is because two micrometer-sized electrodes are very convenient for detection of two electroactive species and for acquirement of dual information in single cells[34].

5.2. Carbon Ultrathin Ring

Investigations for nonplanar electrodes are important because it is easier to construct spherical or conical-shaped microelectrodes than disk-shaped microelectrodes, especially those with a very small tip[39].

Most often, ring electrodes are fabricated by applying a conductor to the walls of an insulating cylindrical support. This is often a glass rod, or for smaller diameter rings, a flame/laser heat drawn glass rod. To fabricate a metal ring, the support can be either painted with organometallic compounds or coated by vapour deposition, sputtering of metal onto a rotating glass rod or pyrolysis of methane. However, the vapor deposition method ensures a uniform metal coating and permits rings of thickness ranging from 10 nm to 5 μm. The coated support is then insulated from solution by sealing into a larger glass tube with resin or collapsing the glass around the rod. The structure is then sectioned and polished to expose the inlaid ring[35].

5.3. Carbon Fiber Line Electrodes

The first carbon fiber microelectrode reported in literature was that fabricated by Ponchon and co-workers in 1979[18]. This procedure involved pulling a glass tube to obtain a diameter of few micrometers. Then the carbon fiber (outside diameter 8 μm, length 20 to 40 mm) was threaded into the capillary, thus enabling the fiber to be pushed a few mm through the capillary. The authors reported that this method minimized the interstitial space between the capillary and the carbon fiber. Then, the capillary was inverted into a mixture of graphite powder and polyester resin to fill 4-5 mm of the body with the paste. A contact wire was then pushed as far as possible into the barrel filled with the paste. Immediately before use, the electrodes were cut to a length of 0.5 mm[18].

The present conventional method for fabricating carbon fiber microelectrodes is as follows. The carbon fiber is aspirated into the glass capillary that is then pulled to the dimensions of the fiber using a vertical puller. The fiber is then sealed in the glass capillary with epoxy and the electrical junction made by back filling the capillary with graphite and inserting a chrome wire for contact. In this method, poor sealing between the fiber/glass interface can often arise from unavoidable bad sealing and leakage of the epoxy. This results in high noise, low sensitivity, short electrode life and sometimes pollution of the solution in which the electrode is immersed. In addition, owing to difficulty in ensuring a successful back filling procedure with graphite, the fabrication efficiency of the method is low. Finally, with most epoxies being organic based, electrode modification or even application in organic solvents can be a challenge[40].

Carbon fiber electrodes tend to have a relatively larger cylindrical surface area, compared to, for example, that of ultrasmall carbon ring electrodes. They are readily accessible to the diffusing species, giving rise to a larger detection current at carbon fiber electrodes. However, owing to the soft mechanical strength of carbon fibers, penetration into soft tissue or frequent vibrations under a microscope often make it a demanding task to manipulate the electrode into the *in vivo* microenvironment.

5.4. Microelectrode Arrays

As the electrode size decreases, especially for point electrodes, Faradaic current generated decreases proportionally to the disk radius, leading to a diminishing ohmic potential drop. In fast experiments, radial diffusion contributes little to the flux of reactant at the electrode. Thus the cell current, which is proportional to the disk area, plummets rapidly as smaller and smaller disks are used. Consequently, it is necessary to use a high-gain current-to-voltage converter, often with two or more stages of amplification, and careful attention must be paid to noise and bandwidth considerations. A direct way of increasing the current to be measured is to use more than one microelectrode, i.e., arrays of N widely separated and non-interacting disks that will provide N times the current from a single disk[38]. This enables exploitation of the advantages of microelectrodes whilst ensuring large total currents by using microelectrode arrays, where each microelectrode has the same function. If these microelectrodes are sufficiently spaced apart, then the array can act as the sum of the individual responses. On the other hand, if they are very close, then the array behaves as a macroelectrode with dimensions equal to that of the assembly. Signal-to-noise ratios can be improved by using such arrays, since the noise levels depend on the active area of the electrodes whereas the signal depends on the total area of the diffusion field[24].

Xiao *et al*[41] have reported the construction of a random array of boron doped diamond nano-disk electrodes, formed by a simple three-step method. Initially, molybdenum(IV) dioxide nanoparticles were electrodeposited on a boron doped diamond substrate. This was then covered in an insulating polymer film by electropolymerizing a 4-nitrophenyldiazonium salt. Next, molybdenum dioxide nanoparticles were dissolved from the boron doped diamond surface (removing the polymer layer directly above them only) using dilute hydrochloric acid etching. This resulted in the exposure of nano-disks of boron doped diamond of 20 nm (with a standard deviation of 10 nm) in diameter surrounded by a polymer insulating the remainder of the boron doped diamond. This method produced up to 650 million (with a standard deviation of 25 million) boron doped diamond nano-disk electrodes per cm[2]. Various random arrays of boron doped diamond nanodisk electrodes were produced using this method with a similar distribution of nano-disk size and number density, confirming that this was a reliable and reproducible method of manufacturing such nanoelectrode arrays. At modest scan rates (10 – 1000 mV s^{-1}) the array was found to produce peak currents approaching that of the Randles-Ševčík limit for the equivalent geometric electrode area, despite the fact that most of the surface was insulated by the polymer as shown by voltammetry and atomic force microscopy. The experimental results were compared with simulations of both ordered and random arrays of nano-disk electrodes, the results of which demonstrated that the maximum current obtainable at such arrays was that predicted by the Randles-Ševčík equation. The array of boron doped diamond nano-disks also showed a significantly reduced capacitive background current compared to the bare boron doped diamond electrode, suggesting that such devices may offer improved signal resolution in electroanalytical measurements.

6. Challenges in Dopamine Detection

Detection of dopamine in a physiological environment with selectivity and sensitivity has been an important topic of electroanalytical research but one that has also experienced great challenges. Direct voltammetric detection of dopamine at naked electrodes such as carbon and metallic electrodes (such as Au, Pt) is ineffective partly because of overlapping signals from interferents in a biological environment such as the brain. These interferents include serotonin, 3,4-dihydroxyphenylacetic acid (DOPAC), uric acid and ascorbic acid. Ascorbic acid is the most commonly encountered interferent and an electroactive species that coexists with dopamine in the central nervous system. In general, dopamine is oxidized at 400 mV versus saturated calomel electrode[25,26], whereas ascorbic acid is at 500 mV[25,29] and both species have comparable sensitivities on known bare electrodes. In the extracellular fluid of the central nervous system, dopamine is present in the concentration range of 0.2 – 2.0 μM[31,42], whereas ascorbic acid level is very much higher at 125 – 420 μM[32,33]. All these make it very difficult to selectively detect dopamine in the presence of ascorbic acid by electrochemical methods.

Another common challenge in electrochemical analysis of dopamine is the phenomenon of fouling. Electrode fouling is the passivation of the electrode surface by the adsorption of non-electroactive species, particularly in the analysis of biological samples. Species such as lipids, peptides and high molecular weight proteins present in biological matrices are major sources of fouling, which results in a decreasing electrode response over time, distorts the voltammetric signal and suppresses the sensitivity of the electrode[43].

6.1. Fast Scan Cyclic Voltammetry

In order to minimize fouling, it is essential that the electrochemical technique be fast enough to detect the analyte and quantify it before severe fouling can take place. One such technique is fast-scan cyclic voltammetry[44]. Voltammetric measurements allow the rapid concentration dynamics of redox-active species to be followed *in situ*. No other method offers this quantitative and qualitative information concerning endogenous substances on a ms time scale. Other electrochemical methods have either less chemical resolution or low time resolution[45]. In particular, dopamine released by short stimulations (<1 s) can be monitored and fast-scan cyclic voltammetry provides a good method for the evaluation of drug actions on dopamine neurons. This, with the added high time resolution of the technique, also allows the kinetics of dopamine release to be followed in greater detail[46]. Fast-scan cyclic voltammetry has been particularly useful for monitoring fluctuations of neurotransmitter concentrations both *in vivo* and *in vitro*[47,48]. However, fast-scan cyclic voltammetry also suffers from the drawback that the very high potential scan rates reduce the sensitivity of the method compared to that of other techniques. This is primarily due to the high background current that exceeds the Faradaic current from redox reactions of dopmaine. The background is composed of current required to charge the double layer and current arising from redox reactions of surface-attached functional groups. The magnitude of both of these is directly proportional to the potential scan rate, whereas the current arising from a diffusion-controlled electrochemical reaction is proportional to the square root of the potential scan rate. Thus optimum ratios of the Faradaic to background current are not achieved with fast-scan cyclic voltammetry[49]. As an example, fast-scan cyclic voltammetry is unable to detect concentrations much below 200 nM[50].

Fast scan cyclic voltammetry also provides only limited chemical resolution. The redox potential (E°) of a substance is insufficiently unique for molecular identification. In addition, to distinguish between chemical species that are involved in diffusion-controlled one-electron electrolysis processes, their E°'s need to differ by at least 0.118 V. in aqueous solution, the potential limits are less than 2.0 V and hence, even under optimum conditions, less than 15 compounds could be resolved[45]

To overcome these issues, as well as to detect dopamine in the presence of interferents such as ascorbic acid and uric acid, several means to improve the sensitivity and selectivity of fast-scan cyclic voltammetry have been adopted. An extension of the anodic scan limit to 1400 mV has been reported to result in a dramatic increase in the sensitivity of the electrodes to dopamine[50]. The electrodes were found to retain their sensitivity in brain tissue and were capable of measuring dopamine concentrations of 50 nM in the presence of DOPAC or ascorbic acid. Recently, an analogue method to subtract the background currents that occur during cyclic voltammetry at high scan rates has been reported[49]. This subtraction enables the use of higher gains before the analogue-to-digital conversion. Furthermore, using principal component regression to account for background changes permitted fast-scan cyclic voltammetric measurements to be made for longer times. This has enabled the monitoring of dopamine over time windows that previously were accessible only to microdialysis experiments but with a 600 times greater time resolution. With such high time resolution, short-term dopamine fluctuations in dopamine concentrations can also be measured.

The most common approach to selective determination of dopamine in the presence of ascorbic acid and other interferents using fast-scan cyclic voltammetry is to prevent the interfering species from accessing the electrode surface. This has been achieved by many studies and approaches ranging from application of selective layers of organic films that repel the interferents, to methods of enhancing the dopamine signal while suppressing that of others.

6.2. Film Coated Electrodes

In 1984, the use of Nafion was as a permselective film coating on small graphite electrodes was reported by Gerhardt and co-workers[51]. This polymer is an ion-exchange perfluoronated derivative film of Teflon, which are highly permeable to cations but almost impermeable to anions. A Nafion-coated electrode will respond minimally to ascorbic acid in extracellular fluid. The membrane strongly rejects passage of anionic metabolites such as DOPAC and 5-hydroxyindoleacetic acid (5-HIAA). It is also insensitive to natural metabolites such as 3,4-dihydroxyphenylethyleneglycol. Thus, it is highly selective for only cationic species such as the primary neurotransmitters dopamine, norepinephrine, and 5-hydrocytryptamine, which are all cationic at physiological pH of ~7.4[51]. Since then, a number of studies have emerged on Nafion-modified electrodes[9,52-56].

However, Nafion-modified electrodes also exhibited several disadvantages. For example, the response time of the Nafion-coated sensors increases due to a reduced diffusion coefficient value in the film[7]. This can pose a serious disadvantage for *in vivo* work where dopamine and other neurotransmitter releases often occur on a sub-second time scale. In addition, Nafion coatings perform well for applications such as stripping analysis, but their use for direct voltammetric analysis is complicated by slow equilibration of the film with solution species[57]. Therefore, there is a need for a modification system that can allow for rapid and selective permeation of the ions of interest.

6.3. Electrochemically Grafted Aryl Films

In recent years, many carbon electrodes were modified by an oxidative procedure that generated oxygen functionalities that are useful for further chemistries[58]. In 1990, Barbier *et al.*[59] argued that electrochemical or chemical oxidation can often damage the carbon surface and oxidation tends to lead to the generation of superficial carboxylic, quinonic, ketonic or hydroxylic groups that then further react with the substance to be attached. The exact nature and number of oxygenated functional groups were thus difficult to ascertain and control, and corrosion of the carbon surface was observed, leading to large background currents. Their study provided an alternative method that was based on the electrochemical reduction of a phenyldiazonium derivative. This carbon surface modification procedure involved the formation of a diazonium radical that forms a covalent bond to the glassy carbon electrode surface. The technique was based on the electrochemical reduction of diazonium salts, which leads to very solid and non-corrosive covalent attachment of aryl groups onto carbon surfaces.

The versatility of the method is founded on the possibility of grafting a variety of functionalised aryl groups. This allows the attachment of a wide spectrum of substances[60]. In 1992, a study by Delamar and co-workers[61] demonstrated that reduction of diazonium salts at carbon surfaces resulted in a strongly attached surface layer. They attributed this to covalent bond formation between the aryl radical and the carbon surface[61,62]. One electron reduction of aryl diazonium salts at carbon electrodes leads to grafting of aryl groups to the surface. Acetonitrile is often used as the modification medium. Reduction of the diazonium salt can be achieved by cyclic voltammetry or controlled potential electrolysis. The coupling reaction is favored both by the adsorption of the diazonium prior to its reduction and by the relatively positive potential of the diazonium prior to its reduction[62].

Numerous studies have now focussed on this technique of using diazonium salts for modifying electrode surfaces for a whole host of applications[9,57,58,63-65]. For example, Hong and Porter[66] have reported the electrochemical reduction of benzenediazonium tetrafluoroborate in acetonitrile containing tetrabutylammonium tetrafluoroborate to incorporate a phenyl layer on glassy carbon electrodes. The phenyl modifier is reported to show strong hydrophobicity and produce the thinnest film, hence the choice of phenyl layer as a film. More recently, Pellissier *et al.*[67] reported the modification of glassy carbon electrodes with phenyl-C_n-H_{2n}-COOH moieties by electrochemical reduction of *in situ* generated diazonium salts bearing carboxylic acid groups. These groups then served as a precursor to grafting of an enzyme layer.

Downard *et al.*[9] have reported the application of a phenylacetate layer to glassy carbon macroelectrodes. Their study determined dopamine levels in the presence of ascorbic acid. Differential pulse voltammetry of dopamine and ascorbic acid at both modified and unmodified electrodes showed almost a six-fold enhancement of dopamine anodic peaks at the modified electrodes. For ascorbic acid, while the magnitude of its anodic current remained similar at modified electrodes, the peaks were no longer as well-resolved as for unmodified electrodes.

6.4. Other Modifying Coatings

In addition to films such as Nafion and phenylacetate, conducting polymers[6,68] including polypyrrole, polythiophene, polyaniline, polyacetylene, and polyindole have attracted considerable attention. Among these, polypyrrole and its derivatives play the leading role because of their versatile applicability and the wide variety of molecular species covalently linked to a pyrrole group[68]. Other polymeric molecules applied to microelectrodes include polycarbazole and poly(carbazole-co-*p*-tolylsulfonyl pyrrole)[69]. Unfortunately, while improving sensor selectivity, the incorporation of conducting polymers render the electrode surface hydrophobic. With high molecular proteins being hydrophobic as well, there is subsequent adsorption of these proteins onto the electrode surface[7]. In addition, considering that covering the electrode with such protective layers is neither reproducible nor effective[70], alternative surface modifications are clearly required.

6.5. Nanoparticle-Modified Electrodes

Jia *et al.*[13] fabricated glassy carbon electrodes (GC) modified with gold nanorods (GN) and gold nanoparticles (GNP) *via* a template technique and then dispersed the electrodes in a saturated sodium citrate solution by ultrasonication to form a gold nanorod and gold nanoparticle suspension, respectively. The electrodes were labeled as GNR/GC and GNP/GC, respectively. For comparison, glassy carbon electrodes were subjected to the same procedure but in a sodium citrate solution without any gold particles. These were labeled as activated electrodes. Dopamine was detected at all the four types of electrodes (GNR/GC, GNP/GC, activated GC and bare GC electrodes) and the resulting anodic peak currents were compared. At the GNR/GC electrode, the dopamine anodic peak current was 5 times larger than that at the GNP/GC electrodes, and 26 times larger than that at the bare GC electrodes. Peak currents similar to the bare GC electrodes were obtained at the activated GC electrodes, indicating that any increase in the peak current was due to the gold nanorods and not activation alone. The study also found that the increase in electrode surface area resulting from the gold nanorod modification was linearly related to the increase in currents. The detection of dopamine in the presence of 1000 fold ascorbic acid was found to be unhindered by the ascorbic acid at GNR/GC electrodes. This selectivity for dopamine over ascorbic acid by GNR/GC electrodes was attributed to the positively charged amine group of dopamine (pK_a = 8.9), whereas the hydroxyl next to the carbonyl group of ascorbic acid (pK_a = 4.10) is negatively charged at pH 7.4, which is similar to the pH of extracellular fluid. As the dispersed gold nanorods are stabilized by citrate ions and thus hold the negative charges, the gold nanorod-modified glassy carbon electrode was electrostatically repelling ascorbic acid and attracting dopamine. Therefore, the oxidation of ascorbic acid is inhibited and the oxidation of dopamine is promoted at the gold nanorod-modified glassy carbon electrode, which improves the selectivity of detection.

6.6. Hydrogenated Electrodes

A strategy to promote the formation of a hydrophobic surface is to directly introduce a hydrogen-terminated layer on carbon electrodes. Moreover, compared to polymeric membranes, hydrogenation reaction is more likely to yield a low-capacitance film with much less severe coverage problems. Recently, Alwarappan *et al.*[44] introduced a hydrogenated film on physically small carbon cylinder electrodes by remote plasma hydrogenation. The modified electrode clearly indicated a minimal fouling effect of 5% at hydrogenated carbon cylinder electrodes. This anti-fouling property is attributed to the hydrophobic hydrogenated layer that is free from oxygen bearing functionalities and other essential sites that facilitate the adsorption of high-molecular weight proteins, peptides and lipids.

6.7. Diamond Electrodes

Diamond is a material exhibiting unique properties such as extraordinary high atomic density, hardness, insulating ability, thermal conductivity, and chemical inertness. Diamond became an object of electrochemical investigation only two decades ago because of serious handicaps including its non-conductivity and accessibility[71]. Since the first article on diamond as an electrochemical material published in 1983 by Iwaki and co-workers[72], and subsequent extensive work by Pleskov and co-workers[71], research into diamond has attracted a lot of attention. This is because the progress in the technology, deposition of diamond films from gas phase at a sub-atmospheric pressure became possible. Furthermore, the performance of doped diamond electrodes can be vastly superior to that of alternative material such as glassy carbon[73]. Notable advantages include an excellent stability and reproducibility as a result of the chemical inertness, a wide potential working window in aqueous solution due to high overpotential for hydrogen and oxygen evolution and fast reaction kinetics for simple electron transfer processes[11]. Another strong factor fuelling the turn towards diamond electrodes was their ultimately strong resistance to surfactant fouling effects reflecting the surface properties of diamond electrodes, particularly the minimal number of oxygen functional groups and other surface sites that are commonly responsible for the adsorption of surface-active agents[70]. Most characterization studies on films have used either a combination of Raman spectroscopy[74,75], scanning electron microscopy[23,76], X-ray diffraction[77], atomic force microscopy[78], or X-ray photoelectric spectroscopy[79], in addition to chemical characterization for surface studies.

There are divergent views among researchers on the role of surface termination on diamond electrode sensitivity and/or background current levels. For example, Park *et al.*[80] have reported that diamond microelectrodes do not possess surface oxides when they are hydrogen-terminated. Therefore, there are no redox waves present and the background is relatively insensitive to changes in solution pH at constant ionic strength. On the other hand, according to Suzuki *et al.*[10] oxygen-terminated boron-doped diamond is more stable than hydrogen-terminated boron-doped diamond.

Although often containing low levels of nitrogen (yellow coloration), boron (blue coloration), and other elements as dopants, natural diamond is essentially electrically insulating. Synthetic high purity diamond is one of the best insulator materials known[81] with a break down voltage of up to 10^9 V m^{-1}[82]. However, enhancing its conductivity by doping with a conducting species allows diamond to be turned into a good electrical conductor.

Boron-doped diamond electrodes have attracted much attention in the past due to their superior properties including low background currents, a wide working potential window, favorable electron transfer kinetics and surface inertness which results in high resistance to deactivation[83-86]. Boron-doped diamond is a near-ideal electrode material for analytical chemistry because it interferes very little with the electrochemistry of the species being measured. The typically used boron-doped diamond films prepared *via* chemical vapor deposition or hot filament deposition are hydrogen terminated. This surface provides relatively high electron transfer rates to many redox couples which involve a single electron transfer[87]. Highly boron-doped diamond couples metallic conductivity with desirable intrinsic material properties of diamond; it is robust, hard, and inert. Boron-doped diamond exhibits an impressive resistance to fouling and electrode deactivation in comparison to other electrode materials[88].

As recently as 2007, few reports on boron-doped diamond microelectrodes in biological tissue had been published. This mainly arises from the difficulties in making boron-doped diamond microelectrodes with very small tips that are less invasive of tissue. The diameter of reported boron-doped diamond microelectrodes (10-30 μm) is still too big for applying them to *in vivo* detection, when a diameter of ~10 μm with a length of 25-500 μm is generally required for minimal tissue damage[10].

A boron-doped diamond microelectrode fabricated for application in *in vivo* detection has been reported in literature[10]. The boron-doped diamond was deposited on tungsten wires through the following procedure. Boron-doped diamond was initially deposited on tungsten wires that were electrochemically etched in 2 M NaOH at 3.0 V (vs Ag|AgCl) for 20 s to produce conical tips with very small tip diameters (~5 μm). Then seeding in an ultrasonic bath containing 2-propanol suspension of diamond particles was conducted for 1 hour. Deposition of diamond was achieved using a microwave plasma assisted chemical vapor deposition system. The carbon source was a mixture of acetone and ethanol (ratio 9:1), while B_2O_3 was the boron source. The diamond grain size was ~2 μm, while the average tip length was ~250 μm. In a hydrogen plasma chemical vapor deposition chamber, electrodes tend to be initially H-terminated, but this procedure went a step further involving an anodic oxidation of the boron-doped diamond electrodes, which resulted in C–O surface bonds, to facilitate peak separation between ascorbic acid and dopamine. The electrostatic repulsion between the negatively charged ascorbic acid and the negative potential of the anodically oxidized electrode surface was reported to shift the potential to more positive values (>1.4 V versus Ag|AgCl). For *in vivo* analysis, the boron-doped diamond electrode exhibited low noise and low standard deviation between analyses[10].

Alternative methods for introducing electrical conductivity into diamond have been developed, which include dopants such as nitrogen[72,78,81,89], sp^2 carbon inclusions in grain boundaries[75], and metal and metal cluster inclusions, and subsurface hydrogen[75]. Other forms of conductive diamond, such as surface conductive[81] or ultracrystalline diamond[78] have also been quoted in literature, suggesting that several types of chemically vapor-deposited diamond may find electrochemical applications[75].

Nitrogenated nanocrystalline diamond with grain sizes ~10 nm is also in use as electrode material in neurotransmitter detection. The nanocrystalline films can be grown in methane (up to 30% volume with nitrogen) and argon microwave plasma. This material is an intermediate between microcrystalline diamond and amorphous diamond-like carbon. The intergrain zones consist of disordered carbon with high mixture of nitrogen. It is these zones (disordered carbon of intergrain boundaries) that impart conductivity to the material[71].

Gruen and co-workers[90] and Fausett *et al.*[81] also discussed about manufacturing smoother diamond films by modifying the growth conditions, but these films usually contain nondiamond intergranular phases. They found that nanocrystalline diamond films produced from C_{60}|Ar gas mixtures demonstrated basic electrochemical properties that were similar to boron-doped microcrystalline diamond films. These include a wide working potential window (~ 3 V), a low voltammetric background current (~1 order of magnitude lower than freshly polished glassy carbon), and a high degree of electrochemical activity for several inorganic redox systems without any conventional pretreatment. Nanocrystalline diamond films produced from such gas mixtures were found to be undoped, yet they possessed semi-metallic electronic properties over a potential range of at least 1.0 to -1.5 V (versus saturated calomel electrode). The conductivity of the film was attributed to charge carriers introduced by grain boundary carbon. Any resistance found in the films was recommended as being possibly reduced through doping. As a consequence of the non-diamond intergranular phases, such films are not as hard, as chemically resistant or as thermally stable as pure diamond.

Gaudin *et al.*[91] have suggested that conductivity in polycrystalline diamond films is due to migration of adsorbates such as water, hydrocarbons, NO_2 and NH_3 through the film grain boundaries. These are believed to be capable of influencing the properties of the near surface of the film.

As Hian *et al.*[73] demonstrated, sub-micron grain sized nanocrystalline diamond films, which display conductivity as a result of graphitic inclusions within the grain boundaries, may be preferred over boron-doped diamond films as a choice in electrochemical applications. Compared to boron-doped diamond, nanocrystalline diamond films demonstrate superior advantages including wider working potential window, more robust nature of electrode, good and reproducible activity, greater activity towards aqueous systems[73].

Diamond-coated metallic microprobes of cylindrical geometry, fabricated by chemical vapor diamond deposition on tungsten wires, using selective growth techniques have also been quoted[82]. The tungsten wires (130 μm diameter, 5.5 cm long) were electrochemically sharpened to a tip diameter of approximately 0.5 μm. The chemical vapor diamond deposition was performed on these sharpened wires. Scanning electron microscopy showed the surface to have a texture with nanoscale features, which increased the surface area. The actual surface exposed per length of microprobe was much greater than as smooth surface, which was attributed as one of the reasons for higher sensitivity of the microprobe in the analyte. The nano-diamond microprobe also demonstrated a large potential window of 3 V suggesting it could be a replacement for metal electrodes for electrochemical analysis and neuron imaging in brains. The sharper the tip the more sensitive the response is, with less background current.

Park *et al.*[92] have shown that a microelectrode for electroanalytical measurements can be formed by depositing boron-doped diamond thin film on a sharpened Pt wire. Response stability, fouling resistance, and low and pH independent background current were highlighted as characteristic features of this new microelectrode. These attractive properties were attributed to the absence of carbon–oxygen functional groups on the hydrogen-terminated diamond surface. Electrochemical and video imaging techniques were used to simultaneously monitor norepinephrine released from sympathetic nerves supplying rat mesenteric artery and vasoconstriction.

A comparative study between a boron-doped diamond coated Pt wire and carbon fiber electrodes to study serotonin and melatonin has recently been reported[93]. In this study, the boron-doped diamond thin film was deposited on a Pt wire by microwave-assisted chemical vapor deposition. The tapered end of this diamond-coated Pt wire was carefully heated inside a polypropylene micropipette tip, which softened the polypropylene and caused it to conformably coat the rough, polycrystalline diamond surface. This procedure resulted in a microelectrode that was cylindrical with a diameter of ~40 μm. The length of the exposed electrode was 100–200 μm. According to the study, this method of fabrication lacks precise control of the exposed electrode length. However, when applied to *in vitro* work in the mucosa in rabbit iliem, the electrodes provided extremely stable responses, with excellent sensitivity and a low limit of detection. There was no significant electrode fouling observed during the experiments, which allowed for long-term repeated measurements compared to carbon fiber electrodes from the same study.

In another study by Patel and co-workers[94], comparisons were again made in the *in vitro* electrochemical behavior of 5-hydroxytryptamine and serotonin (neurotransmitter regulating feeding patterns) at boron-doped diamond coated Pt electrodes and carbon fiber electrodes The diamond microelectrode was found to be attractive for the measurement of these neurotransmitters, and clearly outperformed a bare carbon fiber because of its resistance to fouling by the 5-hyroxytryptamine oxidation reaction products at low analyte concentrations. This is in contrast to the strong adsorption that occurs on the oxygen terminated, sp^2 bonded (i.e., extended *p* electron system) carbon fiber surface. This was attributed to the absence of strong molecular adsorption on the H-terminated, sp^3-bonded diamond surface.

Halpern *et al.*[95] have reported their studies of neurons from the marine mollusc, *Aplysia californica.* In this study, the electrode of choice was a 30-μm diameter diamond microdisk electrode to study feeding patterns in the animal model based on extracellular measurements of 5-hydroxytryptamine. Apart from stable oxidation currents for the electrically-evoked release of serotonin from metacerebral cells, the key finding from this work was that the diamond electrode could be employed in both stimulation and recording of neurotransmitter release.

In another recent study, Suzuki *et al.*[10] reported the application of boron-doped diamond films on tungsten wire. The wire was electrochemically etched while simultaneously being lifted up from the etching solution. Finally, the tip of the wire was conically shaped to leave a tip with a diameter of 3 μm. The sharpened wire was then subjected to a seeding process in an ultrasonic bath containing a 2-propanol suspension of diamond nanoparticles before a boron-doped diamond film was deposited using a microwave. This electrode was used in the *in vivo* detection of dopamine in a rat. It demonstrated a larger electroactive area with lower background current, higher sensitivity, and selectivity for dopamine oxidation was demonstrated. Moreover, the different behavior of the potential dependence between dopamine and ascorbic acid measured by different pulse voltammetry methods suggests a new method for selective detection of dopamine in the presence of ascorbic acid. As an example of an application, *in vivo* detection of dopamine in a mouse brain was also performed. High sensitivity and stability of the peak currents were found following medial forebrain stimulation. Selective *in vivo* detection of dopamine was confirmed by the inhibition of the dopamine uptake process by nomefensine.

7. Concluding Remarks

In a complex environment such as the brain, analysis of selected neurotransmitters present at a lower concentration than most other species has its challenges. While electrochemistry is not without limitations, it does present significant advantages over other techniques. It provides a platform for neurotransmitter sensing and monitoring *via* a wide range of techniques depending on the information needed. However, its greatest contribution is the continuously and rapidly improving advancements in sensor fabrications and design, facilitating *in vivo* chemistry in continually smaller environments.

The various designs and sizes of microelectrodes in existence today and the improvements being made to them are the foundation supporting these advancements in *in vivo* and *in vitro* analyses. Each design has its strengths and weaknesses, and research is continually exploring ways to make smaller, more sensitive and selective sensors that can deliver information at a similar rate to the release and flux of the neurotransmitters in the brain. Fast scan cyclic voltammetry is often used to accomplish these rapid analyses. However, the high potential scan rates themselves lead to reduced sensitivities, high background current and limited chemical resolution. Then, the interference at a bare carbon surface from other neurotransmitters masks the signal from the neurotransmitter of choice. To overcome these difficulties, the electrode surface can be coated with protective coatings such as that of permselctive polymers and conducting polymers.

However, while electrodes modified with various films, such as Nafion, clay, conducting polymers, and others, at a physiological pH of 7.4 could absorb and even preconcentrate the cationic dopamine while effectively rejecting the negatively charged ascorbic acid and other anionic interfering agents, some disadvantages exist in the previously reported modified electrodes. For example, the response time of the Nafion-coated sensors increases due to a smaller diffusion coefficient value in the film, whereas conducting polymer-modified sensors have hydrophobic surfaces that would adsorb proteins easily. The adsorption of protein on the electrode surface is undesirable because the sensors would need renewal frequently due to the fouling effect. In most cases, a simple polymer or polymer-complex layer have been coated on the electrode surface, which plays the role of separating the voltammetric peaks other than showing electrocatalytic activity to these interested species.

Alternatively, hydrogenated electrodes have been successfully applied to electrode surfaces to suppress interferents of some unwanted neurotransmitter signals (such as that of ascorbic acid when analyzing for DA). More recently, attention has turned to doped diamond as an electrode material with dopants ranging from boron, nitrogen, to intergranular sp^2 carbon in the film. Apart from retaining its uniquely advantageous properties such as high atomic density, hardness and chemical inertness, doped-diamond is an excellent electrical conductor and has a H-terminated sp^3-bonded surface that leads to absence of strong molecular adsorption of fouling species on its surface. With anodic oxidation of the H-terminated surface, the introduction of C—O surface bonds has been employed to facilitate separation of ascorbic acid and dopamine peaks. Perhaps, the next course of research should focus on preparing a surface that can repel both ascorbic acid (in the case of dopamine) and fouling species at a diamond electrode. With its versatility, doped diamond can be applied to a range of substrates such as carbon, metals, and in cases of bigger electrodes, even silicon wafers. This new electrode material has significant promise for even greater capabilities such as complete resistance to interferents. Future research is likely to engage in this pursuit for some time to come yet.

REFERENCES

[1] Andrew H. Evans; Pavese, N.; Lawrence, A. D.; Tai, Y. F.; Appel, S.; Doder, M.; Brooks, D. J.; Lees, A. J.; Piccini, P. *Annals of Neurology* 2006, *59*, 852-858.

[2] Michael, D. J.; Wightman, R. M. *Journal of Pharmaceutical and Biomedical Analysis* 1999, *19*, 33-46.

[3] Venton, B. J.; Troyer, K. P.; Wightman, R. M. *Analytical Chemistry* 2002, *74*, 539-546.

[4] Arya, S. K., Singh, S. P. and Malhotra, B. D., Ed. *Electrochemical techniques in biosensors.*; John Wiley & Sons, Ltd.: Chichester, 2007.

[5] Troyer, K. P.; Heien, M. L. A. V.; Venton, B. J.; Wightman, R. M. *Current Opinion in Chemical Biology* 2002, *6*, 696-703.

[6] Wang, J. *Analytical Electrochemistry*, Third Edition ed.; John Wiley & Sons: Hoboken, 2006.

[7] Xiao, Y.; Guo, C.; Li, C. M.; Li, Y.; Zhang, J.; Xue, R.; Zhang, S. *Analytical Biochemistry* 2007, *371*, 229-237.

[8] Robinson, D. L.; Venton, B. J.; Heien, M. L. A. V.; Wightman, R. M. *Clinical Chemistry (Washington, DC, United States)* 2003, *49*, 1763-1773.

[9] Downard, A. J.; Roddick, A. D.; Bond, A. M. *Analytica Chimica Acta* 1995, *317*, 303-310.

[10] Suzuki, A.; Ivandini, T. A.; Yoshimi, K.; Fujishima, A.; Oyama, G.; Nakazato, T.; Hattori, N.; Kitazawa, S.; Einaga, Y. *Anal. Chem.* 2007, *79*, 8608-8615.

[11] Hiramatsu, M.; Lau, C. H.; Bennett, A.; Foord, J. S. *Thin Solid Films* 2002, *407*, 18-25.

[12] Chen, L.-C.; Chang, C.-C.; Chang, H.-C. *Electrochimica Acta, In Press, Accepted Manuscript.*

[13] Jia, Z.; Liu, J.; Shen, Y. *Electrochemistry Communications* 2007, *9*, 2739-2743.
[14] Xu, R. D.; Huang, X.; Kramer, K. J.; Hawley, M. D. *Analytical Biochemistry* 1995, *231*, 72-81.
[15] Smythies, J.; De Iuliis, A.; Zanatta, L.; Galzigna, L. *Neurotoxicity Research* 2002, *4*, 77 - 81.
[16] Hasegawa, T.; Matsuzaki, M.; Takeda, A.; Kikuchi, A.; Furukawa, K.; Shibahara, S.; Itoyama, Y. *Journal of Neurochemistry* 2003, *87*, 470.
[17] Alhasan, R.; Njus, D. *Analytical Biochemistry* 2008, *381*, 142-147.
[18] Ponchon, J.; Cespuglio, R.; Gonon, F.; Jouvet, M.; Pujol, J. *Analytical Chemistry* 1979, *51*, 1483-1486.
[19] Hermans, A.; Seipel, A. T.; Miller, C. E.; Wightman, R. M. *Langmuir* 2006, *22*, 1964-1969.
[20] Westerink, R. H. S. *NeuroToxicology* 2004, *25*, 461-470.
[21] Sulzer, D.; Edwards, R. *Neuron* 2000, *28*, 1-9.
[22] Suaud-Chagny, M.-F. *Methods* 2004, *33*, 322-329.
[23] McNally, M.; Wong, D. K. Y. *Anal. Chem.* 2001, *73*, 4793-4800.
[24] Fungaro, D., A.; Brett, C. M. A. *Analytica Chimica Acta* 1999, *385*, 257-264.
[25] Xu, G.-R.; Xu, M.-L.; Zhang, J.-M.; Kim, S.; Bae, Z.-U. *Bioelectrochemistry* 2008, *72*, 87-93.
[26] Sun, W.; Yang, M.; Jiao, K. *Anal. Bioanal. Chem.* 2007, *389*, 1283-1291.
[27] Laschi, S.; Mascini, M. *Medical Engineering & Physics* 2006, *28*, 934-943.
[28] Wang, J. *Electroanalysis* 1991, *3*, 255-259.
[29] Ambrosi, A.; Morrin, A.; Smyth, M. R.; Killard, A. J. *Analytica Chimica Acta* 2008, *609*, 37-43.
[30] Jiao, S.; Li, M.; Wang, C.; Chen, D.; Fang, B. *Electrochimica Acta* 2007, *52*, 5939-5944.
[31] Schenk, J. O.; Miller, E.; Rice, M. E.; Adams, R. N. *Brain Research* 1983, *277*, 1-8.
[32] Brazell, M. P.; Marsden, C. A. *Brain Research* 1982, *249*, 167-172.
[33] Miele, M.; Fillenz, M. *Journal of Neuroscience Methods* 1996, *70*, 15-19.
[34] Gao, N.; Lin, X.; Jia, W.; Zhang, X.; Jin, W. *Talanta* 2007, *73*, 589-593.
[35] Wong, D. K. Y.; Xu, L. Y. F. *Anal. Chem.* 1995, *67*, 4086-4090.
[36] Lee, Y.; Amemiya, S.; Bard, A. J. *Anal. Chem.* 2001, *73*, 2261-2267.
[37] Koichi, A. *Electroanalysis* 1993, *5*, 627-639.
[38] Strohben, W. E.; Smith, D. E.; Evans, D. H. *Analytical Chemistry* 1990, *62*, 1709-1712.
[39] Correia, A. N.; Machado, S. A. S.; Sampaio, J. C. V.; Avaca, L. A. *Journal of Electroanalytical Chemistry* 1996, *407*, 37-43.
[40] Huang, W. H.; Pang, D. W.; Tong, H.; Wang, Z. L.; Cheng, J. K. *Anal. Chem.* 2001, *73*, 1048-1052.
[41] Xiao, L.; Streeter, I.; Wildgoose, G. G.; Compton, R. G. *Sensors and Actuators B: Chemical* 2008, *133*, 118-127.
[42] Lane, R. F.; Blaha, C. D.; Hari, S. P. *Brain Research Bulletin* 1987, *19*, 19-27.
[43] Park, J.; Quaiserova-Mocko, V.; Patel, B. A.; Novotny, M.; Liu, A.; Bian, X.; Galligan, J. J.; Swain, G. M. *The Analyst* 2008, *133*, 17-24.
[44] Alwarappan, S.; Butcher, K. S. A.; Wong, D. K. Y. *Sensors and Actuators B: Chemical* 2007, *128*, 299-305.

[45] Heien, M. L. A. V.; Johnson, M. A.; Wightman, R. M. *Anal. Chem.* 2004, *76*, 5697-5704.
[46] Stamford, J. A.; Kruk, Z. L.; Millar, J. *Brain Research* 1986, *381*, 351-355.
[47] Bath, B. D.; Michael, D. J.; Trafton, B. J.; Joseph, J. D.; Runnels, P. L.; Wightman, R. M. *Analytical Chemistry* 2000, *72*, 5994-6002.
[48] Kuhr, W. G.; Wightman, R. M. *Brain Research* 1986, *381*, 168-171.
[49] Hermans, A.; Keithley, R. B.; Kita, J. M.; Sombers, L. A.; Wightman, R. M. *Anal. Chem.* 2008, *80*, 4040-4048.
[50] Hafizi, S.; Kruk, Z. L.; Stamford, J. A. *Journal of Neuroscience Methods* 1990, *33*, 41-49.
[51] Gerhardt, G. A.; Oke, A. F.; Nagy, G.; Moghaddam, B.; Adams, R. N. *Brain Research* 1984, *290*, 390-395.
[52] Santos, R. M.; Lourenço, C. F.; Piedade, A. P.; Andrews, R.; Pomerleau, F.; Huettl, P.; Gerhardt, G. A.; Laranjinha, J.; Barbosa, R. M. *Biosensors and Bioelectronics* 2008, *24*, 704-709.
[53] Selvaraju, T.; Ramaraj, R. *Journal of Electroanalytical Chemistry* 2005, *585*, 290-300.
[54] Wiedemann, D. J.; Basse-Tomusk, A.; Wilson, R. L.; Rebec, G. V.; Wightman, R. M. *Journal of Neuroscience Methods* 1990, *35*, 9-18.
[55] Wiedemann, D. J.; Kawagoe, K. T.; Kennedy, R. T.; Ciolkowski, E. L.; Wightman, R. M. *Analytical Chemistry* 1991, *63*, 2965-2970.
[56] Xiang-Qin, L.; Guang-Feng, K.; Ying, C. *Chinese Journal of Analytical Chemistry* 2008, *36*, 157-161.
[57] Alison J. Downard, A. D. R. *Electroanalysis* 1995, *7*, 376-378.
[58] Saby, C.; Ortiz, B.; Champagne, G. Y.; Belanger, D. *Langmuir* 1997, *13*, 6805-6813.
[59] Barbier, B.; Pinson, J.; Desarmot, G.; Sanchez, M. *Journal of The Electrochemical Society* 1990, *137*, 1757-1764.
[60] Blaha, C. D.; Lane, R. F. *Brain Research Bulletin* 1983, *10*, 861-864.
[61] Delamar, M.; Hitmi, R.; Pinson, J.; Saveant, J. M. *J. Am. Chem. Soc.* 1992, *114*, 5883-5884.
[62] Alison, J. D. *Electroanalysis* 2000, *12*, 1085-1096.
[63] Bourdillon, C.; Delamar, M.; Demaille, C.; Hitmi, R.; Moiroux, J.; Pinson, J. *Journal of Electroanalytical Chemistry* 1992, *336*, 113-123.
[64] Alison J. Downard, A. b. M. *Electroanalysis* 1999, *11*, 418-423.
[65] Alison J. Downard, A. D. R. *Electroanalysis* 1997, *9*, 693-698.
[66] Hong, H.-G.; Porter, M. D. *Journal of Electroanalytical Chemistry* 2005, *578*, 113-119.
[67] Pellissier, M.; Barrière, F.; Downard, A. J.; Leech, D. *Electrochemistry Communications* 2008, *10*, 835-838.
[68] Cosnier, S. In *Handbook of Biosensors and Biochips*; Marks, R. S., Cullen, D.C., Karube, I. Lowe, C.R. and Weetall, H.H., Ed.; John Wiley & Sons Ltd.: Chichester, 2007; Vol. 1, pp 237-249.
[69] Ates, M.; Castillo, J.; Sezai Sarac, A.; Schuhmann, W. *Microchimica Acta* 2008, *160*, 247-251.
[70] Dongchan Shin, Donald A. T., Akira Fujishima, Arben Merkoçi, Joseph Wang *Electroanalysis* 2005, *17*, 305-311.
[71] Pleskov, Y. V. In *Electroanalytical Chemistry Research Developments*; Jiang, P. N., Ed.; Nova Science Publishers Inc: Hauppauge, 2007, pp 183-227.

[72] Iwaki, M.; Sato, S.; Takahashi, K.; Sakairi, H. *Nuclear Instruments and Methods in Physics Research*, *209-210*, 1129-1133.

[73] Hian, L. C.; Grehan, K. J.; Compton, R. G.; Foord, J. S.; Marken, F. *Diamond and Related Materials* 2003, *12*, 590-595.

[74] Ferreira, N. G.; Azevedo, A. F.; Beloto, A. F.; Amaral, M.; Almeida, F. A.; Oliveira, F. J.; Silva, R. F. *Diamond and Related Materials* 2005, *14*, 441-445.

[75] Lau Chi Hian, Kieron J. G. Christiaan H. G. Richard G. C. John S. F. F. M. *Electroanalysis* 2003, *15*, 169-174.

[76] Olivia, H.; Sarada, B. V.; Shin, D.; Rao, T. N.; Fujishima, A. *The Analyst* 2002, *127*, 1572-1575.

[77] Yan, X.-b.; Xu, T.; Chen, G.; Xue, Q.-j.; Yang, S.-r. *Electrochemistry Communications* 2004, *6*, 1159-1162.

[78] Achatz, P.; Williams, O. A.; Bruno, P.; Gruen, D. M.; Garrido, J. A.; Stutzmann, M. *Physical Review B (Condensed Matter and Materials Physics)* 2006, *74*, 155429.

[79] Saw, K. G.; du Plessis, J. *Materials Letters* 2004, *58*, 1344-1348.

[80] Park, J.; Show, Y.; Quaiserova, V.; Galligan, J. J.; Fink, G. D.; Swain, G. M. *Journal of Electroanalytical Chemistry* 2005, *583*, 56-68.

[81] Bryan Fausett; Michael C. Granger; Mateusz L. Hupert; Jian Wang; Greg M. Swain; Gruen, D. M. *Electroanalysis* 2000, *12*, 7-15.

[82] Richard G. Compton, John S. F. F. M. *Electroanalysis* 2003, *15*, 1349-1363.

[83] Pickles, C. S. J.; Hall, C. E.; Jiang, L.; Perkins, N.; Kleijhorst, R. A.; (Element Six Limited, UK; Kemp, Mark). 2005, 24 pp.

[84] Tsunozaki, K.; Einaga, Y.; Rao, T. N.; Fujishima, A. *Chemistry Letters* 2002, 502-503.

[85] Sarada, B. V.; Rao, T. N.; Tryk, D. A.; Fujishima, A. *Journal of the Electrochemical Society* 1999, *146*, 1469-1471.

[86] Murilo Sérgio da Silva Julião, Érica C. A. M. Aquiles La S. Neidenêi G. F. Richard G. C. Sílvia H. Pires S. *Electroanalysis* 2005, *17*, 269-274.

[87] Tryk, D. A.; Tachibana, H.; Inoue, H.; Fujishima, A. *Diamond and Related Materials* 2007, *16*, 881-887.

[88] Holt, K. B.; Hu, J.; Foord, J. S. *Anal. Chem.* 2007, *79*, 2556-2561.

[89] Chen, G. *Talanta* 2007, *74*, 326-332.

[90] Gruen, D. M.; Shengzhong, L. *Applied Physics Letters* 1994, *64*, 1502.

[91] Gaudin, O.; Whitfield, M. D.; Foord, J. S.; Jackman, R. B. *Diamond and Related Materials* 2001, *10*, 610-614.

[92] Park, J.; Quaiserova-Mocko, V.; Peckova, K.; Galligan, J. J.; Fink, G. D.; Swain, G. M. *Diamond and Related Materials* 2006, *15*, 761-772.

[93] Patel, B. A. *The Analyst* 2008, *133*, 516-524.

[94] Patel, B. A.; Bian, X.; Quaiserova-Mocko, V.; Galligan, J. J.; Swain, G. M. *The Analyst* 2007, *132*, 41-47.

[95] Halpern, J. M.; Xie, S.; Sutton, G. P.; Higashikubo, B. T.; Chestek, C. A.; Lu, H.; Chiel, H. J.; Martin, H. B. *Diamond and Related Materials* 2006, *15*, 183-187.

INDEX

3

A

B

C

D

E

F

G

H

I

J

K

L

M

N

O

P

Q

T

U

V

W

X

Y

Z